Handbook of Asian American Health

Grace J. Yoo • Mai-Nhung Le
Alan Y. Oda
Editors

Handbook of Asian American Health

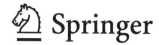

Editors
Grace J. Yoo
Department of Asian American Studies
San Francisco State University
San Francisco, CA, USA

Mai-Nhung Le
Department of Asian American Studies
San Francisco State University
San Francisco, CA, USA

Alan Y. Oda
Department of Undergraduate
  Psychology
Azusa Pacific University
Azusa, CA, USA

ISBN 978-1-4614-2226-6 (Hardcover)   ISBN 978-1-4614-2227-3 (eBook)
ISBN 978-1-4939-1344-2 (Softcover)
DOI 10.1007/978-1-4614-2227-3
Springer New York Heidelberg Dordrecht London

Library of Congress Control Number: 2012932598

Springer is part of Springer Science+Business Media (www.springer.com)

To my daughter, Kristen, who constantly reminds me of what is truly important in life, and to my life partner, Brad, whose unwavering love and support have made me a better person, friend, partner, and mother.

–MNL

To my loving and patient family Donna, Peter, and Andrew, blessings and better health

–AYO

To my partner-in-life, Jason, and sons, Albert and Jeremy, who support each of my projects with encouragement and enthusiasm. Thank you for always cheering me on!

–GJY

We also dedicate this book to Asian Americans fighting for health and wellness for themselves, their families and their communities

Preface

The health and illness experience of Asian Americans is often disregarded by, if not invisible to, those outside of this community. Rather, if the health and illness of Asian Americans are depicted, Asian Americans are often perceived as a "healthy minority," similar to the stereotype of the "model minority." When the health issues confronting Asian Americans are discussed, conclusions are often based on generalizations that do not consider the diversity of experiences and economic backgrounds that are distinctive to the 30 different Asian ethnicities, all grouped under the one rubric of "Asian American". There is a common stereotype that Asian Americans rarely, if ever, are afflicted with cancer, diabetes or other chronic health conditions. Yet this population confronts numerous health issues, problems of which most of the American public and many policy makers are unaware.

Viewed as a uniformly successful group, Asian Americans are typically assumed to have few social problems or concerns, including medical. Although many ethnic Asians have achieved some successes within American society, many others live in poverty, crowded conditions, and are deprived of even basic health care and other important services. Sixty percent of Asian Americans are foreign-born, so they face various issues and challenges unfamiliar to non-immigrants. Language barriers and cultural differences often affect health care access and the quality of health care received.

The editors of this handbook have been teaching and conducting research on Asian Americans and health for two decades. As such, we are too aware of the difficulty in finding comprehensive, readily available, and accessible scholarship that addresses the number of health issues confronting this American subpopulation today. We present the most current work on the status of health and Asian Americans, providing a broad examination of the various critical issues facing this community. It is presented as to be accessible for students, educators, researchers, and practitioners.

Leading Asian American health experts in fields such as nursing, psychology, medicine, public health, sociology, ethnic studies, and Asian American studies contributed to various chapters. The thematic sections were developed through a thorough review of the different contemporary health issues and concerns in the Asian American community. The thematic sections are:

- Ethnicity and Health
- Social Determinants of Health
- Confronting Critical Health Issues

- Health Care Delivery
- Social Movements and Health

In this volume, Asian Americans as a whole are explored as well as issues impacting various ethnic groups within the community. The first section examines how immigration history, culture, structure and society have impacted the health of various Asian Americans and how many concerns remain salient. We acknowledge the needs of the largest populations within Asian America – those subgroups who have been in the United States over two centuries and ethnic groups numbering over one million in the U.S. In these chapters, we've included changing demographics and key health issues confronting these groups. We also acknowledge smaller subgroups who have shorter histories, generally numbering less than one million in number. We have included chapters focused on these emerging subpopulations among South Asians and Southeast Asian Americans.

In addition, the second section of this volume key social determinants of health and well-being, by exploring the critical health issues facing Asian Americans. The top eight health and wellness issues impacting morbidity and mortality among Asian Americans are the primary focus of this volume. These chapters provide a general overview to specific illnesses and diseases and the various social and cultural challenges associated with treatment, management, and prevention, as well as providing recommendations for future research.

In a third section, this book examines inequality and disparities that Asian Americans face associated with health care delivery. Finally, this book chronicles past and current health social movements including the work of extraordinary grassroots advocates, Ted Fang, Jonathan Leong and Susan M. Shinagawa, who have addressed issues in hepatitis B, bone marrow donor donation and cancer survivorship within the Asian American community.

Each chapter begins with a case study or example of the issue presented. Next, a broad contemporary and sometimes historical overview of the main topic is offered. This is followed by issue-specific discussions of challenges and future directions. The 31 chapters include background information, challenges to health care, and the prospects and outlooks for each of the issues. When relevant, the chapters describe how gender, class, immigrant status, and regionalism impact the different issues. Our goal for this book is that it will contribute to literature on Asian American health but also challenge existing stereotypes and assumptions that are often so prevalent about Asian Americans and the well-being of their human bodies.

San Francisco, CA, USA   Grace J. Yoo
San Francisco, CA, USA   Mai-Nhung Le
Azusa, CA, USA   Alan Y. Oda

Acknowledgements

We would like to thank Jonathan Lee and Holly Raña Lim's assistance with referencing throughout this edited volume. We are also grateful to the department of Asian American Studies at San Francisco State University for their continued support.

Contents

Contributors

Alvin N. Alvarez College of Health and Human Services, Department of Counseling, San Francisco State University, San Francisco, CA

Emily Avera Asian American Donor Program, Alameda, CA

Roshan Bastani Department of Health Services, University of California, Los Angeles (UCLA) School of Public Health, Los Angeles

Nancy J. Burke Department of Anthropology, History, and Social Medicine, Helen Diller Comprehensive Cancer Center, University of California, San Francisco, USA

Moon S. Chen Jr. University of California, Davis Cancer Center, Davis, CA, USA

Serena Chen Department of Sociomedical Sciences, Columbia University Mailman School of Public Health, New York, NY, USA

Ricky Y. Choi Asian Health Services Community Health Center, Oakland, CA, USA

Vy Thuc Dao Department of Sociology, Tulane University, New Orleans, LA, USA

Roderick Raña Daus-Magbual Pin@y Educational Partnerships (PEP), San Francisco, CA, USA

Kira Donnell Department of Ethnic Studies, University of California Berkeley, Berkeley, CA, USA

Ted Fang AsianWeek Foundation, San Francisco Hep B Free, San Francisco, CA, USA

Linda A. Gerdner Stanford Geriatric Education Center, Center for Education in Family and Community Medicine, Stanford University School of Medicine, Palo Alto, CA, USA

Deborah A. Goebert Asian/Pacific Islander Youth Violence Prevention Center, Department of Psychiatry, John A. Burns School of Medicine, University of Hawaii, Honolulu, HI, USA

Fang Gong Department of Sociology, Ball State University, Muncie, IN, USA

Ariel T. Holland Health Policy Research Department, Palo Alto Medical Foundation Research Institute, Palo Alto, CA, USA

Laureen D. Hom Independent Scholar New York, USA

Nadia Islam Department of Medicine, NYU Prevention Research Center, NYU Center for the Study of Asian American Health, New York University School of Medicine, New York, NY

Su Yeong Kim Department of Human Development and Family Sciences, University of Texas at Austin, Austin, TX, USA

Caroline Kuo Department of Psychiatry, Rhode Island Hospital and Alpert Medical School, Brown University, Providence, RI, USA

Simona C. Kwon NYU Institute of Community Health and Research and Department of Medicine, Division of General, Internal Medicine, New York University School of Medicine, New York, NY, USA

Mai-Nhung Le Department of Asian American Studies, San Francisco State University, San Francisco, CA, USA

Thao N. Le College of Tropical Agriculture and Human Resources, Family & Consumer Sciences, University of Hawaii at Manoa, Honolulu, HI, USA

Jonathan Leong Asian American Donor Program, Alameda, CA, USA

Maureen Lichtveld Freeport McMoRan Chair of Environmental Policy, Environmental Health Sciences Department, Tulane University School of Public Health and Tropical Medicine, New Orleans, LA, USA

Russell F. Lim School of Medicine, Department of Psychiatry & Behavioral Sciences, University of California, Sacramento, CA, USA

Jason Liu San Francisco Hep B Free, San Francisco, CA, USA

Francis G. Lu School of Medicine, Department of Psychiatry & Behavioral Sciences, University of California, Sacramento, CA, USA

Richard Sean Magbual Kaiser Permanente Hospital of Riverside, CA, USA

Annette E. Maxwell School of Public Health, University of California, Los Angeles, CA, USA

Ranjita Misra College of Education and Human Development, Department of Health and Kinesiology, Texas A&M University, College Station, TX, USA

Heather Ngai Department of Health and Human Services, Data Branch, Office of Quality and Data, Bureau of Primary Health Care, Health Resources and Services Administration, Rockville, MD, USA

Quyen Ngo-Metzger Department of Health and Human Services, Data Branch, Office of Quality and Data, Bureau of Primary Health Care, Health Resources and Services Administration, Rockville, MD, USA

Giang T. Nguyen Department of Family Medicine and Community Health, Center for Public Health Initiatives, University of Pennsylvania, Philadelphia, PA, USA

Tung T. Nguyen Vietnamese Community Health Promotion Project, School of Medicine, University of California, Asian American Network Research, and Training (AANCART), San Francisco, CA, USA

Tu-Uyen Nguyen Asian American Studies Program, California State University, Fullerton, CA, USA

Alan Y. Oda Department of Undergraduate Psychology, Azusa Pacific University, Azusa, CA, USA

Don Operario Program in Public Health, Brown University, Providence, RI, USA

Latha P. Palaniappan Health Policy Research Department, Palo Alto Medical Foundation Research Institute, Palo Alto, CA, USA

Shilpa Patel NYU School of Medicine, NYU Prevention Research Center, NYU Center for the Study of Asian American Health, New York, USA

Tazuko Shibusawa Silver School of Social Work, New York University, New York, NY, USA

Jaeyoun Shin Pyramid Alternatives, Inc, Pacifica California, CA, USA

Susan M. Shinagawa Asian and Pacific Islander National Cancer Survivors Network (Asian & Pacific Islander American Health Forum, San Francisco, CA), Intercultural Cancer Council (Baylor College of Medicine, Houston, TX), Spring Valley, CA, USA

Dara H. Sorkin Division of General Internal Medicine, Health Policy Research Institute, University of California, Irvine, CA, USA

Susan Stewart School of Medicine, UCSF Helen Diller Family Comprehensive Cancer Center Biostatistics Core, University of California, San Francisco, USA

Jeanelle J. Sugimoto-Matsuda Asian/Pacific Islander Youth Violence Prevention Center, Department of Psychiatry, John A. Burns School of Medicine, University of Hawaii, Honolulu, HI, USA

Angela Sun Chinese Community Health Resource Center (CCHRC), San Francisco, CA, USA

David T. Takeuchi School of Social Work and Department of Sociology, University of Washington, Seattle, WA, USA

Judy Tan Center for AIDS Prevention Studies, University of California San Francisco, San Francisco, CA, USA

Cathy J. Tashiro Nursing Program, University of Washington Tacoma, Tacoma, WA, USA

Vicky Taylor Department of Health Services, Cancer Prevention Program at Fred Hutchinson Cancer Research Center, University of Washington, Seattle, WA, USA

Khatharya Um Asian American and Asian Diaspora Program, Department of Ethnic Studies, University of California, Berkeley, CA, USA

Stephen Vong San Francisco State University, San Francisco, CA, USA

May C. Wang Department of Community Health Sciences, UCLA School of Public Health, Los Angeles, CA, USA

Yijie Wang Department of Human Development and Family Sciences, University of Texas at Austin, Austin, TX, USA

Isha Weerasinghe NYU Institute of Community Health and Research, Center of the Study of Asian American Health, New York University School of Medicine, New York, NY, USA

Evaon Wong-Kim Department of Social Work, California State University, East Bay, Hayward, CA, USA

Sachiko Wood Cancer Disparities Research Group, San Francisco State University, San Francisco, CA, USA

Gwen Yeo Stanford Geriatric Education Center, Center for Education in Family and Community Medicine, Stanford University School of Medicine, Palo Alto, CA, USA

Grace J. Yoo Department of Asian American Studies, San Francisco State University, San Francisco, CA, USA

Lixin Zhang San Francisco State University, CA, USA

Wei Zhang College of Social Sciences, Sociology Department, University of Hawaii at Manoa, Honolulu, HI, USA

Ethnicity and Health

1

Fang Gong and David T. Takeuchi

Introduction

It has demonstrated repeatedly that socially disadvantaged and marginalized racial and ethnic groups are more likely to suffer from poorer health than groups who have distinct economic, social, and political resource advantages (Williams & Sternthal, 2010). Despite such well-documented trends, patterns of health disparities between Asian Americans and Whites as well as disparities within Asian subgroups remain less clear and underexplored. With the fast growth of the Asian American population, it is both surprising and problematic that the health within Asian American communities is not better understood.

Along with White, Black or African American, American Indian or Alaska Native, and Pacific Islander, Asian American is one of the major racial categories included in the 2010 U.S. Census (U.S. Census Bureau, 2010c). The Asian population in the United States is growing at a rapid rate. The most recent census estimates show that there are 15.5 million Asian Americans, comprising

5% of the total population. It had grown 2.7% between 2007 and 2008, the highest of any other group. It is projected that between 2008 and 2050, ethnic Asian residents will almost triple, reaching 40.6 million people (or 9% of the total population) in the United States (U.S. Census Bureau, 2010b).

The rapid growth is largely due to immigration. Recent census estimates indicate that immigrants from Asian countries have accounted for over a quarter of immigrants in the United States since 1990s (Grieco, 2010). Such rapid increase of Asians, particularly immigrants, will exert a strong influence on health policies and profiles of the United States.

The Asian American population is exceedingly heterogeneous, encompassing a diversity of ethnic groups. Chinese are the biggest subgroup, followed by Filipinos, Indians, Vietnamese, Koreans, and Japanese. Additionally, there are other significant subgroups, including Cambodian/Khmer, Pakistanis, Laotians, Hmong, Thais, and Bangladeshi (U.S. Census Bureau, 2010a). The extreme diversity presents a tremendous challenge for researchers to investigate health disparities both within the Asian American population and across Asians and other racial/ethnic groups. Accordingly, the research on Asian Americans and health has been underdeveloped at best.

The present chapter reviews existing literature and highlights the relationship between ethnicity and health among Asian Americans. We begin the chapter by defining several terms and theoretical perspectives that are important to

F. Gong (✉)
Department of Sociology, Ball State University,
Muncie, IN, USA
e-mail: fgong@bsu.edu

D.T. Takeuchi
School of Social Work and Department of Sociology,
University of Washington, Seattle, WA, USA
e-mail: dt5@u.washington.edu

G.J. Yoo et al. (eds.), *Handbook of Asian American Health*,
DOI 10.1007/978-1-4614-2227-3_1, © Springer Science+Business Media, LLC 2013

3

understand ethnicity and health. Next, we review current literature on patterns of physical and mental health among Asian ethnic groups. We conclude the chapter with recommendations for future directions.

Terms and Definitions

When studying ethnicity and health, it is of foremost importance to distinguish between race and ethnicity. Whereas race and ethnicity are often used interchangeably, they are two overlapping, yet distinct concepts. *Race* refers to "groups of people with shared biological traits that are often reflected by phenotype as a marker or some underlying shared genetic attribute" (Boykin & Williams, 2010, p. 322). *Ethnicity* is a broader term, including common ancestry and characteristics of groups such as culture, language, religion, physical traits and other factors (Boykin & Williams, 2010). One defining characteristic that distinguishes ethnicity from race is *culture*. Members of an ethnic group have common cultural origin and share norms, values, attitudes and behaviors that are typical of the ethnic group.

A major debate in the race/ethnicity literature considers whether race as a construct is still meaningful. Historically, race was regarded to reflect underlying genetic homogeneity. Yet recent analysis of DNA and genetics demonstrates that conventional "racial" groups only account for 6% of the human genetic variations whereas the other 94% exists *within* so-called racial groups (Williams & Harris-Reid, 1999). Such evidence suggests that race, rather than a genetic category, is instead socially constructed. Given the controversy, some anthropologists have lobbied to phase out data collection on race and urged to collect data on ethnicity only (Omi, 2001). Although this argument is undoubtedly contentious, it implies the importance of ethnicity research.

The *ethnicity-oriented race theory* provides an integrative framework linking both race and ethnicity. The perspective views race as a collection of identities that are culturally grounded, highlighting the importance of cultural factors and

variations among ethnic groups within a single racial category (Winant, 2000). A key construct within this theoretical framework is *ethnic identity*, which refers to "the sharing of cultural heritage, a sense of social relatedness, and symbolic cultural ties" (Sodowsky, Kwan, & Pannu, 1995). It is often measured using multidimensional components including ethnic identification, sense of belonging to one's ethnic group, ethnic pride/hatred toward one's ethnic group, and participation in ethnic activities (Phinney, 1990).

Prior research on the health and well-being of Asian Americans has not fully utilized the ethnicity-oriented race perspective. A review of recent literature reveals some major gaps in this line of work, including limited research on Asian American health and minimal data available on Asian subgroups.

Ethnicity and Health

There had been a profound lack of research on Asian American health prior to 2000. Ghosh (2003) reported that only 0.01% of published research involved Asian and Pacific Islander health, among over 5,000 publications in the MEDLINE database from 1966 to 2000. The very early work on Asian American health tended to regard Asian Americans as a "model minority," having more favorable health outcomes than Whites and other racial/ethnic minorities (Petersen, 1966). Subsequent empirical research has dispelled the notion of Asian Americans as universally "healthy, wealthy, and wise;" rather, Asian Americans are heterogeneous with respect to health risks (Chen & Hawks, 1995).

Data from the National Center for Health Statistics (NCHS) showed that compared with Whites, Asian Americans consistently had lower mortality rates across multiple indicators of chronic (heart, cancer, diabetes, and liver diseases) and infectious (pneumonia/influenza, HIV/AIDS) diseases (Williams, 2001). Such aggregate data, however, may obscure serious health disparities between ethnic subgroups (Ghosh, 2009). While the overall percentage of deaths attributable to heart disease was 24.6% for Asian

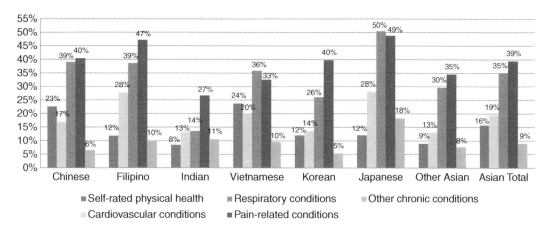

Fig. 1.1 Weighted percentage distribution of physical health conditions by Asian ethnic groups: the National Latino and Asian American Study (N = 2,095)

Americans and Pacific Islanders in 2004, the range for different subgroups was from 19.5% in Vietnamese to 34.6% in Indians (Heron, 2007). Asian Indians had much higher rate of diabetes (14.2%) than other Asian ethnic groups which ranged from 4% for Koreans and 8.9% for Filipinos (Barnes, Adams, & Powell-Griner, 2008).

The National Latino and Asian American Study (NLAAS) was one of the first and most comprehensive studies of the health (especially mental health) status of Asians and Latinos based on nationally representative samples (Alegria et al., 2004). The study surveyed a national sample of 2,095 Asian adults in 2002 and 2003 from the following ethnic categories: Chinese, Filipinos, Vietnamese, Indians, Koreans, Japanese, and other Asians.[1] Figure 1.1 presents relevant findings on self-rated physical health and various chronic health conditions obtained from weighted analyses of the NLAAS data.

The figures demonstrate significant health disparities across ethnic groups. For example, on average 16% of Asian Americans reported their physical health as poor or fair, ranging from 8% among Asian Indians and 24% of Vietnamese Americans. Nearly 30% of Filipinos and Japanese

reported cardiovascular conditions (including heart attack, stroke, heart disease, high blood pressure) whereas other Asian ethnic groups had much lower rates. There was also a huge difference between Japanese (50%) and Indians (14%) on respiratory ailments (including hay fever, asthma, tuberculosis, and other chronic lung diseases such as emphysema and chronic obstructive pulmonary disease).

Cancer researchers found that many Asian ethnic groups had higher rates of liver, breast, cervix and stomach cancers compared to other American ethnicities, as well as demonstrating intragroup variations. For example, the stomach cancer rate for Korean men was 54.6%, more than doubled the average rate of 20.1% for other Asian Americans and Pacific Islanders (McCracken et al., 2007). Further, Korean Americans were 5–7 times more likely to develop stomach cancer (Miller et al., 1996). The cervical cancer rate for Vietnamese women was 14%, much higher than the 8.8% average rate for Asian and Pacific Islander women (McCracken et al., 2007). Vietnamese also had high liver cancer incidence and death rates, approximately seven times higher than Whites (Miller et al., 1996). Despite the high prevalence of such cancers like gastric and liver cancers experienced by some Asian ethnic subgroups, these distinctions were excluded from the minority health focus areas in *Healthy People 2010*, suggesting that the diverse

---

[1] The weighted percentages of each ethnic group are listed in parentheses: Chinese (28.7%), Filipinos (21.6%), Vietnamese (12.9%), Indians (8.9%), Koreans (7.0%), Japanese (7.6%), and other Asians (13.3%).

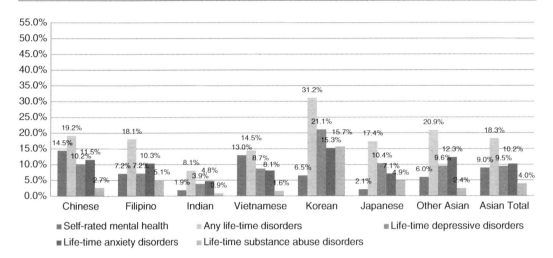

Fig. 1.2 Weighted percentage distribution of mental health conditions by Asian ethnic groups: the National Latino and Asian American Study (N = 2,095)

health needs of Asian Americans have yet to be fully acknowledged (Ghosh, 2009).

There have been important achievements in the study of Asian American mental health. The earliest data based on admission rates to mental hospitals indicated a pattern of underutilization of services by Chinese, Japanese and Filipinos in the 1960s and 1970s (Sue & Morishima, 1982). Later, community studies reviewed ethnic differences in distress and identified major demographic (e.g., socioeconomic status, gender, marital status) and acculturation variables (e.g., bicultural strategies) associated with mental health outcomes among various Asian ethnic groups (Vega & Rumbaut, 1991). Still, the lack of representative samples limits the generalizability of the data.

Takeuchi et al. (1998) has conducted a series of epidemiological studies to gather information on the population estimates of rates of psychiatric disorders among Asian Americans using rigorous probabilistic sampling strategies. In the 1990s, the author conducted two large-scale epidemiological studies on the mental health status of the two largest Asian subgroups, the Chinese American Psychiatric Epidemiological Study (CAPES) (N = 1,747) and the Filipino American Community Epidemiological Study (FACES) (N = 2,285).

These two studies collected data on probability samples of Chinese residing in Los Angeles and Filipinos in Honolulu and San Francisco respectively. The CAPES showed that the rates of mental health problems for Chinese Americans were low when compared with the average rates of the overall U.S. population (Sue, Sue, Sue, & Takeuchi, 1995; Takeuchi et al., 1998). The data from FACES was the first comprehensive documentation about alcohol problems and other health concerns of Filipino Americans (Gee, Delva, & Takeuchi, 2007; Gong, Takeuchi, & Agbayani-Siewert, 2003; Mossakowski, 2003 & 2007). Although these studies generated valuable data on specific Asian groups, national data on Asian Americans were still needed to make broad-level generalizations and recommendations.

The aforementioned NLAAS represents a major landmark in Asian American mental health research, the Asian component of which was again led by Takeuchi et al. (2007). To date, this has been the first large-scale national sample of Asians with wide-ranging measures of psychiatric disorders, service utilization and immigration factors. Weighted analyses by ethnic groups illustrated in Fig. 1.2 reveal significant ethnic differences in self-reported mental health and prevalence rates of lifetime psychiatric disorders.

Interestingly, a similar pattern was found for self-reported mental health as for self-reported physical health: Chinese subjects had the highest rate of self-rated poor and fair mental health (15%) while Indians had the lowest rate (2%). Using the criteria of the DSM-IV and the ICDI-10, Korean Americans had more reports of psychiatric disorders than other ethnic groups. The specific data includes 31% for "any psychiatric disorders," 21% for "any depressive disorders," 15% for "any anxiety disorders," and 16% for "any substance-abuse disorders." However, only 7% of Koreans self-rated their mental health as poor or fair.

Prior scholarship on Asian American health has indicated that perceptions of racial and ethnic discrimination were related to health and well-being. Gee (2002) reported from the CAPES data that both self-perceived discrimination and institutional discrimination (segregation and redlining) were linked to poor health of Chinese Americans. Similarly, the FACES data revealed perceptions of discrimination were associated with depression among Filipino Americans, though strong ethnic identity buffered the stress of discrimination (Mossakowski, 2003).

The NLAAS suggested subgroup differences in reporting of discrimination. Seventy-five percent of Thais reported that they were never disliked because of their race compared to 30% of Laotians (Gee & Ro, 2009). Perceptions of discrimination also affect help-seeking behaviors. Chinese Americans who perceived language discrimination were more likely to use informal medical services (Spencer & Chen, 2004). A limitation of the discrimination and health research is that the measure of discrimination does not always distinguish between racial from ethnic discrimination. It is important to make this distinction to fine-tune our understanding of the relationship between ethnic discrimination and health.

Future Research Directions

Significant progress has been made in documenting Asian ethnic disparities in health, yet much remains to be done to improve this research.

The most urgent need is to collect data on subgroups to more fully reveal the diversity inherent in this population. Ghosh (2009) recommended the largest and fastest-growing ethnicities should be given precedence, as well as the most underserved and vulnerable groups. Identifying and investigating health problems salient among specific Asian ethnic groups is also a priority.

Ethnicity-oriented race theory can serve as a useful theoretical framework to guide researchers to study ethnicity and health among Asian Americans (Winant, 2000). Race and ethnicity are often deemed as control variables by researchers, diminishing some important concerns of Asian subgroups. The ethnicity-based perspective reminds health researchers that there are underlying social and cultural meanings associated with specific ethnicities, and huge variations may exist across numerous subgroups that comprise a racial category. For example, the expression of illness may be different among one ethnic group from another. Some ethnic groups develop "cultural-bound syndromes" (Brown, Sellers, Brown, & Jackson, 1999; U.S. Department of Health and Human Services, 2001). Neurasthenia, chronic weakness and fatigue experienced by Chinese Americans and *hwa-byung*, somatisized anger and sorrow expressed by Korean Americans (Agbayani-Siewert, Takeuchi, & Pangan, 1999; Kleinman, 1986; U.S. Department of Health and Human Services, 2001) are two syndromes that are specific to the respective ethnicities.

Cultural factors may also influence self-reports of health status. The self-rated health reports may be flawed because of inconsistent response styles and diverse cultural values held by different subgroups (Jylhä, 2009). It is intriguing to note the discrepancy between low rates of self-rated poor mental health and the high prevalence rates of life-time disorders among Korean Americans, which warrants further investigation. Future research should examine the important roles that cultural factors play in determining, expressing, and reporting health.

More recently, scholars have proposed a comprehensive approach that focuses on the "context" to understanding Asian American health (Islam, Trinh-Shevrin, & Rey, 2009;

Leung & Takeuchi, 2011). Multiple dimensions such as *structural* (e.g., social policies), *institutional* (e.g., workforces and schools), *historical* (e.g., immigration, political or social histories), *community and family* (e.g., family structures), *geographical* (e.g., environment) and *cultural* (e.g., systems of beliefs and practices) are determinants associated with health behaviors, diseases and well-being (Islam, Trinh-Shevrin, & Rey, 2009).

This contextual approach sheds useful insights into the future study of ethnic discrimination and health. Discrimination experienced by Chinese Americans may be different from that experienced by Filipino Americans given the different structural, institutional, historical, geographical and cultural contexts of these two groups. As a result, the impact of ethnic discrimination on health or mechanisms linking discrimination to health may also be dissimilar.

Research on Asian ethnic groups is needed not only in different contexts, but also at multiple levels. Under the guidance of the community-based participatory research (CBPR), researchers can engage with local community organizations to capture the health needs of Asian subgroups and thus better document ethnic disparities in health. At the broader level, state and national health agenda targeting specific Asian ethnic groups and overseeing organizations are necessary to guide the study on Asian American health (Ghosh, 2009).

In summary, it is crucially important to investigate the health of the specific ethnic subgroups within the Asian population, given the rapid growth of this population overall. Research and practice on Asian ethnicity and health requires collaborative efforts from scholars, practitioners, and activists in various disciplines (e.g., medicine, social epidemiology, medical sociology, medical anthropology, and medical psychology) and across multiple domains (e.g., academia, medical practice, community advocacy groups, and local and federal government agencies). Such cooperative work will lead to the collection of high-quality subgroup data, the transformation of data into effective research and policy recommendations, and ultimately the elimination of ethnic disparities and improvement in health among Asian Americans.

References

Agbayani-Siewert, P., Takeuchi, D. T., & Pangan, R. W. (1999). Mental illness in a multicultural context. In C. S. Aneshensel & J. C. Phelan (Eds.), *Handbook of the sociology of mental health* (pp. 19–36). New York: Kluwer Academic/Plenum.

Alegria, M., Takeuchi, D. T., Ganino, G., Duan, N., Shrout, P., Meng, X.-L., et al. (2004). Considering context, place, and culture: The national Latino and Asian American Study. *International Journal of Methods in Psychiatric Research, 13,* 208–220.

Barnes, P. M., Adams, P. F., & Powell-Griner, E. (2008). *Health characteristics of the Asian adult population: United States, 2004–2006.* Hyattsville, MD: National Center for Health Statistics.

Boykin, S. D., & Williams, D. R. (2010). Race, ethnicity, and health in a global context: Methods and applications. In A. Steptoe (Ed.), *Handbook of behavioral medicine* (pp. 321–339). New York: Springer.

Brown, T. N., Sellers, S. L., Brown, K. T., & Jackson, J. S. (1999). Race, ethnicity and culture in the sociology of mental health. In C. S. Aneshensel & J. C. Phelan (Eds.), *Handbook of the sociology of mental health* (pp. 167–182). New York: Kluwer Academic/Plenum.

Chen, M. S., Jr., & Hawks, B. L. (1995). A Debunking of the myth of healthy Asian Americans and Pacific Islanders. *American Journal of Health Promotion, 9,* 261–268.

Gee, G. C. (2002). A multilevel analysis of the relationship between institutional and individual racial discrimination and health status. *American Journal of Public Health, 92,* 615–623.

Gee, G. C., Delva, J., & Takeuchi, D. T. (2007). Relationships between self-reported unfair treatment and prescription medication use, illicit drug use, and alcohol dependence among Filipino Americans. *American Journal of Public Health, 97,* 933–940.

Gee, G. C., & Ro, A. (2009). Racism and discrimination. In C. Trinh-Shevrin, N. S. Islam, & M. J. Rey (Eds.), *Asian American communities and health: Context, research, policy, and action* (pp. 364–402). San Francisco: Jossey-Bass.

Ghosh, C. (2003). Healthy People 2010 and Asian Americans/Pacific Islanders: Defining a baseline of information. *American Journal of Public Health, 93,* 2093–2098.

Ghosh, C. (2009). Asian American health research: Baseline data and funding. In C. Trinh-Shevrin, N. S. Islam, & M. J. Rey (Eds.), *Asian American communities and health: Context, research, policy, and action* (pp. 73–103). San Francisco: Jossey-Bass.

Gong, F., Takeuchi, D. T., & Agbayani-Siewert, P. (2003). Acculturation, psychological distress and alcohol use: Investigating the effects of ethnic identity and religiosity. In K. M. Chun, P. B. Organista, & G. Marin (Eds.), *Acculturation: Advances in theory, measurement, and applied research* (pp. 189–206). Washington, DC: American Psychological Association.

Grieco, E. M. (2010). "Race and Hispanic origin of the foreign-born population in the United States: 2007. Retrieved March 18, 2011, from http://www.census.gov/prod/2010pubs/acs-11.pdf.

Heron, M. (2007). *Deaths: Leading causes for 2004.* Hyattsville, MD: National Center for Health Statistics.

Islam, N. S., Trinh-Shevrin, C., & Rey, M. J. (2009). Toward a contextual understanding of Asian American health. In C. Trinh-Shevrin, N. S. Islam, & M. J. Rey (Eds.), *Asian American communities and health: Context, research, policy, and action* (pp. 3–22). San Francisco: Jossey-Bass.

Jylhä, M. (2009). What is self-rated health and why does it predict mortality? Towards a unified conceptual model. *Social Science & Medicine, 69,* 307–316.

Kleinman, A. (1986). *Social origins of distress and disease: Depression, Neurasthenia and pain in the modern China.* New Haven, CT: Yale University Press.

Leung, M. C., & Takeuchi, D. T. (2011). Race, place and health. In L. M. Burton, S. P. Kemp, M. C. Leung, S. A. Matthews, & D. T. Takeuchi (Eds.), *Communities, neighborhoods, and health: Expanding the boundaries of place* (pp. 73–88). New York: Springer.

McCracken, M., Olsen, M., Chen, M. S., Jr., Jemal, A., Thun, M., Cokkinides, V., et al. (2007). Cancer incidence, mortality, and associated risk factors among Asian Americans of Chinese, Filipino, Vietnamese, Korean, and Japanese ethnicities. *CA: A Cancer Journal for Clinicians, 57,* 190–205.

Miller, B. A., Kolonel, L. N., Bernstein, L., Young, J. L., Swanson, G. M., West, D. W., et al. (1996). *Racial/ethnic patterns of cancer in the United States, 1988–1992.* Bethesda, MD: National Cancer Institute. NIH Pub. No. 96-4104.

Mossakowski, K. N. (2003). Coping with perceived discrimination: Does ethnic identity protect mental health? *Journal of Health and Social Behavior, 44,* 318–333.

Mossakowski, K. N. (2007). Are immigrants healthier? The case of depression among Filipino Americans. *Social Psychology Quarterly, 70,* 290–304.

Omi, M. (2001). The changing meaning of race. In N. J. Smelser, W. J. Wilson, & F. Mitchell (Eds.), *America becoming: Racial trends and their consequences* (Vol. 1, pp. 243–263). Washington, DC: National Academy Press.

Petersen, W. (1966, January 9). Success story, Japanese-American style. *The New York Times.*

Phinney, J. S. (1990). Ethnic identity in adolescents and adults: Review of research. *Psychological Bulletin, 108,* 499–514.

Sodowsky, G. R., Kwan, K.-L. K., & Pannu, R. (1995). Ethnic identity of Asians in the United States. In J. G. Ponterotto, J. M. Casas, L. A. Suzuki, & C. M. Alexander (Eds.), *Handbook of multicultural counseling* (2nd ed., pp. 123–154). Thousand Oaks, CA: Sage.

Spencer, M. S., & Chen, J. (2004). Effect of discrimination on mental health service utilization among Chinese Americans. *American Journal of Public Health, 94,* 809–814.

Sue, S., & Morishima, J. K. (1982). *The mental health of Asian Americans: Contemporary issues in identifying and treating mental problems.* San Francisco: Jossey-Bass.

Sue, S., Sue, D. W., Sue, L., & Takeuchi, D. T. (1995). Psychopathology among Asian Americans: A model minority? *Cultural Diversity and Mental Health, 1,* 39–51.

Takeuchi, D. T., Chung, R. C.-Y., Lin, K.-M., Shen, H., Kuraski, K., Chun, C.-A., et al. (1998). Lifetime and twelve-month prevalence rates of major depressive episodes and Dysthymia among Chinese Americans in Los Angeles. *The American Journal of Psychiatry, 155,* 1407–1414.

Takeuchi, D. T., Zane, N., Hong, S., Chae, D. H., Gong, F., Gee, G. C., et al. (2007). Immigration-related factors and mental disorders among Asian Americans. *American Journal of Public Health, 97,* 84–90.

U.S. Census Bureau. (2010a). 2009 American Community Survey. Retrieved March 18, 2011, from http://factfinder.census.gov/home/saff/main.html?_lang=en.

U.S. Census Bureau. (2010b). Asian/Pacific American Heritage Month: May 2010. Retrieved March 18, 2011, from http://www.census.gov/newsroom/releases/archives/facts_for_features_special_editions/cb10-ff07.html

U.S. Census Bureau. (2010c). U.S. census form 2010. Retrieved March 18, 2011, from http://2010.census.gov/2010census/pdf/2010_Questionnaire_Info.pdf.

U.S. Department of Health and Human Services. (2001). *Mental health: Culture, race, and ethnicity-a supplement to mental health: A report of the surgeon general.* Rockville, MD: U.S. Department of Health and Human Services/Substance Abuse and Mental Health Services Administration/Center for Mental Health Services.

Vega, W. A., & Rumbaut, R. G. (1991). Ethnic minorities and mental health. *Annual Review of Sociology, 17,* 351–383.

Williams, D. R. (2001). Racial variations in adult health status: Patterns, paradoxes and prospects. In N. J. Smelser, W. J. Wilson, & F. Mitchell (Eds.), *America becoming: Racial trends and their consequences* (Vol. 2, pp. 371–410). Washington, DC: National Academy Press.

Williams, D. R., & Harris-Reid, M. (1999). Race and mental health: Emerging patterns and promising approaches. In A. V. Horwitz & T. L. Scheid (Eds.), *A handbook for the study of mental health: Social contexts, theories and systems* (pp. 295–314). New York: Cambridge University Press.

Williams, D. R., & Sternthal, M. (2010). Understanding racial-ethnic disparities in health: Sociological contributions. *Journal of Health and Social Behavior, 51,* S15–S27.

Winant, H. (2000). Race and race theory. *Annual Review of Sociology, 26,* 169–185.

Critical Health Issues Impacting Asian Indian Americans

Ranjita Misra

Demographics

Asian Indians or Indian Americans are individuals of Indian ancestry. They are represented under the broader classification of Asian Americans (AA) or Asian American and Pacific Islanders (AAPI) (Office of Minority Health [OMH], 2006). Sometimes they are also referred to as South Asians which denotes people belonging to various countries from the Indian subcontinent (India, Pakistan, Sri Lanka, Bangladesh, and Nepal). India is the seventh-largest country by geographical area, the second-most populous country with 1.18 billion people, and the most populous democracy in the world (Baggett et al., 2009).

Asian Americans are a heterogeneous collection of over 50 Asian American subgroups, comprising 5% (13.9 million) of the U.S. population (Yagalla, Hoerr, Song, Enas, & Garg, 1996). According to the U.S. Census Bureau population estimate, Asian Americans are the fastest growing racial/ethnic group and are expected to reach 22 million by 2050 (212% increase) (OMH, 2006). Asian Americans, whether they are immigrants or U.S.- born, represent a diverse and rich mixture of cultures, languages, beliefs and practices.

R. Misra (✉)
Department of Health and Kinesiology,
Center for the Study of Health Disparities (CSHD),
Texas A&M University, College Station, TX, USA
e-mail: Ranjita.misra@osumc.edu

Immigrant Patterns and Asian Indian Population in the United States

Currently, Asian Indians comprise 16.4% of the Asian Americans living in the United States. Seventy-one percent of them are 18–64 years old, and 77% are immigrants (Misra et al., 2010).

Most Asian Indian immigrants entered the United States within the last 30 years, following the passage of the Immigration Act of 1965 which allowed increasing numbers of Asian Indians to enter the United States (Ruy, Young, & Kwak, 2002). A number of Asian Indians immigrated to the United States via other countries such as the United Kingdom (where 2% of the population is of Indian origin), Canada, Mauritius, South Africa and nations of Southeast Asia such as Malaysia and Singapore.

Asian Indians are the third largest Asian American subgroup in the United States, following Chinese Americans and Filipino Americans (U.S. Census Bureau, 2000a). They are also one of the fastest growing Asian American subgroups. For example, between 1980 and 1990, the Asian Indian population in the United States grew by 126% as compared to the 108% growth of all Asian Americans combined. According to the U.S. Census Bureau, between 1990 and 2000, the Indian population in the U.S. grew 130% – 10 times the national average of 13%, and according to the American Community Survey of the U.S. Census Bureau, the Asian Indian population increased from 1,679,000 in 2000 to 2,570,000 in

G.J. Yoo et al. (eds.), *Handbook of Asian American Health*,
DOI 10.1007/978-1-4614-2227-3_2, © Springer Science+Business Media, LLC 2013

11

2007 with a growth rate of 53%, putting it among the fastest growing Asian subgroups in the United States (U.S. Census Bureau, 2000a).

In 2006, legal immigrants to the United States from all countries totaled 1,266,264, of which 58,072 were from India. Immigration from India is currently at its highest level in history. It is noted that between 2000 and 2006, 421,006 Indian immigrants were admitted to the United States (an increase from 352,278 during the 1990–1999 period) (Misra et al., 2010).

Despite their increasing numbers, current research on Asian American health does not adequately address the health needs of Asian Indians. The literature on health behaviors and chronic diseases indicates an increase in behavioral risk factors (e.g., consumption of high fat diet and more animal products, sedentary lifestyle) as well as biological risk factors (e.g., obesity, hypertension) for chronic diseases when individuals migrate to more prosperous countries (South Asian Public Health Association [SAPHA], 2002). This is true among Japanese and Hispanic immigrants to the United States. A review of current health literature shows that while there has been a fair amount of research focused on some groups of immigrants such as the Japanese, Chinese, and Filipinos, other immigrants, particularly Asian Indians, have been less studied. Current national surveys are incapable of assessing preventive health behaviors and disease prevalence in specific Asian subpopulations because multiple ethnic groups are aggregated into the general category of "Asian and Pacific Islander," and because sample sizes of individual Asian subgroups are small (Misra et al., 2010).

Key Features of this Ethnic Group

Diversity

Asian Indians comprise more distinct and diverse subgroups than other Asian immigrants originating from a single nation. This is due to differences in their primary languages, provincialism, religious affiliations, and India's caste system. India has 14 official languages and Indians come from

28 different provinces or states. Additionally, there are at least four distinct racial types and five major religions represented in this group. This diversity hinders Asian Indians in forming clusters like the Chinese, Japanese, and Filipinos and contributes to their lack of social and political visibility in this country. Furthermore, Asian Indians, unlike many other Asian and South American immigrant groups, do not depend highly on local ethnic networks for financial and/or occupational support due to their high educational status and professional careers. Consequently they are geographically dispersed. This geographic dispersion, combined with extreme internal diversities, does not encourage them to form ethnic clusters in defined geographic areas as seen among Chinese and other immigrants (Sharma, Malarcher, Giles, & Myers, 2004). First generation Asian Indians tend to retain the distinct languages, culture, and religious practices of their subgroups. This tends to inhibit the development of ethnic solidarity as seen among Chinese, Japanese, or Filipino immigrants.

Religions

While the majority of Asian Indian immigrants in the United States are Hindus, there are significant numbers of Indian Sikhs, Muslims, Christians, and Jains that enter the country also. As of 2000, the American Hindu population was approximately one million. Religious diversity among Asian Indians is evident in the numerous cultural and religious associations and organizations that have been established in the United States by Hindus, Sikhs, Jains, Buddhists, Muslims, Christians, Parsis, and Jews from India. The first Indian religious center to be established in the U.S. was a Sikh Gurudwaras in Stockton, California in 1912. However, Asian Indians who follow the Hindu religion believe themselves to be quite different from Sikhs from the state of Punjab. Today there are many Sikh Gurudwaras, Hindu, Buddhist and Jain temples in all 50 states. Additionally, many sects such as ISKCON, Swaminarayan Sampraday, BAPS Swaminarayan Sanstha, Chinmaya Mission, and Swadhyay

Pariwar are well established in the United States. Yoga is practiced and promoted by many Indian religious leaders. More than 18 million Americans are now practicing some form of Yoga.

Muslim Indian Americans generally congregate with other South Asian and American Muslims, including those from Pakistan and Bangladesh (Nan et al., 1991). The United States had several immigrant Muslim organizations for Asian Indians, such as the Indian Muslim Council. Christians, who comprise approximately 6% of the Indian population in India, are concentrated in the states of Kerala and Maharashtra (Goa). Asian Indian immigrant Christians have several Indian Christian churches across the United States such as the Syro-Malabar Catholic Church, Syro-Malankara Catholic Church, Indian Orthodox Church, and Church of South India to name a few. There are also a number of Asian Indian Christians who attend mainstream American churches (Agarwal, Lee, Raju, & Stephen, 2009). The Federation of Indian American Christian Organizations of North America (FIACONA) was formed to represent a network of Indian Christian Organizations in the United States and Canada. The Parsi community and Indian Jews are perhaps the smallest Asian Indian minority communities in the United States.

Language

India has 14 official languages, and Asian Indians from different states typically speak different languages. Hindi is the official national language in India. According to the Census of India, there are approximately 90 million Indian English speakers (as a second or third language) due to the colonial rule of Britain in India (Misra, Patel, Davies, & Russo, 2000). With the exception of some families who communicate primarily in English, as well as members of the relatively small Anglo–Indian community numbering less than half a million, speakers of Indian English use it as a second or third language, after their indigenous Indian language(s), such as, Assamese, Oriya, Urdu, Gujarati, Punjabi, Hindi, Sindhi, Bengali, Kannada, Telugu, Marathi, Tamil, and Malayalam.

Socioeconomic Status

Education

Asian Indians, along with some other Asian subgroups, have among the highest levels of educational qualifications when compared to other racial and ethnic groups in the United States. A national study on Asian Indians in the United States showed 86% Indians have at least a bachelor's degree compared to 28% nationally and 44% average for all Asian American groups. Almost 40% of all Asian Indians in the United States have a master's, doctorate or other professional degree, which is five times the national average (Misra et al., 2010). Among Indian Americans, 72.3% participate in the U.S. workforce, of which 57.7% are employed in managerial and professional specialties (Snehalatha, Viswanathan, & Ramachandran, 2003).

A joint Duke University – University of California, Berkeley study revealed that Asian Indian immigrants have founded more engineering and technology companies from 1995 to 2005 than immigrants from the U.K., China, Taiwan and Japan combined (Assisi, 2007). Another study from UC Berkeley reported that one-third of the engineers in Silicon Valley are of Indian descent, while 7% of Silicon Valley high-tech firms are led by Asian Indian CEOs (Saxenian, 1999).

Asian Indians also represent a disproportionately higher percentage of medical students and physicians in the United States (OMH, 2006). Ten to twelve percent of medical students entering US schools are of Indian origin (Singh, 2012). According to the American Association of Physicians of Indian Origin (AAPIO), there are approximately 50,000 Indian American physicians and about 15,000 medical students/residents of Indian heritage in this country, making them the largest ethnic minority of physicians in the United States. Indian physicians make significant contributions to health care, not only practicing in inner cities, rural areas and peripheral communities but also at top medical schools and other academic centers in the U.S. (Jonnalagadda & Diwan, 2002a).

Income

Asian Indians in the United States tend to be highly educated professionals, prosperous, and English speaking. Their mean income level is 25% above the national average, and the median income is $60,093, compared to $41,110 for non-Hispanic Whites (Misra et al., 2010). Hence, the economic power of Asian Indians in the U.S. is indisputable. Furthermore, 67% of foreign-born Asian Indians have a college education as compared to 21% of Caucasians. Hence, Asian Indians are perceived as having good access to health care. However, there are marked variations in educational attainment, income, and wealth among Asian Indians (Misra et al., 2000). Recent immigrant cohorts comprise both highly-educated professionals as well as individuals who lack education and job skills. The latter are mostly family members of earlier immigrants.

According to the 2000 U.S. Census, Asian Indian men had "the highest year-round, full-time median earning ($51,094)," while Asian Indian women had a median income of $35,173. This phenomenon has been linked to the "brain drain" of the Indian intelligence from India. (The trend of the best and brightest students and professionals immigrating to the U.S. and other westernized countries in order to seek better financial opportunities is termed 'brain drain.') Recently, however, there has been a drop in immigration of Indians from India to the U.S. This is generally attributed to the improving economy of India. This trend, along with the long history of immigration from India, leads to a growing percentage of Asian Indians who are second or third generation. Although the majority of Asian Indians are professionals (doctors, computer scientists, academics, etc.), a significant number are business owners or involved with the lodging industry. Indian Americans own 50% of all economy lodges and 35% of all hotels in the United States (Dhingra, 2012). In 2002, there were over 223,000 Asian Indian owned firms in the U.S., employing more than 610,000 workers, and generating more than $88 billion in revenue (Huang & Carrasquillo, 2008).

Culture

Food

Throughout history, the culture and cuisines of India have been influenced by other civilizations such as the Moghuls, the British and now the Americans (Enas & Senthilkumar, 2001). Asian Indians have popularized the Asian Indian cuisine in the United States, and there are hundreds of Indian restaurants and eateries nationwide. Currently, there are many Indian markets and ethnic grocery stores in the United States, especially in cities with a large Asian Indian population (Raj, Ganganna, & Bowering, 1999). Some of the biggest Indian markets are in Silicon Valley, Chicago, New York City, the Philadelphia metropolitan area, and Edison, New Jersey. Areas with a significant Indian market presence also include the Devon Avenue neighborhood in Chicago, Pioneer Boulevard in the Los Angeles region, and University Avenue in Berkeley, California. Other predominantly Indian neighborhoods are Journal Square in Jersey City, New Jersey, Jackson Heights in Queens, New York, Hillcroft Avenue in Houston, Texas and Richardson near Dallas, Texas. Asian Indians of different religions observe different dietary laws and codes for fasting and feasting which influence their eating patterns.

Entertainment

Hindi radio and television stations are available in areas with high Asian Indian populations. Several cable and satellite providers offer Asian Indian channels such as Sony TV, Zee TV, and Star Plus. Furthermore, many metropolitan areas with high Asian Indian populations now have movie theatres specializing in Indian movies produced by Bollywood (named after Hollywood). Bollywood is the informal term popularly used for the Hindi language film industry based in Mumbai, Maharashtra, India. Since 2000, Bollywood films are believed to have influenced musical films in the United States and the world. The Bollywood film industry has been credited for the success of individuals such as

A.R. Rahman, an Indian film composer who wrote the music for Danny Boyle's Slumdog Millionaire (2008) – winner of four Golden Globes and eight Academy Awards. The influence of Bollywood music can also be seen in popular music around the world.

Geographical Concentration

In the United States, the states with the largest Asian Indian populations, in order, are California, New York, New Jersey, Texas, and Illinois (Chandalia, Mohan, Adams-Huet, Deepa, & Abate, 2008). There are also large Asian Indian populations in Pennsylvania, Florida, Michigan, Maryland, Virginia, Georgia, and Ohio. The New York metropolitan area, consisting of New York City and adjacent areas within the state of New York as well as nearby areas within New Jersey, Connecticut, and Pennsylvania, is home to approximately 600,000 Asian Indians as of 2009, comprising by far the largest Asian Indian population of any metropolitan area in the United States (Misra et al., 2010). At least 17 Asian Indian enclaves characterized as "Little India" have emerged in the New York metropolitan area.

Other metropolitan areas with large Asian Indian populations include San Francisco/San Jose/Oakland, Chicago, Los Angeles, Washington/Baltimore, Philadelphia, Boston, Detroit, Houston, Dallas/Ft. Worth, Charlotte, North Carolina and Atlanta. The town of Edison, New Jersey (total population 100,499) is 17.5% Asian Indian – the highest percentage of any municipality in the United States. The mostly agrarian Imperial Valley, California near the Mexican border has a long history of Asian Indians (an estimated 21,000 live in Imperial County, California alone) since the first arrivals to the California desert in the early 1900s. The first American Sikh temples were in the Sacramento (Marysville and Yuba City) and San Joaquin Valleys (Lodi and Stockton) to serve the early wave of Sikh Indian workers arrived there. In contrast with East Asian Americans, who tend to be concentrated in California and other areas near the Pacific coast, Asian Indians are more evenly distributed throughout the United States (U.S. Census, 2000b).

Established and Emerging Health Issues

In 2003, the Institute of Medicine (IOM, 2003) released a report documenting disparities in access to health care and quality of care that impact the health and health care of racial/ethnic minorities as compared with non-Hispanic Whites (NHWs). Numerous studies indicate diabetes and cardiovascular disease disproportionately affect Asian Indians (Enas & Senthilkumar, 2001; Misra et al., 2010; Mohanty, Woolhandler, Himmelstein, & Bor, 2005).

Cancer is the leading cause of death for Asian Indians, followed by heart disease and stroke (Misra & Vadaparampil, 2004; Misra, Menon, Vadaparampil, & Belue, 2011). Invasive cancer among South Asian women is much higher as compared to other ethnic groups. Among Asian Indian men, cardiovascular disease (e.g., diseases of the heart and stroke) is the leading cause of death; Asian Indian women, however, are afflicted by cancer significantly more than their male counterparts. Among Asian Indian men the top five cancer sites were lung, prostate, pancreas, leukemia, and liver; for Asian Indian women the five main cancer sites were breast, lung, colorectum, ovary, and pancreas.

While cancer incidence and mortality are currently lower among Asian Indians than the U.S. Caucasian population, with increasing acculturation the cancer rates are expected to increase to match rates among Americans as has been seen with other Asian subgroups such as the Japanese and Chinese (Misra, Rastogi, & Joshi, 2009).

High Risk for Chronic Diseases

The burden of diabetes and cardiovascular disease among Asian Indians living in the United States is well documented. For example, Asian Indians with type II diabetes have five times higher risk of cardiovascular disease than the general U.S. population. Results from the Diabetes among Indian Americans (DIA) study show Asian Indian immigrants have a prevalence of diabetes and pre-diabetes at 17.4% and 33% - much higher than any other ethnic groups in the United States (Misra et al., 2010). Asian Indians are also reported to have high rates of metabolic syndrome (a clustering of risk factors for diabetes and cardiovascular disease) and coronary heart disease or coronary artery disease (CAD) and related complications (Anand et al., 2000; Balasubramanyam, Rao, Misra, Sekhar, & Ballantyne, 2008; Chandie Shaw et al., 2002; Enas et al., 1996; Hughes, Aw, Kuperan, & Choo, 1997; McKeigue, Ferrie, Pierpoint, & Marmot, 1993; McKeigue, Pierpoint, Ferrie, & Marmot, 1992; Misra et al., 2009; Mohanty et al., 2005; Omar et al., 1985; Ramaiya, Denver, & Yudkin, 1995; Samanta, Burden, & Jagger, 1991). Insulin resistance is prevalent in Asian Indian immigrants, despite low rates of obesity (McKeigue, 1996; McKeigue et al., 1992; Whincup et al., 2002). In the United States, Asian Indians have the highest ethnic-specific prevalence of cardiovascular disease (CVD), with age-specific mortality two to three times higher than Caucasians (Enas & Senthilkumar, 2001; Enas et al., 1996; Wild, Laws, Fortmann, Varady, & Byrne, 1995). Traditional risk factors such as hypertension, obesity and hypercholesterolemia do not account completely for these high rates. Data from national surveys are limited due to small sample sizes or aggregation of ethnic data into a heterogeneous group of "Asian Americans" or "Asian and Pacific Islanders" (Mohanty et al., 2005).

The rate of CVD and diabetes among Asian Indians is among the highest in the world for both men and women. The relative risk of Coronary Artery Disease (CAD) mortality is about 1.4 for Asian Indians compared with the general U.S. population. Enas and his colleagues (2001) reported Asian Indians have the highest rate of heart attacks of any ethnic group in the world. Similarly, the prevalence of diabetes is strikingly high in Asian Indian immigrants to the U.S., and is estimated to be two to three times higher than in the general U.S. population. Diabetes may be a contributing factor in up to 20% of cardiovascular deaths in Asian Indians. It is unclear why the CAD rate is so much higher in this population given that risk factors such as hypertension, smoking, and obesity are actually less prevalent than in the Caucasian population. However, many Asian Indians have abdominal/visceral adiposity without BMI obesity.

The prevalence of a high triglyceride (TG)/low density lipoprotein (HDL) pattern in Asian Indians is also high in both India and in Britain, and this pattern is associated with excess cardiovascular risk. Lipoprotein has been shown to be an independent risk factor for CAD, and this has also been reported to be especially prevalent in Asian Indians. Inactivity, commonly found in Asian Indians in the U.S., and dietary patterns that are high in carbohydrates and low in fat, exacerbate the high TG/low HDL pattern even further. Paradoxically, vegetarians appear to be an especially high-risk group because of the high carbohydrate dietary pattern, and some preliminary reports suggest an even higher CAD risk in vegetarians. Healthy diet and regular physical activity could help control these abnormalities. These factors warrant further research into disease prevalence and health behavior patterns of this high-risk ethnic Asian subgroup.

Mental Illness

While Asian Americans in general, and Asian Indians in particular, are underrepresented or unreported in most studies of mental illness, the effects of mental illness, such as racism, suicide, substance abuse, and poor access to health care are prevalent in this group (Smokowski, David-Ferdon, & Stroupe, 2009).

Social and Cultural Factors

Diversity among Asian Indians extends to their religions, language, dietary habits, and cultural practices. Most Asian Indians are Hindus, and their religious beliefs, spirituality, and faith play roles in their support and coping mechanisms and recovery from health related problems, as well as in the personal and social adjustments they must make to adapt to the new culture of the United States.

A small percentage of Asian Indians are Muslims, and Islamic customs influence everyday life for this minority group. For example, tobacco and alcohol use are prohibited in the Koran. A study of Muslim immigrant women found women declined cervical cancer screening because they perceived the screening services to be threatening to their religious values (Martin, 2005; Rajaram & Rashidi, 1999). Asian Islamic women were also found to have lower rates of mammography and clinical breast exams which researchers attributed in large part to the religious influence of Islam (Rajaram & Rashidi, 1999).

Educational level and health outcomes are highly correlated for all immigrants, including Asian Indians. However, not all Asian Indians have high socio-economic levels, for example, recent immigrants who are family members of green card holders. Hence, programs for this group need to be tailored by health literacy levels of the participants. The clustering of an individual's educational level with socio-economic status, access to health care, knowledge of disease and health promoting lifestyle serve as a strong basis for health professionals to be cognizant of the lifestyle of the Asian Indian community they serve. It is not surprising that higher all-cause morbidity and mortality occurs among people who are at the lowest socio-economic status levels.

Recent scholarship indicates immigration status is important in health insurance coverage and access to care. As a result, children of immigrants are less likely to have well child care, and wellness screening rates are lower among immigrants if documentation is required. Undocumented persons tend to have poorer health and are less likely to seek health care, and also receive worse care than those who have better access to care (Derose, Escarce, & Lurie, 2007). The use of complementary and alternative medicine, chronic and infectious diseases, mental health concerns, end of life issues, health behaviors and general lifestyle all have important effects on Asian Indian immigrants.

Culture is a major determinant of lifestyle behavior and corresponding health outcomes. Cultural beliefs influence perceptions of illness and health management and are more pronounced among Asian Indians given their more recent immigration history. Acculturation, defined as the process by which immigrants adopt the customs, beliefs and behaviors of a new culture, can have either a positive or a negative influence on health enhancing behaviors as these immigrants become more westernized (Sundquist & Winkleby, 2000). Literature indicates that being acculturated is linked to use of health services. Less acculturated Asian Indians utilize less wellness screenings, and engage in more tobacco use compared to their more acculturated peers. Being more acculturated, however, may also lead to lifestyle and behavioral practices that override the protective cultural influences experienced by a group. These include changes to the dietary practices that encourage the development of obesity and chronic diseases, and a more sedentary lifestyle (Gomez, Kelsey, Glaser, Lee, & Sidney, 2004). Acculturation, however, is a multidimensional construct and usually measured by generational status, language and food preference, and the number of years of U.S. residence. Given the diversity of experiences and exposures to mainstream society based on the diversity within the Asian Indian community, acculturation experiences within this ethnic group may not be similar. Despite these inconsistencies, acculturation is often used by researchers as a predictor of health beliefs, attitudes, behaviors, and outcomes (Lv & Cason, 2004).

Trends and Emerging Concerns Impacting Asian Indians

Lifestyle Changes

There are several growing issues that impact Asian Indian lifestyles and behaviors. As Asian Indians acculturate, their eating habits become increasingly westernized (Jonnalagadda & Diwan, 2002b). There is a general shift from vegetarianism to non-vegetarianism, and ethnic foods are consumed along with traditional ingredients found in American supermarkets. Consequently, diets of immigrants living in the United States have changed from being low in fat and rich in fiber to being high in saturated fat and animal protein and low in fiber (Esperat, Inouye, Gonzalez, Owen, & Feng, 2004). There is also an increased tendency to consume fast foods and convenience foods. These dietary changes, along with sedentary and stressful lifestyles, and genetic predisposition to diabetes and CVD may increase their risk for chronic diseases among acculturated and second- and third-generation immigrants. Overweight and obesity research indicates that obesity is linked to migration patterns with the individual's length of stay in the United States. For Asian Indian immigrants, food is a vital part of the social matrix and changes from traditional Asian Indian diet to western/fast foods results in a higher consumption of fatty meats, dairy products and processed snacks and desserts. Asian Indians are experiencing the same trend of increasing overweight and obesity observed in other ethnic groups in the United States. While it is difficult to specify what has caused this trend, physical inactivity and poor eating habits are certainly contributors. Asian Indians are less physically active with higher levels of inactivity and obesity among women. Although highly educated, many Asian Indians do not read food labels to monitor their caloric and nutrient intake (Misra et al., 2010). Minimally nutritional and calorie dense foods are readily available and inexpensive in the United States, and the automobile is the preferred mode of transportation even for short distances. Additional compounding factors are fatalism, lack of knowledge, and perceived barriers that prohibit behavior change (Pasick & Burke, 2008).

Overweight and Obesity

Research indicates that obesity is linked to migration patterns with the individual's length of stay in the United States. For Asian Indian immigrants,

food is a vital part of the social matrix and changes from traditional Asian Indian diet to western/fast foods resulting in a higher consumption of fatty meats, dairy products and processed snacks and desserts. Asian Indians are experiencing the same trend of increasing overweight and obesity observed in other ethnic groups in the United States. While it is difficult to specify what has caused the trend but physical inactivity and poor eating habits are certainly contributors. Asian Indians are less physically active with higher levels of inactivity and obesity among women. Although highly educated, many Asian Indians do not read food labels for keeping track of their calories and nutrient intake (Misra et al., 2010). Minimally nutritional and calorie dense foods are readily available and inexpensive in the United States, and the automobile is the preferred mode of transportation even for short distances. Additional confounding factors are fatalism, lack of knowledge, and perceived barriers that prohibit behavior change.

Health Problems and Nutritional Status of Asian Indians in the US

Some of the important health problems faced by Asian Indian immigrants include chronic degenerative diseases such as diabetes, hypertension, CVD and complications arising from any of these conditions. In fact, Asian Indian immigrants have a significantly higher risk of cardiovascular disease with heart disease rates estimated to be one and one half to four times greater than Whites. In addition to the genetic susceptibility in developing type II diabetes and cardiovascular disease, risk factors such as abnormal lipid levels, increased abdominal fat, diets high in fat, saturated and trans-fats, simple carbohydrates and sedentary lifestyles contribute to the development of chronic disease (Jonnalagadda & Diwan, 2002b).

Research on health issues of Asian Indians has been limited. National studies are of little value since Asian Indians comprise a relatively small percentage of the U.S. population. Most research studies specifically targeting Asian Indians have been conducted in specific areas with high concentrations of Asian Indians such as New York and California, with little attention to other geographic regions which have growing Asian American populations such as Texas and Illinois.

Conclusion

Asian Indians have a wide variety of classes, social habits, cultural practices, diets, and lifestyles that characterize the Asian Indian diversity. They are generally well-educated with the highest annual income among all Asian American immigrants. Hence, Asian Indians are perceived as having good access to health care. However, there are marked variations within this growing ethnic subgroup in terms of educational attainment, income, and access to care. Further, they have a genetic predisposition to chronic diseases such as diabetes and cardiovascular disease. Hence, primary and secondary prevention programs can help improve their health outcomes and quality of life. Although Asian Indians retain a high level of ethnic identity, they are known to assimilate into American culture while at the same time preserving the culture of their ancestors. They assimilate more easily than many other Asian immigrant groups due to the lack of language barrier (English is widely spoken in India), their high educational level, and their professional jobs.

References

Agarwal, S., Lee, A. D., Raju, R. S., & Stephen, E. (2009). Venous thromboembolism: A problem in the Indian/Asian population? *Indian Journal of Urology, 25*, 11–16. doi:10.4103/0970-1591.45531.

Anand, S. S., Yusuf, S., Vuksan, V., Devanesen, S., Teo, K. K., Montague, P. A., et al. (2000). Differences in risk factors, atherosclerosis and cardiovascular disease between ethnic groups in Canada: The study of health assessment and risk in ethnic groups (SHARE). *Indian Heart Journal, 52*, S35–S43.

Asian Americans Profile - The Office of Minority Health (OMH). (2006). *Home Page - The Office of Minority Health - OMH*. Retrieved from http://minorityhealth.hhs.gov/templates/browse.aspx?lvl=3&lvlid=29.

Assisi, F. C. (2007). *News & analysis:* Skilled Indian immigrants create wealth for America. *INDOlink* Retrieved from INDOlink http://www.indolink.com/displayArticleS.php?id=010307105012.

Baggett, H. C., Graham, S., Kozarsky, P. E., Gallagher, N., Blumensaadt, S., Bateman, J., et al. (2009). Pretravel health preparation among US residents traveling to India to VFRs: Importance of ethnicity in defining VFRs. *Journal of Travel Medicine, 16*, 112–118. doi:doi:10.1111/j.1708-8305.2008.00284.x.

Balasubramanyam, A., Rao, S., Misra, R., Sekhar, R. V., & Ballantyne, C. M. (2008). Prevalence of metabolic syndrome and associated risk factors in Asian Indians. *Journal of Immigrant and Minority Health, 10*, 313–323. doi:10.1007/s10903-007-9092-4.

Chandalia, M., Mohan, V., Adams-Huet, B., Deepa, R., & Abate, N. (2008). Ethnic difference in sex gap in high-density lipoprotein cholesterol between Asian Indians and Whites. *Journal of Investigative Medicine, 56*, 574–580. doi:10.231/JIM.0b013e31816716fd0004287 1-200803000-00005 [pii].

Chandie Shaw, P. K., Vandenbroucke, J. P., Tjandra, Y. I., Rosendaal, F. R., Rosman, J. B., Geerlings, W., et al. (2002). Increased end-stage diabetic nephropathy in Indo-Asian immigrants living in the Netherlands. *Diabetologia, 45*, 337–341.

Derose, K. P., Escarce, J. J., & Lurie, N. (2007). Immigrants and health care: Sources of vulnerability. *Health Affairs, 26*(5), 1258–1268.

Dhingra, P. (2012). *Life beyond the lobby: Indian American motel owners and the American dream* (pp. 50–88). Stanford: Stanford University Press.

Enas, E. A., & Senthilkumar, A. (2001). Coronary artery disease in Asian Indians: an update and review. *The Internet Journal of Cardiology, 1*.

Enas, E. A., Garg, A., Davidson, M. A., Nair, V. M., Huet, B. A., & Yusuf, S. (1996). Coronary heart disease and its risk factors in first-generation immigrant Asian Indians to the United States of America. *Indian Heart Journal, 48*, 343–353.

Esperat, M. C., Inouye, J., Gonzalez, E. W., Owen, D. C., & Feng, D. (2004). Health disparities among Asian Americans and Pacific Islanders. *Annual Review of Nursing Research, 22*, 135–159.

Gomez, S. L., Kelsey, J. L., Glaser, S. L., Lee, M. M., & Sidney, S. (2004). Immigration and acculturation in relation to health and health-related risk factors among specific Asian subgroups in a health maintenance organization. *American Journal of Public Health, 94*, 1977–1984.

Gungabissoon, U., Andrews, N., & Crowcroft, N. S. (2007). Hepatitis A virus infection in people of South Asian origin in England and Wales: Analysis of laboratory reports between 1992 and 2004. *Epidemiology and Infection, 135*, 549–554. doi:S0950268806007242 [pii]10.1017/S0950268806007242.

Huang, K., & Carrasquillo, O. (2008). The role of citizenship, employment, and socioeconomic characteristics in health insurance coverage among Asian subgroups in the United States. *Medical Care, 46*, 1093–1098. doi:10.1097/MLR.0b013e318185ce0a00005650-2008 10000-00016 [pii].

Hughes, K., Aw, T. C., Kuperan, P., & Choo, M. (1997). Central obesity, insulin resistance, syndrome X, lipoprotein(a), and cardiovascular risk in Indians,

Malays, and Chinese in Singapore. *Journal of Epidemiology and Community Health, 51*, 394–399.

Institute of Medicine (IOM). (2003). In B. D. Smedley, A. Y. Stith, & A. R. Nelson (Eds.), *Unequal treatment: Confronting racial and ethnic disparities in healthcare.* Washington, DC: The National Academies Press.

Institute of Medicine (IOM). (2008). *Challenges and successes in reducing health disparities: Workshop summary.* Washington, DC: The National Academies Press.

Jonnalagadda, S. S., & Diwan, S. (2002a). Nutrient intake of first generation Gujarati Asian Indian immigrants in the U.S. *Journal of the American College of Nutrition, 21*, 372–380.

Jonnalagadda, S. S., & Diwan, S. (2002b). Regional variations in dietary intake and body mass index of first-generation Asian-Indian immigrants in the United States. *Journal of the American Dietetic Association, 102*, 1286–1289.

Lv, N., & Cason, K. L. (2004). Dietary pattern change and acculturation of Chinese Americans in Pennsylvania. *Journal of the American Dietetic Association, 104*, 771–778.

Martin, M. Y. (2005). Community health advisors effectively promote cancer screening. *Ethnicity & Disease, 15*, S14–S16.

McKeigue, P. M. (1996). Metabolic consequences of obesity and body fat pattern: Lessons from migrant studies. *Ciba Foundation Symposium, 201*, 54–64. Discussion 64–67, 188–193.

McKeigue, P. M., Ferrie, J. E., Pierpoint, T., & Marmot, M. G. (1993). Association of early-onset coronary heart disease in South Asian men with glucose intolerance and hyperinsulinemia. *Circulation, 87*, 152–161.

McKeigue, P. M., Pierpoint, T., Ferrie, J. E., & Marmot, M. G. (1992). Relationship of glucose intolerance and hyperinsulinaemia to body fat pattern in South Asians and Europeans. *Diabetologia, 35*, 785–791.

Misra, R., Menon, U., Vadaparampil, S. T., & Belue, R. (2011). Age- and sex-specific cancer prevention and screening practices among Asian Indian immigrants in the United States. *Journal of Investigative Medicine.* doi:10.231/JIM.0b013e3182160d5d.

Misra, R., Patel, T. G., Davies, D., & Russo, T. (2000). Health promotion behaviors of Gujurati Asian Indian immigrants in the United States. *Journal of Immigrant Health, 2*, 223–230.

Misra, R., Patel, T., Kotha, P., Raji, A., Ganda, O., Banerji, M., et al. (2010). Prevalence of diabetes, metabolic syndrome, and cardiovascular risk factors in US Asian Indians: Results from a national study. *Journal of Diabetes and its Complications, 24*, 145–153. doi:S1056-8727(09)00002-6 [pii]10.1016/j.jdiacomp. 2009.01.003.

Misra, A., Rastogi, K., & Joshi, S. R. (2009). Whole grains and health: Perspective for Asian Indians. *The Journal of the Association of Physicians of India, 57*, 155–162.

Misra, R., & Vadaparampil, S. T. (2004). Personal cancer prevention and screening practices among Asian Indian physicians in the United States. *Cancer Detection and Prevention, 28*, 269–276. doi:10.1016/j.cdp. 2004.02. 004S0361090X04000765 [pii].

Mohanty, S. A., Woolhandler, S., Himmelstein, D. U., & Bor, D. H. (2005). Diabetes and cardiovascular disease among Asian Indians in the United States. *Journal of General Internal Medicine, 20*, 474–478.

Nan, L., Tuomilehto, J., Dowse, G., Zimmet, P., Gareeboo, H., Chitson, P., et al. (1991). Prevalence and medical care of hypertension in four ethnic groups in the newly-industrialized nation of Mauritius. *Journal of Hypertension, 9*, 859–866.

Omar, M. A., Seedat, M. A., Dyer, R. B., Rajput, M. C., Motala, A. A., & Joubert, S. M. (1985). The prevalence of diabetes mellitus in a large group of South African Indians. *South African Medical Journal, 67*, 924–926.

Pasick, R. J., & Burke, N. J. (2008). A critical review of theory in breast cancer screening promotion across cultures. *Annual Review of Public Health, 29*, 351–368.

Raj, S., Ganganna, P., & Bowering, J. (1999). Dietary habits of Asian Indians in relation to length of residence in the United States. *Journal of the American Dietetic Association, 99*, 1106–1108.

Rajaram, S. S., & Rashidi, A. (1998). Minority women and breast cancer screening: The role of cultural explanatory models. *Preventive Medicine, 27*, 757–764. doi:S0091-7435(98)90355-3 [pii]10.1006/ pmed.1998.0355.

Rajaram, S. S., & Rashidi, A. (1999). Asian-Islamic women and breast cancer screening: A socio-cultural analysis. *Women & Health, 28*, 45–58.

Raleigh, V. S. (1996). Suicide patterns and trends in people of Indian subcontinent and Caribbean origin in England and Wales. *Ethnicity & Health, 1*, 55–63. doi: 10.1080/13557858.1996.9961770.

Ramaiya, K. L., Denver, E., & Yudkin, J. S. (1995). Diabetes, impaired glucose tolerance and cardiovascular disease risk factors in the Asian Indian Bhatia community living in Tanzania and in the United Kingdom. *Diabetic Medicine, 12*, 904–910.

Ruy, H., Young, W. B., & Kwak, H. (2002). Differences in health insurance and health service utilization among Asian Americans: Method for using the NHIS to identify unique patterns between ethnic groups. *The International Journal of Health Planning and Management, 17*, 55–68.

Samanta, A., Burden, A. C., & Jagger, C. (1991). A comparison of the clinical features and vascular complications of diabetes between migrant Asians and Caucasians in Leicester, U.K. *Diabetes Research and Clinical Practice, 14*, 205–213.

Saxenian, A. (1999). *Silicon valley's new immigrant entrepreneurs* (pp. 9–21). San Francisco: Public Policy Institute of California.

Sharma, S., Malarcher, A. M., Giles, W. H., & Myers, G. (2004). Racial, ethnic and socioeconomic disparities in the clustering of cardiovascular disease risk factors. *Ethnicity & Disease, 14*, 43–48.

Singh, T. (2012). For the patients: Indian or U.S. trained physicians? *Asian Student Medical Journal, 11*: 7.

Smokowski, P. R., David-Ferdon, C., & Stroupe, N. (2009). Acculturation and violence in minority adolescents: A review of the empirical literature. Journal of Primary Prevention, 30, 215–263. doi:10.1007/s10935-009-0173-0.

Snehalatha, C., Viswanathan, V., & Ramachandran, A. (2003). Cutoff values for normal anthropometric variables in Asian Indian adults. *Diabetes Care, 26*, 1380–1384.

South Asian Public Health Association (SAPHA). (2002) *A brown paper: The health of South Asians in the United States* (1st ed.). Baltimore, MD: SAPHA.

Sundquist, J., & Winkleby, M. (2000). Country of birth, acculturation status and abdominal obesity in a national sample of Mexican-American women and men. *International Journal of Epidemiology, 29*, 470–477.

U.S. Census Bureau. (2000a). *Statistical abstract of the United States*. Washington, DC: Author.

U.S. Census Bureau. (2000b). *Statistical abstract of the United States*. Washington, DC: Author.

U.S. Department of Health and Human Services. Asian American/Pacific Islander profile. Accessed December 27, 2011, from http://minorityhealth.hhs.gov/templates/browse.aspx?lvl=2&lvlid=53.

Whincup, P. H., Gilg, J. A., Papacosta, O., Seymour, C., Miller, G. J., Alberti, K. G., et al. (2002). Early evidence of ethnic differences in cardiovascular risk: Cross sectional comparison of British South Asian and white children. *BMJ, 324*, 635.

Wild, S. H., Laws, A., Fortmann, S. P., Varady, A. N., & Byrne, C. D. (1995). Mortality from coronary heart disease and stroke for six ethnic groups in California, 1985 to 1990. *Annals of Epidemiology, 5*, 432–439.

Yagalla, M. V., Hoerr, S. L., Song, W. O., Enas, E., & Garg, A. (1996). Relationship of diet, abdominal obesity, and physical activity to plasma lipoprotein levels in Asian Indian physicians residing in the United States. *Journal of the American Dietetic Association, 96*, 257–261.

Chinese Americans and Health: The Impact of Culture on Disease Prevention and Management

Angela Sun

Introduction

Cultural perceptions and health beliefs can greatly affect health promotion, care and early detection of disease. Mr. Wong, a 40-year-old Chinese immigrant, arrived in tears at a local community cancer information center. He went to the center to seek services for his mother, who was undergoing treatment for cancer. Mr. Wong's mother had been living with him, his wife, and their two young children in a low-income, one-bedroom housing unit. The wife feared that her mother-in-law's cancer would spread to her children, and she believed that the cancer was caused by previous wrongdoings. Such comments hurt Mr. Wong greatly because he understood that it is his responsibility to take care of his ailing mother. Quarrels regarding the mother's condition escalated to the point of divorce. Although Mr. Wong did not want to divorce his wife, his mother's cancer diagnosis changed his wife's attitude, and she had become hostile toward her mother-in-law because of cultural stigma.

Scenarios such as Mr. Wong's are commonly seen in the Chinese American community concerning health. The following chapter will focus on Chinese culture and its effects on health as well as future areas of research.

A. Sun (✉)
Chinese Community Health Resource Center (CCHRC), San Francisco, CA, USA
e-mail: angelas@chasf.org

Immigration Patterns

Chinese American immigration began in the early nineteenth century, with only a handful of Chinese immigrants, mostly merchants, students, and sailors. When gold was discovered in California in 1848, the number of Chinese immigrants increased dramatically. These Chinese fled their own country because of economic and political crisis. The new immigrants sought work in sugar plantations, railroad, gold mines, agriculture, and fisheries to fulfill the labor shortage in the United States (Wong, 2005). There were three notable waves of Chinese migration to the United States (Tsai, 2008).

The First Wave (1800s–1949)

The first immigrants came mainly from the Canton province of China, working as laborers. These immigrants received little education from their native country, came with very little (if any) English proficiency, faced great challenges in assimilation, and experienced a great deal of racial discrimination.

In 1882, the Chinese Exclusion Act greatly limited the number of Chinese immigrants entering the United States. During this period, Chinese immigrants were segregated, forced to relocate, and restricted to live within geographic locations known today as *Chinatowns*. During this wave, Chinese merchants and district associations – which later evolved into networks known as Chinese Benevolent Associations and Chinese surname associations – provided much-needed services and social welfare, including health care, to the Chinese community (Wong, 2005).

The Second Wave: 1949–1980s

Immigrants of the second wave came mainly from Taiwan. These immigrants established the Taiwanese American subgroup. The majority was affluent, well-educated and skilled, had some English proficiency, and primarily spoke Mandarin. The Taiwanese Americans formed their own Chinese communities in some of America's major metropolitan cities (Wong, 2005).

The Third Wave: 1980s–Present

The third wave of immigrants came from various social economic backgrounds. After the Tiananmen Square incident in 1989, many foreign students from China were granted permanent residency in the United States under the Chinese Student Protection Act of 1992 (Fu, 1995). Additionally, an influx of undocumented aliens, primarily from Fujian Province, came to America with little or no education seeking manual work. Some of these undocumented Fuzhounese eventually sought political asylum and subsequently gained permanent resident status (Wong, 2005).

Demographics

Chinese-Populated Urban Areas

With 3.8 million people, Chinese Americans make up the largest ethnic group in the United States (U.S. Census Bureau, 2009). Ten of the most Chinese-populated metropolitan urban areas (Table 3.1) in the United States include New York City, San Francisco Bay Area, Los Angeles, Boston, Chicago, Washington, DC, Houston, Seattle, Philadelphia, and Dallas (U.S. Census Bureau, 2009).

Key Features

The Chinese population is heterogeneous in culture and beliefs. The following is a snapshot of some key features (i.e., language, cuisine, religion/philosophy, holidays/festivals, etc.) affecting health promotion, disease management, detection of illness, health-seeking pathway, and utilization of health information and services.

Language

- *Spoken*: There are 10 major Chinese language groups and 196 dialects. In the United States, the two major spoken dialects are Mandarin (Putonghua) and Cantonese (Yue). Mandarin-speaking immigrants typically originate from the northern regions of China and Taiwan, and the Cantonese-speaking immigrants originate from Canton (GuangDong), Hong Kong, and Macau.
- *Written*: Unlike spoken Chinese, the single written language uses either traditional or simplified characters. After the Cultural Revolution, simplified Chinese characters were practiced in mainland China.

Religion/Philosophy

The percentage of Chinese who classify themselves as religious is ranked lowest internationally (Grim, 2008). However, five religions are recognized: Buddhism, Christianity (Protestantism, Catholicism), Islam, Confucianism, and Taoism (Bhattacharji, 2008; Grim, 2008). The latter two are considered philosophies rather than religions by some.

Cuisine

Chinese cuisine is extremely heterogeneous. The two major classifications of cuisines are based on spices used and food staples. Northern Chinese cuisine is spicy, with a main staple of wheat products such as noodles, buns, and dumplings,

Table 3.1 Population profile of Chinese descent in the United States[a]

Category	Subcategory	Total US population 307,006,556	White alone or in combination with one or more races 236,287,989	Asian alone or in any combination 15,733,402 (5.1% of total population)	Chinese alone or in any combination 3,796,796 (1.24% of total population)
Gender	Male	49.3%	49.4%	48.3%	47.5%
	Female	50.7%	50.6%	51.7%	52.5%
Age	0–17 years	24.3%	23.1%	26.3%	24.7%
	18–64	62.9%	62.5%	64.9%	65.4%
	65+	12.9%	14.3%	8.8%	9.9%
Marital status	Married, except separated	49.3%	52.1%	57.6%	57.8%
	Widowed	2.5%	6.4%	1.4%	4.3%
	Divorced	10.6%	11.0%	5.3%	5.0%
	Separated	2.2%	1.8%	1.3%	1.1%
	Never married	35.2%	28.7%	35.7%	31.9%
Educational attainment	High school graduate and below	43.2%	41.5%	30.5%	30.0%
	Some college or Associate's degree	28.9%	29.3%	20.6%	15.9%
	Bachelor's degree	17.6%	18.4%	29.1%	25.7%
	Graduate or professional degree	10.3%	10.8%	19.8%	25.1%
Median household income	Individuals and families	$50,221	$52,976	$68,103	$69,037
	Family income (married couple family)	$61,082	$65,096	$78,064	$81,154
	Individual per capita income	$26,409	$28,548	$28,000	$30,044
Poverty rates	All people	14.3%	11.9%	11.2%	12.2%
	Under 18 years	20.0%	15.9%	11.5%	10.3%
	18–64	13.1%	11.2%	10.8%	12.0%
	65+	9.5%	8.1%	13.1%	18.0%
	All families	10.5%	8.2%	8.7%	9.7%
Health insurance coverage	Private health insurance coverage	67.4%	71.8%	71.7%	72.4%
	Public health coverage	28.5%	27.4%	19.4%	20.3%
	No health insurance	15.1%	13.3%	14.1%	12.3%
Place of birth	The United States	87.5%	91.8%	40.4%	39.3%
	Foreign born	12.5%	8.2%	59.6%	60.7%
Language spoken at home	English only	80.0%	85.4%	29.4%	24.7%
	Language other than English	20.0%	14.6%	70.6%	75.3%
	Speak English less than "very well"	8.6%	6.0%	32.3%	41.1%

[a]U.S. Census Bureau (2009)

whereas southern Chinese cuisine is mild, with a main staple of rice products.

Holidays and Festivals

Major Chinese festivals celebrated in the United States:

- *Lunar New Year*: The gathering of all family members at the New Year's Eve dinner brings good luck and family unity in the new year. Chinese individuals usually avoid medical facilities and appointments during the first 7 days of the Lunar New Year to avoid bad luck (Chinese Spring Festival, 2011).
- *Mid-autumn (Moon) Festival*: This holiday celebrates the end of the autumn harvest season. Traditionally, families gather together to admire the full moon and share moon cakes (Beijing International, n.d.).
- *Dragon Boat Festival*: This festival honors the life and death of Qu Yuan, a loyal Chinese minister. Activities include preparing and eating zongzi and watching or participating in dragon boat races (China Internet Information Center, n.d.).

Numbers and Colors Associated with Either Life and Prosperity or Death

Numbers:
- *Lucky*: Three sounds similar to life, eight to prosperity, and nine to longevity.
- *Unlucky*: Four rhymes with death and seven is associated with death.

Colors:
- *Lucky*: Red signifies happiness, prosperity, and life.
- *Unlucky*: White, black, and blue are associated with death, funerals, and hospitals. Medical facilities should avoid decorations (i.e., flowers) in these colors.

Contributions/Inventions:

The four major inventions of ancient China (Jin, Fan, Fan, & Liu, 1986) are papermaking (100 BC), compass (Warring States Period), gunpowder (Tang Dynasty 618–907 AD), and printing (Tang Dynasty 1020 AD). Other contributions include, silk, noodle, millet cultivation, and soybeans.

Chinese Cultural Values and Health

Contrary to the Asian minority myth model for health, every Asian ethnic group faces particular health challenges and diseases. Some illnesses occur across all races, whereas others are more prevalent in specific ethnicities due partially to genetics, cultural practices, and epidemiologic differences (Table 3.2). To better understand how such differences in diseases can occur among various ethnicities, it is important to understand the concepts and influences of culture and tradition on health.

Definitions of Culture

Spector (1991) defined culture as "the sum of beliefs, practices, habits, likes, dislikes, norms, customs, and rituals shared by a group of people" (p. 61). Culture is conveyed through the unique shared values, beliefs, and practices in a population or subgroup that are directly or indirectly associated with health-related behavior (Pasick, D'Onofrio, & Otero-Sabogal, 1996). Bowman and Singer (2001) stated "cultures are maps of meaning through which people understand the world and interpret the things around them" (p. 455). Understanding the Chinese cultural "map" concerning health and healing can greatly enhance communication and/or treatment plans in caring for Chinese Americans.

Chinese culture has a long history and tradition distinct from Western culture because of the philosophical teachings of Buddhism, Confucianism, and Taoism (Chen, 1996; Ino & Glicken, 1999; Uba, 1994). In contrast to Western values – which encourage confrontation, independence, and autonomy in individual behavior (Ma, 1999) – Chinese culture has modeled health to emphasize harmony, respect, self-control, yin–yang balance, interdependency, collectivism, and community (Ino & Glicken, 1999; Spector, 1991). These cultural values are achieved by balancing the state of the mind and body, parent–child interactions, social relationships, individual and

Table 3.2 Concept of health and disease prevention: east versus west

Concept	East	West

Diet	• BALANCED DIET based on: *warming and cooling properties*
	• SPECIFIC DIETARY RECOMMENDATIONS with major food groups: *Hot, cold, and toxic*
	• Hot and cold related to energy warming and cooling properties. Excess intake of:
	  Hot foods results in: Acne, bad breath, constipation, dry mouth, nosebleeds, sore throat
	  Cold foods results in: Weakened immune system [EX: Foods high in antioxidants (melons and green leafy vegetables) may be avoided during illness because they are "cold foods"]
	  Toxic foods are not suitable for patients with cancer, arthritis, or postsurgery
	• Consumption of particular part of an animal will restore health of corresponding human part
		• BALANCED DIET based on: major food groups and *number of servings* per group
		• NO SPECIFIC DIETARY RECOMMENDATIONS for many conditions, except for a few, such as diabetes, heart disease, cancer prevention, gout, etc. Recommendations are based on nutritional values

Disease and healing	CONCEPT: • Harmony, respect, self-control, yin-yang balance, interdependency, collectiveness, and community (Ino & Glicken, 1999; Spector, 1991) • *Disease*: Result of imbalance in the body's own internal energy; controlled by energy levels (Hoeman, Ku, & Ohl, 1996). The following *imbalances* promote disease: • Five phases/elements: Wood, fire, earth, metal, and water • Yin-Yang HEALING: • Use traditional Chinese medicine (herbal remedies, acupuncture) and food to balance the body's energy level, strengthen the immune system to promote self-healing, resist disease, and improve health and physical well-being (EX: cupping therapy) • Unfamiliar with the Western concept of preventive care (EX: Diagnostic tests are viewed as treatment, not screening)	CONCEPT: • Encourage forwardness, independence and autonomy in individual decision making (Ma, 1999) • Value preventive care (health screenings and vaccinations) HEALING: • Use antibiotics and drugs to fight and treat diseases • May choose Eastern medicine as an alternative or in conjunction with Western methods
Decision-making process	• Heavily based on family discussion and agreement (Jenkins & Kagawa-Singer, 1994) • Elderly parents usually leave important life decision to their adult children (i.e., son)	• Individual usually makes final decision
Death and dying	CONCEPT: • Illness: Fate, destiny or punishment for wrongdoings by their ancestors • Discussion of serious illness and death impolite and cruel because it can cause undue stress, depression, and a sense of helplessness and hopelessness ACTION: • Refrain from discussing serious illness with patient • Bad news communicated to family, not patient • Talking about death and dying might cause death to become a reality	CONCEPT: • Patient rights are highly valued ACTION: • Bad news is communicated directly to the patient in order to make an informed decision

group aspirations, and health-seeking behaviors (Wu, 1995). The three major philosophies influencing health are Buddhism, Confucianism, and Holism.

Buddhism: The basic tenet of Buddhism is that "all life is suffering, and that suffering originates from inappropriate desires" (Ino & Glicken, 1999). All living beings are doomed to ride the "wheel of life" through endless cycles of birth, growth, maturity, aging, illness, and death, unless they seek the enlightenment of Buddhism (Carter, 1993). Enlightenment can be attained by avoiding inappropriate desires and adhering to diligence and selflessness (Ino & Glicken, 1999). With this philosophy, Chinese view engaging in emotional restraint and coping with suffering, such as terminal illness, as ways to improve the quality of one's next life (Ino & Glicken, 1999). This belief is contrary to the basic philosophy of the American health care system that no one should suffer (Kagawa-Singer, 1996).

Confucianism: Among all traditional Chinese teachings, Confucianism may be the most influential on Chinese culture because of its detailed rules and regulations for social, interpersonal, and familial relationships (Liu, 1959; Shih, 1996). Confucianism values the importance of family (filial piety and respect for elders), the virtue of the individual, and the preservation of social harmony at all levels of society (Ino & Glicken, 1999; Spector, 1991). Confucianists emphasize collectivism, in which the common good and community pursuits and needs take precedence over individual pursuits and needs. Collectivist values, in contrast to individualism in the West, affect the Chinese Americans' health beliefs and behaviors. They believe in the group identity, interdependency, and consensus modes of decision making. Therefore, health behavior is greatly influenced by family members (Jenkins & Kagawa-Singer, 1994).

Holism: Chinese tend to view health holistically, with the ultimate goal of harmonizing with nature (Chen, 1996). Holism has two major features. First, the human body is regarded as an organism.

Local pathological changes such as diseases are considered to be in conjunction with other organs and tissues of the entire body rather than ailing individual parts. Second, the human body is viewed as an internal organism integrated with the external environment. The onset and development of disease are considered in conjunction with social and environmental changes experienced in the life of an individual (Spector, 1991).

Based on this holistic concept, traditional Chinese believe that diseases are preventable or controllable only through the maintenance of balanced energy levels and proper eating habits (Hoeman, Ku, & Ohl, 1996). Chinese immigrants accept some health measures, such as herbal remedies, acupuncture, and other traditional medical treatments, in order to strengthen the body, resist disease, and improve health and physical well-being (Ma, 1999; Spector, 1991). For many Chinese immigrants, Western diagnostic procedures are not used for screening purposes, but for health problems only. Therefore, they may not understand why so many diagnostic tests are necessary (Spector). Chinese immigrants who have no experience with preventive care may not comprehend the concept of screening for a disease that they do not have. They may follow some recommended health treatments, but may not necessarily accept the Western approach to disease prevention.

Language Barriers and Health

The Chinese population in America rates higher on many socioeconomic status measures. However, this group has the one of the highest rates of low English proficiency as well as linguistic isolation (Huang, Yu, Liu, Young, & Wong, 2009; U.S. Census Bureau, 2009). Language proficiency impacts levels of utilization rates of healthcare services (Huang et al.). In studies assessing health-related needs among low-income residents of San Francisco's Chinatown, access and use of health care services were hindered by the residents' limited English skills (Dube, 2003; Jang, Lee, & Woo, 1998). After interviewing Chinese immigrants living in metropolitan

Houston, Ma (2000) reported that acculturation levels were associated with access to and utilization of health services. Data from the California Health Interview Survey (McCracken et al., 2007) suggested that limited English proficiency may contribute to low cancer screening rates among Asian Americans.

Although low literacy among American adults could result from a lack of education, reading and/or comprehension problems, or specific learning disabilities, low literacy among Chinese immigrant groups is associated with the basic difficulty of learning English as a second language (Michielutte, Alciati, & el Arculli, 1999). As Liang, Yuan, Mandelblatt, and Pasick (2004) and Schneider (2006) commented, health guidelines delivered in ways that are linguistically sensitive and respectful of one's cultural background are more likely to achieve compliance with recommendations, despite the complexity of the American health care system.

Technology Barriers and Health

Based on the US Census Bureau's American Community Survey in 2009, Asian Americans are the fastest growing ethnic group in the United States. The Internet has been recognized as a viable and easily accessible resource for health information. Asian Americans reportedly have the highest rates of Internet access (82%) among all racial groups in the United States (75% for Whites, 59% for Blacks, 55% for Hispanics) (Rainie, 2011). However, access does not always translate to usage because of their lack of technological skills. Choi (2011) indicated that older (65+) non-Hispanic Asians had significantly lower health information technology usage compared to non-Hispanic Whites.

Discussion of Current Health Issues

As immigrants advance in their socioeconomic conditions and acculturation into the Western lifestyle, changes in disease prevalence and patterns occur (Birch, 1991; Yeung, 1999, 2000;

Yeung, Ko, & Ho, 2002). The processes Chinese Americans – as well as other minority Americans – underlying adaptation to residency in the United States are complex, yet invaluable in assessing and understanding the health needs of a subpopulation.

Major Health Concerns in the Chinese Community

Major health issues that impact the Chinese American community include chronic diseases and their management, childhood obesity, osteoporosis, tuberculosis, cancer, clinical trial participation, end of life care, smoking, mental health issues, and domestic violence. Limited data are available on the prevalence of and successful management strategies for most health conditions among Chinese Americans because many of data collected have been categorized under Asian Americans.

Kim et al. (2010) commented that the generalization of findings under the aggregated Asian category may not accurately reflect the true status of health in specific Asian groups. Having disaggregated data available on specific Asian groups would help policymakers and providers better serve their respective Asian groups.

Chronic Diseases

In the United States, chronic diseases are the leading causes of mortality and disability (Lui & Wallace, 2010). Conditions including arthritis, diabetes, cancer, heart disease, and stroke are among the most common and costly, yet preventable health conditions in the United States. Lack of physical activity, poor nutrition, tobacco use, and excessive alcohol consumption are preventable risk factors associated with the development of cardiovascular disease (Centers for Disease Control and Prevention [CDC], 2010). Mui and Shibusawa (2008) stated that among their study participants, older Chinese Americans comprised one of the two Asian groups reported living with the most chronic conditions.

The major chronic illnesses that impact the Chinese American community disproportionately are diabetes mellitus, cardiovascular diseases, hepatitis B (see discussion in another chapter), tuberculosis, and cancer.

Diabetes

Asian Americans as a population are believed to be at a higher risk for diabetes mellitus (DM). Diabetes is the fifth leading cause of illness and death for this population (Office of Women's Health, 2010). It is a debilitating disease that can lead to serious heart, blood vessel, eye, kidney, and nerve problems if not well controlled. Major complications of DM may result in blindness, limb amputation, kidney failure, heart disease, and stroke (World Health Organization [WHO], 2011), which are the leading causes of death among individuals with DM.

The increased incidence of overweight or obesity and the decline in physical activity are the major risk factors associated with diabetes (WHO, 2011). A 2004 study using data from the 2001 Behavioral Risk Factor Surveillance System (BRFSS) found that, although age- and sex-adjusted DM rates were the same among Asian Americans and White Americans, rates among Asian American populations were nearly 60% higher after adjusting for body mass index (BMI) (McNeely & Boyko, 2004). Moreover, at any particular BMI, Asian Americans were more likely to develop DM than their White counterparts.

Despite the growing Chinese population in the United States, limited national and statewide data exist for this group. Studies estimate that diabetes prevalence among Chinese American adults ranges from 12% to 21%, compared to 6.86% among non-Hispanic White Americans (Chen & Wong, 2010). The Chinese population has higher prevalence of Type 2 diabetes compared to non-Hispanic Whites, despite having lower age- and sex-adjusted BMI (Lee, Brancati, & Yeh, 2011). Select reports (Caballero, 2005) and studies (McNeely & Boyko, 2004) have also reported that Type 2 diabetes prevalence is almost twice as prevalent for Chinese Americans compared to the general national population. Studies have further indicated a strong correlation between incidence of diabetes, and poor diabetes management and depressive symptoms among all ethnic groups, including Chinese Americans (Jayne & Rankin, 2001; Maraldi et al., 2007).

Diabetes self-management programs have mainly been available for individuals with higher socioeconomic status, whose primary language spoken at home is English, and who strongly connect with individualistic values (Hardin, Leong, & Bhagwat, 2004). In contrast to Western values, Chinese culture encourages group identity, interdependency, and consensual modes of decision-making (Jenkins & Kagawa-Singer, 1994; Ma, 1999; Matsumoto, Yoo, & Fontaine, 2008). Such differences in language and culture complicate diabetes management for Chinese American immigrants (Chesla, Chun, & Kwan, 2009). Limited data exists on whether Chinese Americans diabetics successfully engage with diabetes self-management and medication compliance (Chan & Molassiotis, 1999; Xu, Pan, & Liu, 2010).

Cardiovascular Disease

Cardiovascular disease (CV) is the leading cause of death in the United States. Heart disease and stroke are the first and third leading causes of mortality among Asian and Asian Pacific Islanders (APIs) ages 65 and older (CDC, 2008). Chinese are disproportionately affected by this disease compared to other ethnic populations in United States (Wong, Dixon, Cilbride, Chin, & Kwan, 2010). Kim et al. (2010) analyzed data drawn from California Health Interview Survey collected between July 2007 and early March 2008. The rate of Chinese Americans living with CV was reported at 69.5%, with hypertension being the most common risk factor. Even at a lower BMI and waist circumference, Chinese American adults have a higher risk for CV when compared to their White counterparts (Wildman, Gu, Reynolds, Duan, & He, 2004), and a significantly higher level of uncontrolled hypertension (Kramer et al., 2004). Similar to DM, obesity and physical inactivity are risk factors associated with the onset of CV (Chaturvedi, 2003; Mokdad, Marks, Stroup, & Gerberding, 2004). Acculturation to and adaptation of Western lifestyle and food choices have found to be associated with an increased risk for CV (Diez Roux et al., 2005; Goel, McCarthy, Phillips, & Wee, 2004; Kandula et al., 2008; Liu et al., 2010; Lv & Cason, 2004; Singh, Siahpush, Hiatt, & Timsina, 2010; Unger et al., 2004).

The control of chronic health conditions such as DM and CV requires not only fundamental lifestyle changes in diet and physical activity but also adherence to medication and regular doctor visits. The complex management of chronic illness, particularly DM, among Chinese Americans is complicated by above-mentioned cultural and linguistic factors (Ton et al., 2010). More than 40% of Chinese Americans have reported having limited English proficiency (U.S. Census Bureau, 2009). Access to multidisciplinary care often is limited by the lack of available resources that are culturally and linguistically appropriate. Medication compliance is particularly challenging in the management of chronic diseases because treatment can require multiple medications and complicated dosing regimens. Factors that can lead to noncompliance include the expense of medications, difficulty remembering doses or reading prescription labels, and difficulty obtaining refills (Odegard & Capoccia, 2007; Odegard & Gray, 2008). To address such concerns, culturally appropriate interventions for chronic disease prevention and management must be identified and investigated.

In addition to these barriers, evidence shows that Chinese Americans may hold cultural beliefs and behaviors which influence their adherence to medications prescribed by practitioners of Western medicine. These beliefs include perceptions of the disease and its consequences, and the relative risks and benefits of using Western medicine (Hsu, Mao, & Wey, 2010).

In addition, the use of Chinese traditional medicine and herbal medicines may compete with, not complement, Western medication use (Ma, 1999). Further research is needed to test the efficacy of integrated (Eastern and Western) medication and therapies.

Childhood Obesity

Obesity in children is associated with immediate and long-term physical and psychological disorders such as CV, hypertension, Type 2 DM, sleep disorders, depression, social withdrawal, and premature death (Buiten & Metzger, 2000; CDC, 2007a; Datar, Sturm, & Magnabosco, 2004; Friedland, Nemet, Gorodnitsky, Wolach, & Eliakim, 2002; Swallen, Reither, Haas, & Meier, 2005). Prevention of childhood obesity has been recognized as a public health priority because of the long-term adverse complications of obesity later in adulthood (Goran, Ball, & Cruz, 2003; Young, Dean, Flett, & Wood-Steiman, 2000).

Waist circumference is significantly associated with insulin resistance and high systolic blood pressure among Chinese American children (Sung et al., 2007). Lower maternal acculturation and poor food choices can contribute to obesity and high blood pressure (Chen, Weiss, Heyman, & Lusting, 2009; Chen & Wu, 2008). Culturally tailored interventions have been shown to improve children's BMI, physical activity levels, and food choices (Chen, Weiss, Heyman, Vittinghoff, & Lusting, 2008). Further research is needed to determine the role culture plays in childhood obesity.

Osteoporosis

Osteoporosis is a common debilitating chronic disease among the aging population worldwide. The condition is characterized by low bone mineral density (BMD) which can lead to bone fracture (National Institutes of Health Osteoporosis and Related Bone Diseases National Resource Center [NIH], 2009). Most data on osteoporosis are grouped under Asian Americans, and specific data among Asian subethnic groups such as Chinese American are extremely scarce. The National Osteoporosis Foundation (n.d.) estimates 20% of Asian American women ages 50 and older will develop osteoporosis. With Chinese Americans being the largest Asian group, its elderly population will be greatly impacted. Lauderdale, Kuohung, Chang, & Chin (2003) conducted a study of 469 Chinese Americans and reported that the Chinese foreign-born women age 50 or older had a lower average BMD value than US-born American and White females. The smaller stature of most Asians, including Chinese individuals, contributes to the prevalence of lower BMD among Asians when compared to Whites (Bhudhikanok et al., 1996; National Osteoporosis Foundation, n.d.; Ross et al., 1996).

Osteoporosis often is undetected until bone fracture occurs, however the condition can be screened and detected by the defined T-score (WHO, 1994). Factors associated with osteoporosis include age, nutrition, weight-bearing activity, and genetics (Pothiwala, Evans, & Novakofski, 2006); The National Osteoporosis Foundation (n.d.) estimates that about 90% of Asian American adults are lactose intolerant and have difficulty consuming adequate dietary calcium. Jackson and Savaiano (2001) revealed that Asian Americans and other ethnicities may have a higher risk for low calcium intake, which may increase their risk for osteoporosis.

Dark green leafy vegetables, calcium-fortified foods and beverages, canned fish with bones, calcium supplements, are among other alternative good sources of calcium (National Osteoporosis Foundation, n.d.). Culturally appropriate programs on osteoporosis awareness can help to improve bone mass and muscle strength in Chinese Americans (Qi, Resnick, Smeltzer, & Bausell, 2011). Nutrition education introducing ethnic foods high in calcium and physical activities such as Tai Chi, a popular exercise practiced by Chinese elders, can be incorporated as part of osteoporosis awareness programs for the Chinese immigrant community (Lui, Qin, & Chan, 2008).

Tuberculosis

Mycobacterium tuberculosis (TB) infected nearly one third of the global population, accounting for 1.6 million TB-related deaths in 2005 (WHO, 2007). In the United States, foreign-born individuals have contributed to more than half of all cases of TB since 2001, with more cases among APIs than any other racial ethnic group (CDC, 2006). Between 1993 and 2004, the number of US-born TB cases dropped by 62%, but the number of foreign-born TB cases increased by 5% (CDC, 2005).

Manangan et al. (2009) reported that being foreign-born is significantly associated with the risk for TB. Other risk factors for TB include poor housing environment, inadequate nutrition, homelessness, and drug abuse (CDC, 1989). Studies have also identified an association between lower socioeconomic status and an array of diseases, including TB (Cantwell, Snider, Cauthen, & Onorato, 1994; Lerner, 1993; Spence, Hotchkiss, Williams, & Davies, 1993). Based on U.S. Census Bureau data (2009), approximately 60.7% of Chinese Americans are foreign born, and China has been identified as one of the top ten countries with the most foreign-born TB cases (Cain et al., 2007). Screening immigrants, especially from countries such as China has proven to be effective in TB control (Gounder, Driver, Scholten, Shen, & Munsiff, 2003; Verver, van Soolingen, & Borgdorff, 2002).

Involving family members as guardians, rather than officials from public health TB treatment programs, attained more desirable results in TB treatments (Manders et al., 2001). In the social marketing of TB education and treatment programs, the involvement of Chinese individuals from a similar social status as the target population, and collaboration with local community partners and health care providers, can be effective (Ho, 2004). Therefore, strategies used must be culturally sensitive and appropriate to successfully detect, track, treat, and monitor TB cases among Chinese Americans.

Cancer

Cancer is the leading cause of death among APIs (U.S. Department of Health and Human Services [USDHHS], 2011a, 2011b). Breast cancer is the leading cause of cancer death and accountable for the highest incidence rate of all cancers within the Chinese American population (American Cancer

Society [ACS], 2012). According to the ACS (2012), culture contributes to cancer disparities. Although cultural factors can enhance or impede participation in cancer education and control activities, several researchers have found that barriers to cancer screening and early detection are more common among cultural minority groups (Kagawa-Singer, 1995; Liang Yuan, Mandelbatt, & Pasick, 2004; Pourat, Singer, Breen, & Sripipatana, 2010; Spector, 1991; Yi, 1994).

Many factors influence the extent to which members of a specific culture participate in cancer prevention and screening. These factors include a patient's birthplace and the level of acculturation or assimilation to the new host society (Hedeen, White, & Taylor, 1999; Pourat, Singer, & Sripipatana, 2010); cultural attitudes toward bodily functions and the power attributed to indigenous healers (McBride et al., 1998); general and cancer-specific beliefs; practices concerning health; diet and access to screening; as well as expectations concerning the quality of patient–provider interaction and communication in the health care setting (Liang et al., 2004; Olsen & Stromborg, 1993). Underutilization of cancer screening services among ethnic minorities often is attributed to factors such as language difficulties, cultural values and beliefs, and fear of cancer (Hoeman, Ku, & Ohl, 1996).

Cancer has a negative connotation within Chinese culture (Sun, Wong-Kim, Stearman, & Chow, 2005a). Beliefs about the causes of cancer may determine what interventions are preferred and considered appropriate for cancer treatment. For example, some Chinese Americans may believe that cancer is a punishment for transgressions in this life or in past lives. These beliefs may cause Chinese immigrants who suspect cancer themselves to delay seeking diagnosis and treatment from a physician (Jenkins & Kagawa-Singer, 1994; Lin, Finlay, Tu, & Gray, 2005). The belief that cancer is a form of retribution for past transgressions may make traditional Chinese families reluctant to admit openly that they have cancer and seek treatment promptly. This reluctance may explain why Chinese Americans and other Asian women often are diagnosed with late-stage cancer of the cervix and breast (Jenkins & Kagawa-Singer, 1994).

Clinical Trial Participation

Clinical trials are studies designed to test and evaluate new approaches toward the prevention, detection, and treatment of diseases and illness. In order for the established effective interventions to be applicable to Asian Americans, including Chinese Americans, it is crucial to have adequate representation from this population. Like many diseases, different variables exist genetically, epidemiologically, prognostically by gender or ethnic group in the treatment of disease (Tu et al., 2005).

Nevertheless, participation in clinical trials has been low from minority populations, including Asian Americans. Federal legislation has been established in the United States to encourage and fund research on the recruitment of minorities and women into clinical trials (U.S. Department of Health and Human Services [USDHHS], 2001).

Data on clinical trials concerning Chinese Americans have been scarce. Barriers to clinical trial participation include language; apprehension about the risks involved; the lack of accurate concepts about the research; the fear of being experimented; the complexity of the protocol; insufficient financial and social support; lack of recommendations by their physicians; and the family-based decision-making process (Nguyen, Somkin, & Ma, 2005a, 2005b; Tu et al., 2005). Further studies are necessary to assess effective strategies in clinical trial recruitment, organ donation, and biobanking among Chinese Americans.

Smoking

Tobacco use among Chinese adults is a serious problem in China and the United States. The rate of smoking among Chinese American men ranges from 22% to 38%, as compared to 23.9% among US-born males (CDC, 2006; Fu, Ma, Tu, Siu, & Metlay, 2003; Hu et al., 2006; Shelley et al., 2004). Lower levels of acculturation, English proficiency, educational level, socioeconomic status, and recent immigration status are associated with the prevalence of smoking (Fu et al., 2003;

Hu et al.; Spigner, Yip, Huang, & Tu, 2007; Tang, Shimizu, & Chen, 2005). Smoking among Chinese American immigrant women is much lower than among foreign-born Chinese males. As Chinese immigrant females become more acculturated, they have been found to be more likely to smoke (Maxwell, Bernaards, & McCarthy, 2005; Tang et al., 2005). In addition depression is prevalent among Chinese American smokers (Luk & Tsoh, 2010; Tsoh, Lam, Delucchi, & Hall, 2003).

Smoking cessation interventions involving local Chinese media physicians and culturally tailored intensive behavior counseling, combined with pharmacological interventions; culturally appropriate community-based tailored programs; and public policies have been shown to effectively reduce the smoking rate among Chinese Americans (Ferketich et al., 2004; Shelley et al., 2008; Tsoh et al., 2003; Wu et al., 2009). More research is needed to identify a possible association between acculturation and smoking rates among Chinese females, and test effective and culturally appropriate smoking cessation interventions for Chinese American smokers.

Smoking and Adolescents

The prevalence of smoking among Chinese American adolescents is lower than other non-Asian ethnic groups (Chen, Unger, Cruz, & Johnson, 1999). However, the smoking rate among Chinese American adolescents is positively correlated with Western acculturation. Their smoking rate also increases concomitantly with language acculturation (Chen, Unger, & Johnson, 1999). Chinese adolescent males are more likely than their female counterparts to smoke. Adolescent smokers are less likely to become nonsmokers later in life (Kaplan, Nguyen, & Weinberg, 2008). Smoking also increases as depression rates increase among Asian American youth, including Chinese American adolescents (Hahm, Lahiff, & Guterman, 2003; Rosario-Sim & O'Connell, 2009). Given the established association between stress and depression, smoking cessation interventions targeting Chinese American youth should incorporate strategies on

depression prevention and stress management (Hammen, 2005; Mazure, 1998).

End-of-Life Care

Planning for one's death is significantly associated with one's perceptions about death and dying. Most Chinese Americans and their views on death and dying are greatly influenced by the cultural values of Confucianism, Buddhism, and Taoism (Hsiang & Ferrans, 2007; Hsu, O'Connor, & Lee, 2009; Yick & Gupta, 2002). Looking through the lens of Chinese cultural values can help one to understand the values and attitudes they about planning for end-of-life care.

According to Chinese beliefs, the future is preordained and beyond one's control; suffering is part of life; prolonging one's life becomes a burden to society and family; end-of-life planning does not impact one's life cycle; any discussion about death is considered a bad omen; and refusal to treat and care for one's parents is contrary to the teaching of filial piety (Hall, 1976; Bowman & Singer, 2001). Chinese culture prizes the interdependence of family members, which takes priority over one's autonomy, whereas the Western health care culture is autonomy-based and values the dignity, sovereignty, and uniqueness of the individual (Harwood, 1981).

Discussions of end-of-life care issues are particularly difficult among less acculturated Chinese Americans. Thus, end-of-life care plans are not well promoted (Chou, Stokes, Citko, & Davies, 2008; Medvene et al., 2003; Tse, Chong, & Fok, 2003). Children usually become the caretakers of their aging parents within Chinese families. It is difficult for children to bring up issues related to advance directives or decisions to remove their parents from life support apparatuses for fear that others will consider this a violation of the principle of filial piety. Therefore, children prefer that social workers or doctors raise such issues with sick parents (Braun & Nichols, 1997).

Hospice care in the United States is considered the "gold standard" for care of dying individuals (American Hospice Foundation, n.d.) because it provides not only effective pain management and other physical comfort measures, but also psychological and spiritual support as well as bereavement counseling for family and friends who are left behind (Hospice Foundation of America, n.d.; USDHHS, 2011c). In some states, hospice is fully funded by Medicare and MediCal, as well as most private insurances (USDHHS, 2011c). Care can be provided in the patient's home, where a primary caregiver is available, or in a hospital, nursing home, or privately run facility (USDHHS, 2011c). Americans have increasingly selected this alternative since the hospice movement began in the United States more than 30 years ago, with over 1.3 million receiving hospice care in 2006, an increase of 162% over the last 10 years (National Hospice and Palliative Care Organization [NHPCO], 2008).

The growing use of hospice has not been uniform across all ethnic groups. Minority groups have been less inclined than Whites to choose this option due to misconceptions and fears (Yeo & Hikoyeda, 2000). Although APIs represent about 5% of the US population, they comprise less than 2% of hospice patients (Ngo-Metzger, Phillips, & McCarthy, 2008). Additional research is necessary to properly assess barriers and effective interventions for end-of-life care for Chinese Americans will require further study.

Mental Health

Immigrants are at an increased risk for depression and other mental health conditions because of conflicts resulting from immigration including cultural changes, language and employment challenges, discrimination, economic and social status changes, and isolation from family and familiar social surroundings (Abe & Zane, 1990; Kuo, 1984; Leu, Walton, & Takeuchi, 2010; Ying, 1988). Researchers (Escobar, 1998; Vega et al., 1998) have suggested that even through immigrants face stressful and challenging situations, the elements of their native cultures may serve as protective mechanisms in preventing the development of psychiatric disorders. As immigrants become more acculturated to the host culture, such protective mechanisms may be lessened or

lost (Escobar, 1998; Vega et al., 1998). Studies (Hwang, Chun, Takeuchi, Myers, & Siddarth, 2005) have suggested that the risk for developing the first episode of depression decreases as the length of stay in United States increases, whereas others (Burnam, Hough, Karno, Escobar, & Telles, 1987; Golding, Karno, & Rutter, 1990; Hwang, Myers, & Takeuchi, 2000; Leu et al., 2010) have identified higher acculturation as an important predictor of the first onset of depressive episodes.

Utilization of mental health services is low among Asian Americans, including the Chinese immigrant community (Fogel & Ford, 2005; Sue, Fujino, Hu, Takeuchi, & Zane, 1991; Ying & Hu, 1994; Yeung et al., 2004a). This underutilization may reflect the stigma associated with mental health (Ho, 1976; Tabora & Flashkerud, 1997). *Face saving*, the maintenance of the family's good reputation or name, is deeply ingrained in Chinese culture. Traditionally, mental illness is considered as "craziness" and shameful to the family name.

The family is regarded as the basic unit of society in Chinese culture, which carries the responsibility of caring for its members (Kleinman & Kleinman, 1993; Lin, Miller, Poland, Nuccio, & Yamaguichi, 1991). Thus, most Chinese families will take care of family members who are mentally ill at home rather than seek medical help. Hsu et al. (2008) reported the stigma of mental health issues such as depression was worse among Chinese Americans compared to Caucasians, regardless of whether depression was viewed as either a psychosis or perceived as a physical illness.

Compared to Latinos and Caucasians, more Asians, including Chinese Americans, are diagnosed with major psychotic disorders (Flaskerud & Hu, 1992). Abe-Kim, Takeuchi, and Hwang (2002) found that family conflict often predicted the use of mental health services among Chinese Americans. This reluctance to seek mental health treatment at an early stage has been demonstrated by the significantly delayed treatment for many Chinese patients with mental disorders (Ho & Chung, 1996; Shin, 1999; Yeung et al., 2004b). Reasons for underutilization include cost of treatment, lack of awareness of mental health service availability, lower levels of acculturation (Tabora & Flashkerud, 1997; Stokes, Thompson, Murphy, & Gallagher-Thompson, 2001), and the scarcity of culturally and linguistically appropriate mental health services and providers (Shin, 1999; Spencer & Chen, 2004; Sue et al., 1991).

Depression Among Adolescents

Cultural and language dissonance between parents and children as well as high parental pressure on academic performance are related to depression and mental health disorders among Chinese American adolescents. Studies reveal that foreign-born youth who are proficient in their heritage language experience less cultural dissonance, fewer family conflicts, and fewer depressive symptoms than their U.S.-born counterparts who lack proficiency in their heritage language (Costigan & Dokis, 2006; Liu, Benner, Lau, & Kim, 2009; Tardif & Geva, 2006).

Kim, Chen, Li, Huang, and Moon (2009) reported that the father-adolescent cultural discrepancy in American orientation within Chinese immigrant families contributes to unsupportive parenting practices and family conflicts. These conflicts are associated with increased adolescent depressive symptoms. Portes and Rumbaut (1996) stated acculturation similarities shared between parents and children result in generational consonance within the family, whereas a parent–child acculturation discrepancy leads to generational dissonance. For example, Western culture values the parental expression of emotions and the autonomy of children, whereas Chinese culture emphasizes emotional restraint and strict parental control. Family conflict results when Chinese American parents who demand strict parental authority are faced with acculturated adolescents who demand independence (Juang, Syed, & Takagi, 2007). Adolescents living in households with generational dissonance tend to avoid seeking guidance from their parents during difficult times, and that the parents are less likely to use inductive reasoning techniques. Both adolescent and parental behaviors have been associated with lower self-esteem and increased

depressive symptoms among adolescents of immigrant families (Costigan & Dokis, 2006; Farver, Narang, & Bhadha, 2002; Ge, Conger, Lorenz, & Simons, 1994; Juang et al., 2007; Weaver & Kim, 2008).

Additionally, in Chinese culture, children's academic success is the primary responsibility of the parents and is indicative of effective parenting (Chao & Tseng, 2002). Failure to achieve academically not only reflects poor parenting skills but also results in the "loss of face" for the family (Stevenson & Lee, 1996). Inability to meet the high expectations of Chinese parents is associated with depression among Chinese adolescents (Costigan & Costigan, 2006).

Domestic Violence

Domestic violence is an abusive behavior by one individual against another within a relationship. This relationship could be between husbands and wives, parents and their children, and gay or lesbian partners. Domestic violence can be physical, emotional, verbal, or financial abuse. It can occur across all types of relationships, ethnicities, economic classes, ages, and religious groups. Domestic violence is a global problem among all communities, including the Chinese community. However, limited research that assesses the prevalence of and effective interventions for domestic violence is available within the Chinese American population.

Chinese Culture and Domestic Violence

Numerous factors contribute to domestic violence in the Chinese community, including cultural values, language barriers, racism, discrimination, prejudice, parental stress, and acculturative stress (Wang, Probst, Moore, Martin, & Bennett, 2010; Yick, 2000). Acculturative stress refers to the economic, social, familial, and other cultural stressors experienced by individuals as they adapt to a new environment (Lee, Choe, Kim, & Ngo, 2000; Smart & Smart, 1995; Ward & Kennedy, 1999).

Historically, domestic violence – particularly wife beating or child beating – has been culturally and institutionally legitimized within Chinese society (Dobash & Dobash, 1978; Yoshioka, DiNoia, & Ullah, 2001). Women were considered the possessions of their husbands, and children were the properties of their parents (Tang, 1999). The Chinese theory of *xiao* (Hsiao), or filial piety may, in some cases, promote child abuse. Children can be treated in any way that the parents wish, with little interference from "outsiders" (Tang, 1998).

Many Chinese American victims of domestic violence are ashamed of abuse and fear that disclosure of the abuse will bring shame to the entire family (Torres, 1991; Chang, Shen, & Takeuchi, 2009). The cultural values of "loss of face," shame, and language barriers may contribute to the lack of data and action taken to combat domestic violence in the Chinese community. Over the last two decades, researchers and advocates have begun to collect data on domestic violence within the API population. However, most collected data have not been separated by ethnicity, but congregated together with other APIs. This congregated data collection method has further led to the scarcity of data on domestic violence, specifically in the Chinese population (Xu, Campbell, & Zhu, 2001; Leung, Kung, Lam, Leung, & Ho, 2002).

Theories Associated with Domestic Violence

Many theories, such as feminism, patriarchal, and acculturation, have been postulated to explain the etiology of domestic violence. The feminism and patriarchal theories support the contention that the primary cause of domestic violence is the societal norm that asserts the subordination of women (Kurz, 1989; Yick, 2000). Traditionally, males within Chinese families are expected to be the head of the household and in a position of authority. Women are to be subservient and nurturing, and complement men's roles. This imbalance of power may have contributed to domestic violence in Chinese families.

The theory of acculturation supports the controversy that the stressors experienced in the process of adaptation to a new country may increase a family's vulnerability to domestic violence. Moreover, language barriers, the lack of culturally and linguistically competent social support systems, unemployment or underemployment, and the experience of discrimination and racism can escalate existing family conflicts that can result in domestic violence (Sluzki, 1979).

Adverse mental health conditions (Leung et al., 2002), poor health, and behavior problems are well documented as symptoms of posttraumatic stress resulting from domestic violence (Graffunder, Noonan, Cox, & Wheaton, 2004). Yick, Shibusawa, and Agbayani-Siewert (2003) indicated that posttraumatic anxiety of domestic violence results in four times the rate of depression and 5.5 times the rate of suicidal attempts when compared to nonvictimized counterparts.

One of the commonly recommended interventions used is empowerment of domestic violence victims. However, Yick (2001) indicated that, although the intervention of empowerment often is the focus of treatment, it is important for practitioners to remember that empowerment is a Western concept that focuses on individualism and may not be congruent with traditional Chinese values. These values emphasize the importance of family and suppressing one's own needs for the sake of keeping the family unit together. When applying the intervention of empowerment to Chinese victims of domestic violence, practitioners should explore informal and formal resources, respect their cultural beliefs, and support their decision in working with domestic violence victims.

Verbal Abuse

Verbal abuse is another form of abuse that occurs in all communities. This form of abuse commonly occurs among Chinese Americans because many do not recognize verbal abuse as a form of violence. Based on limited studies available, Yick (2001) reported that among a sample of 262 Chinese American immigrants, more than 80% of the participants reported having experienced some type of verbal abuse from their intimate partners in the last 12 months.

Furthermore, a study conducted by Yick and Agbayani-Siewert (1997) reported Chinese Americans were less likely to label non-physical abusive behaviors as a type of psychological abuse or domestic violence. Another study, using a convenience sample of 588 Chinese immigrants residing in the San Francisco Bay Area, revealed that 82.7% of the participants did not consider emotionally based acts, such as name-calling or putdowns, as a form of violence. The findings indicated a need to educate the Chinese community that verbal abuse is indeed a form of violence (Sun, Tsoi, Stearman, & Chow, 2005b), as well as develop a culturally appropriate tool for assessing abuse in the Chinese community (Yick & Berthold, 2005).

Child Sexual Abuse

Sexual abuse among children is demoralizing, yet more common than expected. Children who experience sexual abuse may develop low self-esteem, feelings of worthlessness, and abnormal or distorted views of sex. Some children may become withdrawn and mistrustful of adults, and can become suicidal. The victims of child sexual abuse tend to repeat the pattern of abuse with their own children. As adults, they may have trouble establishing and maintaining close relationships and are at greater risk for anxiety, depression, substance abuse, medical illness, and problems at work (American Academy of Child and Adolescent Psychiatry [AACAP], 2008).

Statistics on child sexual abuse within the Chinese American community have been even more limited, partially because of the congregated data collection method. Studies have suggested that Asians are the least likely to report family violence because of the lack of awareness of the definition of violence, cultural shame and stigma associated with violence, protection of the family name, and the desire for privacy (Chan, Chun, & Chung, 2008; Hicks, 2006). According to Kenny and McEachern (2000) many Asian families may choose to ignore and/or cover up cases of child sexual abuse in order to preserve the family honor. Underreporting of

child sexual abuse cases may also be due to stigma and taboo associated with any discussion of sexuality issues (Rhee, Chang, Weaver, & Wong, 2008). In examining Chinese immigrant families in the Los Angeles area, Rhee et al. reported that Chinese immigrant families had higher rates of child physical abuse compared to the general population.

Additionally, Asian American victims and their families are more likely to be immigrants than Caucasian victims (Kenny & McEachern, 2000). Additionally, Asian and Asian American parents generally are not supportive of the victim, as they are less likely to report the abuse and do not believe abuse has actually occurred (Chan et al., 2008; Hicks, 2006). Furthermore, the researchers reported that although Asian American children who are sexually abused are the least likely to display inappropriate sexual behaviors and anger when compared to Caucasians and African Americans, they often are suicidal and display behavioral disturbances and nonspecific psychosomatic signs (Rao, DiClemente, & Ponton, 1992).

Future Recommendations

Documented research has been noted in the areas of health, disease, and disease prevalence, particularly in relation to acculturation, cultural beliefs and practices, language, socioeconomic status, access to and search for health services and information, and its respective barriers. The role of culture and its impact on health care decision-making and health promotion has been a resonating theme throughout this chapter. Nevertheless, many issues remain to be further investigated and explored. Areas of additional recommended research for Chinese Americans are as follows:
• Oral health.
• Eye care and early detection of eye diseases among seniors.
• Utilization of benevolent and surname associations as platforms for senior health promotion.
• Pain management.

- Palliative care.
- Attitudes and perceptions of disabilities and quality of life for those who are disabled.
- Involvement of young children in health promotion activities.
- Complement strengths between seniors and youth to improve health outcomes.

Acknowledgments Special thanks to the following staff and student interns from the Chinese Community Health Resource Center in San Francisco for their assistance in editing, formatting, and locating references: Teresa Ai, Joanne Chan, Joyce Cheng, Cynthia Huang, Yvonne Liang, and Dorothy Tao.

References

Abe, J. S., & Zane, N. W. S. (1990). Psychological maladjustment among Asian and White American College Students: Controlling for confounds. *Journal of Counseling Psychology, 37*(4), 437–444.

Abe-Kim, J., Takeuchi, D., & Hwang, W.-C. (2002). Predictors of help seeking for emotional distress among Chinese Americans: Family matters. *Journal of Consulting and Clinical Psychology, 70*, 1186–1190.

American Academy of Child & Adolescent Psychiatry (AACAP). (2008). *Facts for families: Child sexual abuse.* Washington, DC: American Academy of Child & Adolescent Psychiatry. Retrieved December 27, 2010, from http://www.aacap.org/galleries/FactsFor Families/09_child_sexual_abuse.pdf.

American Cancer Society. (2010). *Cancer facts & figures 2010.* Atlanta, GA: American Cancer Society. Retrieved January 28, 2011, from http://www.cancer.org/acs/groups/content/@nho/documents/document/acspc-024113.pdf.

American Cancer Society. (2012). *Cancer facts & figures 2012.* Atlanta, GA: American Cancer Society. Retrieved December 27, 2011, from http://www.ccrcal.org/pdf/Reports/ACS_2012.pdf.

American Hospice Foundation. (n.d.). *Share your story.* American Hospice Foundation. Retrieved December 28, 2011, from http://www.americanhospice.org/share-your-story.

Beijing International. (n.d.). *Mid-autumn festival: A time for reunion.* Retrieved December 30, 2011, from http://www.ebeijing.gov.cn/Culture/EnjoyBJ/t950624.htm.

Bhattacharji, P. (2008). *Religion in China.* The Council on Foreign Relations, Inc. Retrieved December 30, 2011, from http://www.cfr.org/china/religion-china/p16272.

Bhudhikanok, G. S., Wang, M.-C., Eckert, K., Matkin, C., Marcus, R., & Bachrach, L. K. (1996). Differences in bone mineral in young Asian and Caucasian Americans may reflect differences in bone size. *Journal of Bone and Mineral Research, 11*(10), 1545–1556.

Birch, A. (1991). *Hong Kong: The colony that never was.* Hong Kong: Hong Kong Sing Cheong Printing.

Bowman, K. W., & Singer, P. A. (2001). Chinese seniors' perspectives on end-of-life decisions. *Social Science & Medicine, 53*(4), 455–464.

Braun, K. L., & Nichols, R. (1997). Death and dying in four Asian American cultures: A descriptive study. *Death Studies, 21*(4), 327–359.

Buiten, C., & Metzger, B. (2000). Childhood obesity and risk of cardiovascular disease: A review of the science. *Pediatric Nursing, 26*(1), 13–18.

Burnam, M. A., Hough, R. L., Karno, M., Escobar, J. I., & Telles, C. A. (1987). Acculturation and lifetime prevalence of psychiatric disorders among Mexican Americans in Los Angeles. *Journal of Health and Social Behavior, 28*(1), 89–102.

Caballero, A. E. (2005). Diabetes in minority populations. In C. R. Kahn, G. C. Weir, G. L. King, A. M. Jacobson, A. C. Moses, & R. J. Smith (Eds.), *Joslin's diabetes mellitus* (14th ed., pp. 505–524). Philadelphia: Lippincott Williams & Wilkins.

Cain, K. P., Connie, H. A., Armstrong, L. R., Garman, K. N., Wells, C. D., Iademarco, M. F., et al. (2007). Tuberculosis among foreign-born persons in the United States. Achieving tuberculosis elimination. *American Journal of Respiratory and Critical Care Medicine, 175*, 75–79. doi:10.1164/rccm.200608-1178OC.

Cantwell, M. F., Snider, D. E., Cauthen, G. M., & Onorato, I. M. (1994). Epidemiology of tuberculosis in the United States, 1985 through 1992. *Journal of the American Medical Association, 272*(7), 535–539.

Carter, J. R. (1993). *On understanding Buddhists: Essays on the Theravada tradition in Sri Lanka.* Albany, NY: State University of New York Press.

Centers for Disease Control and Prevention (CDC). (1989). A strategic plan for the elimination of tuberculosis in the United States. *Morbidity and Mortality Weekly Report, 38*(Suppl no. S-3), 1–25.

Centers for Disease Control and Prevention (CDC). (2006). Tobacco use among adults – United States, 2005. *Morbidity and Mortality Weekly Report, 55*(42), 1145–1148. Retrieved January 10, 2011, from http://www.cdc.gov/chronicdisease/overview/index.htm.

Centers for Disease Control and Prevention (CDC). (2007a). *Childhood obesity.* Atlanta, GA, USA: Department of Health and Human Services, Center for Disease Control and Prevention, National Center for Chronic Disease Prevention and Health Promotion, Division of Adolescent and School Health. Retrieved January 17, 2011, from http://www.cdc.gov/HealthyYouth/obesity/.

Centers for Disease Control and Prevention (CDC). (2008). *Behavioral risk factor surveillance system.* Atlanta, GA: U.S. Department of Health and Human Services. Retrieved January 19, 2011, from http://apps.nccd.cdc.gov/brfss/list.asp?cat=PA&yr=2007&qkey=4418&state=All.

Centers for Disease Control and Prevention (CDC). (n.d). Adult cigarette smoking in the United States: Current estimate. Atlanta, GA: US Department of Health and Human Services, CDC. Retrieved January 28, 2011, from http://www.cdc.gov/tobacco/data_statistics/fact_sheets/adult_data/cig_smoking/index.htm.

Chan, Y-c, Chun, P.-k. R., & Chung, K-w. (2008). Public perception and reporting of different kinds of family abuse in Hong Kong. *Journal of Family Violence, 23*, 253–263.

Chan, Y. M., & Molassiotis, A. (1999). The relationship between diabetes knowledge and compliance among Chinese with non-insulin dependent diabetes mellitus in Hong Kong. *Journal of Advanced Nursing, 30*, 431–438.

Chang, D. F., Shen, B.-J., & Takeuchi, D. T. (2009). Prevalence and demographic correlates of intimate partner violence in Asian Americans. *International Journal of Law and Psychiatry, 32*(3), 167–175.

Chao, R. K., & Tseng, V. (2002). Parenting of Asians. In M. H. Bornstein (Ed.), *Handbook of parenting* (Social conditions and applied parenting 2nd ed., Vol. 4, pp. 59–93). Mahwah, NJ: Lawrence Erlbaum Associates.

Chaturvedi, N. (2003). Ethnic differences in cardiovascular disease. *Heart, 89*(6), 681–686.

Chen, Y.-L. D. (1996). Conformity with nature: A theory of Chinese American elders' health promotion and illness prevention processes. *Advances in Nursing Science, 19*(2), 17–26.

Chen, X., Unger, J. B., Cruz, T. B., & Johnson, C. A. (1999). Smoking patterns of Asian-American youth in California and their relationship with acculturation. *Journal of Adolescent Health, 24*(5), 321–328.

Chen, X., Unger, J. B., & Johnson, C. A. (1999). Is acculturation a risk factor for early smoking initiation among Chinese American minors? A comparative perspective. *Tobacco Control, 8*(4), 402–410.

Chen, J.-L., Weiss, S., Heyman, M. B., & Lusting, R. (2009). Risk factors for obesity and high blood pressure in Chinese American children: Maternal acculturation and children food choices. *Journal of Immigrant and Minority Health*. doi:10.1007/s10903-009-9288-x.

Chen, J.-L., Weiss, S., Heyman, M. B., Vittinghoff, E., & Lusting, R. (2008). Pilot study of an individual tailored educational program by mail to promote healthy weight in Chinese American children. *Journal for Specialists in Pediatric Nursing, 13*(3), 212–222.

Chen, J. Y., & Wong, C. C. (2010). Cardiovascular health. In *The encyclopedia of Asian American issues today* (Vol. 1, pp. 289–299). Santa Barbara, CA: Greenwood Press/ABC-CLIO/LLC.

Chen, J.-L., & Wu, Y. (2008). Cardiovascular risk factors in Chinese American children: Association between overweight, acculturation, and physical activity. *Journal of Pediatric Health Care, 22*(2), 103–110. doi:10.1016/j.pedhc.2007.03.002.

Chesla, C. A., Chun, K. M., & Kwan, C. M. L. (2009). Cultural and family challenges to managing type 2 diabetes in immigrant Chinese Americans. *Diabetes Care, 32*(10), 1812–1816.

China Internet Information Center. (n.d.). *Traditional Chinese festival – dragon boat festival*. Retrieved December 30, 2011, from http://www.china.org.cn/english/features/Festivals/78316.htm.

Chinese Spring Festival. (2011). *Chinatravel.com*. Retrieved December 30, 2011, from http://www.chinatravel.com/facts/chinese-culture-and-history/chinese-festivals/traditional-chinese-festival/chinese-spring-festival.htm.

Choi, N. (2011). Relationship between health service use and health information technology use among older adults: Analysis of the US National Health Interview Survey. *Journal of Medical Internet Research, 13*(2), 1–13.

Chou, W.-Y. S., Stokes, S. C., Citko, J., & Davies, B. (2008). Improving end-of life care through community-based grassroots collaboration: Development of the Chinese-American coalition for compassionate care. *Journal of Palliative Care, 24*(1), 31–40.

Costigan, C. L., & Dokis, D. P. (2006). Relations between parent–child acculturation differences and adjustment with immigrant families. *Child Development, 77*(5), 1252–1267.

Datar, A., Sturm, R., & Magnabosco, J. L. (2004). Childhood overweight and academic performance: National study of kindergartners and first-graders. *Obesity Research, 12*(1), 58–68.

Diez Roux, A. V., Detrano, R., Jackson, S., Jacobs, D. R., Schreiner, P. J., Shea, S., et al. (2005). Acculturation and socioeconomic position as predictors of coronary calcification in a multiethnic sample. *Circulation, 112*, 1557–1565.

Dobash, R. E., & Dobash, R. P. (1978). Wives: The 'appropriate' victims of marital violence. *Victimology: An International Journal, 2*(3/4), 426–442.

Dube, A. (2003). *San Francisco restaurant industry analysis*. Berkeley: Center for Labor Research and Education, University of California.

Escobar, J. I. (1998). Immigration and mental health: Why are immigrants better off? *Archives of General Psychiatry, 55*, 781–782.

Farver, J. A. M., Narang, S. K., & Bhadha, B. R. (2002). East meets west: Ethnic identity, acculturation, and conflict in Asian Indian families. *Journal of Family Psychology, 16*, 338–350.

Ferketich, A. K., Wewers, M. E., Kwong, K., Louie, E., Moeschberger, M. L., Tso, A., et al. (2004). Smoking cessation interventions among Chinese Americans: The role of families, physicians, and the media. *Nicotine & Tobacco Research, 6*(2), 241–248.

Flaskerud, J. H., & Hu, L.-T. (1992). Relationship of ethnicity to psychiatric diagnosis. *The Journal of Mental and Nervous Disease, 180*(5), 296–303.

Fogel, J., & Ford, D. E. (2005). Stigma beliefs of Asian Americans with depression in an internet sample. *Canadian Journal of Psychiatry, 50*(8), 470–478.

Friedland, O., Nemet, D., Gorodnitsky, N., Wolach, B., & Eliakim, A. (2002). Obesity and lipid profiles in children and adolescents. *Journal of Pediatric Endocrinology & Metabolism, 15*(7), 1011–1016.

Fu, X. (1995). Impact of the 1993 Chinese student protection act on American and Chinese societies. *East Asia, 14*(2), 3–22. doi:10.1007/BF03023431.

Fu, S. S., Ma, G. X., Tu, X. M., Siu, P. T., & Metlay, J. P. (2003). Cigarette smoking among Chinese Americans and the influence of linguistic acculturation. *Nicotine & Tobacco Research, 5*(6), 803–811.

Ge, X., Conger, R. D., Lorenz, F. O., & Simons, R. L. (1994). Parents' stressful life events and adolescent depressed mood. *Journal of Health and Social Behavior, 35*, 28–44.

Goel, M. S., McCarthy, E. P., Phillips, R. S., & Wee, C. C. (2004). Obesity among US immigrant subgroups by duration of residence. *Journal of the American Medical Association, 292*, 2860–2867.

Golding, J. M., Karno, M., & Rutter, C. M. (1990). Symptoms of major depression among Mexican-Americans and Non-Hispanic Whites. *The American Journal of Psychiatry, 147*(7), 861–866.

Goran, M. I., Ball, G. D. C., & Cruz, M. L. (2003). Obesity and risk of type 2 diabetes and cardiovascular disease in children and adolescents. *The Journal of Clinical Endocrinology and Metabolism, 88*(4), 1417–1427.

Gounder, C. R., Driver, C. R., Scholten, J. N., Shen, H., & Munsiff, S. S. (2003). Tuberculin testing and risk of tuberculosis infection among New York city schoolchildren. *Pediatrics, 111*(4), e309–e315.

Graffunder, C. M., Noonan, R. K., Cox, P., & Wheaton, J. (2004). Through a public health lens. Preventing violence against women: An update from the US Centers for Disease Control and Prevention. *Journal of Women's Health, 13*(1), 5–16. doi:10.1089/154099904322836401.

Grim, B. (2008). *Religion in China on the eve of the 2008 Beijing olympics*. Pew Research Center Publications. Retrieved December 30, 2011, from http://pewforum.org/Importance-of-Religion/Religion-in-China-on-the-Eve-of-the-2008-Beijing-Olympics.aspx.

Hahm, H. C., Lahiff, M., & Guterman, N. B. (2003). Acculturation and parental attachment in Asian-American adolescents' alcohol use. *Journal of Adolescent Health, 33*(2), 119–129.

Hall, E. T. (1976). *Beyond culture*. New York: Anchor Books.

Hammen, C. (2005). Stress and depression. *Annual Review of Clinical Psychology, 1*, 293–319.

Hardin, E. E., Leong, F. T. L., & Bhagwat, A. A. (2004). Factor structure of the self construal scale revisited. *Journal of Cross-Cultural Psychology, 35*(3), 327–345.

Harwood, A. (1981). *Ethnicity and medical care*. Cambridge, MA: Harvard University Press.

Hedeen, A. N., White, E., & Taylor, V. (1999). Ethnicity and birthplace in relation to tumor size and stage in Asian American women with breast cancer. *American Journal of Public Health, 89*(8), 1248–1252.

Hicks, M. H. (2006). The prevalence and characteristics of intimate partner violence in a community study of Chinese American women. *Journal of Interpersonal Violence, 21*(10), 1249–1269.

Ho, D. Y. (1976). On the concepts of face. *The American Journal of Sociology, 81*(4), 867–884.

Ho, M.-J. (2004). Health-seeking patterns among Chinese immigrant patients enrolled in the directly observed therapy program in New York city. *International Journal of Tuberculosis and Lung Disease, 8*(11), 1355–1359.

Ho, T.-P., & Chung, S. Y. (1996). Help-seeking behaviours among child psychiatric clinic attenders in Hong Kong. *Social Psychiatry and Psychiatric Epidemiology, 31*(5), 292–298.

Hoeman, S. P., Ku, Y. L., & Ohl, D. R. (1996). Healthy beliefs and early detection among Chinese women. *Western Journal of Nursing Research, 18*(5), 518–533.

Hospice Foundation of America. (n.d.). *What is hospice?* Hospice Foundation of America. Retrieved December 28, 2011, from http://www.hospicefoundation.org/.

Hsiung, Y.-F. Y., & Ferrans, C. E. (2007). Recognizing Chinese Americans cultural needs in making end-of-life treatment decisions. *Journal of Hospice and Palliative Nursing, 9*(3), 132- 140. doi:10.1097/01.NJH.0000269993.13625.49.

Hsu, Y. H., Mao, C.-L., & Wey, M. (2010). Antihypertensive medication adherence among elderly Chinese Americans. *Journal of Transcultural Nursing, 21*(4), 297–305.

Hsu, C.-Y., O'Connor, M., & Lee, S. (2009). Understandings of death and dying for people of Chinese origin. *Death Studies, 33*(2), 153–174.

Hsu, G. L. K., Wan, Y. M., Chang, H., Summergrad, P., Tsang, B. Y. P., & Chen, H. (2008). Stigma of depression is more severe in Chinese Americans than Caucasian Americans. *Psychiatry, 71*(3), 210–218.

Hu, K. K., Woodall, E. D., Do, H. H., Tu, S.-P., Thompson, B., Acorda, E., et al. (2006). Tobacco knowledge and beliefs in Chinese American men. *Asian Pacific Journal of Cancer Prevention, 7*(3), 434–438.

Huang, Z. J., Yu, S. M., Liu, X. W., Young, D., & Wong, F. Y. (2009). Beyond medical insurance: Delayed or forgone care among children in Chinese immigrant families. *Journal of Health Care for the Poor and Underserved, 20*(2), 364–377.

Hwang, W.-C., Chun, C.-A., Takeuchi, D. T., Myers, H. F., & Siddarth, P. (2005). Age of first onset major depression in Chinese Americans. *Cultural Diversity and Ethnic Minority Psychology, 11*(1), 16–27.

Hwang, W.-C., Myers, H. F., & Takeuchi, D. T. (2000). Psychosocial predictors of first-onset depression in Chinese Americans. *Social Psychiatry and Psychiatric Epidemiology, 35*(3), 133–145.

Ino, S. M., & Glicken, M. D. (1999). Treating Asian American clients in crisis: A collectivist approach. *Smith College Studies in Social Work, 96*(3), 525–540.

Jackson, K. A., & Savaiano, D. A. (2001). Lactose maldigestion, calcium intake and osteoporosis in African-, Asian-, and Hispanic-American. *Journal of the American College of Nutrition, 20*(Suppl), S198–207S.

Jang, M., Lee, E., & Woo, K. (1998). Income, language, and citizenship status: Factors affecting the health care access and utilization of Chinese Americans. *Health and Social Work, 23*(2), 136–145.

Jayne, R. L., & Rankin, S. H. (2001). Application of Leventhal's self-regulation model to Chinese immigrants with type 2 diabetes. *Journal of Nursing Scholarship, 33*(1), 53–59.

Jenkins, C. H., & Kagawa-Singer, M. (1994). *Confronting health issues of Asian and Pacific Islander Americans.* Thousand Oaks, CA: Sage.

Jin, G., Fan, D., Fan, H., & Liu, Q. (1986). The evolution of Chinese science and technology. In J. T. Fraser, N. Lawrence, & F. C. Haber (Eds.), *Time, science, and society in China and the West* (pp. 170–180). Amherst, MA: University of Masaschusetts.

Juang, L. P., Syed, M., & Takagi, M. (2007). Intergenerational discrepancies of parental control among Chinese American families: Links to family conflict and adolescent depressive symptoms. *Journal of Adolescence, 30,* 965–975.

Kagawa-Singer, M. (1995). Socioeconomic and cultural influences on cancer care of women. *Seminars in Oncology Nursing, 11*(2), 109–119.

Kagawa-Singer, M. (1996). Cultural systems related to cancer. In R. McCorkle, M. Frank-Stromborg, & S. B. Baird (Eds.), *Cancer nursing – A comprehensive textbook* (2nd ed., pp. 38–52). Philadelphia: W. B. Saunders.

Kandula, N. R., Diez-Roux, A. V., Chan, C., Daviglus, M. L., Jackson, S. A., Ni, H., et al. (2008). Association of acculturation levels and prevalence of diabetes in the multi-ethnic study of atherosclerosis (MESA). *Diabetes Care, 31,* 1621–1628.

Kaplan, C. P., Nguyen, T. T., & Weinberg, V. (2008). Longitudinal study of smoking progression in Chinese and Vietnamese American adolescents. *Asian Pacific Journal of Cancer Prevention, 9,* 335–342.

Kenny, M. C., & McEachern, A. G. (2000). Racial, ethnic, and cultural factors of childhood sexual abuse: A selected review of the literature. *Clinical Psychology Review, 20*(7), 905–922.

Kim, S. Y., Chen, Q., Li, J., Huang, X., & Moon, U. J. (2009). Parent–child acculturation, parenting, and adolescent depressive symptoms in Chinese immigrant families. *Journal of Family Psychology, 23*(3), 426–437. doi:10-1037-a0016019.

Kim, G., Chiriboga, D. A., Jang, Y., Lee, S., Huang, C.-H., & Parmelee, P. (2010). Health status of older Asian Americans in California. *Journal of American Geriatrics Society, 58*(10), 2003–2008. doi:10.1111/j.1532-5415.2010.03034.x.

Kleinman, A., & Kleinman, J. (1993). Face, favor and families: The social course of mental health problems in Chinese and American societies. *Chinese Journal of Mental Health, 6,* 37–47.

Kramer, H., Han, C., Post, W., Goff, D., Diez-Roux, A., Cooper, R., et al. (2004). Racial/ethnic differences in hypertension and hypertension treatment and control in the multi-ethnic study of atherosclerosis (NESA). *American Journal of Hypertension, 17*(10), 963–970.

Kuo, W.-H. (1984). Prevalence of depression among Asian-Americans. *The Journal of Nervous and Mental Disorders, 172*(8), 449–457.

Kurz, D. (1989). Social science perspectives on wife abuse: Current debates and future direction. *Gender and Society, 3*(4), 489–505.

Lauderdale, D. S., Kuohung, V., Chang, S.-L., & Chin, M. H. (2003). Identifying older Chinese immigrants at high risk for osteoporosis. *Journal of General Internal Medicine, 18,* 508–515.

Lee, J. W., Brancati, F. L., & Yeh, H. C. (2011). Trends in the prevalence of type 2 diabetes in Asians versus whites: Results from the United States National Health Interview Survey, 1997–2008. *Diabetes Care, 34*(2), 353–357.

Lee, R. M., Choe, J., Kim, G., & Ngo, V. (2000). Construction of the Asian American family conflicts scale. *Journal of Counseling Psychology, 47,* 211–222.

Lerner, B. H. (1993). New York city's tuberculosis control efforts: The historical limitations of the 'war on consumption'. *American Journal of Public Health, 83*(5), 758–766.

Leu, J., Walton, E., & Takeuchi, D. (2010). Contextualizing acculturation: Gender, family, and community reception influences on Asian Immigrant mental health. *American Journal of Community Psychology.* doi:10.1007/s10464-010-9360-7

Leung, W. C., Kung, F., Lam, J., Leung, T. W. H., & Ho, P. C. (2002). Domestic violence and postnatal depression in a Chinese community. *International Journal of Gynecology & Obstetrics, 79*(2), 159–166.

Liang, W., Yuan, E., Mandelblatt, J. S., & Pasick, R. J. (2004). How do older Chinese women view health and cancer screening? Results from focus groups and implications for interventions. *Ethnicity and Health, 9*(3), 283–304.

Lin, J. S., Finlay, A., Tu, A., & Gray, F. M. (2005). Understanding immigrant Chinese Americans' participation in cancer screening and clinical trials. *Journal of Community Health, 30*(6), 451–466.

Lin, K.-M., Miller, M. H., Poland, R. E., Nuccio, I., & Yamaguichi, M. (1991). Ethnicity and family involvement in the treatment of schizophrenic patients. *The Journal of Nervous and Mental Disease, 179*(10), 631–633.

Liu, J. T. C. (1959). *Reform in Sung China: Wang An-shih (1021–1086) and his new policies.* Cambridge, MA: Harvard University Press.

Liu, L. L., Benner, A. D., Lau, A. S., & Kim, S. Y. (2009). Mother-adolescent language proficiency and adolescent academic and emotional adjustment among Chinese American families. *Journal of Youth and Adolescence, 38,* 572–586. doi:10.1007/s10964-008-9358-8.

Liu, A., Berhane, Z., & Tseng, M. (2010). Improved dietary variety and adequacy but lower dietary moderation with acculturation in Chinese women in the United States. *Journal of the American Dietetic Association, 110*(3), 457–462.

Lui, C., & Wallace, S. P. (2010). *Chronic conditions of Californians. 2007 California Health Interview Survey.* Oakland, CA: California HealthCare Foundation. Retrieved January 10, 2011, from http://data.chcf.org/pdf/Chronic_Conditions_of_Californians_2007.pdf.

Lui, P. P. Y., Qin, L., & Chan, K. M. (2008). Tai Chi Chuan exercises in enhancing bone mineral density in active seniors. *Clinics in Sports Medicine, 27,* 75–86.

Luk, J. W., & Tsoh, J. Y. (2010). Moderation of gender on smoking and depression in Chinese Americans. *Addictive Behaviors, 35*(11), 1040–1043.

Lv, N., & Cason, K. L. (2004). Dietary pattern change and acculturation of Chinese Americans in Pennsylvania. *Journal of the American Dietetic Association, 104*(5), 771–778.

Ma, G. X. (1999). Between two worlds: The use of traditional and western health services by Chinese immigrants. *Journal of Community Health, 24*(6), 421–437.

Ma, G. X. (2000). Barriers to the use of health services by Chinese Americans. *Journal of Allied Health, 29*(2), 64–70.

Manangan, L. P., Elmore, K., Lewis, B., Pratt, R., Armstrong, L., Davison, J., et al. (2009). Disparities in tuberculosis between Asian/Pacific Islanders and Non-Hispanic Whites, United States, 1993–2006. *The International Journal of Tuberculosis and Lung Disease, 13*(9), 1077–1085.

Manders, A. J., Banerjee, A., van den Borne, H. W., Harries, A. D., Kok, G. J., & Salaniponi, F. M. L. (2001). Can guardians supervise TB treatment as well as health workers? A study on adherence during the intensive phase. *The International Journal of Tuberculosis and Lung Disease, 5*(9), 838–842.

Maraldi, C., Volpato, S., Penninx, B., Yaffe, K., Simonsick, E. M., Strotmeyer, E. S., et al. (2007). Diabetes mellitus, glycemic control, and incident depressive symptoms among 70- to 79-year-old persons: The health, aging and body composition study. *Archives of Internal Medicine, 167*, 1137–1144.

Matsumoto, D., Yoo, S. H., & Fontaine, J. (2008). Mapping expressive differences around the world: the relationship between emotional display rules and individualism versus collectivism. *Journal of Cross-Cultural Psychology, 39*(1), 55–74.

Maxwell, A. E., Bernaards, C. A., & McCarthy, W. J. (2005). Smoking prevalence and correlates among Chinese-and Filipino-American adults: Findings from the 2001 California Health Interview Survey. *Journal of Preventive Medicine, 41*(2), 693–699.

Mazure, C. M. (1998). Life stressors as risk factors in depression. *Clinical Psychology: Science and Practice, 5*(3), 291–313.

McBride, M. R., Pasick, R. J., Stewart, S., Tuason, N., Sabogal, F., & Duenas, G. (1998). Factors associated with cervical cancer screening among Filipino women in California. *Asian American and Pacific Islander Journal of Health, 6*(2), 358–367.

McCracken, M., Olsen, M., Chen, M. S., Jemal, A., Thun, M., Cokkinides, V., et al. (2007). Cancer incidence, mortality, and associated risk factors among Asian Americans of Chinese, Filipino, Vietnamese, Korean, and Japanese ethnicities. *CA: A Cancer Journal for Clinicians, 57*, 190–205. doi:10.3322/canjclin.57.4.190.

McNeely, M. J., & Boyko, E. J. (2004). Type 2 diabetes prevalence in Asian Americans: Results of a National Healthy Survey. *Diabetes Care, 27*(5), 66–69.

Medvene, L. J., Wescott, J. V., Huckstadt, A., Ludlum, J., Langel, S., Mick, K., et al. (2003). Promoting signing of advance directives in faith community. *Journal of General Internal Medicine, 18*(2), 914–920.

Michielutte, R., Alciati, M. H., & el Arculli, R. (1999). Cancer control and literacy. *Journal of Health Care for the Poor and Underserved, 10*, 281–297.

Mokdad, A. H., Marks, J. S., Stroup, D. F., & Gerberding, J. L. (2004). Actual causes of death in the United States, 2000. *Journal of the American Medical Association, 291*, 1238–1245.

Mui, A. C., & Shibusawa, T. (2008). *Asian American elders in the twenty-first century: Key indicators of well-being*. New York: Columbia University Press. http://www.cancer.gov/clinicaltrials/education/outreach-education-advocacy.

National Hospice and Palliative Care Organization. (2008). *NHPCO facts and figures: Hospice care in America*. Alexandria, VA: National Hospice and Palliative Care Organization. Retrieved January 26, 2011, from http://www.mass.gov/Ihqcc/docs/expert_panel/2008_NHPCO_Facts%20and%20Figures.pdf.

National Institutes of Health Osteoporosis and Related Bone Diseases National Resource Center. (2009). *Bone mass measurement: What the numbers mean*. Washington, DC. Retrieved December 27, 2010, from http://www.niams.nih.gov/Health_Info/Bone/Bone_Health/bone_mass_measure.asp.

National Osteoporosis Foundation. (2010). *Osteoporosis and Asian American women*. Washington, DC. Retrieved December 27, 2010, from http://www.nof.org/aboutosteoporosis/whatwomencando/asianamericanwomen.

National Osteoporosis Foundation. (n.d.). *Osteoporosis and Asian American women*. National Osteoporosis Foundation. Retrieved December 27, 2010, from http://www.nof.org/aboutosteoporosis/whatwomencando/asianamericanwomen.

Ngo-Metzger, Q., Phillips, R. S., & McCarthy, E. P. (2008). Ethnic disparities in hospice use among Asian-American and Pacific Islander patients dying with cancer. *Journal of the American Geriatrics Society, 56*(1), 139–144.

Nguyen, T. T., Somkin, C. P., & Ma, Y. (2005a). Participation of Asian-American women in cancer chemoprevention research. Physician perspectives. *Cancer Supplement, 104*(12), 3006–3014.

Nguyen, T. T., Somkin, C. P., Ma, Y., Fung, L.-C., & Nguyen, T. (2005b). Participation of Asian-American women in cancer treatment research: A pilot study. *Journal of the National Cancer Institute. Monographs, 35*, 102–105.

Odegard, P. S., & Capoccia, K. (2007). Medication taking and diabetes: A systematic review of the literature. *The Diabetes Educator, 33*(6), 1014–1029.

Odegard, P. S., & Gray, S. L. (2008). Barriers to medication adherence in poorly controlled diabetes mellitus. *The Diabetes Educator, 34*(4), 692–697.

Office of Women's Health. (2010). *Minority women's health: Diabetes, 2010*. Atlanta, GA: U.S. Department of Health and Human Services, Office of Women's Health.

Olsen, S. J., & Frank-Stromborg, M. (1993). Cancer prevention and early detection in ethnically diverse populations. *Seminars in Oncology Nursing, 9*(3), 198–209.

Pan, S., & Jordan-Marsh, M. (2010). Internet use intention and adoption among Chinese older adults: From the expanded technology acceptance model perspective. *Computers in human behavior 26*(5), 1111–1119. Retrieved from Sciencedirect on December 30, 2011, from http://www.sciencedirect.com/science/article/pii/S0747563210000555.

Pasick, R. P., D'Onofrio, C. N., & Otero-Sabogal, R. (1996). Similarities and differences across cultures: Questions to inform a third generation for health promotion research. *Health Education Quarterly, 23*(Suppl), S142–S161.

Portes, A., & Rumbaut, R. G. (1996). *Immigrant American: A portrait* (2nd ed.). Berkeley, CA: University of California Press.

Pothiwala, P., Evans, E. M., & Novakofski, K. M. C. (2006). Ethnic variation in risk for osteoporosis among women: A review of biological and behavioral factors. *Journal of Women's Health, 15*(6), 709–719.

Pourat, N., Singer, M. K., Breen, N., & Sripipatana, A. (2010). Access versus acculturation: Identifying modifiable factors to promote cancer screening among Asian American women. *Medical care, 48*(12), 1088–1096.

Qi, B.-B., Resnick, B., Smeltzer, S. C., & Bausell, B. (2011). Self-efficacy program to prevent osteoporosis among Chinese immigrants: A randomized controlled trial. *Nursing Research, 60*(6), 393–404.

Rainie, L. (2011). Asian Americans and technology [powerpoint slides]. Retrieved from the Pew Research Center web site http://www.pewinternet.org/Presentations/2011/Jan/Organization-for-Chinese-Americans.asp.

Rao, K., DiClemente, R. J., & Ponton, L. E. (1992). Child sexual abuse of Asians compared with other populations. *Journal of the American Academy of Child and Adolescent Psychiatry, 31*, 880–886.

Rhee, S., Chang, J., Weaver, D., & Wong, D. (2008). Child maltreatment among immigrant Chinese families: Characteristics and patterns of placement. *Child Maltreatment, 13*(3), 269–279.

Rosario-Sim, M. G., & O'Connell, K. A. (2009). Depression and language acculturation correlate with smoking among older Asian American adolescents in New York city. *Public Health Nursing, 26*(6), 532–542.

Ross, P. D., He, Y., Yates, A. J., Coupland, C., Ravn, P., McClung, M., et al. (1996). Body size accounts for most differences in bone density between Asian and Caucasian women. *Calcified Tissue International, 59*(5), 339–343.

Schneider, T. R. (2006). Getting the biggest bang for your health education buck: Message framing and reducing health disparities. *American Behavioral Scientist, 49*(6), 812–822.

Shelley, D., Fahs, M. C., Scheinmann, R., Swain, S., Qu, J., & Burton, D. (2004). Acculturation and tobacoo use among Chinese Americans. *American Journal of Public Health, 94*(2), 300–307.

Shelley, D., Fahs, M. C., Yerneni, R., Das, D., Nguyen, N., Hung, D., et al. (2008). Effectiveness of tobacco control among Chinese Americans: A comparative analysis of policy approaches versus community-based programs. *Preventive Medicine, 47*(5), 530–536.

Shih, F. J. (1996). Concepts related to Chinese patients' perceptions of health, illness and person: Issues of conceptual clarity. *Accident and Emergency Nursing, 4*(4), 208–215.

Shin, J. K. (1999). Help-seeking behaviors by Korean immigrants for their depression. *Dissertation Abstracts International, 60*, 2064B.

Singh, G. K., Siahpush, M., Hiatt, R. A., & Timsina, L. R. (2010). Dramatic increases in obesity and overweight prevalence and body mass index among ethnic-immigrant and social class groups in the United States, 1976–2008. *Journal of Community Health, 36*(1), 94–110. doi:10.1007/s10900-001-9287-9.

Singh, G. K., Siahpush, M., Hiatt, R. A., & Timsina, L. R. (2011). Dramatic increases in obesity and overweight prevalence and body mass index among ethnic-immigrant and social class groups in the United States, 1976–2008. *Journal of Community Health, 36*(1), 94–110. doi:10.1007/s10900-001-9287-9.

Sluzki, C. E. (1979). Migration and family conflict. *Family Process, 18*(4), 381–394.

Smart, J. F., & Smart, D. W. (1995). Acculturative stress: The experience of the Hispanic immigrant. *The Counseling Psychologist, 23*, 25–42.

Spector, R. E. (1991). *Cultural diversity in health and illness* (3rd ed.). East Norwalk, CT: Appleton and Lance.

Spence, D. P., Hotchkiss, J., Williams, C. S., & Davies, P. D. O. (1993). Tuberculosis and poverty. *British Medical Journal, 307*(6907), 759–761.

Spencer, M. S., & Chen, J. (2004). Effect of discrimination on mental health service utilization among Chinese Americans. *American Journal of Public Health, 94*, 809–814.

Spigner, C., Yip, M.-P., Huang, B., & Tu, S. P. (2007). Chinese and Vietnamese adult male smokers' perspectives regarding facilitators of tobacco cessation behavior. *Asian Pacific Journal of Cancer Prevention, 8*(3), 429–435.

Stevenson, H. W., & Lee, S-y. (1996). The academic achievement of Chinese students. In M. H. Bond (Ed.), *The handbook of Chinese psychology* (pp. 124–142). New York: Oxford University Press.

Stokes, S. C., Thompson, L. W., Murphy, S., & Gallagher-Thompson, D. (2001). Screening for depression in immigrant Chinese-American elders: Results of a pilot study. *Journal of Gerontological Social Work, 36*, 27–44.

Sue, S., Fujino, D. C., Hu, L. T., Takeuchi, D. T., & Zane, N. W. S. (1991). Community mental health services for ethnic minority groups: A test of the cultural responsiveness hypothesis. *Journal of Consulting and Clinical Psychology, 59*(4), 533–540.

Sun, A., Tsoi, E., Stearman, S. M., & Chow, E. (2005). *Perception of family violence in the Chinese community.* Presented at the American Public Health Association 133rd annual meeting & exposition, New Orleans, LA.

Sun, A., Wong-Kim, E., Stearman, S., & Chow, E. A. (2005). Quality of life in Chinese patients with breast cancer. *Cancer Supplement, 104*(12), 2952–2954.

Sung, R. Y. T., Yu, C. C., Choi, K. C., Xu, S. L. Y., Chan, D., Lo, A. F. C., et al. (2007). Waist circumference and body mass index in Chinese children: Cutoff values for predicting cardiovascular risk factors. *International Journal of Obesity, 31*(3), 550–558.

Swallen, K. C., Reither, E. N., Haas, S. A., & Meier, A. M. (2005). Overweight, obesity, and health-related quality of life among adolescents: The National Longitudinal Study of Adolescent Health. *Pediatrics, 115*(2), 340–347.

Tabora, B. L., & Flashkerud, J. H. (1997). Mental health beliefs, practices and knowledge of Chinese American immigrant women. *Mental Health Nursing, 18,* 173–189.

Tang, C. S.-K. (1998). The rate of physical child abuse in Chinese families: A community survey in Hong Kong. *Child Abuse & Neglect, 22*(5), 381–391.

Tang, C. S.-K. (1999). Wife abuse in Hong Kong Chinese families: A community survey. *Journal of Family Violence, 14*(2), 173–191.

Tang, H., Shimizu, R., & Chen, M. S., Jr. (2005). English language proficiency and smoking prevalence among California's Asian Americans. *Cancer, 104*(12 Suppl), 2982–2988.

Tardif, C. Y., & Geva, E. (2006). The link between acculturation disparity and conflict among Chinese Canadian immigrant mother-adolescent dyads. *Journal of Cross-Cultural Psychology, 37,* 191–211. doi:1177/0022022105284496.

Ton, T. G. N., Steinman, L., Yip, M.-P., Ly, K. A., Sin, M.-K., Fitzpatrick, A. L., et al. (2010). Knowledge of cardiovascular health among Chinese, Korean and Vietnamese immigrants to the US. *Journal of Immigrant and Minority Health, 13*(1), 127–139. doi:10.1007/s10903-010-9340-x.

Torres, S. (1991). A comparison of wife abuse between two cultures: Perceptions, attitudes, nature and extent. *Issues in Mental Health Nursing, 12*(1), 113–131.

Tsai, S. (2008). The Chinese family: Historical roots & modern American existence. Stanford.edu. Retrieved January 28, 2011, from http://www.standford.edu/~stsai417/the_chinese_family/index.html.

Tse, C. Y., Chong, A., & Fok, S. Y. (2003). Breaking bad news: A Chinese perspective. *Palliative Medicine, 17,* 339–343.

Tsoh, J. Y., Lam, J. N., Delucchi, K. L., & Hall, S. M. (2003). Smoking and depression in Chinese Americans. *The American Journal of the Medical Sciences, 326*(4), 187–191.

Tu, S.-P., Chen, H., Chen, A., Lim, J., May, S., & Drescher, C. (2005). Clinical trials. Understanding and perceptions of female Chinese-American cancer patients. *Cancer Supplement, 104*(12), 2999–3005.

U.S. Census Bureau. (2009). Selected population profile in the United State, Chinese alone or in any combination. American Community Survey 1-Year Estimates. Retrieved December 29, 2010, from http://factfinder.census.gov.

U.S. Department of Health and Human Services. (2001). NIH guidelines on the inclusion of women and minorities as subjects in clinical research. The Office of Minority Health. *Fed Regist* 1994(59), 14508–14513.

U.S. Department of Health and Human Services. (2011a). Cancer data/statistics. The Office of Minority Health. Retrieved January 28, 2011, from http://minorityhealth.hhs.gov/templates/browse.aspx?lvl=3&lvlid=4.

U.S. Department of Health and Human Services. (2011b). Cancer and Asians/Pacific Islanders. The Office of Minority Health. Retrieved January 28, 2011, from http://minorityhealth.hhs.gov/templates/content.aspx?lvl=3&lvlID=4&ID=3055.

U.S. Department of Health and Human Services, The Office of Minority Health, Centers for Medicare and Medicaid. (2011c). *Medicare hospice benefits.* Retrieved December 28, 2011, from http://www.medicare.gov/Publications/Pubs/pdf/02154.pdf.

Uba, L. (1994). *Asian Americans: Personality patterns, identity, and mental health.* New York: Guilford Press.

Unger, J. B., Reynolds, K., Shakib, S., Spruitz-Metz, D., Sun, P., & Johnson, C. A. (2004). Acculturation, physical activity, and fast food consumption among Asian American and Hispanic adolescents. *Journal of Community Health, 29*(6), 467–481.

Vega, W. A., Kolody, B., Aguilar-Gaxiola, S., Alderet, E., Catalano, R., & Caraveo-Anduaga, J. (1998). Lifetime prevalence of DSM-III-R psychiatric disorders among urban and rural Mexican Americans in California. *Archives of General Psychiatry, 55*(9), 771–778.

Verver, S., van Soolingen, D., & Borgdorff, M. W. (2002). Effect of screening of immigrants on tuberculosis transmission. *The International Journal of Tuberculosis and Lung Disease, 6*(2), 0121–0129.

Wang, J.-Y., Probst, J. C., Moore, C. G., Martin, A. B., & Bennett, K. J. (2010). Place of origin and violent disagreement among Asian American families: Analysis across five states. *Journal of Immigrant and Minority Health.* doi:10.1007/s10903-010-9398-5.

Ward, C., & Kennedy, A. (1999). The measurement of sociocultural adaptation. *International Journal of Intercultural Relations, 23,* 659–677.

Weaver, S. W., & Kim, S. Y. (2008). A person-centered approach on the linkages among parent–child differences in cultural orientation, supportive parenting, and adolescent depressive symptoms in Chinese American families. *Journal of Youth and Adolescence, 37*(1), 36–49.

Wildman, R. P., Gu, D., Reynolds, K., Duan, X., & He, J. (2004). Appropriate body mass index and waist circumference cutoffs for categorization of overweight and central adiposity among Chinese adults. *American Journal of Clinical Nutrition, 80*(5), 1129–1136.

Wong, M. G. (2005). Chinese-Americans. In E. W.-C. Chen & G. J. Yoo (Eds.), *Encyclopedia of Asian American issues today* (Vol. 1, pp. 110–145). Santa Barbara, CA: ABC-CLIO/LLC.

Wong, S. S., Dixon, L. B., Cilbride, J. A., Chin, W. W., & Kwan, T. W. (2010). Diet, physical activity, and cardiovascular disease risk factors among older Chinese Americans living in New York city. *Journal of*

Community Health, 80(5), 1129–1136. doi:10.1007/s10900-010-9323-6.

World Health Organization. (1994). Assessment of fracture risk and its application to screening for postmenopausal osteoporosis. Report of a WHO Study Group. World Health Organization Technical Report Series, 843, 1–129.

World Health Organization. (2007). Global tuberculosis control: Key findings. Geneva, Switzerland: WHO. Retrieved January 17, 2011, from http://www.who.int/tb/publications/global_report/2007/key_findings/en/index.html.

World Health Organization. (2011). Diabetes – Fact sheet N. 312. Geneva, Switzerland: WHO. Retrieved January 28, 2011, from http://www.who.int/mediacentre/factsheets/fs312/en/index.html.

Wu, Y. (1995). The Chinese virago: A literary theme. Cambridge, MA: Harvard University Press.

Wu, D., Ma, G. X., Zhou, K., Zhou, D., Liu, A., & Poon, A. N. (2009). The effect of a culturally tailored smoking cessation for Chinese American smokers. Nicotine & Tobacco Research, 11(12), 1448–1457.

Xu, X., Campbell, J. C., & Zhu, F. C. (2001). Intimate partner violence against Chinese women. Trauma, Violence & Abuse, 2(4), 296–315.

Xu, Y., Pan, W., & Liu, H. (2010). Self-management practices of Chinese Americans with type 2 diabetes. Nursing and Health Sciences, 12(2), 228–234.

Yeo, G., & Hikoyeda, N. (2000). Cultural issues in end of life decision making among Asians and Pacific Islanders in the United States. In K. L. Braun, J. H. Pietsch, & P. L. Blanchette (Eds.), Cultural issues in end-of-life decision making (pp. 101–126). Thousand Oaks, CA: Safe Publications Inc.

Yeung, C. Y. (1999). Changing pattern of childhood diseases in Hong Kong – A rapidly developing community. Current Pediatrics, 9, 209–214.

Yeung, C. Y. (2000). Changing pattern of neonatal disease in Hong Kong. Journal of Paediatrics, Obsterics & Gynecology (Honk Kong Edition), 26(1), 5–12.

Yeung, A., Chan, R., Mischoulon, D., Sonawalla, S., Wong, E., Nierenberg, A. A., et al. (2004a). Prevalence of major depressive disorder among Chinese-Americans in primary care. General Hospital Psychiatry, 26(1), 24–30.

Yeung, A., Kung, W. W., Chung, H., Rubenstein, G., Roffi, P., Mischoulon, D., et al. (2004b). Integrating psychiatry and primary care improves treatment acceptability among Asian Americans. General Hospital Psychiatry, 26(4), 256–260.

Yeung, C. Y., Ko, P. Y. S., & Ho, F. (Eds.). (2002). Chinese children are different. Chinese Child Health International web-site http://www.cchi.com.hk.

Yi, J. K. (1994). Factors associated with cervical cancer screening behavior among Vietnamese women. Journal of Community Health, 19(3), 189–200.

Yick, A. G. (1997). Chinese-Americans' perceptions of and experiences with domestic violence and factors related to their psychological well-being. Ph.D. dissertation, School of Public Policy and Social Research, University of California, Los Angeles.

Yick, A. G. (2000). Predicators of physical spousal/intimate violence in Chinese American families. Journal of Family Violence, 15(3), 249–267.

Yick, A. G. (2001). Feminist theory and status inconsistence theory: Application to domestic violence in Chinese immigrant families. Violence Against Women, 7(8), 900–926.

Yick, A. G., & Agbayani-Siewert, P. (1997). Perceptions of domestic violence in a Chinese American community. Journal of Interpersonal Violence, 12(6), 832–846. doi:10.1177/088626097012006004.

Yick, A. G., & Berthold, S. M. (2005). Conducting research on violence in Asian American communities: Methodological issues. Violence and Victims, 20(6), 661–677.

Yick, A. G., & Rashmi, G. (2002). Chinese cultural dimensions of death, dying, and bereavement: Focus group findings. Journal of cultural diversity, 9(2), 32–42.

Yick, A. G., Shibusawa, T., & Agbayani-Siewert, P. (2003). Partner violence, depression, and practice implications with families of Chinese descent. Journal of Cultural Diversity, 10(3), 96–104.

Ying, Y.-W. (1988). Depressive symptomatology among Chinese-Americans as measured by the CES-D. Journal of Clinical Psychology, 44(5), 739–746.

Ying, Y.-W., & Hu, L-t. (1994). Public outpatient mental health services: Use and outcome among Asian Americans. The American Journal of Orthopsychiatry, 64(3), 448–455.

Yoshioka, M. R., DiNoia, J., & Ullah, K. (2001). Attitudes toward marital violence. Violence Against Women, 7(8), 900–926.

Young, T. K., Dean, H. J., Flett, B., & Wood-Steiman, P. (2000). Childhood obesity in a population at high risk for type 2 diabetes. The Journal of Pediatrics, 136(3), 365–369.

The Health of Filipina/o America: Challenges and Opportunities for Change

Introduction

After a 12-hour graveyard shift, Virginia Lacuesta Raña Magbual would make the 1-hour traffic ridden commute to her tract home. Her work caring for others provided for her and her family, and helped them pursue the American dream they had been seeking. As a registered nurse for 40 years, she personifies a generation of post-1965 Filipina nurses who sent money from the United States to their families in the Philippines, sponsored relatives to migrate to America and sacrificed many nights of sleep to provide for loved ones. While caring for others as a nurse, Virginia was also living with type II diabetes, caring for both her father and son, who were also battling type II diabetes.

In 2010, Virginia was diagnosed with a rare form of stage IV metastatic melanoma brain cancer and passed shortly after her diagnosis. Many Filipina and Filipino Americans, like Virginia, have worked tirelessly to care for others and their families, and for themselves.

Although Filipina/o Americans are heavily involved in the care of others, many of these same individuals face numerous cultural, structural and social barriers to maintaining good health. Diabetes, heart disease, and cancer are all leading causes of death for Filipina/o Americans (Dalusung-Angosta, 2010; de Castro, Gee, & Takeuchi, 2008; Harle et al., 2007). Race, class, and gender all provide strong explanatory models of why Filipina/o Americans face great health risks (Brown & James, 2000; de Castro et al., 2008; Frisbee, Cho, & Hubber, 2002).

Like Virginia's story, many Filipina/o Americans play a significant role in the health care industry as caregivers, technicians, nurse assistants, nurses, and physicians, but when it comes to dealing with their own health they face many challenges and barriers including occupational stress, access to affordable healthcare, culturally sensitive services, and language barriers (Abesamis-Mendoza et al., 2007; California Asian Pacific Islander Joint Legislative Caucus, 2009; David, 2011; Montano, Acosta-Deprez, & Sinay, 2009; Semics, 2007).

Profile of Filipina/o America

To understand the Filipina/o American community, it is important to trace the history of colonization, diaspora, and issues of this population. Spain's desire for resources such as land, markets, raw materials, and slave labor reached the Philippines with the arrival of Ferdinand Magellan in 1521. In the late nineteenth century, the colonial relationship of the Philippines with Spain

R.R. Daus-Magbual (✉)
Pin@y Educational Partnerships (PEP),
San Francisco, CA, USA
e-mail: rodmagbual@gmail.com

R.S. Magbual
Kaiser Permanente Hospital of Riverside, CA, USA
e-mail: richmagbual@gmail.com

G.J. Yoo et al. (eds.), *Handbook of Asian American Health*,
DOI 10.1007/978-1-4614-2227-3_4, © Springer Science+Business Media, LLC 2013

and the United States led to rampant poverty and to the diaspora of the Filipina/o from their native country (Chua, 2009; Parrenas, 2001; San Juan, 2006). Filipina/o migration to the Americas spans more than 500 years. The earliest migrants traveled through the Manila-Acapulco Galleon Trade Route, landing in Morro Bay, California, and later creating early Filipino settlements in Louisiana (Cordova, 1983; Crouchett, 1982, Espina, 1988).

From 1905 to 1945, many Filipinos – mostly men – arrived on the shores of Hawaii and the California coast (Morales, 1998; Takaki, 1989). These Filipinas/os served America's labor demand for cheap manual labor, especially in the agricultural industry. As a result, many Filipinos were subjected to explicit racial violence and exclusion including anti-miscegenation laws, poor working conditions, low wages, and racial violence, making the Filipino as "the other." The irony behind this exclusion, given the long history of Filipinos in the United States, from American colonization was particularly evident for Filipinos. They organized mass numbers of farm laborers to participate in demonstrations in Hawaii and California, taking advantage of their American education and upbringing. These Filipino farm workers played an instrumental role in developing labor unions to increase wages and introduce fair labor practices in the agriculture industry (Mabalon, Reyes, & Filipino American National Historic Society, 2008; Scharlin & Villanueva, 1994).

A new wave of Filipinas/os migrated to the United States between 1945 and 1965. In the aftermath of World War II, the Philippines achieved independence. Independence significantly improved access to naturalized citizenship, the formation and reunification of families, and the creation of Filipina/o American communities throughout California and the West coast, including the arrival of new professionals alongside the maturation of first and second generation Filipina/o Americans (Mabalon et al., 2008; Posadas, 1999). Previous waves of Filipino migration helped initiate subsequent and substantial migration of Filipinas/os, especially Filipinas, during the 1960s.

The passage of the Immigration and Nationality Act of 1965 transformed the landscape of Filipino American communities in the United States. This legislation fulfilled two goals, specifically relieving occupational shortages and achieving more family reunifications (Morales, 1998; Posadas, 1999). Many physicians and nurses arrived to fulfill the shortage of health care providers in underserved areas (Choy, 2003). By the 1980s, Filipino nurses represented 75% of all foreign nurses in the nursing field (Brush, Sochalski, & Berger, 2004). The post 1965 immigration wave constituted the major influx of Filipina/o professionals arriving in America and helped form many of today's Filipina/o communities throughout the United States.

The Civil Rights movement of the 1960s and early 1970s sparked the creation of Filipina/o American Studies and the emergence of various Filipina/o American organizations within labor, colleges, housing, and the arts. Activist organizations were visible throughout the West Coast (Geron, de la Cruz, Saito, & Singh, 2001). In the 1970s and 1980s, the fight against Martial Law in the Philippines served as a platform that influenced many young Filipina/o and Filipina/o Americans to engage in organizing local Filipina/o American communities throughout the United States (Toribio, 1998). The legacies of these movements have played a critical role in shaping today's Filipina/o American social movements. Currently, Filipina/o Americans represent the second largest Asian immigrant population, second only to the Chinese (Lai & Arguelles, 2003). An estimated four million Filipina/o Americans live in the United States, constituting 1.4% of the American population (Chua, 2009; U.S. Department of State, 2010). About half of the population are permanent residents, while the rest of the demographic consists of undocumented immigrants (24%), and American citizens (26%) (Chua, 2009). Geographically, West Coast cities such as greater Los Angeles, San Francisco Bay Area, San Diego, and Seattle, as well as Honolulu, have of the largest numbers of Filipina/o Americans (Lai & Arguelles, 2003). On the East Coast, the New York City area represents the fourth largest region where Filipina/o Americans reside (Lai & Arguelles, 2003).

Despite their long history in the United States, Filipina/o Americans face many issues such as poverty, immigration, the pressure to assimilate, and access to affordable and quality healthcare (Abesamis-Mendoza et al., 2007; Daus-Magbual & Molina, 2009; Javier, Huffman, & Mendoza, 2007; Lee, 2005; Nadal, 2008; Unemoto & Ong, 2006). Filipinas/os, like many immigrant groups before them, were left to integrate into communities that lacked the necessary culturally appropriate services and resources. The absence of such health resources and a lack of access to affordable quality healthcare, as well as discrimination and racism all help prevent Filipina/o Americans from getting needed medical services (Abesamis-Mendoza et al., 2007; Javier et al., 2007). The social pressures to survive through adversity have likely contributed to the high stress levels related to diabetes, cancer, and cardiovascular diseases (Abesamis-Mendoza et al., 2007; Grunbaum, Lowry, Kann, & Pateman, 2000; Montano et al., 2009; National Heart, Lung, and Blood Institute [NHLBI], 2003; Semics LLC, 2007).

Filipina/o Americans and Health

Information specifically focused on Filipina/o Americans is limited and often misconstrued, since Filipinas/os are generally masked under the larger umbrella of Asian America (Espiritu, 1992; Siu, 1996; Strobel, 1996). Yet when data on Asian Americans are disaggregated, Filipina/o Americans rank amongst the highest in youth incarceration, high school dropout rates, teenage pregnancy, risk for contracting sexual transmitted diseases, obesity, and teenage suicide (Daus-Magbual & Molina, 2009; Doan, 2006; Javier et al., 2007; Nadal, 2008). The result is high rates of chronic health diseases, cardiovascular diseases, stress, mental health issues, and cultural mistrust to find treatment (Abesamis-Mendoza et al., 2007; David, 2011; Nadal, 2009).

Although research and statistics focused on Filipina/o Americans are relatively scarce, the available literature reveals that the top health issues affecting the Filipna/o American community are cardiovascular diseases, cancer, and diabetes (Abesamis-Mendoza et al., 2007; Barnes, Adams, & Powell-Griner, 2008; Choi, Chow, Chung, & Wong, 2010; Dalusung-Angosta, 2010; Giyeon et al., 2010; Kao, 2010; Montano et al., 2009;

NHLBI, 2003; Palaniappan et al., 2010). Research to date provides a foundation to explore and discuss the urgency of the growing phenomenon of health issues in the Filipina/o American community.

Cardiovascular Health

Previous studies of different metropolitan cities including Los Angeles, San Francisco, and New York all identified cardiovascular disease as the leading health concern and cause of death within the Filipina/o American community (Abesamis-Mendoza et al., 2007; Klatsky & Armstrong, 1991; Montano et al., 2009; NHLBI, 2003; Semics LLC, 2007). According to the National Vital Statistics Report (2006), cardiovascular disease is the leading cause of death in the United States. Worth noting is Filipina/o Americans are one of the most affected subpopulations for cardiac related issues (Dalusung-Angosta, 2010).

One particularly extensive study, based on data from 87,029 interviews among Asian American adults, found that Filipinas/os had the highest incidence of obesity (14%) and hypertension (27%) (Barnes et al., 2008). Studies of Filipina/o immigrants and Filipina/o Americans reveal the health consequences associated with years of living in America and the associated accumulation of stress, leading to chronic health risks and conditions (Brown & James, 2000; Castro et al., 2008). Brown & James, (2000) reported that Filipino American immigrant nurses who relocated to the American mainland from Hilo, Hawaii developed higher levels of norepinephrine levels and hypertension.

Based on focus groups and interviews with Filipina/o American community leaders in San Francisco and Daly City, a common observation was heredity plus Filipino foods containing high levels of fat, cholesterol, and sodium contribute to the prevalence of cardiovascular diseases (NHLBI, 2003). More than 60% of Filipina/o adults in California consume less than the recommended five fruits and vegetables per day (California Asian Pacific Islander Joint Legislative Caucus, 2009).

A report by the National Heart, Lung, and Blood Institute (2003) concluded socioeconomic status often takes precedence over personal health for many Americans, resulting in less time devoted to health maintenance and improvement. The same study expressed that socioeconomic status in surviving in America played a critical role in high rates of stress resulting in hypertension. High levels of stress have led to the consumption of available and affordable comfort foods, which tend to be high in fat and sodium. The conclusions in the report are reflected in the Filipina/o population. High stress levels have also led many Filipina/o Americans, both youth and adults, to partake in various health vices such as smoking, alcohol, and other drugs to relieve stress, anxiety, and depression (Nadal, 2011).

A major factor contributing to the high rates of cardiovascular disease within the Filipina/o American community is delayed care and treatment. Several studies shared a common theme, that Filipinas/os forgo preventive health services and only seek care when conditions are life-threatening (Abesamis-Mendoza et al., 2007; David, 2010; Semics, 2007).

The delay in care and treatment was associated with lack of insurance and denial/fear of diagnosis, issues that affect many ethnic populations. Perhaps unique to Filipinas/os is the notion that prevention is not a priority nor commonly accepted practice. Silencing health issues is also a prevalent issue in delaying care and treatment. Filipina/o immigrant and American adults and elderly hide their health concerns from their families to prevent stress and burden amongst their families (Semics, 2007).

Physical fitness appears to be inconsequential. A study based on Filipina/o Americans in New York City reported a lack of exercise due to time constraints, unavailability of facilities, and a perception that fitness is an American phenomenon (Abesamis-Mendoza et al., 2007). Working Filipina/o and Filipina/o Americans bear the burden to simultaneously earn income and run a household that prevents them from having the capacity to pursue fitness. Making exercise a priority is not any more imperative on the West Coast. The California Asian Pacific Islander Joint Legislative Caucus (2009) stated that 46% of Filipina/o American adults are obese or overweight. The report describes the Health Fitness Zone (HFZ), used to evaluate whether a student meets the goal of physical activity and body composition that offers protection against diseases. It appears that sedentary living is the lifestyle for many youth, since 29.6% of Filipina/o American 5th graders are not in the desirable HFZ (California Asian Pacific Islander Joint Legislative Caucus, 2009). A cycle of obesity continues to future generations, propagating a lifestyle of unhealthy living and a lack of physical activity, potentially increasing the incidence of cardiovascular diseases for years to come (Nadal, 2011).

Cancer

Cancer is another prevalent health concern in the Filipina/o American community, the second leading cause of death for Filipino Americans (Hoyert & Kung, 1997). Prostate, lung, colorectum, non-Hodgkin, and liver cancer are the top five illnesses for Filipino American men (Miller, Chu, Hankey, & Ries, 2007). Filipino Americans had the highest incidence and death rate from prostate cancer at 15.7% among Asian Americans (McCraken et al., 2007). Filipino American men ranked second in incidence (71.9%) and mortality rates (49.8%) from lung cancer. Interestingly, the rate of lung cancer is significant among Filipino American men (23.7%) even though they had a lower prevalence of being current smokers compared to Korean (36.2%) and Vietnamese American men (30.9%) (McCraken et al., 2007).

Cancer rates are also significant and even alarming for Filipinas. Miller et al. (2007) reported breast, colorectal, lung, endometrial, and thyroid cancers were the top five manifestations of the disease for American born Filipinas. Rossing, Schwartz, and Weiss (1995) found that Filipinas born in the Philippines had 3.2 times the rate of thyroid cancer compared to American born white females, while American born Filipinas did not demonstrate the same increased risk. Among Asian American women, Filipinas had the second highest incidence (102.4/100,000) and the highest mortality rate (17.5/100,000) for breast cancer (McCraken et al., 2007). Asian Americans have demonstrated poor colorectal cancer screening rates in California, though Filipinas/os rank second (59%) to Koreans with 70% in undergoing the necessary testing (California Asian Pacific Islander Joint Legislative Caucus, 2009).

One relevant detail noted by McCraken et al. (2007) was that being overweight is a key risk factor for postmenopausal breast cancer. Further, the authors stated that 33.5% of Filipina Americans were categorized as overweight, higher than any other Asian ethnic group. The same study also reported that the incidence rate of cervical cancer among Filipina Americans (8.5/100,000) is higher than white females (7.3/100,000), but not as high compared to Korean (11.4/100,000) and Vietnamese women (14.0/100,000).

Diabetes

Several studies document a high rate of diabetes affecting Filipina/o Americans (Asian Pacific Islander American Health Forum [APIAHF], 2008; Araneta, Wingard, & Barrett-Connor, 2002; Choi et al., 2010; Cuasay, Lee, Orlander, Steffen-Batey, & Hanis, 2001; Langenberg, Araneta, Bergstrom, Marmot, & Barrett-Connor, 2007). The APIAHF (2008) reported that Filipino Americans have the highest prevalence of diabetes rates in comparison to those from their country of origin. Measuring the prevalence of Diabetes Mellitus (DM) amongst Asian American adults in California, Filipina/o Americans ranked the highest with 8.05% followed by Japanese (7.07%), Vietnamese (7.03%), and Koreans (6.3%) (Choi et al., 2010). The same study reported that the prevalence of DM amongst Filipina/o Americans, compared to Caucasians, is associated with socioeconomic status, lifestyle behaviors, and co-morbidities that place Filipina/o Americans at high risk.

The researchers added that increased age, being male, having hypertension, lack of vegetables intake, lack of vigorous exercise, and increased body mass index were all factors that led to the greater likelihood of diabetes. Such risk factors are prevalent within the Filipina/o American community.

Filipinas also present disturbing numbers associated with diabetes-related ailments. Araneta et al. (2002) studied diabetes and metabolic syndrome in Filipina Americans versus Caucasian females. The researchers reported that Filipinas had a higher prevalence of diabetes despite being non-obese. Additional information also appeared counterintuitive. Compared to the Caucasian women, Filipina Americans were less likely to smoke and drink, yet were still more likely to use antihypertensive medications. Javier et al. (2007) stated that Filipino mothers had the highest rate of gestational diabetes, and that Philippine born Filipino mothers are significantly more likely to have diabetes during pregnancy than U.S. born Filipino mothers.

The causative link may be socioeconomic factors. Langenberg et al. (2007) reported that the odds of diabetes, among Filipino American women, were significantly lower with those with better childhood financial conditions, greater education, and higher adult income. Issues of stress, work, money, and taking care of children and family were indicators that contributed to the challenges of obtaining and managing diabetes (Langenberg et al., 2007; NHLBI, 2003).

Mental Health and Seeking Help

Filipina/o Americans reportedly have relatively high rates of depression and suicide, yet have low rates of seeking mental health treatment (Barnes et al., 2008; David, 2010; Nadal, 2009; Sanchez & Gaw, 2007). Some possible risk factors identified include low socio-economic status, lack of employment, gender, immigration status, and cultural and linguistic barriers (Javier et al., 2007; Sanchez & Gaw, 2007). Montano et al. (2009), studied Filipino American health in the greater Long Beach (California) area. The researchers found that half of the respondents expressed statements reflecting various negative emotions, including feeling "downhearted" or "sometimes blue." About one-third of respondents reported not being able to work or participate in physical activities because of emotional issues.

There are also concerns among youth. More than two-thirds (70.9%) of Filipina/o American middle school students stated they experienced depression during the previous 12 months and/or felt bad or hopeless almost daily for 2 weeks or more (Youth Risk and Behavior Survey [YRBS], 2001). Gender differences were also noted, specifically children of Filipina/o immigrants found that Filipina American college-aged students spoke of suicidal ideation (Maramba, 2008). As a headline story in a local newspaper, 45.6% of Filipina American high school students stated they considered suicide, later reported by the *San Diego Union Tribune* as the highest percentage among different ethnicities (Lau, 1995). The same article also reported that Filipina youths indicated that culture and family expectations led to a variety of stressors, related to their consideration of suicide.

Social and Cultural Practices That Affect Filipina/o American Health

Socio-economic status, immigrant status, levels of education, job stress and duration, diet and exercise, gender, acculturation, and colonial mentality are cited as contributing factors negatively affecting the health of the Filipina/o American community (Brown & James, 2000; Choi et al., 2010; David, 2010; Langenberg et al., 2007; LaVeist, 2002). The earlier review of Filipinas/os in America points to some possible sources for some of the stated factors.

Exploring the historical oppression of Filipina/o Americans and mechanisms they use to cope with a hostile environment, the community challenged stereotypes about race, class, gender, and sexuality on a daily basis. Such ongoing trials can be considered as *micro aggressions*, frequent verbal, behavioral, and/or environmental indignities, which are either intentional or unintentional. Micro aggressions can create hostilities and incite derogatory comments and insults towards historically oppressed groups (Nadal, 2008). Sue (2010) described that micro aggressive stress can cause biological and physical effects, noting that high rates of stress accumulate that strongly correlates to increased illness. The long term effects of colonialism, cultural and linguistic barriers to health care, job intensity and duration, and immigrant constant struggle to survive are likely examples that have resulted in ongoing insults to the health of Filipina/o Americans.

Socio-economic status plays a considerable role in the health of Filipina/o Americans. Langenberg et al. (2007) reported that factors such as substandard financial conditions during childhood, lack of adequate education, and lower wage jobs significantly increased the risk of diabetes among Filipina Americans. A study of Los Angeles residents discovered there is a general reluctance by many Filipina/o immigrants to use hospital and doctors services' because of the perceived expense. This perception is derived from experiences with the generally costly medical services in the Philippines. Consequently, medical services may not be considered unless the individual is acutely sick (Semics LLC, 2007). This was a common trend among Filipina/o Americans, as 50% of Filipina/o Americans in a New York City report indicated that financial barriers to care, particularly over the cost and/or lack of availability of insurance, influenced their decision to not seek health care (Abesamis-Mendoza et al., 2007).

Cultural and language barriers may also prevent elder Filipinas/os and Filipina/o immigrants from accessing proper health care services. Abesamis-Mendoza et al. (2007) stated that although many Filipina/o immigrants have high English proficiency, communication and cultural misunderstanding were nonetheless obstacles for health care. Language and cultural barriers created an uncomfortable environment to seek medical services or communicate openly with their providers (Semics LLC, 2007). However, longer residency in America and more frequent visits to providers did assist Filipina/o immigrants in becoming more comfortable with their doctor (Semics LLC, 2007).

Cultural mistrust also plays a significant role in preventing Filipina/o immigrant and Filipina/o Americans from accessing mental health services. David (2010) stated the historic and contemporary experiences of oppression towards Filipinas/os and Filipina/o Americans create a culture of mistrust, extending to available therapists and counselors. Cultural mistrust is apparently a consequence of both historical and contemporary oppression, influencing the attitudes of Filipino Americans toward seeking professional assistance. An indigenous Filipino trait such as *hiya* (devastating shame) – which can be incurred by those seeking mental health interventions – is another critical factor that prevents Filipina/o Americans from seeking mental health services (Sanchez & Gaw, 2007). The desire to avoid a sense of shame in the family could lead to stigmatizing mental illness, creating a potential barrier to appropriate health care (Semics LLC, 2007).

Diet and nutrition of Filipina/o Americans may contribute to the prevalence of chronic disease in the Filipina/o American community. Ingredients such as *Patis* (fish sauce), *Bagoong* (shrimp paste), anchovies and anchovy paste, and soy sauce are common ingredients in the Filipino diet. The overuse of salt in various Filipina/o dishes is linked to high rates in cardiovascular diseases. In a San Francisco and Daly City assessment on Filipina/o Americans and cardiovascular risk found that research participants understood that eating less salt is better for their blood pressure and health in general, but are not likely to reduce their salt intake (NHLBI, 2003). Popular Filipino dishes are also deep fried and high in starch and sugars.

Future Directions

Health care providers and services should take into account the historic and cultural complexity of the Filipina/o American experience. Understanding the social, historical, cultural, and political nature of Filipina/o Americans provide insight on the behaviors and health issues of this community. Sanchez and Gaw (2007) provided essential guidelines for a culturally sensitive approach for mental health practitioners in working with Filipino American clients. Some of the highlighted points of their recommendations were: to understand the immigration and regional orientation of Filipina/o Americans; incorporate culturally sensitive practices to ensure adequate and proper understanding of diagnosis and treatment; consider social inhibitions and nonverbal cues that may mislead practitioners; and engage family and patient's power

hierarchy (Sanchez & Gaw, 2007). Although these recommendations were created for mental health providers, general health service providers can and should also consider these guidelines. David (2010) added the importance of cultural mistrust as a factor in the underutilization of mental health services, again likely generalizable to all health care providers.

Many Filipina/o Americans are aware that current health problems could be addressed through adopting westernized traditions of health such as better nutrition, exercise, and routine prescriptive medicine. At the same time, embracing alternative health care may also be worthwhile (Semics LLC, 2007). Exploring traditional cultural views of medicine, through an indigenous Filipino orientation, encompasses a metaphysical dimension (de Guia, 2010). Semics LLC (2007) reported that Filipinas/os and Filipina/o Americans see traditional medicine, with holistic remedies, as promoting better well-being and health. Such alternatives to western medicine include prayer, meditation, and return to Philippine cultural and regional diets (de guia, 2010). Worth noting is traditional Filipina/o regional diets such as the Ilocano diet that emphasizes fish, rice, and a plethora of vegetables and fruit provide a healthier choice for Filipina/o Americans, in contrast to the high fat, salt, and starch items that are normally associated with Filipino cuisine (Fernandez, 2002).

The power of family and community are critical influences that promote the health and well being of Filipina/o Americans. Abesamis-Mendoza et al. (2007) expressed the necessity of capturing the needs and resources of Filipina/o Americans. Such engagements can help encourage the advancement of community assessments and research studies, community education, and appropriate mental health services. Developing Filipina/o American partnerships to advocate for more resources, funding, and policy changes that address specific needs should also be a priority. These recommendations share common strategies and approaches utilized by Filipina/o American communities across the nation (Aguilar et al., 2010; Montano et al., 2009; Semics LLC, 2007).

Future research should continue to disaggregate health data from the larger Asian American umbrella. The need to examine specific Asian ethnic subgroups provides a better understanding of health risks, incidence, and mortality. As the Filipina/o American population continues to grow, there will be a need to examine and address health issues of chronic and infectious diseases, substance abuse, and mental health specific to this community.

Another area that has been understudied is the large number of Filipino immigrant health care providers and their personal health. Numerous Filipino immigrant health care providers have experienced prejudice and discrimination in the workplace. Over the last four decades, lawsuits have been commonplace with Filipino plaintiffs filing for discrimination in hiring, workplace issues, and wage discrimination. Presently there are no studies on the occupational stresses that health care providers face and the deleterious effects of these stressors. Limited research shows that Filipina/o health care providers experience undesirably higher rates of overload and burn-out (Bacharach, Bamberger, & Conley, 1991). As health care providers, many Filipino immigrants lead stressful lives supporting their families and caring for their loves ones, but also others. Health care delivery is changing, with more being expected out of health care providers. How does this impact those who are paid to care for the sick and ill? Moreover, how are Filipino immigrants as care providers treated in terms of hiring, wages, and workplace environment? With so many Filipino Americans concentrated in the health care industry, further research needs to explore these areas.

The health status of children of the post 1965-generation of Filipina/o American health workers is worthy of discussion. The vast amount of research on Filipinas/os and Filipna/o Americans are examined through a cultural deficit model that points to culture as being one of the primary factors towards unhealthy living in America. A more productive perspective may be to examine the larger social and cultural factors that play into the health, illness, and mortality of Filipina/o and Filipina/o Americans. Although there is a significant amount of Filipina/o

Americans in the health profession, this current article has shown there is significant, albeit limited research on health risks, incidence, and mortality rates of Filipina/o Americans.

There is also a need for further research on Filipina/o American community partnerships that promote education, health, and well-being. Studying organizations that provide health education and advocacy such as New York City's Kalusugan Collection (KC) and Pilipino American Physical Activity Youth Assessment (PAPAYA Project); Filipino American Service Group, inc. (FASGI); Search to Involve Pilipino Americans (SIPA) in Los Angeles; the Filipino Mental Health Initiative (FMHI) in San Mateo County in the Bay Area; and Filipino American Community Health Initiative of Chicago (FACHIC). These organizations are examples of resources addressing the health and well-being of the Filipina/o American community. By examining their approaches of outreach, advocacy, and services, these community-based coalitions have become an effective channel to address various health problems within specific ethnic communities (Wynn et al., 2007). The development of more Filipina/o American healthcare coalitions across the nation can provide aid in overcoming cultural barriers and make the community aware of medical concerns, thus getting individuals appropriate healthcare in a more timely fashion and hopefully saving lives.

Conclusion

With a population of more than 2.4 million, Filipina/o Americans are not only the second largest Asian immigrant population in the United States, but they are the third largest immigrant population overall, behind only Mexican Americans and Chinese Americans. Despite this large and ever growing Filipina/o American population, research on the healthcare needs of Filipina/o Americans is still lacking. More research is needed to study not only prevalent diseases – including cardiovascular issues, cancer, and diabetes – but also corresponding behaviors that increase risk, including obesity, stress, and mentality poly-substance abuse. STDs and HIV are other concerns which can affect general well-being and subsequent mortality.

As we discussed in this chapter from our own literature review, we have re-confirmed that the most pressing social and cultural practices, which affect health and illness in the Filipino American community, include immigration stress and relocation, socio-economic status, and loss of self-esteem due to discrimination, all correlated with cultural alienation. The silence about health issues among working Filipina/o American youth, working adults, and elderly, can be considered the result of cultural challenges that emphasize the desire to avert burden on their families (Semics, 2007). Barriers to accessing affordable healthcare and lack of health insurance lead to a general reluctance of Filipinas/os and Filipina/o Americans to utilize health services (Abesamis-Mendoza et al., 2007; Langenberg et al., 2007; Semics, 2007). The future well-being of the Filipinas/os, including both current and future generations, will be determined by how these concerns are addressed.

Acknowledgments This chapter is dedicated to our mother, Virginia Lacuesta Raña Magbual. Writing this chapter has provided us a sense of healing and understanding to come to terms with our mother's death Our mother's life represents so many other Filipino immigrant women in this country struggling to provide for their family through caring for others through countless graveyard shifts, hour-long commutes, while caring for family responsibilities as a wife and mother. It is our hope that this chapter will provide reflection, understanding, and action to create change in the Filipino American community through a critical lens towards understanding fully healthy living.

References

Abesamis-Mendoza, N., Cadag, K., Nadal, K., Ursua, R., Gavin, N., & Divino, L. A. (2007). *Community health needs & resource assessment: An exploratory study of Filipino Americans in the New York metropolitan area.* New York: New York University School of Medicine Institute of Community Health and Research.

Aguilar, D. E., Abesamis-Mendoza, N., Ursua, R., Divino, L. A. M., Cadag, D., & Gavin, N. P. (2010). Lessons learned and challenges in building a Filipino health coalition. *Health Promotion Practice, 1*(3), 428–436.

Asian & Pacific Islander American Health Forum (APIAHF). (2008). Health brief: Asian Americans, Native Hawaiians & Pacific Islanders and diabetes. *San Francisco Asian Pacific Islander American Health Forum.*

Araneta, M. R., Wingard, D. L., & Barrett-Connor, E. (2002). Type 2 diabetes and metabolic syndrome in Filipina-American women: A high-risk nonobese population. *Diabetes Care, 25*(3), 494–499.

Bacharach, S. B., Bamberger, P., & Conley, S. (1991). Work-home conflict among nurses and engineers: Mediating the impact of role stress on burnout and satisfaction at work. *Journal of Organizational Behavior, 12*, 39–53. doi:10.1002/job.4030120104.

Barnes, P. M., Adams, P. F., & Powell-Griner, E. (2008). *Health characteristics of the Asian adult population: United States, 2004–2006.* Advance Data From Vital and Health Statistics 394: U.S. Department Of Health and Human Services Centers for Disease Control and Prevention National Center for Health Statistics.

Brown, D. E., & James, G. D. (2000). Physiological stress responses in Filipino-American immigrant nurses: The effects of residence time, lifestyle and job strain. *Psychosomatic Medicine, 62*, 394–400.

Brush, B. L., Sochalski, J., & Berger, A. M. (2004). Imported care: Recruiting foreign nurses to U.S. health care facilities. *Health Affairs, 23*(3), 78–87.

California Asian Pacific Islander Joint Legislative Caucus. (2009). *The State of Asian American, Native Hawaiian and Pacific Islander health in California report.*

Choi, S. E., Chow, V.H., Chung, S. J., & Wong N. D. (2010). Do risk factors explain the increased prevalence of type 2 diabetes among California Asian adults? Published online 2010 October 9. doi: 10.1007/s10903-010-9397-6

Choy, C. C. (2003). *Empire of care: Nursing and migration in Filipino American history.* Durham, NC: Duke University Press.

Chua, P. (2009). *Ating Kalagayan: The social and economic profile of U.S. Filipinos.* Woodside, NY: National Bulosan Center.

Cordova, F. (1983). *Filipinos: Forgotten Asian Americans.* Dubuque, IA: Kendall/Hunt Publishing Company.

Crouchett, L. J. (1982). *Filipinos in California: From the days of the galleons to the present.* El Cerrito, CA: Downey Place Pub House.

Cuasay, L. C., Lee, E. S., Orlander, P. P., Steffen-Batey, L., & Hanis, C. L. (2001). Prevalence and determinants of type 2 diabetes among Filipino-Americans in the Houston, Texas metropolitan statistical area. *Diabetes Care, 24*, 2054–2058.

Dalusung-Angosta, A. (2010). Concept analysis of risk in relation to coronary heart disease among Filipino-Americans. *Nursing Forum, 45*, 253–259.

Daus-Magbual, R., & Molina, J. (2009). At-risk youth. In G. Yoo & E. W. C. Chen (Eds.), *Encyclopedia of Asian American issues today* (pp. 228–230). Santa Barbara, CA: Greenwood Publishing Group.

David, E. J. R. (2010). Cultural mistrust and mental health help-seeking attitudes among Filipino Americans. *Asian American Journal of Psychology, 1*(1), 57–66.

David, E. J. R. (2011). *Filipino-/American American post-colonial psychology: Oppression, colonial mentality, and decolonization.* Bloomington, IN: AuthorHouse.

Doan, K. (2006). A sociocultural perspective on at-risk Asian American students. *Teacher Education and Special Education, 29*(3), 157–167.

de Castro, B., Gee, G. C., & Takeuchi, D. T. (2008). Job-related stress and chronic health conditions among Filipino immigrants. *Journal of Immigrant and Minority Health, 10*(6), 551–558.

de Guia, K. (2010). An ancient reed of wholeness – the Babaylan. In L. Mendoza-Strobel (Ed.), *Babaylan: Filipinos and the call of the indigenous* (pp. 69–108). Davao City, Philippines: Ateneo de Davao University-Research and Publication Office.

Espiritu, Y. L. (1992). *Asian American panethnicity: Bridging institutions and identities.* Philadelphia: Temple University Press.

Espina, M. E. (1988). *Filipinos in Louisiana.* New Orleans: Laborde.

Fernandez, D. G. (2002). Food and war. In A. V. Shaw & L. H. Francia (Eds.), *Vestiges of war: The Philippine-American war and the aftermath of an imperial dream* (pp. 237–246). New York: New York University Press.

Frisbee, W. P., Cho, Y., & Hubber, R. A. (2002). Immigration and the health of Asian and Pacific Islander adults in the United States. In T. La Veis (Ed.), *Race, ethnicity, and health: A public reader* (pp. 231–251). San Francisco: Jossey-Bass.

Geron, K., de la Cruz, E., Saito, L. T., & Singh, J. (2001). Asian Pacific Americans: Social movements and interest groups. *Political Science & Politics, 34*, 619–624.

Giyeon, K., Chiriboga, D. A., Jang, Y., Lee, S., Huang, C.-H., & Parmelee, P. (2010). Health status of older Asian Americans in California. *Journal of the American Geriatrics Society, 58*, 2003–2008.

Grunbaum, J. A., Lowry, R., Kann, L., & Pateman, B. (2000). Prevalence of health risk behaviors among Asian American/Pacific Islander high school students. *Journal of Adolescent Health, 27*(5), 322–330.

Harle, M., Dela, R. F., Veloso, C. G., Rock, J., Faulkner, J., & Cohen, M. Z. (2007). The experiences of Filipino American patients with cancer. *Oncology Nursing Forum, 34*(6), 1170–1175.

Hoyert, D., & Kung, H.-C. (1997). Asian or Pacific Islander mortality, selected states, 1992. In *Monthly vital statistics report* (Vol. 6, p. 1). Hyattsville, MD: National Center for Health.

Javier, J. R., Huffman, L. C., & Mendoza, F. S. (2007). Filipino child health in the United States: Do health and health care disparities exist? *Preventing Chronic Disease, 4*(2), 1–8.

Kao, D. (2010). Factors associated with ethnic differences in health insurance coverage and type among Asian Americans. *Journal of Community Health, 35*(2), 142–155.

Klatsky, A. L., & Armstrong, M. A. (1991). Cardiovascular risk among Asian American living in Northern California. *American Journal of Public Health, 81*(11), 1423–1428.

Langenberg, C., Araneta, M. R. G., Bergstrom, J., Marmot, M., & Barrett-Connor, E. (2007). Diabetes and coronary heart disease in Filipino-American women role of growth and life-course socioeconomic factors. *Diabetes Care, 30*(3), 535–541.

Lai, E. Y. P., & Arguelles, D. (Eds.). (2003). *The new face of Asian Pacific America: Numbers, diversity, & change in the 21st century.* Los Angeles: UCLA Asian American Studies Center Press.

Lau, A. (1995, February 11). "Filipino girls think suicide at No. 1 rate". *San Diego Union-Tribune*, A-1.

LaVeist, T. (2002). *Minority populations and health: An introduction to health disparities in the United States.* San Francisco: Jossey-Bass.

Lee, S. J. (2005). *Up against whiteness: Race, school, and immigrant youth.* New York: Teachers College Columbia University.

Mabalon, D. B., Reyes, R., & Filipino American National Historic Society. (2008). *Images of America: Filipinos in Stockton.* San Francisco: Arcadia Publishing.

Maramba, D. (2008). Immigrant families and the college experience: Perspectives of Filipina Americans. *Journal of College Student Development, 49*(4), 336–350.

McCraken, M., Olsen, M., Chen, M. S., Jr., Jemal, A., Thun, M., Cokkinides, V., Deapen, D., & Ward, E. (2007). Cancer incidence, mortality, and associated risk factors among Asian Americans of Chinese, Filipino, Vietnamese, Korean, and Japanese ethnicities. *CA: A Cancer Journal for Clinicians, 57*, 190–205.

Miller, B. A., Chu, K. C., Hankey, B. F., & Ries, L. A. G. (2007). Cancer incidence and mortality patterns among specific Asian and Pacific Islander populations in the U.S. *Cancer Causes and Control, 19*(3), 227–256.

Montano, J. J., Acosta-Deprez, V., & Sinay, T. (2009). Accessing the health care needs of Filipina/o American in greater long beach. *Public Administration & Management, 13*(3), 156–190.

Morales, R. (1998). *Makibaka 2: The Pilipino American struggle* (2nd ed.). Philippines: Crown Printers.

Nadal, K. L. (2008). A culturally competent classroom for Filipino Americans. *Multicultural Perspectives, 10*(3), 155–161.

Nadal, K. L. (2009). *Filipino American psychology: A handbook of theory, research, and clinical practice.* Bloomington, IN: Authorhouse.

Nadal, K. L. (2011). *The PAPAYA PROJECT: Physical activity and Pilipino America youth assessment.* New York: The PAPAYA Project.

National Heart, Lung, and Blood Institute (NHLBI). (2003). *Cardiovascular risk in the Filipino community: Formative research from Daly City and San Francisco, California.* San Francisco: National Heart, Lung, and Blood Institute/Asian & Pacific Islander American Health Forum/West Bay Pilipino Multi-Services.

National Vital Statistics Report. (2006). Centers for Disease Control and Prevention, National Center for Health Statistics, National Vital Statistics System.

Palaniappan, L. P., Araneta, M. R. G., Assimes, T. L., Barrett-Connor, E. L., Carnethon, M. R., Criqui, M. H., et al. (2010). Call to action: Cardiovascular disease in

Asian Americans. *American Heart Association* [epub ahead of print].

Parrenas, R. S. (2001). *Servants of globalization: Women, migration, and domestic work.* Stanford, CA: Stanford University Press.

Posadas, B. M. (1999). *The Filipino Americans.* Westport: Greenwood Press.

Rossing, M. A., Schwartz, S. M., & Weiss, N. S. (1995). Thyroid cancer incidence in Asian migrants to the United States and their descendants. *Cancer Causes and Control, 6,* 439–444.

San Juan, E., Jr. (2006). *On the presence of Filipinos in the United States.* Salinas: SRMNK Publishers.

Sanchez, F., & Gaw, A. (2007). Mental health care of Filipino Americans. *Psychiatric Services, 58*(6), 810–815.

Scharlin, C., & Villanueva, L. V. (1994). *Philip Vera Cruz: A personal history of Filipino immigrants and the farmworkers movement* (Memorialth ed.). Los Angeles: UCLA Labor Center of Industrial Relations/UCLA Asian American Studies Center.

Siu, S-F. (1996). Asian American students at risk: A literature review (Crespar Rep. No. 8). Baltimore, MD: Johns Hopkins University. ED404406. http://www.csos.jhu.edu/crespar/reports.htm.

Semics LLC. (2007). *Culture and health among Filipinos and Filipino-Americans in Central Los Angeles.* Los Angeles: The Historic Filipinotown Health Network and Semics LLC.

Strobel, L. (1996). Filipino American identity and Asian American panethnicity. *Ameriasia Journal, 22*(2), 31–54. Los Angeles: Asian American Studies Center, University of California Los Angeles.

Sue, D. W. (2010). *Microaggressions and marginality: Manifestation, dynamics, and impact.* Hoboken, NJ: Wiley.

Takaki, R. (1989). *Strangers from a different shore: A history of Asian Americans.* Boston: Little Brown and Company.

Toribio, H. C. (1998). We are revolution: A reflective history of the union of democratic Filipinos (KDP). *Amerasia Journal, 24*(2), 155–178.

U.S. Department of State: Background Note – Philippines. (2010). U.S. Department of State Website. Retrieved January 29, 2011, from http://www.state.gov/r/pa/ei/bgn/2794.htm.

Unemoto, K., & Ong, P. (2006). Asian American Pacific Islander Youth: Risks, Challenges, and Opportunities. *aapi nexus, 4*(2), v–ix.

Wynn, T. A., Johnson, R. E., Fouad, M., Holt, C., Scarinci, I., Nagy, A., et al. (2007). Addressing disparities through coalition building: Alabama REACH 2010 lesson learned. *Journal of Health Care for the Poor and Underserved, 17,* 55–77.

Youth Risk and Behavior Survey (YRBS). (2001). Depression among San Francisco Unified School District Middle School Students. *San Francisco Unified School District (SFUSD).*

Japanese Americans: Current Health Issues and Directions for Future Research

5

Tazuko Shibusawa

Introduction

It was 1947, during the height of anti-Japanese sentiment in the United States. V.S. McClatchy, co-owner of the *Sacramento Bee* newspaper and a strong proponent of anti-Japanese immigration laws, pronounced that because of "great pride of race, [the Japanese] have no idea of assimilation in the sense of amalgamation [i.e., intermarriage and disappearance as a biologically distinct group.]" (Spikard, 2009, p. 63). Ironically, because of decades of acculturation and a high incidence of intermarriage, today many would argue that Japanese Americans are the most assimilated among Asian Americans. This is not because other Asian groups have not had a comparably long history in the United States, but because unlike the Japanese, these groups continue to immigrate to the United States in significant numbers, leaving a higher percentage to learn the ways of their adopted country. Compared to other Asian groups, Japanese Americans have the highest percentage of people who were born in the United States, who speak English as a first language, and who follow a Westernized life style. The health issues of Japanese Americans, therefore, reflect the impact of their significant acculturation and assimilation into US society. This chapter presents a background of the history of Japanese immigrants in the United States, followed by a review of epidemiological studies, discussion of emerging health issues, and directions for future research.

Historical Background and Immigration Patterns

The majority of Japanese immigrants came to the United States between the late 1800s and early 1920s. They first immigrated to Hawaii to work on sugar plantations. After Hawaii was annexed by the United States in 1898, many Japanese moved to the West Coast where they were initially employed in agriculture, railroad construction, mining, lumbering, and canning (Spikard, 2009). Japanese immigrated during an era of intense anti-Asian sentiment. As an ethnic group, they were not allowed to become US citizens, with Alien Land Laws prohibiting them from owning land. The Chinese Exclusion Act, which banned immigration from China, had been enacted in 1882. Consequently, many anti-Japanese groups also lobbied to ban immigration from Japan. In 1907, under mounting pressure from the United States, the Japanese government agreed not to send any more immigrants. The so-called *Gentleman's Agreement* limited immigration from Japan to family members of those already living in the United States. By 1924, an immigration law was enacted that prohibited all Japanese along with other Asian groups from immigrating to the United States. It was not until

T. Shibusawa, Ph.D. (✉)
Silver School of Social Work, New York University,
New York, NY, USA
e-mail: tazuko.shibusawa@nyu.edu

G.J. Yoo et al. (eds.), *Handbook of Asian American Health*,
DOI 10.1007/978-1-4614-2227-3_5, © Springer Science+Business Media, LLC 2013

the 1965 Immigration Act that the majority of Asians were able to again immigrate to the United States without severe restrictions.

It is estimated that 450,000 Japanese immigrated to the United States before the 1924 exclusion act (Lai & Arguelles, 2003). The first immigrants from Japan were men who had expected to return to Japan after they made their fortune. However, even earning a decent living proved difficult, so many settled in Hawaii, California, Oregon, and Washington. Some men returned to Japan to find wives, while others married through proxy so that their wives could enter the United States as family members under the Gentlemen's Agreement. The women who arrived in the United States through these arranged marriages were known as *picture brides*. As a result of these arranged marriages, between 1907 and 1924, some 15,000 women immigrated to be with their husbands (Takaki, 1983; Tanaka, 2004).

The anti-Japanese sentiment that had long been present on the west coast culminated in the internment of Japanese Americans after the outbreak of World War II. Over 110,000 Japanese Americans were classified as "enemy aliens" and incarcerated in concentration camps in remote areas of Arizona, Arkansas, California, Colorado, Idaho, Utah, and Wyoming. Two-thirds of the internees, many of whom were children, were second-generation Japanese Americans as well as being US citizens. Some families were torn apart even further since men who were community leaders were incarcerated in POW camps.

As Japanese Americans were released from these camps, most had lost their property and businesses while they were interned and had to start over again. The internment experience left an indelible mark on subsequent generations of Japanese Americans. Researchers note that many second generation Japanese Americans experienced feelings of shame and humiliation about being Japanese as a result of internment, and pressure to prove their loyalty to the United States accelerated a push towards assimilation following World War II (Nagata, Trierweiler, & Talbot, 1999).

The immigration ban against Japanese was lifted for spouses and adopted children of US servicemen in 1945 after the end of World War II. As a result, it is estimated that over 50,000 Japanese "war brides" immigrated between 1946 and 1965 (Crawford, Hayashi, & Suenaga, 2010). As noted previously, the number of Japanese immigrants to the United States following the 1965 Immigration Act has been low compared to immigrants from China, Korea, India, the Philippines, and Southeast Asia. The lower rate of Japanese immigration may be attributed to the relatively stable economy and political situation in Japan in contrast to some other Asian nations. Still, although small in number, there continues to be a steady influx of immigrants from Japan. Between 1965 and 2000, 176,000 new Japanese immigrants entered the United States (Lai & Arguelles, 2003). The current Japanese American population is a heterogeneous group, representing new immigrants as well as descendants of those who immigrated in the early 1900s.

Demographic Characteristics

The 2009 American Community Survey reported 766,875 people who identify as ethnically Japanese, plus 1.3 million who identify as Japanese or in combination with one or more other racial group (U.S. Bureau of the Census, 2011). The majority of Japanese (60%) live in two states, Hawaii and California (Niiya, 2010).

There are several features that distinguish Japanese Americans from other Asian American groups. Because of the small number of new immigrants, a large number of Japanese Americans are US-born, with nearly 60% of Japanese Americans born in the United States in contrast to Asian Indian (27%), Chinese (31%), Filipino (33%), Korean (26%), and Vietnamese (31%). Over 54% of Japanese Americans speak only English, significantly higher than the five other major Asian American groups (which average 20.4%).

Another characteristic that distinguishes Japanese Americans from other Asian American communities is the high proportion of people who identify as biracial or multiracial. Since the 1990s, there have been more Japanese/White births than mono-racial Japanese American births

(Root, 1996). Currently, about one-third of Japanese Americans report that they are of mixed race heritage, which is significantly higher than Asian Indians (6%), Chinese (11%), Filipinos (20%), Koreans (13%), and Vietnamese (7%).

In the general population of the United States, 12.9% of the population is 65 and older. The proportion of older adults among Filipinos (12.2%) and Chinese (11%) are similar to that of the general US population because of the long residence of these groups in the United States despite the continued influx of new immigrants. Asian Indians (6.3%), Koreans (9.3%) and Vietnamese (9.6%) have much smaller number of older adults because new immigrants tend to arrive to the United States before reaching mid-life. By contrast, Japanese Americans have close to twice the number of older adults (23.6%) than the overall US population (U.S. Bureau of the Census, 2011). In fact, if the current demographic trend continues, in the next few years, one out of four Japanese Americans will be 65 years of age or older. Fewer Japanese Americans (2.4%) live in culturally traditional three-generational households, compared to Asian Indians (6.4%), Chinese (5.5%), Filipinos (7.3%), and Vietnamese (6.6%) (U.S. Bureau of the Census). Such findings have implications for caregiving of seniors within each of these ethnic groups. Health issues among Japanese Americans, therefore, need to be considered in light of this aging population.

The poverty rate among Japanese Americans is reportedly 8.6%. More Japanese Americans than Asian Indians (7.5%) and Filipinos (5.8%) live under the poverty line. At the same time, the poverty rate among Japanese is lower than Chinese (12.7%), Koreans (14.9%), Vietnamese (15.5%), and the overall US population (14.3%) (U.S. Bureau of the Census).

Another unique characteristic of Japanese Americans is that they self-identify by generations, age cohorts who share common experiences and cultural values. Immigration from Japan took place during a short period of time because of the Exclusion Act of 1924. As a result there was basically one age cohort that emigrated from Japan, identified as the *Issei*, which means first generation. The children of *Issei* who were born in the US identify as *Nisei* or second-generation. A subgroup of *Nisei* are known as *Kibei Nisei*, which means "return to the United States. This particular cohort returned to the United States after being sent back to be educated in Japan during childhood. Each subsequent generation is defined by its relationship to the original immigrants. The grandchildren of the *Issei* (children of the *Nisei*) are the *Sansei*, or third generation, while the great grandchildren (children of the *Sansei*) are the *Yonsei* (fourth generation). The great-great grandchildren of the first immigrants (children of the (children of the *Yonsei*) are known as the *Gosei* (fifth generation). There is a distinctive title for Japanese who immigrated after World War II, these individuals are known as the *Shin Issei* ("new" *Issei*). Some of the new immigrants came as students or for business and stayed in the United States. Others immigrated to be reunited with their families who had immigrated to the United States earlier. Most of the original *Issei* have now passed away, and the majority of *Nisei* who were born between 1915 and 1940 are now older adults (Meredith, Wenger, Liu, Harada, & Kahn, 2000). The third generation *Sansei* belong to the baby boom generation and they too are becoming senior citizens.

Research on Japanese American Health

Two extensive cross-national and longitudinal studies have provided valuable information on the health status of Japanese Americans. The first study, known as the *Ni-Hon-San* study (acronym for *Ni*hon, *Hon*olulu, and *San* Francisco), was initiated in 1965 to compare rates of coronary heart disease, cerebral vascular disease, and different types of cancers among Japanese men born between 1900 and 1919 in Hiroshima, Honolulu, and San Francisco (Robertson et al., 1977). By studying Japanese residing in three different geographical areas, researchers have been able to examine genetic, environmental, and cultural factors associated with the development of diseases.

Perhaps the central finding of the study has been the significant differences in rates of coronary heart disease among Japanese in Japan and those who reside in Honolulu and San Francisco. Japanese Americans in San Francisco had a much higher rate of coronary heart disease than their cohorts in Japan, while the rates for ethnic Japanese in Hawaii were in-between individuals living in Japan and San Francisco. A Westernized diet consisting of large amounts of meat and lower amounts of vegetables along with a more sedentary lifestyle are considered to increase risk factors for coronary heart disease among Japanese who immigrated to the United States. The mortality rate from cerebrovascular diseases, however, was lower among Japanese Americans than Japanese in Japan, attributed by medical researchers to higher intake of salt inherent in the traditional Japanese diet.

The *Honolulu Heart Program*, a study that examines heart disease among Japanese American men in Hawaii, grew out of the *Ni-Hon-San* study in response to the high rates of coronary heart disease among this population, particularly as the cohorts become older. In addition to a longitudinal follow-up of over 8,000 Japanese men who were in the Honolulu arm of the *Ni-Hon-San* study, the *Honolulu Heart Program* includes 400 offspring of the original study participants, extending the scope of examination to two generational cohorts.

A second large scale cross-national study, the *Ni-Hon-Sea* study (1991–2000) (acronym for *Ni*hon, *Hon*olulu, and *Sea*ttle), examined the relationship between lifestyle and cognitive aspects of aging among elders, including the development of dementia, among Japanese in Hiroshima, Honolulu, and Seattle (Larson et al., 1998). The Honolulu arm of the study consisted of participants enrolled in the aforementioned *Honolulu-Asia Aging Study*. The study revealed difference in types of dementia between Japanese elders in Japan and the United States. The rates of Alzheimer's disease among Japanese Americans were more similar to the rates of the overall US population and higher than their cohort in Japan. On the other hand, compared to elders in Japan, older Japanese Americans had lower rates of vascular dementia caused by strokes (Graves et al., 1999; Rodriguez et al., 1996).

The Seattle portion of the study, individually known as the *Kame Project*, included more than 2,000 study participants, mostly *Nisei*. *Kame* means turtle in Japanese, symbolizing longevity. An important finding from the Seattle portion of the study is the possible relationship between bilingualism/biculturalism and later cognitive function. Elders who learned Japanese as a child, and who maintained a Japanese lifestyle, experienced lower rates of cognitive decline than Japanese elders who lived a less traditional Japanese lifestyle. The researchers attribute the findings to increased brain reserve, which results from increased connections among brain cells that developed from speaking Japanese and English. Greater social support among Japanese Americans who retained traditional Japanese culture is also considered to be a protective factor from cognitive decline (Graves et al., 1999).

Current Health Issues

The findings of the *Ni-Hon-San* and *Ni-Hon-Sea* studies demonstrate the impact of both genetic factors and acculturation on the health of immigrants. The study findings may be attributed to the "healthy migrant effect" in which recent immigrants or migrants whose home countries' lifestyles are healthier than those of the host country. Additionally, current health issues among Japanese Americans reflect the influence of genetic factors, changes in life style and environment on the health of immigrant populations.

Cancer

Japanese Americans have higher rates of breast, colorectal, stomach, prostate, and uterine cancer compared to Chinese, Korean, Filipinos, and Vietnamese in the United States (McCracken et al., 2007). In California, Japanese Americans have the highest mortality rates from colorectal cancer (57.5 per 100,000), female breast cancer (105.5 per 100,000), and uterine cancer compared to other Asian Americans groups (16.7 per 100,000) (Kwong, Chen, Snipes, Dileep, &

Wright, 2005). Despite high rates of cancer screening, Japanese women have twice the rate of breast cancer than Chinese and Korean Americans (Deapen, Liu, Perkins, Bernstein, & Ross, 2002).

As in the case with cardiovascular diseases, high cancer rates among Japanese Americans are attributed to adapting to Western diet and life-style. Typical risk factors for colorectal cancer include a high consumption of processed meats and red meats, low fruit and vegetable intake, lack of physical inactivity, obesity, and alcohol use. Similarly, the increase in breast cancer among Japanese Americans has also been attributed to comparable changes in lifestyle from traditional Japanese behaviors. A study of nutrition among second- and third-generation Japanese American women found that third generation women ate fewer times a day, ate out more often, and dined on more take-out food, saltier snacks, soft drinks and alcohol, which is a variance from second generation Japanese women who consumed more tra-ditional foods such as fish, vegetables, and beans (Kudo, Falciglia, & Couch, 2000). Japanese American women have the highest rates of post-menopausal treatment among Asian American women, which may be associated with high rates of breast cancer. Japanese American women have the highest rate of smoking among Asian women also contributing to higher rates of cancer (15.6%) (McCracken et al., 2007).

It is important to note that the incidence of cancer increases with age. In the United States, approximately 60% of all cancers occur among people over 65 years of age (Ershler, 2003). Since Japanese Americans have a high proportion of older adults, prevention and early detection of cancer are crucial for improving the health status of this population.

Diabetes

Acculturation towards a Western diet and life-style not only affects risks for coronary heart dis-ease and cancer, but also affects the incidence of diabetes. Japanese Americans have higher rates of type II diabetes than non-Hispanic Whites and Japanese residing in Japan (Fujimoto, 1992). The rates of diabetes among Japanese Americans in Seattle are two to three times higher than that of Japanese in Japan (Hara, Egusa, & Yamakido, 1996). Higher risks for diabetes are observed among Japanese Americans who follow a more Westernized diet which includes higher intake of animal fat and simple carbohydrates. Specifically, Japanese American men in Seattle had twice the intake of fat than Japanese men in Japan.

Weight gain and increase in intra-abdominal fat are associated with diabetes risk. Japanese Americans, in general, are not overweight com-pared to other populations in the United States. Yet a study of Type II diabetes among second and third generation Japanese Americans found risks factors among people with body mass index (BMI) of 25–29, which is lower than the criteria for obesity set forth by the National Heart, Lung, and Blood Institute States (McNeely et al., 2001). Although obesity rates among Japanese Americans are lower than people of other races in the United States, weight gain is nonetheless a concern for this population. Studies indicate that Japanese in the United States are heavier than Japanese in Japan. Research in California also suggest that among Asian Americans, Japanese American men have the highest prevalence of being overweight (52.5%), while women have the second highest prevalence (28.3%) following Filipinas (McCracken et al., 2007). Furthermore, post-menopausal Japanese American women are at risk for diabetes because of increased intra-abdominal fat.

Mental Health

Population-based studies on the mental health status of Japanese American are not available. Some information can be gleaned from available research. In Hawaii, Japanese American female adolescents report higher depressive symptoms compared to boys (Williams et al., 2005). Risk factors for depression among Japanese American youth include lower self-concept and poorer body image compared with non-Hispanic Whites (Pang, Mizokawa, Morishima, & Olstad, 1985).

Japanese American parents hold higher educational expectations for their children than European Americans. School pressure from parents can also be a risk factor for depression (Goyette & Xie, 1999).

Aging is associated with depression, with an estimate that 20% of community dwelling elders in the United States experience depressive symptoms. Studies based on convenience samples indicate higher rates of depressive symptoms among Japanese Americans than non-Hispanic White American elders (Shibusawa & Mui, 2001). As is common with other populations, poor health and lack of social support are risk factors for depression among older Japanese Americans (Shibusawa & Mui). Depression is a concern among older Japanese Americans because of high suicide rates. Among Japanese American women between ages 75 and 84, the suicide rate is 2.5 times higher than those of white women. For Japanese men age 85 and over, the suicide rate is almost three times greater than those of white men (Baker, 1994).

Some studies indicate that Japanese American elders who are more acculturated are at higher risk for depression than those who retain their Japanese culture. In the Honolulu-Asia Aging Study, second generation Japanese American men who were more Westernized reported increased depressive symptoms. Differences are noted among Japanese Americans who retain a more Japanese life style in reporting less depressive symptoms due to having a social support network that serves as protective factors. Such results may be circumspect, as higher reports of depressive symptoms among acculturated Japanese Americans may be due to the fact that they are more open to discuss mental health symptoms and because depression scales pick up more depressive items among people who are more Westernized (Harada et al., 2011).

Conflicting data is presented in a study of Japanese American elders in Los Angeles, reporting elders who are primarily Japanese-speaking and less acculturated are at higher risk for depression. Compared to English-speaking Japanese American elders, those who were Japanese-speaking were more distressed towards becoming dependent on their adult children and reported higher depressive symptoms (Shibusawa & Mui, 2001).

Alcohol and Substance Abuse

Cross-national studies indicate that drinking patterns among Japanese Americans are more similar to those of non-Hispanic Whites than to Japanese who live in Japan (Higuchi, Parrish, Dufour, Towle, & Harford, 1994). While the highest proportion of heavy drinkers in Japan are among middle-aged (30–59) men, the highest number of Japanese Americans who consume large amounts of alcohol are younger men between the ages of 18 and 29 years. According to the 2004–2008 National Survey on Drug Use and Health (NSDUH), Japanese Americans report lower rates of alcohol use (48.5%) than Korean Americans (51.9%). However, Japanese American adolescents report the highest use of illicit drugs including marijuana, inhalants, and cocaine (6.2%) among all Asian American groups (Price, Risk, Wong, & Klingle, 2002). Higher rates of illicit substance among Japanese American youth may be attributed to greater acculturation plus access to the same drugs as the majority population. Since biracial and multiracial Asians also have higher risks of substance abuse, it follows that higher rates of drug use exist among Japanese American adolescents because of the large proportion of biracial and multiracial individuals among this group (Price et al.).

Health Beliefs and Health Service Utilization

Health Beliefs

Beliefs about health and illness in traditional Japanese culture derive from Buddhism and Taoism introduced from China and Korea, and the ancient indigenous religion of *Shintoism*. These spiritual traditions have shaped how Japanese (1) believe in the importance of co-existing with nature and natural forces, (2) respect a natural order that is greater than individual will, and (3) believe in the importance of balance and harmony between the mind and body. Traditional Chinese medicine was introduced to Japan in the sixth century. It is known in Japanese as *kanpo,* which means the "Chinese Way" (Lock, 1985). An important influence of Chinese medicine is the concept of *ki* (or *qi* in Chinese), a form of energy, which connects the mind and body. An old Japanese saying, "illness comes from *ki*" (*yamai wa ki kara*), points to the importance of *ki* in sustaining health.

Some Japanese Americans seek indigenous healing practices, such as herbal medicine, acupuncture, and moxibustion, which are believed to restore the flow of *qi* and enhance the body's immune system. While individuals are thought to be responsible for maintaining physical and psychological health through self-discipline, Japanese also pray for protection from ill health from the Buddha, Shinto deities or spiritual forces (*kami*), and ancestral spirits (Roemer, 2010). At the same time, serious and terminal illnesses are often viewed as something to be accepted as part of one's faith (Shibusawa & Chung, 2009). While Buddhism views death as a part of life, until recently most physicians respected the traditional practice of not disclosing terminal illnesses openly to patients.

Health Service Utilization

In the United States, the use of health care services is generally determined by patients' needs with at least some respect to structural, social, and cultural factors (Andersen, 1995; Damon-Rodriguez et al., 1994). Structural factors include accessibility, affordability, availability, and knowledge about services. Financial resources, access to health insurance, transportation, family and social support that enable access to services are also important structural factors that determine health service use. Cultural factors include health beliefs such as the perception and explanation of physical symptoms, beliefs about care, and acceptability of services (Damon-Rodriguez,

Wallace, & Kington, 1994). Patients' needs refer to physical and psychological conditions for which services are sought (Andersen).

Among Asian Americans, several factors including social stigma, limited English language proficiency, low socioeconomic status, lack of health insurance, fragmented health care systems, inability to access and navigate the health care system, and lack of culturally appropriate services inhibit service utilization (Damon-Rodriguez et al., 1994; Jang, Lee, & Woo, 1998; Shibusawa and Chung 2009). Although specific research on health care utilization among Japanese Americans is limited, available data suggests a relationship between acculturation and service use. For example, Japanese American women have higher rates of breast cancer screening than other Asian American women, perhaps not surprising given the larger number of US-born and English-speaking Japanese compared to other Asian groups. Japanese American children in California also have better access to health care compared to Filipino, Korean and Vietnamese children (Yu, Huang, & Singh, 2010). In addition, Japanese American mothers receive better prenatal care than Chinese, Korean and Vietnamese women (Yu, Alexander, Schwalberg, & Kogan, 2001).

As previously noted, Japanese Americans are a heterogeneous group whose acculturation patterns result in a variety of attitudes towards health care. English-speaking Japanese Americans as a group have more trust towards their physicians than do Japanese-speaking individuals. Japanese Americans who speak English are better able to communicate with physicians and may be more comfortable with the physician's Westernized mannerisms (Tarn et al., 2005). Those who are Japanese-speaking may be less comfortable interacting with physicians because Japanese culture dictates that patients be deferential to physicians and not question their authority (McDonald-Scott, Machizawa, & Sato, 1992).

Attitudes towards end-of-life care among Japanese Americans are also influenced by acculturation processes (Braun, Onaka, & Horiuchi, 2001; Matsumura et al., 2002). When an individual is considered to be in terminal condition, there are differences in the response between American and Japanese cultures. In the United States, patient autonomy is a priority. Individuals are expected to be informed of their medical status and treatment options, and make decisions regarding their own advance care directives (Kagawa-Singer & Blackhall, 2001). Traditional Japanese culture, on the other hand, emphasizes the interdependent nature of human relationships, so that decisions about the utilization and cessation of treatment consider the welfare of the group or family over the needs of the individual. In a study of English-speaking and Japanese-speaking Japanese Americans, the former expressed preference for autonomy in end-of-life decision making, while the latter favored family-centered decision making in advance care planning. Both English-speaking and Japanese-speaking respondents, however, preferred to have family and/or friends make decisions as a group rather than designate a single individual in the event that they themselves were not able to make decisions about using life-sustaining machines (Matsumura et al., 2002).

Mental Health Service Utilization

Mental illness is a source of shame and sigma for many Japanese Americans. Their preference is to resolve problems on their own before seeking assistance from a professional (Shibusawa, 2005). For example, unlike non-Hispanic Whites, Japanese American youth prefer talking to friends rather than seeking help from a mental health counselor (Suan & Tyler, 1990). The reluctance to seek outside help also extends to issues other than psychiatric problems, such as domestic violence (Yoshihama, 2000) and substance abuse (Substance Abuse and Mental Health Services Administration, 2010). The unwillingness among Japanese American families to acknowledge psychological disorders also inhibits elders who are depressed or who have early stages of dementia from receiving appropriate and preventive interventions (Fugita, Ito, Abe, & Takeuchi, 1991).

Although somatization is a common manifestation of emotional distress among the population at large, the problem is acute among all American Asian populations, including Japanese Americans. Specifically, psychological distress is expressed through somatic complaints such as insomnia, loss of appetite, migraine, body pain, dizziness, and feelings of physical weakness among Japanese Americans. Mental illness is often conceptualized as an imbalance in the autonomic nervous system, which is believed to be caused by irregular life styles and life habits, which in turn, trigger vulnerability to stress (Munakata, 1989).

Reluctance to seek mental health treatment has led Japanese Americans (as well as other Asian Americans) to utilize psychiatric emergency services during full-blown crises more than other American ethnic groups (Sakayue, 1989). Mental health utilization is higher when ethnic-specific mental health programs are available (Kugaya, 2007), yet a challenge for mental health services for Japanese Americans is the shortage of Japanese American mental health professionals. A recent study of Los Angeles County, confirms the lack of Japanese American counselors and other mental health practitioners in an area with the largest number of Japanese Americans in the country. There is less than one-third the US average of available psychiatrists and less than one-fifth the US average of mental health professionals available for this ethnic community (Kugaya, 2007).

Geriatric Care

Earlier, a review was presented of Japanese American elderly and mental health issues. In addition to mental health, concerns regarding Japanese Americans and care for the elderly have also been reviewed. Japanese American elders have traditionally been reluctant to use long term care services such as nursing homes and home health care because of language barriers, lack of culturally appropriate services, and fear of prejudicial treatment (Sakayue, 1989). It is worth noting that in traditional Japanese culture, adult children are expected to be the caretakers for elderly parents. Japanese American men with dementia in Hawaii have twice the rate of dying in hospitals but half the rate of dying in nursing homes compared to the national average (Bell et al., 2009). The value of filial obligation (*oyakoko*) in which adult children believe that they need to care for their elders at home, may account for the low rates of mortality in residential nursing homes. Expectations for families to care for frail elders, however, are diminishing in Japanese American communities, especially on the mainland US. The rate of institutionalization in geriatric facilities among Japanese American elderly is 1.6%, while the prevalence of nursing home use among all elders in the United States is 5% (Himes, Hogan, & Eggebeen, 1996). Institutionalization rates, however, are higher in geographical areas where Japanese facilities and long-term care programs are available. In Seattle, where there is a Japanese nursing home, the institutionalization rate is 5% (McCormick et al., 1996). There are a number of Japanese American long-term care facilities available in California, which are generally the facilities of choice for adult children compared to non-Japanese American facilities (Hikoyeda & Wallace, 2001).

Relationships between adult children and older parents by and large remain close. One study suggests that Japanese American elders who are English-speaking are more comfortable depending on their adult children than Japanese-speaking children (Shibusawa & Mui, 2001). Japanese-speaking elders worry about being a burden on their children because they are not capable of reciprocating their children's assistance. In Japanese culture, people who are not able to give in return the help they receive are expected to accept the care passively without voicing complaints or asserting their desires (Shibusawa & Mui 2001). Those receiving care are expected to practice "*enryo*," which means "hold back" or "restrain" ones wishes. Dependence or being a burden on others in Japanese culture comes with a cost – one must passively accept the help, and not assert oneself or negotiate for the kind of assistance one wants lest being perceived as ungrateful to caregivers. A study of Japanese Canadians found that elders would prefer to pay for formal services than burden family members (Matsuoka, 1999).

Another factor that affects eldercare among Japanese American families is the high rate of out-marriages. The rate of interracial marriages among Japanese Americans has been increasing over the years, so that an increasing number of Japanese American elders will have children-in-law and grandchildren of diverse cultural backgrounds. Both Japanese American elders and their offspring will need to learn to negotiate through a diverse and perhaps disparate set of cultural expectations regarding eldercare.

Directions for Future Research

Racial Discrimination and Health

A large number of Japanese in the United States are third-, fourth-, fifth- and even sixth-generation Americans. Some researchers contend that ethnic groups reach a point where a group becomes acculturated to the point where differences in subsequent generations are minimal (Wooden, Leon, & Toshima, 1988). Acculturation patterns of Japanese Americans, however, differ from those of people of European ancestry because of their skin color and other non-White physical features. While second and third generation European immigrants are rarely questioned about their nativity status, Japanese Americans – no matter what generation – are often asked about their country of origin. According to data from the 2003 to 2005 California Health Interview Survey, close to 30% of Japanese Americans reported experiencing racial discrimination where they felt that they were treated unfairly because of their race (Gee & Ponce, 2010).

There is increasing evidence that suggests an association between racial discrimination and health status. Experiences of discrimination are linked to heart disease, hypertension, respiratory illnesses, chronic health conditions, and depressive symptoms (Gee, Spencer, Chen, & Takeuchi, 2007). Furthermore, substance abuse, in particular may be an unhealthful way to cope with racial discrimination (Yoo, Gee, Lowthrop, & Robertson, 2010).

Japanese Americans live with the legacy of the internment experience of World War II. They are aware of the way in which minority groups can quickly become targets of racial attacks by the dominant society. Some decades later, in the 1980s and 1990s, the derogatory term "Jap" that was used before and during World War II was again used to attack Japanese during trade conflicts between Japan and the United States (Ng, 2005). The treatment of Muslim Americans following the 9–11 terrorist attacks is a chilling reminder of the discrimination Japanese Americans experienced following Pearl Harbor (Nikkei for Civil Rights and Redress, 2010).

Many Japanese Americans along with other Asians have high levels of education and hold professional positions. However, Asian Americans hold fewer managerial or executive-level positions than non-Hispanic Whites. Although Asian Americans, as a group, have higher rates of college graduates than non-White Hispanics, only 1.5% of Fortune 1,000 company executives are of Asian descent (Shibusawa, 2008). The apparent glass ceiling (referred to by Asians as the "bamboo ceiling") in the corporate world is just one example of racial discrimination that is experienced by Japanese and other Asian Americans, suggesting the need for further studies on the impact of racial discrimination on health.

Health of Biracial and Multiracial People

To reiterate, approximately one-third of Japanese Americans report that they belong to more than one race (U.S. Bureau of the Census, 2011). The majority of the US population, however, identify as monoracial, resulting in a paucity of research on the health of biracial and multiracial people (Collins, 2000; Tashiro, 2002). According to the 2009 American Community Survey, only 3% of Whites, 7% of Blacks, and 4% of Hispanics or Latinos of any race reported being of more than one race. On the other hand, 12% of Asian Americans, 50% of American Indian and Alaska Natives, and 50% of Native Hawaiian and other

Pacific Islanders identify as being more than one race (U.S. Bureau of the Census, 2011).

Most studies of biracial and multiracial people have focused on psychological aspects of identity development. Some studies suggest that biracial and multiracial adolescents face more challenges than monoracial individuals during the stage of identity formation because of conflicting cultural backgrounds. Not knowing which group to belong to can lead to identity confusion, self-hatred, alienation, feelings of guilt and disloyalty (Williams et al., 2005). Confusion on the part of others such as teachers and peers can also be stressful for biracial and multiracial adolescents (Campbell & Troyer, 2007). The challenges during identity formation can contribute to anxiety and depression (Williams et al., 2005). Research on substance abuse among adolescents consistently demonstrated higher use among biracial and multiracial individuals (Chavez & Sanchez, 2010). Still, the consequences of difficulties with identity development are not conclusive. Mass (1992) who studied the psychological adjustment among biracial Japanese Americans who have a white and a Japanese parent did not find any differences compared to monoracial Japanese (Mass).

Tashiro (2006) points to the negative consequences of the monoracial assumptions of race categories on biracial and multiracial individuals. There are various health conditions that are associated with race, so the lack of data on health risks of multiracial individuals can have negative consequences on their physical and psychological well-being. Graham (2008) noted that biracial and multiracial individuals have remained invisible in the health research. Biracial and multiracial individuals have been excluded from clinical trials for medications, which can put them at risk for overdosing or underdosing (Graham, 2008). For example, we do not know if BiDil, the first drug that was developed to treat heart failure among African Americans, is effective for Japanese Americans who are part African American. Neither do we know the extent to which biracial Japanese have ALDH2 (which causes face flushing when consuming alcohol), a protective factor against heavy drinking. The effects of psychotropic medicines on biracial and multiracial Japanese Americans are another area that warrants review and analysis. Recent studies suggest that physicians need to be cautious about overmedicating Asians with psychotropic medications such as tricyclic anti-depressants, lithium, and benzodiazepines because they require lower does than White Americans (Lin & Cheung, 1999).

There has also been an increase in Asian inter-ethnic marriages, such as Chinese-Japanese and Korean-Japanese pairings, among other possibilities, especially among those born in the United States. In fact, some researchers predict that intermarriage among Asians may lead to the development of a pan-Asian ethnicity, similar to the way intermarriage among various European immigrant groups led to the formation of a broader "White" category in the United States (Qian & Lichter, 2001). Although this process may take several generations, health research must take into account health factors of biracial and multiracial among not only Japanese, but other Asians as well.

Conclusion

This chapter presented the health issues of Japanese Americans and directions for future research. Japanese Americans are a heterogeneous group including a large number who are second, third, and fourth generation who are acculturated, a smaller group who are recent immigrants, and a rapidly growing group of individuals who are biracial and multiracial. The prevalence of specific health issues among Japanese Americans reflects the impact of acculturation and health risks that are a result of changes in diet and lifestyle, and speak to the importance of examining factors that are beyond heredity and physiological predispositions. The health consequences of acculturation and the need for preventive health care and early detection of symptoms among Japanese Americans also have implications for newer immigrant populations.

References

Andersen, Ronald M. 1995. "Revisiting the behavioral model and access to medical care: Does it matter?" *Journal of Health and Social Behavior* 36:1–10.

Baker, F. M. 1994. "Suicide among ethnic minority elderly: A statistical and psychosocial perspective." *Journal of Geriatric Psychiatry* 27:241–264.

Bell, Christina L., James Davis, Rosanne C. Harrigan, Ernese Somogyi-Zalud, Marianne K.G. Tanabe, and Kamal H. Masaki. 2009. "Factors associated with place of death for elderly Japanese-American men: The Honolulu Heart Program and Honolulu-Asia Aging Study." *Journal of the American Geriatrics Society* 57:714–18.

Braun, Kathryn L., Alvin T. Onaka, and Brian Y. Horiuchi. 2001. "Advance directive completion rates and end-of-life preferences in Hawaii." *Journal of the American Geriatrics Society* 49(12):1708–13.

Campbell, Mary E., and Lisa Troyer. 2007. "The implications of racial misclassification by observers." *American Sociological Review* 72:750–65.

Chavez, Geroge F., and Diana T. Sanchez. 2010. "A clearer picture of multiracial substance abuse: Rates and correlates of alcohol and tobacco use in multiracial adolescents and adults." *Race and Social Problems* (2):1–18.

Collins, J. Fuji 2000. "Biracial Japanese American identity: An evolving process " *Cultural Diversity and Ethnic Minority Psychology* 6(2):115–33.

Crawford, Miki Ward, Katie Kaori Hayashi, and Shizuko Suenaga. 2010. *Japanese war brides in America: An oral history*. Santa Barbara, CA: Praeger.

Damon-Rodriguez, Joanne, Steven Wallace, and Ronald Kington. 1994. "Service utilization and minority elderly: Appropriateness, accessibility and accessibility." *Gerontology & Geriatrics Education* 15:45–63.

Deapen, Dennis, Lihua Liu, Carin Perkins, Leslie Bernstein, and Ronald K. Ross. 2002. "Rapidly rising breast cancer rates among Asian American women." *International Journal of Cancer* 99(6):747–50.

Ershler, William B. 2003. "Cancer: A disease in the elderly." *Journal of Supportive Oncology* 1(Supplement 2):5–10.

Fugita, Stephen, Karen L. Ito, Jennifer Abe, and David T. Takeuchi. 1991. "Japanese Americans." Pp. 61–96 in *Handbook of social services for Asian and Pacific Islanders*, edited by N. Mokuau. New York: Greenwood.

Fujimoto, Wilfred Y. 1992. "The growing prevalence of non-insulin-dependent diabetes in migrant Asian populations and its implications for Asia." *Diabetes Research and Clinical Practice* 15(167–183).

Gee, Gilbert C., and Ninenz Ponce. 2010. "Associations between racial discrimination, limited English proficiency, and health-related quality of life among 6 Asian ethnic groups in California." *American Journal of Public Health* 100(5):888–95.

Gee, Gilbert C., Michael S. Spencer, J. Chen, and David Takeuchi. 2007. "A nationwide study of discrimination and chronic health conditions among Asian Americans " *American Journal of Public Health* 97(7):1275–82.

Goyette, K., and Y. Xie. 1999. "Educational expectations of Asian American youths: Determinants of ethnic differences." *Sociology of Education* 72(1): 22–36.

Graham, Susan. 2008. "The Obama racial identify factor an saving multiracial lives. Accessed Marched 12, 2011 from http://www.projectrace.com/fromthedirector/archive/060708_obama_racial_identity_saving_multiracial_lives.php."

Graves, Amy B., Lakshminarayan Rajaram, James D. Bowen, Wayne C. McCormick, Susan M. McCurry, and Eric B. Larson. 1999. "Cognitive decline and Japanese culture in a cohort of older Japanese Americans in King County, WA: The Kame Project." *Journals of Gerontology* 54:S154–S61.

Hara, Hitoshi, Genshi Egusa, and Michio Yamakido. 1996. "Incidence of non-insulin dependent diabetes mellitus and its risk factors in Japanese Americans living in Hawaii and Los Angeles." *Diabetic Medicine* 13:S133–S42.

Harada, Nobuharu, Junji Takeshita, Iqbal Ahmed, Randi Chen, Helen Petrovitch, Webster Ross, G., and Kamal Masaki. 2011. "Does cultural assimilation influence prevalence and presentation of depressive symptoms in older Japanese American men? The Honolulu-Asia Aging Study." *American Journal of Geriatric Psychiatry* [Epub ahead of print]

Higuchi, Susumu, Kyoko M. Parrish, Mary C. Dufour, Leland H. Towle, and Thomas C. Harford. 1994. "Relationship between age and drinking patterns and drinking problems among Japanese, Japanese-Americans, and Caucasians." *Alcoholism: Clinical and Experimental Research* 18(2):305–10.

Hikoyeda, N., and S.P. Wallace. 2001. "Do ethnic-specific long term care facilities improve resident quality of life?: Findings from the Japanese American community." *Journal of Gerontological Social Work* 36(1/2):83–106.

Himes, Christine L., Dennis P. Hogan, and David J. Eggebeen. 1996. "Living arrangements of minority elders. Journals of Gerontology." *Journals of Gerontology* 51:542–548.

Jang, Michael, Evelyn Lee, and Kent Woo. 1998. "Income, language, and citizenship status: Factors affecting the health care access and utilization of Chinese Americans." *Health & Social Work* 23(2):136–45.

Kagawa-Singer, Marjorie, and Leslie J. Blackhall. 2001. "Negotiating cross-cultural issues at the end of life: You got to go where he lives." *Journal of the American Medical Association* 286(23):2993–3001.

Kudo, Y., G.A. Falciglia, and S.C. Couch. 2000. "Evolution of meal patterns and food choices of Japanese-American females in the United States." *European Journal of Clinical Nutrition* 54(8):665–70.

Kugaya, Akira. 2007. "Japanese Americans in the US: An 'undoctored' minority in an overdoctored area." *Transcultural Psychiatry* 44(1):162–65.

Kwong, Sandy L., Moon S. Chen, Kurt P. Snipes, G. Bal Dileep, and WIlliam E. Wright. 2005. "Asian subgroups and cancer incidence and mortality rates in California." *Cancer* 104(Supplement 12):2975–081.

Lai, Eric and Dennis Arguelles, eds. 2003. *The new faces of Asian Pacific America: Numbers, diversity and change in the 21st century.* Los Angeles, CA: Asian Week/UCLA Asian American Studies Center.

Larson, Eric B., Susan M. McCurry, Amy B. Graves, James D. Bowen, Madeline M. Rice, Wayne C. McCormick, Nancy Zee, Akira Honma, Yukimichi Imai, Lon R. White, Kamal Masaki, Helen Petrovitch, Webb Ross, Michiko Yamada, Yasuyo Mimori, and Hideo Sasaki. 1998. "Standardization of the clinical diagnosis of dementia syndrome and its subtypes in a cross-national study: The Ni-Hon-Sea experience." *The Journals of Gerontology* 53A(4):M313–M19.

Lin, Keh-Ming, and Freda Cheung. 1999. "Mental health issues for Asian Americans." *Psychiatric Services* 50:774–80.

Lock, Margaret. 1985. "The impact of the Chinese medical model on Japan or, how the younger brother comes of age." *Social Science & Medicine* 21(8):945–50.

Mass, Amy Iwasaki. 1992. "Interracial Japanese Americans: The best of both worlds or the end of the Japanese American community?" Pp. 265–79 in *Racially mixed people in America*, edited by Maria Root. Newbury Park, CA: Sage Publications.

Matsumura, Shinji, Seiji Bito, Honghu Liu, Katherine Kahn, Shunichi Fukuhara, Marjorie Kagawa-Singer, and Neil Wenger. 2002. "Acculturation and attitudes toward end-of-life care: A cross-cultural survey of Japanese Americans and Japanese." *Journal of General Internal Medicine* 17:531–39.

Matsuoka, Akiko K. 1999. "Preferred care in later life among Japanese Canadians." *Journal of Multicultural Social Work* 7:127–148.

McCormick, Wayne C., Jay Uomoto, Heather Young, A.B. Graves, W. Kukull, L. Terri, P. Vitaliano, J.A. Mortimer, S.M. McCurry, J.D. Bowen, and E.B. Larson. 1996. "Attitudes toward use of nursing homes and home care in older Japanese-Americans." *Journal of the American Geriatrics Society* 44:769–777.

McCracken, Melissa, Miho Olsen, Moon S. Chen, Ahmedin Jemal, Michael Thun, Vilma Cokkinides, Dennis Deapen, and Elizabeth Ward. 2007. "Cancer incidence, mortality, and associated risk factors among Asian Americans of Chinese, Filipino, Vietnamese, Korean, and Japanese ethnicities." *CA Cancer Journal of Clinicians* 57:190–205.

McDonald-Scott, Patricia, Shizuo Machizawa, and Hiroyuki Sato. 1992. "Diagnositic disclosure: A tale in two cultures." *Psychological Medicine* 22: 147–57.

McNeely, Marguerite J., Edward J. Boyko, Jane B. Shofer, Laura Newell-Morris, Donna L. Leonetti, and Wilfred

Y. Fujimoto. 2001. "Standard definitions of overweight and central adiposity for determining diabetes risk in Japanese Americans." *American Journal of Clinical Nutrition* 74:101–07.

Meredith, Lisa S., Neil Wenger, Honghu Liu, Nancy Harada, and Katherine Kahn. 2000. "Development of a brief scale to measure acculturation among Japanese Americans." *Journal of Community Psychology* 28:103–113.

Munakata, Tsunetsugu. 1989. "The socio-cultural significance of the diagnostic label 'neurasthenia' in Japan's mental health care system." *Culture, Medicine & Psychiatry* 13(2):203–213

Nagata, Donna K., Steven J. Trierweiler, and Rebecca Talbot. 1999. "Long-term effects of internment during early childhood on third generation Japanese Americans." *American Journal of Orthopsychiatry* 69(1):19–29.

Ng, Wendy. 2005. "Japanese in the United States." In *Encyclopedia of diasporas: Immigrant and refugee cultures around the world*, edited by Marvin Ember, Carol Ember, and Ian Skoggrad. New York: Springer.

Niiya, Brian. 2010. "Japanese Americans." In *Encyclopedia of Asian American issues today* edited by Edith Wen-Chu Chen and Grace J. Yoo. Santa Barbara, CA: ABC-CLIO.

Nikkei for Civil Rights & Redress. 2010. "Vigil in Little Tokyo to support Muslim Americans and religious freedom. Accessed March 23 from http://www.ncrr-la.org/news/9-19-10/3.html."

Pang, Valerie O., Donald T. Mizokawa, John K. Morishima, and Roger G. Olstad. 1985. "Self-concepts of Japanese-American children." *Journal of Cross-Cultural Psychology* 16:99–109.

Price, Rumi Kato, Nathan K. Risk, Mamie Mee Wong, and Renee Storm Klingle. 2002. "Substance use and abuse by Asian Americans and Pacific Islanders: Preliminary results from four national epidemiologic studies." *Public Health Reports* 117 (Suppl 1): S39–S50.

Qian, Zhenchao, and Daniel T. Lichter. 2001. "Measuring marital assimilation: Intermarriage among natives and immigrants." *Social Science Research* 30:289–312.

Robertson, Thomas L., Hiroo Kato, George G. Rhoads, Abraham Kagan, Michael Marmot, Leonard Syme, Tavia Gordon, Robert M. Worth, Joseph L. Belsky, Donald S. Dock, Michihisa Miyanishi, and Sadahisa Kawamoto. 1977. "Epidemiologic studies of coronary heart disease and stroke in Japanese men living in Japan, Hawaii and California." *American Journal of Cardiology* 39(2):239–43.

Rodriguez, Beatriz L, Patricia L. Blanchette, Richard J. Havlick, Gilbert Wergowske, Darryl Chiru, Daniel Foley, C. Murdaugh, and J.D. Curb. 1996. "Prevalence of dementia in older Japanese American men in Hawaii." *Journal of the American Medical Association* 276(12):955–60.

Roemer, Michael. 2010. "Religion and psychological distress in Japan." *Social Forces* 89(2):559–83.

Root, Maria P.P. 1996. "The multiracial experience: Racial borders as a significant frontier in race relations." In *The multiracial experience: Racial borders as the new frontier*, edited by M.P.P. Root Thousand Oaks, CA: Sage Publications.

Sakayue, Kenneth M. 1989. "Ethnic variations in family support of the frail elderly." Pp. 65–106 in *Family involvement in treatment of the frail elderly*, edited by M.Z. Goldstein. Washington, DC. American Psychiatric Press.

Shibusawa, Tazuko, and Irene W. Chung. 2009. "Health issues of Asian American elderly." Pp. 199–225 in *Health issues in the Asian American community*, edited by Mariano Rey, Chao Trin-Shevrin, and Nadia Islam. New York: Jossey Bass.

Shibusawa, Tazuko, and Ada C. Mui. 2001. "Stress, coping, and depression among Japanese American elders." *Journal of Gerontological Social Work* 36(1–2):63–81.

Shibusawa, Tazuko. 2005. "Japanese families." Pp. 339–48 in *Ethnicity and family therapy*, edited by M. Mcgoldrick, J. Giordano, and N. Garcia-Preto. New York: Guilford Publications.

Shibusawa, Tazuko. 2008. "Living up to the American dream: The price of being the model immigrants." *Psychotherapy Networker* May/June:41–57.

Spikard, Paul. 2009 *Japanese Americans: The formation and transformation of an ethnic group (Revised Edition)*. New Brunswick, NJ: Rutgers University Press.

Suan, Lance V, and John D. Tyler. 1990. "Mental health values and preferences for mental health resources for Japanese-American and Caucasian-American students." *Professional Psychology: Research and Practice* 21(4):291–96.

Substance Abuse and Mental Health Services Administration. 2010. "Substance use among Asian adults." In *The NSDUH Report*. Rockville, MD: U.S. Department of Health and Human Services.

Takaki, Ronald. 1983. *Pau hana: Plantation life and labor in Hawaii 1835–1920*. Honolulu, HI: University of Hawaii Press.

Tanaka, Kei. 2004. "Japanese picture marriage and the image of immigrant women in early twentieth California." *The Japanese Journal of American Studies* 15:115–38.

Tarn, Derjung M., Lisa S. Meredith, M. Kagawa-Singer, Shinji Matsumura, Seiji Bito, Robert K. Oye, Honghu Liu, Katherine Kahn, Shunichi Fukuhara, and Neil Wenger. 2005. "Trust in one's physician: The role of ethnic match, autonomy, acculturation, and religiosity among Japanese and Japanese Americans." *Annals of Family Medicine* 3:339–47.

Tashiro, Cathy J. 2002. "Considering the significance of ancestry through the prism of mixed-race identity." *Advances in Nursing Science* 25:1–21.

U.S. Bureau of the Census. 2011. "2009 American Community Survey 1-Year Estimates. Accessed May 4, 2011 from http://factfinder.census.gov."

Williams, John Kino Yamaguchi, Iwalani R. N. Else, Earl S. Hishinuma, Deborah A. Goebert, Janice Y. Chang, Naleen N. Andrade, and Stephanie T. Nishimura. 2005. "A confirmatory model for depression among Japanese American and Part-Japanese American adolescents." *Cultural Diversity and Ethnic Minority Psychology* 11(1):41–56.

Wooden, Wayne S., Joseph Leon, J., and Michelle T. Toshima. 1988. "Ethnic identity among Sansei and Yonsei church-affiliated youth in Los Angeles and Honolulu." *Psychological Reports* 62:268–70.

Yoo, Hyung Chol, Gilbert C. Gee, Craig K. Lowthrop, and Joane Robertson. 2010. "Self-reported racial discrimination and substance use among Asian Americans in Arizona." *Journal of Immigrant and Minority Health* 12:683–60.

Yoshihama, Mieko. 2000. "Reinterpreting strength and safety in a socioc-cultural context: Dynamics of domestic violence and experiences of women of Japanese descent." *Children and Youth Services Review* 22(3–4):207–29.

Yu, Stella M, Gregg R Alexander, Renee Schwalberg, and Michael D. Kogan. 2001. "Prenatal care use among selected Asian American groups." *American Journal of Public Health* 91(11):1865–68.

Yu, Stella M., Zhihuan J. Huang, and Gopal K. Singh. 2010. "Health status and health services acess and utilization among Chinese, Filipino, Japanese, Korean, South Asian, and Vietnamese children in California." *American Journal of Public Health* 100(5):823–30.

Challenges and Opportunities for Improving Health in the Korean American Community

Grace J. Yoo and Sachiko Wood

Fifty-five year old Mr. Kim, a thriving Korean immigrant small business owner, experiences a heart attack. He ends up in the ER. He is uninsured, too young to qualify for Medicare, and is unable to qualify for Medicaid because he owns his own small business. With no savings and no state or government assistance, Mr. Kim charges his hospital bill on his credit card. Because he is uninsured, he declines follow-up care. He survives his heart attack and heads back to work the next day.

In the Korean immigrant community, stories like this are not uncommon. Compared to any other racial/ethnic group in the U.S., Korean Americans continue to have the highest uninsured rates. Korean Americans' high self-employment rates often means they lack job-based health insurance and often are uninsured or under-insured (Kim & Yoo, 2009; Yoo & Kim, 2008). Without access to health care services, many Korean immigrants are not able to receive standard or preventative care including cancer screenings and immunizations (Ryu, Young, & Park, 2001; Yoo & Kim, 2008). Reduced access to care can have serious conse-quences for health including delayed diagnosis of life threatening illnesses, and the inability to manage chronic health conditions which often leads to increased morbidity and mortality (Institute of Medicine, 2002).

This chapter will provide a brief overview in terms of Korean immigration history to the U.S. and will also provide an overview of the latest research on current health issues and concerns facing the Korean American community today.

Korean Migration to the United States

For over 100 years Korean immigrants have found home in the United States. They represent the fifth largest ethnic group among Asian American populations. In 2010, the U.S. Census reported over 1.7 million Korean Americans residing in the United States with the majority residing in states such as California, New York, Hawaii, and Texas. Korean immigration to the United States can be divided into three different waves. The first wave (1903–1905) of Koreans were mostly men who migrated to the U.S. as contract laborers to work in the sugar cane fields in Hawaii and the farmlands along the West Coast. Many first wave immigrants were also Christians seeking to escape persecution and economic hardship under Japanese colonial rule. Under the Gentlemen's Agreement of 1908 between Japan and the U.S., all migration of Korean laborers were halted.

G.J. Yoo (✉)
Department of Asian American Studies,
San Francisco State University,
San Francisco, CA, USA
e-mail: gracey@sfsu.edu

S. Wood
Cancer Disparities Research Group, San Francisco State University, San Francisco, CA, USA

G.J. Yoo et al. (eds.), *Handbook of Asian American Health*,
DOI 10.1007/978-1-4614-2227-3_6, © Springer Science+Business Media, LLC 2013

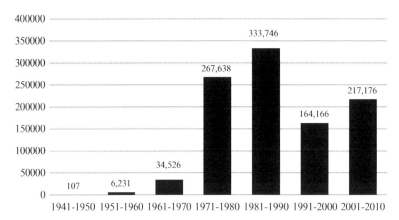

Fig. 6.1 Korean Immigration the U.S. 1941–2000
Source: U.S. Department of Homeland Security (2010).

However, between 1910 and 1924, Korean picture brides arrived to meet and live with their Korean laborer spouses. With the passage of the Immigration Act of 1924, all Koreans were barred from migrating to the United States.

With the outbreak of the Korean War in 1950, "the second wave of Korean immigrants arrived." Korean women came to the United States as "war brides" of American soldiers, and South Korean students came to the United States in the 1950s. Over 150,000 Korean children have been internationally adopted to families in the United States since the 1950s, accounting for nearly 8% of the total Korean population in America (U.S. Department of Homeland Security, 2011).

With the passage of the 1965 Immigration Act, the community started to grow, prompting the third wave of Korean immigration (Figure 6.1). A key reason for the growth of the Korean American community was the passage of the Immigration Act of 1965 which allowed permanent residents and U.S. citizens to petition relatives, and gave special preferences to professionals in short supply such as health care workers and technical workers. In fact, as part of this immigration wave, many physicians and nurses arrived and worked in under-staffed hospitals, clinics and nursing homes across the U.S. Many who arrived after 1965 were highly educated, but faced language barriers and downward mobility,

and subsequently were steered towards self-employment.

Many Korean immigrants employed in small business work have experienced difficulties with not only purchasing health insurance but also issues such as long work hours and sometimes violence. Korean American small business owners in Los Angeles experienced "Sa-I-Gu" (which translates to 4/29) also known as the 1992 Los Angeles Civil Unrest. In response to the acquittal of Los Angeles police officers in the Rodney King beating, African Americans and other Los Angeles residents took to the streets in protest, which soon escalated into chaos and destruction. As a result, the Los Angeles Koreatown area experienced 850 million dollars in material loss and damage and many businesses were permanently closed (Kim, 2000).

Background and Current Research

This section describes current health issues impacting the Korean American community today. Utilizing research published in the last ten years, this section explores key health issues within the Korean American community including access to health care; acculturation and lifestyle as well as tobacco use, obesity and diet; cancer; management of chronic health conditions such as diabetes and high blood pressure; and mental health including education, awareness and access to mental health services.

Access to Health Care

In 2010, there were over 49.1 million people in the United States without health insurance (Kaiser Family Foundation, 2011). Over the last two decades, Korean Americans have had one of the lowest rates of health insurance coverage among all racial and ethnic groups (Yoo & Kim, 2008). In 2003 and 2005, in the state of California, where Korean Americans are most highly concentrated, 35% Korean American adults lacked health insurance (Brown et al., 2007). Furthermore, a 2000 Korean American Health Survey of Koreans living in Los Angeles County found that 46% of the respondents did not have health insurance (Shin, Song, Kim, & Probst, 2005). Most Korean immigrants do not carry health insurance for themselves which is attributed to high rates of self-employment and lack of access to employment-based insurance (Kim & Yoo, 2009; Yoo & Kim, 2008). Many Korean immigrants and their families are stuck in the middle – not poor enough to qualify for Medicaid, and not old enough to qualify for Medicare. Since many Korean immigrants do not have access to health insurance, this also means that these immigrants do not have a regular source of health care through which they can access preventative health care screenings such as cancer screenings, immunizations and physical checkups (Ryu et al., 2001; Shin et al., 2005).

Making ends meet for immigrant families becomes a barrier not only to acquiring health insurance, but in buying quality, accessible health insurance (Kim & Yoo, 2009; Yoo & Kim, 2008). Kim and Yoo's study (2009, 2008), "Saving for Health and the Future," surveyed 269 Korean immigrant small business owners in the San Francisco Bay Area and in the Los Angeles area. Kim and Yoo found in their study, 29% of immigrants in the sample were uninsured, while 71% of this sample had health insurance coverage. Even with obtaining a modest amount of health insurance, financial difficulties and barriers still posed a challenge to accessing health care services. The high costs associated with accessing health insurance did not translate into the receipt of care among the insured in this study. Further, there were no significant differences in different types of health care utilization between the insured and uninsured.

These study results (Yoo & Kim, 2008) on Korean immigrant small business owners found that many with health insurance could be classified as under-insured; although they had access to some health insurance, they had inadequate health insurance coverage and had medical bill problems. This study illustrates that even when Korean immigrants purchase private health insurance, costs to use such health services are still a barrier to needed health services. Private health plans often had higher deductibles, co-payments and premiums, which often meant that these immigrants were reluctant to use their privately purchased health insurance plans. With high deductibles and co-payments, Korean immigrants used medical care for emergencies rather than for preventive care. In this study, individuals with a high deductible experienced greater difficulty accessing care due to cost compared to those with a lower or no deductible. 38% of adults with deductibles of $1,000 or more reported problems with health care access, not filling prescriptions, not accessing specialist care, and forgoing recommended tests and needed care.

Despite the previous difficulties of privately obtaining health insurance for many Korean Americans, the 2010 Patient Protection and Affordable Care Act, signed by President Obama offers some solutions by increasing the number of the medically insured. In 2014, all U.S. citizens and legal residents will be required to have health insurance or pay a fine. Individuals who do not have access to insurance coverage through their employer will be able to purchase affordable coverage through a state health insurance plan that will be affordable. Medicaid will also be expanded to individuals. Moreover, this law states that all health insurers will be required to sell coverage to all regardless of any preexisting condition.

Acculturation, Lifestyle and Behavior

Not only is health care access a huge issue, but Korean Americans are also experiencing changes to lifestyle and behavior that is impacting health. Among Korean Americans, acculturation impacts lifestyle and health behaviors. Acculturation involves evolving from one culture to another. For Korean Americans, acculturation entails adopting and making changes to various aspects of their lives including cultural, social, economic, and/or political views (Song et al., 2004), and often these changes in behavior impact health both positively and negatively.

Acculturation appears to operate in complex ways, influencing Korean American men and women differently. Lee, Sobal, and Frongillo (2000) investigated how acculturation was linked to health behaviors such as smoking, recreational physical activity, fat in diet, weight, and reported health among Korean American men and women. Among Korean Americans, gender and acculturation impacted health behaviors. Three-hundred-fifty-six Korean Americans participated in surveys which showed that acculturated and bi-cultural women had a greater likelihood to smoke than newly-immigrated Korean women, while bi-cultural men had lower tendencies to smoke. Among both men and women, acculturation was not associated with fat in diets or vigorous exercise, but those more acculturated reported more low impact physical activity, higher body weight and more positive self-reported health related than those with less acculturation.

Acculturation also seems to change dietary behavior for Korean Americans. In a study comparing Korean and Korean American adolescents, researchers found that Korean Americans consumed more cookies, sweets, and soda and consumed less rice and kimchi (Park, Paik, Skinner, Spindler, & Park, 2004). Others have found similar results. Yang, Chung, Kim, Bianchi, and Song (2007) examined the dietary changes and chronic diseases of 497 first-generation Korean American immigrants in relation to their length of residence in the U.S. Men who had longer residency in the U.S. (26 years or more) also consumed less rice, kimchi and potatoes while consuming more breakfast cereal, pasta, burritos, salted snacks and wine than Korean men living in the U.S. for 15 years or less. Women living in the U.S. aged 26 years or more consumed less rice/rice dishes, fried fish paste, soybean paste stew, kimchi, and increased consumption of high fat dairy products, sweets, and fresh vegetables and fruits than participants who lived in U.S. less than 15 years. The longer women lived in the U.S., the lower the consumption of Korean traditional foods such as rice and kimchee.

Several studies have shown that there is a correlation between acculturation and smoking habits by Korean American men. A study of 333 Korean American men residing in Maryland showed an association of length of stay in U.S. and smoking. Participants who lived in the U.S. for at least 20 years were not as likely to be currently smoking as those who lived in the U.S. for less than 10 years. Another association with smoking was alcohol; participants who consumed alcohol were more likely to smoke or have had previously smoked (Joun, Kim, Han, Ryu, & Han, 2003). Therefore, newer immigrants were more likely to smoke than immigrants who had been in the U.S for more than 20 years.

Other studies have found similar results with not only smoking, but also with alcohol use and obesity. A study that compared 2,830 Korean Americans in California and 500 Koreans in Seoul (Song et al., 2004) showed that among Korean Americans, acculturated men tended to be more overweight while acculturated women tended to drink alcohol and smoke more. In contrast to Koreans in Seoul, Korean American men were less likely to smoke and drink. Acculturation among Korean American men and women were related to a decreased amount of eating traditional Korean food and an increased amount of American foods. Higher levels of acculturation often related to more health risk, including eating at fast food restaurants, alcohol drinking and smoking for women.

Cancer

Compared to other Asian Americans, Korean American men and women had the highest occurrence and mortality rates from stomach cancer (McCracken et al., 2007). Korean American men (54.6) have almost twice the rate of stomach cancer than Vietnamese American men (28.1) and over five times higher than non-Hispanic whites (9.5) (McCracken et al., 2007). Similarly, Korean American women have almost twice the rates of stomach cancer than Vietnamese women and seven times more than non-Hispanic whites. Helicobacter pylori may be a main factor in causing stomach cancer. Higher stomach cancer rates among Korean Americans might be attributed to diets that contain high levels of salt and nitrites/nitrates (McCracken et al., 2007).

In addition to stomach cancer, Korean Americans seem to have higher rates of various cancers than their Asian American peers. Liver cancer occurrence and mortality was highest for Korean American women in California compared to other Asian groups and second highest among men (McCracken et al., 2007). Likely due to hepatitis B (HBV) infection in Korea, liver cancer rates are third highest in the world for men and 15th for women McCracken et al., 2007). Korean women had second highest occurrence and mortality rate for cervical cancer (McCracken et al., 2007). Compared to other Asian Americans, Korean American men had the highest lung cancer death incidences and the highest smoking occurrence among other Asian American groups in study.

When looking at cancer incidence rates worldwide, cancer rates among Korean Americans look quite different from those residing in Korea. Data from the Surveillance, Epidemiology, and End Results (SEER) show that prostate, colon, and rectum cancer risk increased for Korean American men while risk of stomach, liver, gallbladder, larynx, and esophageal cancer has strongly decreased compared to Koreans residing in Korea. In comparison to whites in the U.S. and to Korean Americans, native Koreans have more cases of stomach, liver, gallbladder, and esophagus cancer. While for Korean American women, there is an increase of breast, lung, colon, rectum and endometrial cancer, and decrease in stomach, liver, gallbladder and cervical cancer incidence (Lee, Demissie, Lu, & Rhoads, 2007).

Korean Americans face tremendous barriers in terms of access to early detection cancer screenings. Early detection in cancer is crucial because detection at a later stage may mean higher mortality and lower survival rates. Several studies have shown that access to various kinds of cancer screenings among Korean Americans is significantly low (McCracken et al., 2007; Jo, Maxwell, Wong, & Bastani, 2008). Screenings for colorectal cancer are critical as they remove precancerous polyps in examinations. Jo et al. (2008) researched the use of colorectal cancer screening among 151 Korean Americans in Southern California and found the biggest challenges to access for screenings included the lack of heath care coverage and not being able to afford testing; lack of knowledge of where to go for testing; language and cultural barriers; and not wanting to burden family. Participants in the study reported that community-based educational workshops, Korean media promotions for outreaching and educational pamphlets in Korean about colorectal cancer might helped increase the use of colorectal screenings. Catalysts for screening included having a doctor referral, affordability of test, hearing helpful things about test, having family or friends make recommendations, and understanding that screenings can decrease mortality rates.

In addition, Korean American women are diagnosed with cervical carcinoma at later stages than White women (Bates, Hofer, & Parikh-Patel, 2008). Korean American women compared to other Asian American women were less likely to have had a Pap test, a cervical cancer screening (Yoo, Le, Vong, Lagman, & Lam, 2011). Many Korean American women have never had a Pap smear (Yoo et al., 2011). A study of Korean American women has shown that 34% of women over the age of 18 have not had a Pap Smear (Lin et al., 2009).

There are several barriers that prevent Korean American women from attaining breast and cervical cancer screenings. The lack of health insurance (Ma et al., 2009b) and fear and discomfort (Yoo et al., 2011) prevent many Korean American women from getting screened (Ma et al., 2009b). From cancer screenings to diagnosis to treatment, support is needed for Korean Americans. One way in which to promote preventative health measures in Korean Americans is to provide language support and health information in Korean. In cancer screenings directed towards Korean immigrant women, language support for patients with limited English proficiency, often meant that women were more likely to receive mammograms, clinical breast exams and Pap smears (Dang et al., 2010). Once diagnosed with cancer, support is continually needed as patients navigate a cancer diagnosis and it's subsequent treatments. Lim and Yi (2009) have found religiosity and spirituality played important roles functioning as survival strategies in the lives of Korean immigrants diagnosed with cancer. In their study of 161 Korean immigrant cancer patients, they found that those with higher levels of religiosity, through church involvement, experienced lower levels of depression, and overall better quality of life.

Management of Chronic Health Conditions

For anyone diagnosed with a chronic illness, there are often complex adjustments one needs to make including understanding medications, adjusting to symptoms, and making changes to one's lifestyle. Effective management of one's chronic illness often means regular medication use, prevention and self-care practices. Poorly managed chronic health issues can lead to increased mortality and morbidity. Past research of Korean Americans and chronic health conditions indicates that this population faces challenges in managing chronic health conditions like diabetes and high blood pressure (Kim et al., 2007; Kang, Han, Kim, & Kim, 2006; Song et al., 2010).

The challenges that Korean Americans face in terms of management of chronic health conditions includes access to care and a bilingual provider, but also information on how to manage their illness effectively. Song et al. (2010) examined 445 hypertensive Korean American immigrants who were involved in a self-help intervention for high

blood pressure care. Results showed having access to health insurance status and high blood pressure-related medical history appeared to be critical components for the management of their illness. Recent immigrants tended to not prioritize their health, nor have health insurance, and therefore did not seek health care services to manage their high blood pressure (HBP). Other studies have indicated that Korean Americans often lack the knowledge to manage their chronic illness. Among Korean Americans, non-adherence to medications like high blood pressure has been related to incomplete knowledge of high blood pressure treatment, including the benefits and side effects of hypertensive medication (Kim et al., 2007).

Several studies have used innovative, culturally and linguistically tailored community interventions to help build better self care, increased informational support and ultimately management of chronic health conditions. Kim, Han, Park, Lee, and Kim (2006) tested the significance of an intervention program for 49 HBP patients of Korean descent and who were at least 60 years old. The study included education on behavior and management of HBP, blood pressure monitoring at home, and support groups once a month facilitated by a bilingual nurse. Results showed that increased bilingual information on how to manage their blood pressure through a self-help intervention program enhanced individuals blood pressure levels and general health. The intervention program included weekly two hours educational classes for 6 weeks at an elderly housing center, neighborhood library and a senior center. Two nurses facilitated these sessions focusing on informing participants of HBP and its management, reducing heart risk causes, and providing health resources for Korean American elders. Nurses also provided education on eating healthy, exercising and discussed ways to deal with life challenges that HBP patients and senior immigrants encounter.

Another effective component in the Kim et al. (2006) study was Korean Americans monitoring blood pressure at home for a period of 6 months, once in the morning and once at night, for two or more days per week. Participants felt empowered by consistently and independently monitoring their own blood pressure levels that subsequently, encouraged them to achieve or strive for ideal blood pressure levels. Home monitoring systems were also helpful for Korean elders, as they tended to express lower comfort levels with Western health care services which often resulted in inaccurate or exaggerated blood pressure measurements at a hospital. Lastly, bilingual nurses facilitated hour-long support groups once a month. Participants discussed challenges they were facing; support groups allowed for problem-solving and seeking and providing informational and emotional support.

Although researchers have proposed self-help interventions for management of chronic health conditions in the Korean American community, very few have studied family support. The limited research on family support and diabetes shows that family plays a vital role in educating and supporting loved ones around lifestyle changes necessary for managing diabetes. Among Korean immigrants, family support provided to be vital in diabetes management, specifically, supporting diet restrictions. Choi (2009) interviewed 143 Korean immigrant men and women with Type II diabetes and found that family support around diet (managing glucose control) resulted in lower levels of glycosylated hemoglobin. Family support was measured by level of involvement in areas including: medication compliance, glucose testing, exercise, and diet. Examples of support reported in the study included family members praising diabetic patients for their diet and eating suggested foods together. Research shows, family support, both emotional and practical (life-style changes) is critical to managing diabetes for Korean Americans (Choi, 2009).

Mental Health

Compared to other U.S. populations, immigrant Asian Americans have the lowest rates of seeking mental health services, though U.S. born individuals were more likely to utilize mental health services than foreign born (Abe-Kim et al., 2007). The Surgeon General's Report on Mental Health noted almost half of Asian Americans' low use of mental health services is due to lack of bilingual providers and/or patients' ability to speak English (U.S. Department of Health and Human Services, 2001). Past research identifies language barriers, lack of culturally-sensitive health care providers, stigmas related to mental illnesses, lack of awareness of mental health disorders in community and belief in traditional medicine as challenges for Korean Americans in accessing mental health services (Lee, Hanner, Cho, Han, & Kim, 2008). Other barriers specific to Koreans accessing mental health services were beliefs that mental disorders are hereditary (often perceived as a "shameful inherited" trait) and being self-reliant when it pertains to emotional problems.

Stigma and the lack of education regarding mental illness continue to plague the Korean American community. Jang, Gum, and Chiriboga (2010) study demonstrated a need for more outreach and education regarding depression among Korean Americans. In the study, Jang et al. investigated 675 Korean Americans' awareness of depression. Results showed that participants who were less aware of depression were not as acculturated as those who were more knowledgeable. Interestingly, there was no association between educational level and knowledge of depression. Further, those that showed less knowledge of depression displayed more symptoms of depression. Jang, Kim, and Chiriboga (2010) explained that this phenomena might be due to the fact that those who exhibit depressive symptoms also tend to be hesitant or disinclined to come forward and learn about their mental illness.

In another study with 209 Korean Americans aged 20–25 and 462 Korean Americans aged 60 and above, researchers found varying attitudes toward mental health services (Jang, Chiriboga, & Okazaki, 2009). The study demonstrated older Korean participants were more inclined to have cultural stigma and misconceptions of mental illness. Further, their often negative perceptions toward health services were influenced by their preconceived notions of mental illness as a social stigma. While older participants tended to view depression as a sign of weakness that brings shame to the family, younger participants were more likely to accept and view depression as a medical condition. Participants who acknowledged a medical model of depression held more positive views toward mental health services.

Other studies have found similar results (Jang, Kim, & Chiriboga 2010). With increased awareness and education, Korean Americans were less likely to have stigma toward mental illnesses and more likely to use needed mental health services. Jang et al. (2008) surveyed 675 Korean American seniors in Tampa and Orlando Florida to measure their awareness of Alzheimer's disease (AD), feelings of shame (should anyone in family have AD), knowledge of AD services, and acculturation. Results showed that participants with higher levels of education and acculturation tended to be more knowledgeable of AD. Participants with lower levels of education reported higher levels of feelings of shame connected with family members having AD. The study also demonstrated that participants who had a family member with AD were more knowledgeable of AD services.

Since the 1980s psychoeducation has become an important tool for individuals and families dealing with mental illnesses. This approach focuses on not only educating patients and families of mental illness, but also learning adaptive skills (Shin, 2004). Psychoeducation works to provide clients an understanding of the illness and treatment, which has proven to be an effective tool in promoting mental health awareness in the Korean American community. Shin (2004) examined the significance of psychoeducation as an intervention method for mental illness among Korean Americans. Dividing 48 Korean Americans with children with mental illnesses into two groups, the study compared the effects of individual counseling and culturally sensitive psychoeducation. The results showed that participants involved in the psychoeducation method drastically enhanced their empowerment, reduced their stigmatized views of mental illness and improved their coping skills. Participants' discussions with social workers about how to cope with their children with mental illnesses and their attendance in workshops with clinicians regarding the navigation of the mental health system proved to be positive as well. Bringing together

Eastern and Western philosophies of mental illness increased the chances of Korean patients accepting and using U.S. mental health services.

Social, Cultural and Community Practices

This section focuses on the social, cultural and community practices of Korean Americans. *Hanyak*, Korean traditional medicine is discussed within the context of the latest research on utilization. In addition, the Korean church is also discussed as a site for education, awareness and support for various health concerns and issues impacting Korean Americans.

Hanyak

Previous research has shown that among older Korean immigrants, traditional health care is still widely practiced, but that those without insurance were more likely to utilize traditional Asian medicine (Yoo & Kim, 2008). Dating back as far as 3000 B.C., *hanyak* is the practice of traditional Korean medicine, which has been influenced by other traditional Asian medicine customs. Some examples of treatment use are herbs and acupuncture. Awareness of *hanyak* is still important today as Korean immigrants in the U.S. sometimes use *hanyak* in combination with Western medicine.

Among Korean Americans, uninsured immigrants and older immigrants were more likely to use *hanyak* to treat ailments. Yoo and Kim (2008) found that for Korean immigrants the financial costs of conventional health care were not accessible, leading them to their cultural reliance on traditional Korean medicine and practices. Research found participants commonly sought traditional Korean medicine for not only preventive care and health supplements but also for treatments including allergies and backaches (Yoo & Kim, 2008). Participants noted costs to visit a traditional Korean practitioner were more affordable (ranging from $10 for herbal to $50 for acupuncture treatment) than Western medical doctors.

Studies have indicated the importance for health care professionals to be aware of Korean American and Korean immigrants' possible use of traditional Korean medicine to avoid possible medicinal or health concerns (Kim, Han, Kim, & Duong, 2002). A study of 205 Korean senior immigrants' use of health care resources showed participants used a range of services that included, one of or sometimes both, Western and Korean Traditional Medicine. The source of health care and whether Korean Americans had health insurance were connected to the kind of heath care participants used (Kim et al., 2002).

The Korean Church

For Korean Americans, the Korean church continues to be a community force and institution. Korean Americans have had a long historical connection between Christianity in Korea and in the United States. American missionaries were responsible for the initial migration out of Korea to the Hawaiian plantations. Korean immigrant churches became community centers for new immigrants. Compared to any other Asian American group in the U.S., church participation is greatest among Korean Americans. The majority of Korean Americans are protestant. The church provides a sense of community, social support and a cultural center for Koreans in the US. The Korean church has also functioned as a center for newly arrived immigrants.

Research shows that Korean church leaders serve a range of social and health needs to their members and neighboring communities (Jo, Maxwell, Yang, & Bastani, 2010). A study that consisted of open-ended interviews and focus groups with 58 community leaders from 23 Korean American churches and three community organizations shared that some leaders noted that supporting social and medical needs is a crucial part of their church. Historically, the role of the clergy in Korean churches has not only been to be spiritual leaders but to also be forefront support for Korean immigrants arriving to the U.S. Jo et al. (2010) found that pastors and church leaders (e.g., pastor's wife, elders, deacons) devoted

up to 50% of their time to meeting the health and social needs of their members which included translating health and legal questions, and transporting and accompanying members to doctor's appointments (often translating), assisting with transportation and accompanying parishioners to hospitals, schools, and also in directing and implementing health programs at the church. When asked about health needs of their members, pastors cited cancer, heart disease, stroke, high blood pressure, diabetes, lack of exercise, and poor diet. They also mentioned psychosocial problems for their congregational members.

Education in the Korean American community is crucial to accessing mental health services. The Association of Korean American Psychiatrists (AKAP), founded in 1979 by first-generation immigrants, provides community workshops on etiology and treatment of mental disorders. AKAP offer these workshops specifically for Korean clergy as they are seen as community leaders and can be influential in terms of helping Korean and Korean Americans seek mental health services. Due to the significant role and involvement the church plays in the lives of Korean Americans, clergy and pastors if educated around mental illness issues can provide the support individuals need through the church or provide a referral. Korean immigrant clergy are often the first people that families turn to when facing a mental health crisis. The clergy are an important potential link for education and referral to not only general health services but also to mental health services.

In a study of 103 Asian American clergy in California, the findings indicated a strong relationship between clergy making referrals for mental health services and their education level, past mental health knowledge, including mental illness, referring members to general health practitioners and providing one-on-one counseling (Yamada, Lee, & Kim, 2012). The study further found that the more discussion and education clergy have regarding mental health issues, the more likely they would be familiar with possible symptoms and thus, making appropriate referrals.

Recent studies are indicating that Korean church involvement might also play a part in reducing unhealthy behaviors. A telephone survey of 2085 Korean American adults found there was an association with church involvement and tobacco smoke. Results showed that Korean Americans who participated in church were less likely to smoke or be exposed to it and have given up smoking and have a ban on it (compared to non-church goers) (Hofstetter et al., 2010).

Although church attendance plays an important role in health behaviors, differing church views and doctrines regarding alcohol among churches proved to influence Korean American women's alcohol use. One study (Sim et al., 2011) showed that depending on the type of Christian denomination, Korean American women's alcohol consumption level varied. Those belonging to Christian denominations that permitted moderate alcohol use (e.g. Catholic and Independent Christian women) demonstrated higher tendencies of alcohol consumption than those of conservative Christian denominations.

Korean church involvement has also been documented in several studies as being good for ones' health in terms of informational, emotional, spiritual and tangible support. In one study, Kang and Romo (2010) examined the role of church participation in 248 Korean American youth ranging from 7th to 12th grades. Through self-reporting surveys, adolescents reported their length of church involvement, preference to attend, and partaking in activities. Results from this study showed that higher levels of church involvement were associated with lower levels of depressive signs for girls and better grades for boys. This study illustrates the importance of utilizing the church's connection to the larger Korean American community to help provide direct and indirect support in regards to health, mental wellness and behavior.

Other studies are finding that the Korean church can be a site for educational health efforts. Jo et al. (2010) provides recommendations on how Korean churches can be partners for both research and health education interventions which could include (1) interventions for prevention and early detection; (2) collaborating with a local university to offer a health fair or seminar; (3) programs that provide pastors or key church leaders with health

information and resources; (4) interventions that address psychosocial needs; and (5) interventions for the church youth. There have been a few studies that have collaborated with a Korean church to provide such interventions.

Ma et al. (2009a) investigated 167 Korean Americans recruited from churches to participate in a study to measure the affect of culturally relevant cancer intervention program. The intervention program involved bilingual support, counseling, discussing accessibility issues, psychological and social barriers, cancer education, and patient support. The control group simply received health education on cancer-related health issues. After a 12 month follow-up, over 77% of participants received cancer screening compared to only 10% in control group. The study illustrates that it is critical for not only churches to assist in educational programs but also to be part of providing culturally relevant intervention programs that address cultural barriers.

Future Directions: Needed Areas of Research

Traditional research on Korean Americans have focused on the Korean immigrant experience of those who arrived after 1965 and their experiences in the U.S. No research has been done on other cohorts of Korean immigrants or American born generations. Although there are hosts of other health issues impacting Korean Americans, much of the research that has been published on Korean Americans and health has focused on cancer screenings, smoking and depression. There are areas that need further research to understand completely the health experiences of Korean Americans.

Access to Health Care

Accessing health care is still a concern for Korean immigrants. Two areas not unexplored are medical tourism and access to dental care. Because of the high uninsured rates among Korean Americans, it is not surprising that many

Korean immigrants have gone back to Korea to seek health care. This is called medical tourism. This phenomenon has not been studied among Korean immigrants in the U.S., but it is widely known and often depicted in Korean immigrant newspapers as way that Korean immigrants can access and afford needed health care. Lee, Kearns, and Friesen (2010) examined the occurrence of Korean migrants returning to their native country of origin for health care services. Results showed that participants' preference to return to their native country for medical care were linked with not trusting the expertise of doctors abroad and the lack of doctors' cultural understanding of Koreans. Patients were not only seeking knowledgeable health professionals but also sought to be in a familiar and comfortable environment. This study demonstrated how Koreans globally are returning to Korea for affordable and linguistically accessible health care (Lee et al., 2010).

An understudied area of research are Korean Americans access to dental care. Only one study available on Medline discussed the dental care needs of Korean Americans. This older study found that there is a need for educating and providing dental care for senior immigrants who have not seen dentists for preventive oral care in their native countries (Lee & Kiyak, 1992). Senior Korean Americans had higher gingival occurrence and plaque. While seniors had higher rates of seeing dentists, visits were predominantly for emergency and/or prosthodontic care.

Differing Cohorts: Different Korean Populations in the U.S.

Differing cohorts of Korean immigrants face specific issues that have not been fully explored. Another understudied area are the health experiences of Korean students who come abroad to study in the U.S. The United States has experienced a growth of Korean students coming abroad to study in the U.S. Often times, many return to Korea after the completion of their studies. However, despite this increase of Koreans studying abroad, there has been little attention to the stressors this population faces. Past research has shown that up to 70% of Asian international students face discrimination and that this perceived discrimination is a major stressor in the lives of these students (Wei, Ku, Russell, Mallinckrodt, & Liao, 2008).

Furthermore, an understudied area is the mental health needs of Korean adoptees. For the last 50 years, over 150,000 Korean adoptees have been placed in American families (U.S. Department of Homeland Security, 2010). Studies have found that transracial adoptees in the U.S. may encounter difficulties around their racial and ethnic identity and in dealing with racism, and that children may better adjust if parents are responsive and sensitive to such needs (Mohanty & Newhill, 2006). There needs to be further research on post adoption adjustment of Korean adoptees, identity and mental health.

Post 1965, Korean immigrants represent a cohort that have been uninsured and often entering their aging years with chronic health issues. Although most Korean Americans at the age of 65 can qualify for Medicare, the many years without health care often comes at a cost for late detection of cancers and poor management of chronic health conditions. Adult second-generation Korean Americans will be the ones caring and supporting their aging parents. Little research has been done on this next generation of caregivers. However, one study (Yoo & Kim, 2010) examined beliefs and attitudes regarding family support among 124 adult children of Korean Americans (the 1.5 and 2nd generation). The study found that many adult children were primarily motivated by feelings of gratitude and held a strong sense of responsibility toward their parents. In addition, because Korean immigrant parents often face language and financial barriers, adult children were preparing themselves for future support of their parents' finances, health care, and long-term care needs.

This chapter focused on the top health issues impacting Korean Americans today. Although there has been increased research on Korean Americans and health, there is still a need to for more innovative research that is relevant to the lives of Korean Americans. Large national surveys and intervention-based research that provides solutions, and qualitative research that brings voice to the diverse experiences of Korean Americans are all needed. The 2010 U.S. Census shows that the Korean American population is also changing. Research should reflect these changes by exploring these differences including immigration cohorts; generation; and geographical region.

Acknowledgements The completion of this chapter was supported by Award Number P20MD000544 from the National Center On Minority Health And Health Disparities. The content is solely the responsibility of the authors and does not necessarily represent the official views of the National Center On Minority Health And Health Disparities or the National Institutes of Health.

References

Abe-Kim, J., Takeuchi, D. T., Hong, S., Zane, N., Sue, S., Spencer, M. S., et al. (2007). Use of mental health–related services among immigrant and US-Born Asian Americans: Results from the National Latino and Asian American Study. *American Journal of Public Health, 97*(1), 91–98.

Bates, J. H., Hofer, B. M., & Parikh-Patel, A. (2008). Cervical cancer incidence, mortality, and survival among Asian subgroups in California, 1990–2004. *Cancer, 113*(10), 2955–2963.

Brown, E. R., Lavarreda, S. A., Ponce, N., Yoon, J., Cummings, J., & Rice, T. (2007). *The state of health insurance in California: Findings from the 2005 California health interview survey.* Los Angeles: UCLA Center for Health Policy Research.

Choi, S. E. (2009). Diet-specific family support and glucose control among Korean immigrants with type 2 diabetes. *The Diabetes Educator, 35*, 978–985.

Dang, J., Lee, J., Tran, J., Kagawa-Singer, M., Foo, M. A., Nguyen, T., et al. (2010). The role of medical interpretation on breast cancer and cervical cancer screening among Asian American and Pacific Islander women. *Journal of Cancer Education, 25*, 253–262.

Hofstetter, C., Ayers, J., Irvin, V., Kang Sim, D., Hughes, S., Reighard, F., et al. (2010). Does church participation facilitate tobacco control? A report on Korean immigrants. *Journal of Immigrant and Minority Health, 2*, 187–197.

Institute of Medicine. (2002). *Care without coverage.* Washington, DC: The National Academies Press.

Jang, Y., Chiriboga, D., & Okazaki, S. (2009). Attitudes toward mental health services: Age-group differences in Korean American adults. *Aging Men's Health,* Author manuscript, National Institute of Health.

Jang, Y., Gum, A., & Chiriboga, D. (2010). Knowledge of depression among Korean American older adults. *Journal of Applied Gerontology* (epub print).

Jang, Y., Kim, G., & Chiriboga, D. (2010). Knowledge of Alzheimer's disease, feelings of shame, and awareness of services among Korean American elders. *Journal of Aging and Health, 22*(4), 419–433.

Jo, A., Maxwell, A., Wong, W., & Bastani, R. (2008). Colorectal cancer screening among underserved Korean Americans in Los Angeles County. *Journal of Immigrant and Minority Health, 10*(2), 119–126.

Jo, A., Maxwell, A., Yang, B., & Bastani, R. (2010). Conducting health research in Korean American churches: Perspectives from church leaders. *Journal of Community Health, 35*(2), 156–164.

Joun, H., Kim, M., Han, H., Ryu, J., & Han, W. (2003). Acculturation and cigarette smoking among Korean American men. *Yonsei Medical Journal, 44*(5), 875–882.

Kaiser Family Foundation. (2011). *The uninsured: A primer.* Menlo Park: Kaiser Family Foundation.

Kang, J., Han, H., Kim, K., & Kim, M. (2006). Barriers to care and control of high blood pressure in Korean-American elderly. *Ethnicity & Disease, 16*(1), 145–151.

Kang, P., & Romo, L. (2010). The role of religious involvement on depression, risky behavior, and academic performance among Korean American adolescents. *Journal of Adolescence, 34*(4), 767–778.

Kim, E. (2000). Home is where the Han is: A Korean American perspective on the Los Angeles upheavals. In J.Y.W.S. Wu & M. Song (Eds.), *Asian American Studies: A reader* (pp. 270–289). New Brunswick, NJ: Rutgers University Press.

Kim, E. Y., Han, H. R., Jeong, S., Kim, K. B., Park, H., Kang, E., et al. (2007). Does knowledge matter? Intentional medication nonadherence among middle-aged Korean Americans with high blood pressure. *The Journal of Cardiovascular Nursing, 22*(5), 397–404.

Kim, M., Han, H., Kim, K., & Duong, D. (2002). The use of traditional and Western medicine among Korean American elderly. *Journal of Community Health, 27*(2), 109–120.

Kim, M. T., Han, H., Park, H., Lee, H., & Kim, K. B. (2006). Constructing and testing a self-help intervention program for high blood pressure control in Korean American seniors-a pilot study. *Journal of Cardiovascular Nursing, 21*(2), 77–84.

Kim, B., & Yoo, G. (2009). Immigrant entrepreneurs: Saving for health and the future. In E. Yu, H. Kim, K. Park, & M. D. Oh (Eds.), *Korean American economy and community in the 21st century* (pp. 545–570). Los Angeles: Korean American Economic Development Center (KAEDC).

Lee, J., Demissie, K., Lu, S., & Rhoads, G. (2007). Cancer incidence among Korean-American immigrants in the United States and native Koreans in South Korea. *Cancer, Culture and Literacy, 14*(1), 78–85.

Lee, H., Hanner, J., Cho, S., Han, H., & Kim, M. (2008). Improving access to mental health services for Korean American immigrants: Moving toward a community partnership between religious and mental health services. *Psychiatry Invest, 5*, 14–20.

Lee, J., Kearns, R., & Friesen, W. (2010). Seeking affective health care: Korean immigrants' use of homeland services. *Health & Place, 16*, 108–115.

Lee, J., & Kiyak, H. (1992). Oral disease beliefs, behaviors, and health status of Korean-Americans. *Journal of Public Health Dentistry, 52*(3), 131–136.

Lee, S., Sobal, J., & Frongillo, E. (2000). Acculturation and health in Korean Americans. *Social Science & Medicine, 51*(2), 159–173.

Lim, J.-W., & Yi, J. (2009). The effects of religiosity, spirituality, and social support on quality of life: A comparison between Korean American and Korean breast and gynecologic cancer survivors. *Oncology Nursing Forum, 36*(6), 699–708.

Lin, M. K., Moskowitz, J. M., Kazinets, G., Ivey, S. L., Kim, Y. B., & McDonnell, D. D. (2009). Adherence to Pap test guidelines: Variation among Asians in California. *Ethnicity & Disease, 19*(4), 425–432.

Ma, G., Shive, S., Tan, Y., Gao, W., Rhee, J., Park, M., et al. (2009a). Community-based colorectal cancer intervention in underserved Korean Americans. *Cancer Epidemiology, 33*(5), 381–386.

Ma, G. X., Toubbeh, J. I., Wang, M. Q., Shive, S. E., Cooper, L., & Pham, A. (2009b). Factors associated with cervical cancer screening compliance and noncompliance among Chinese, Korean, Vietnamese, and Cambodian women. *Journal of the National Medical Association, 101*(6), 541–551.

McCracken, M., Olsen, M., Chen, M., Jemal, A., Thun, M., Cokkinides, V., et al. (2007). Cancer incidence, mortality, and associated risk factors among Asian Americans of Chinese, Filipino, Vietnamese, Korean, and Japanese ethnicities. *CA: A Cancer Journal for Clinicians, 57*, 190–205.

Mohanty, J., & Newhill, C. (2006). Adjustment of international adoptees: Implications for practice and a future research agenda. *Children and Youth Services Review, 28*(4), 384–395.

Park, S., Paik, H. Y., Skinner, J. D., Spindler, A. A., & Park, H. R. (2004). Nutrient intake of Korean-American, Korean, and American adolescents. *Journal of the American Dietetic Association, 104*(2), 242–245.

Ryu, H., Young, W. B., & Park, C. (2001). Korean American health insurance and health services utilization. *Research in Nursing & Health, 24*(6), 494–505.

Shin, S. (2004). Effects of culturally relevant psychoeducation for Korean American families of persons with chronic mental illness. *Research on Social Work Practice, 14*, 231–239.

Shin, H., Song, H., Kim, J., & Probst, J. C. (2005). Insurance, acculturation, and health service utilization among Korean-Americans. *Journal of Immigrant Health, 7*(2), 65–74.

Sim, D., Hofstetter, C., Irvin, V., Ayers, J., Macera, C., Ji, M., & Hovell, M. F., (2011). Do Christian denominations exhibit higher rates of alcohol consumption? A study of Korean American women in California. *Journal of Religion and Health*. doi:10.1007/s10943-011-9471-y.

Song, H., Han, H., Lee, J., Kim, J., Kim, K., Ryu, J. P., & Kim, M. (2010). Does access to care still affect health care utilization by immigrants? Testing of an empirical explanatory model of health care utilization by Korean American immigrants with high blood pressure. *Journal of Immigrant and Minority Health, 12*(4), 513–519.

Song, Y., Hofstetter, R., Hovell, M., Paik, H., Park, H., Lee, J., & Irvin, V. (2004). Acculturation and health risk behaviors among Californians of Korean descent. *Preventive Medicine, 39*(1), 147–156.

U.S. Census Bureau. (2010). *2010: American factfinder fact sheet: 1-year American Community Survey; Profile of general population and housing characteristics: 2010, Koreans alone or in any other combination*. Washington, DC: U.S. Census Bureau. Accessed October 10, 2011, from www.factfinder2.census.gov

U.S. Department of Homeland Security. *2010 Yearbook of immigration*. Washington, DC: U.S. Department of Homeland Security. Accessed October 10, 2011, from http://www.dhs.gov/files/statistics/publications/yearbook.shtm

US Department of Health and Human Services. (2001). Mental health care for Asian Americans and Pacific Islanders. *In Mental health: Culture, race, and ethnicity a supplement to mental health: A report of the surgeon general*. Rockville, MD: US Department of Health and Human Services, Office of the Surgeon General, Substance Abuse and Mental Health Services Administration.

Wei, M., Ku, T. Y., Russell, D. W., Mallinckrodt, B., & Liao, K. (2008). Moderating effects of three coping strategies and self-esteem on perceived discrimination and depressive symptoms: A minority stress model for Asian international students. *Journal of Counseling Psychology, 55*(4), 451–462.

Yamada, A., Lee, K., & Kim, M. (2012). Community mental health allies: Referral behavior among Asian American immigrant Christian clergy. *Community Mental Health Journal, 48*(1), 107–113.

Yang, E., Chung, H., Kim, W., Bianchi, L., & Song, W. (2007). Chronic diseases and dietary changes in relation to Korean Americans' length of residence in the United States. *Journal of the American Dietetic Association, 107*(6), 942–950.

Yoo, G., & Kim, B. (2008). Korean immigrants and health care access: Implications for the uninsured and underinsured. *Research in the Sociology of Health Care, 25*, 77–94.

Yoo, G., & Kim, B. (2010). Remembering sacrifices: Attitudes and beliefs among second generation Korean Americans regarding family support. *Journal of Cross-Cultural Gerontology, 25*(2), 165–181.

Yoo, G., Le, M. N., Vong, S., Lagman, R., & Lam, A. (2011). Cancer screening: Attitudes and behaviors of young Asian American women. *Journal of Cancer Education, 26*(4), 740–746.

Social and Cultural Influences on the Health of the Vietnamese American Population

7

Mai-Nhung Le and Tu-Uyen Nguyen

Introduction

Ms. Loan was in her mid-fifties when she was first diagnosed with type II diabetes. Her doctor advised her to go to a nutrition/diabetes management course offered through her health maintenance organization. She attended the course once or twice, but her English skills are limited and she did not completely understand the instructor. She said that the course was complicated and lacked visual information. Therefore, she stopped going to class and has been self-managing her condition. Since she was diagnosed with diabetes, Ms. Loan has maintained her regular diet, eating as much rice and as many sweets as she desires. She stated that she would cut down on rice and sweets and also take her diabetes medication when she started to feel tired or dizzy. Her Vietnamese friends tell her to drink a lot of water when her sugar level is low, and her family has tried, unsuccessfully, to monitor her eating patterns and encourage her to exercise. She tells her family that health is a matter of luck and that when it is her time to leave this earth God will

take her. Within the last few years, Ms. Loan has suffered from blurred vision, which has resulted in several falls. She recently had eye surgery to address the problem.

This vignette illustrates a common scenario within the Vietnamese American population: language barriers, cultural attitudes, and beliefs play an important role in the treatment and prevention of disease and the promotion of health care within the Vietnamese American community. Understanding these factors, in addition to other socioeconomic and systemic barriers, would help medical professionals to foster more cooperation among their Vietnamese American patients. In this chapter we: (1) offer a brief profile of the Vietnamese American population, (2) examine the social, political, and cultural factors that affect Vietnamese American health outcomes, (3) describe major health issues faced by Vietnamese Americans, and (4) offer recommendations for medical and public health providers and professionals.

Vietnamese American Population

Vietnamese Americans are one of the fastest-growing Asian ethnic groups in the United States. They represent the fourth largest Asian American population. There are 1,548,449 individuals who identify as Vietnamese solely and 1,651,796 individuals who identify as Vietnamese in combination with other ethnicities residing in this country (American Community Survey [ACS], 2009).

M.-N. Le (✉)
Department of Asian American Studies, San Francisco State University, San Francisco, CA, USA
e-mail: mainhung@sfsu.edu

T.-U. Nguyen
Asian American Studies Program, California State University, Fullerton, CA, USA
e-mail: tunnguyen@exchange.fullerton.edu

G.J. Yoo et al. (eds.), *Handbook of Asian American Health*,
DOI 10.1007/978-1-4614-2227-3_7, © Springer Science+Business Media, LLC 2013

Most Vietnamese Americans live in metropolitan areas. The three states with the largest concentrations of Vietnamese Americans are California, Texas, and Washington. Orange County, California, is the area with the largest concentration of Vietnamese outside of Vietnam (233,573), with the neighborhood of "Little Saigon" as its cultural and civic center (Table 7.1).

Table 7.1 Population profile of Vietnamese descent in the United States (*Source*: U.S. Census Bureau, 2009 American Community Survey [ACS])

Category	Subcategory	Total U.S. population	White alone or in combination with one or more races	Asian alone or in any combination	Vietnamese alone	Vietnamese alone or in any combination
Total population		307,006,556	236,287,989	15, 733,402 (5.1% of total population)	1,481,513 (0.48% of total population)	1,651,796 (0.54% of total population)
Gender	Male	49.3%	49.4%	48.3%	49.4%	49.6%
	Female	50.7%	50.6%	51.7%	50.6%	50.4%
Age	0–17 years	24.3%	23.1%	26.3%	26.1%	28.9%
	18–64	62.9%	62.5%	64.9%	65.6%	63.1%
	65+	12.9%	14.3%	8.8%	8.6%	7.9%
Marital status	Married, but separated	49.3%	52.1%	57.6%	57.3%	56.2%
	Widowed	6.1%	6.4%	1.4%	4.3%	4.1%
	Divorced	10.6%	11.0%	5.3%	5.9%	5.9%
	Separated	2.2%	1.8%	1.3%	1.7%	1.7%
	Never married	31.8%	28.7%	35.7%	30.9%	32.1%
Educational attainment	High school graduate and below	43.2%	41.5%	30.5%	51.8%	51.2%
	Some college or an associate's degree	28.9%	29.3%	20.6%	23.5%	23.6%
	Bachelor's degree	17.6%	18.4%	29.1%	18.1%	18.4%
	Graduate or professional degree	10.3%	10.8%	19.8%	6.6%	6.7%
Median household income	Individuals and families	$50,221	$52,976	$68,103	$51,840	$52,444
	Family income (married couple family)	$61,082	$65,096	$78,064	$56,060	$56,279
	Individual per capita income	$26,409	$28,548	$28,000	$20,794	$20, 100
Poverty rates	All people	14.3%	11.9%	11.2%	15.5%	15.0%
	Under 18 years	20.0%	15.9%	11.5%	18.9%	16.9%
	18–64	13.1%	11.2%	10.8%	13.8%	13.8%
	65+	9.5%	8.1%	13.1%	18.2%	18.0%
	All families	10.5%	8.2%	8.7%	13.7%	13.6%
Health insurance coverage	Private health insurance coverage	67.4%	71.8%	71.7%	57.4%	59%
	Public health coverage	28.5%	27.4%	19.4%	26.2%	25.4%
	No health insurance	15.1%	13.3%	14.1%	19.6%	18.7%
Place of birth	United States	87.5%	91.8%	40.4%	31.0%	35.5%
	Foreign born	12.5%	8.2%	59.6%	69.0%	64.5%
Language spoken at home	English only	80.0%	85.4%	29.4%	10.9%	14.8%
	Language other than English	20.0%	14.6%	70.6%	89.1%	85.2%
	Speak English less than "very well"	8.6%	6.0%	32.3%	54.8%	51.7%

A majority of Vietnamese Americans are either first- or second-generation Americans, with nearly 70% being foreign-born (ACS, 2009). They are more inclined to speak Vietnamese at home. Only 10% of the Vietnamese Americans report speaking only English at home. Moreover, over half of the population (54.8%) does not speak English well.

Vietnamese Americans tend to be young, with more than 90% of the population younger than 65 years of age. The sex ratio is fairly evenly distributed, with 50.6% being females and 49.4% being males. An area of concern for Vietnamese Americans is health care coverage. About 17% of Vietnamese Americans are uninsured, 26% are covered under the public health system, and the remaining 57% are covered under private health insurance. Overall, Vietnamese American poverty rates are slightly higher than overall U.S. poverty rates. Moreover, among persons over 65 years of age, the poverty rate is significantly higher for Vietnamese Americans than for the general population (18.2% and 9.5%, respectively).

Vietnamese Immigration

Unlike other Asian immigrants, most Vietnamese Americans came to the United States as refugees from the Vietnam War. Refugees are individuals who have left their country of nationality and are unwilling to return because they fear persecution (Rutledge, 1992). Refugees typically have little or no time to prepare for their journey. Their migration is not voluntary, and they often leave without a known destination. Prior to the Fall of Saigon in 1975, very few Vietnamese were residing in the United States. In 1952, only eight Vietnamese immigrants were admitted to the United States. By 1969, 3,167 more Vietnamese had immigrated to the United States (Rumbaut, 1995). Most of these immigrants consisted of diplomats, war brides, and university students from elite families. Vietnamese immigration to the United States from 1975 to the present has consisted mostly of Vietnamese seeking political asylum or family reunification. Given differences in the makeup of these waves of Vietnamese

immigration, the Vietnamese American population includes those who have been in the United States for at least three decades as well as those who have just arrived. Knowledge of this history provides a crucial context for understanding the health of Vietnamese Americans.

First Wave of Vietnamese Immigration

The first significant wave of Vietnamese immigration began in 1975, a few months prior to the Fall of Saigon, which marked the end of the Vietnam War. More than 120,000 Vietnamese left the country due to the fear of persecution by the North Vietnamese communist government. The first wave tended to be well-educated, relatively affluent, from the southern part of Vietnam, and with close connections to American servicemen. Many were high-ranking military officers and government officials of the Republic Government of Vietnam, and there were significant numbers of Catholics and urban dwellers. With their high level of skills and education, they adapted to American life more quickly than subsequent waves of Vietnamese refugees. A majority of the first-wave refugees left Vietnam by either cargo ships or airplanes dispatched by the U.S. military. After departing Vietnam, they were flown briefly to U.S. government military bases in the Philippines, Wake Island, and Guam. Then they were transferred to one of four refugee centers in the United States. They were detained in these refugee centers until they were matched with sponsors and flown to their resettlement destination. In order to discourage the development of ethnic enclaves and to minimize their possible negative impact on any particular geographic area, the federal government implemented a dispersal policy so that the first-wave Vietnamese were scattered throughout the United States (Montero, 1979). Thus, many first-wave refugees found themselves in communities with little or no opportunities for contact with other Vietnamese refugees or other Asian Americans. Within a few years of their initial resettlement, however, a significant amount of secondary migration occurred as Vietnamese refugees moved to warmer states, such as California and Texas, with large populations of Vietnamese and Asian Americans.

Second Wave of Vietnamese Immigration

The second wave of Vietnamese immigration occurred from 1977 until the mid-1980s. More than 200,000 Vietnamese left Vietnam during this period (Montero, 1979). Due to political and societal changes in Vietnam, thousands of people fled to neighboring countries. A considerable number of second-wave refugees were ethnic Chinese. They tended to be less-educated and came from rural backgrounds. Many escaped Vietnam on tiny, rickety, poorly constructed fishing boats not equipped for the high seas and came to be known as the "boat people." As a result, many individuals lost their lives at sea. Many were reportedly robbed, raped, and tortured by pirates at sea. Those who survived typically ended up in refugee camps in Thailand, Malaysia, Indonesia, Singapore, Hong Kong, or the Philippines, where they awaited permanent asylum in countries willing to accept them. Many of the second-wave refugees eventually were allowed to immigrate to the United States.

Third Wave of Vietnamese Immigration

The third wave of Vietnamese immigration started shortly after implementation of the Orderly Departure Program (ODP) in 1979. This program allowed individuals to leave Vietnam legally for the United States for family reunion and humanitarian reasons. More than 300,000 Vietnamese had immigrated to the United States under this program by 1992: 161,400 individuals under the family reunification program, 81,500 Amerasians and their accompanying relatives, and 61,000 former political prisoners and their families (Rumbaut, 1995). Since the mid-1990s, the majority of Vietnamese relocating to the United States have

been admitted as immigrants through family-sponsored immigration, not as refugees (Dao & Bankston, 2010).

Key Features of the Vietnamese American Community

The first wave of Vietnamese in the United States was a more homogenous group in terms of their education and socioeconomic status, while subsequent waves consisted of a diverse cross section of Vietnamese society. This section describes some significant features of the Vietnamese American population.

Ethnicity

There are 54 distinct ethnic groups in Vietnam. The Viet (Kinh) people account for approximately 86% of Vietnam's population. They reside primarily in the plains and urban centers of nearly all provinces throughout the country. The remaining 53 ethnic minority groups comprise roughly 12 million people who are scattered throughout remote highlands and mountainous areas, except for the Hoa (ethnic Chinese) who are largely urban-based, and the Khmer group in the South of Vietnam (GSO, 2010). Although the first wave of Vietnamese immigrants consisted mostly of the Viet people, subsequent waves included other ethnic groups, such as Hoa, Khmer, Cham, Amerasian and Eurasian.

Language

The Vietnamese language is heavily influenced by Chinese dialect, particularly Cantonese. Vietnamese Americans predominately speak Quốc Ngữ, the Vietnamese national language, which is a Romanized script. Nearly 90% of Vietnamese living in the United States report speaking a language other than English at home (ACS, 2009). Of these respondents, roughly 53% speak English less than "very well" (ACS, 2009).

Religion

The three major belief systems are Buddhism, Confucianism, and Catholicism. A majority of Vietnamese Americans believe in the Northern School of Buddhism, known as Mahayana Buddhism. Although Catholics comprise only 10% of the population in Vietnam, a third or more of Vietnamese Americans are Catholics. Vietnamese Americans also practice Confucianism, Taoism, Cao-Dai, and Hoa-Hao.

Family Unit

The family plays an important role in Vietnamese society. Most first-generation Vietnamese Americans continue to rely on their family as their main source of support. The traditional Vietnamese family is patriarchal, patrilineal, and patrilocal (Rutledge, 1992). Traditionally, Vietnamese women have had fewer rights than men and are brought up according to strict discipline. The Vietnamese household is multigenerational, with parents, their sons with their wives and children, and unmarried siblings all living together in the same household (Trinh, 2002).

Traditional Health Beliefs

Although the Vietnamese are generally well aware of germ theory and antibiotics and have great respect for medical doctors, they also rely heavily on traditional folk treatments (Gordon, Bernadett, Evans, Shapiro, & Dang, 2009; Tung, 1980; Yee, 2004). According to the Chinese concept of yin and yang, two opposing forces must be in balance to maintain good health. The Am-Duong model is based on this concept and many traditional Vietnamese folk treatments are intended to restore this critical balance.

"Coining" is a traditional Vietnamese folk treatment in which a coin is dipped in a mentholated liquid and rubbed vigorously over sections of skin on the body. Another is "cupping," in which heated glass vials are placed on the skin, creating a suction when they cool. Both coining and cupping can leave marks on the skin, which may be mistaken for abuse or injury. The application of balms to the skin and the ingestion of medicinal herbs are also common.

When given access to Western medical treatment, Vietnamese readily accept pills or injections to treat symptoms, as long as this does not conflict with the internal balance of yin and yang. However, some oral medications are viewed as "hot" (yin) and may be considered counterproductive for treating "hot" illnesses, such as skin irritations.

Major Health Concerns

Diabetes

Diabetes affects many Asian American and Pacific Islander communities, including Vietnamese Americans (Carter, Pugh, & Monterrosa, 1996; Fujimoto, 1995; McNeely & Boyko, 2004), but many Vietnamese have little knowledge about the clinical symptoms of diabetes. For Vietnamese immigrants, lack of familiarity with the disease may stem from a lack of education or simply a lack of contact with diabetic patients. Unlike in the United States, type 2 diabetes is relatively rare in Viet Nam, where it is called *tieu duong*—literally, "urinate sugar." In rural areas of the country, people sometimes diagnose the disease if they see ants attracted to the urine (Mull, Nguyen, & Mull, 2001).

In the United States, diabetes is becoming more prevalent in Vietnamese communities. Research indicates that Vietnamese immigrants have adopted an increasingly sedentary lifestyle and higher-calorie diet, which elevate the likelihood of obesity, a major risk factor for diabetes (Mull et al., 2001). In light of these increasing risks, studies have shown that Vietnamese Americans need more education about diabetes. For example, a telephone survey of 426 Vietnamese in Houston, Texas, found that 60% do not recognize common signs of diabetes, such as frequent urination (Baker, Calvert,

Dols, Payne, & Reyes, 2000). An ethnographic study with 40 low-income, diabetic Vietnamese immigrants and eight Vietnamese health providers in Orange County, California, found that ideas about the cause and proper treatment of the disease are culturally influenced. Many patients in this study said that they have used Eastern (herbal) medicine and have a strong aversion to insulin injections. Some patients also said that they lower their dose of oral medications or stop them completely when they feel "out of balance." Almost two-thirds of participants said they have used traditional home remedies, and some expressed a preference for Vietnamese physicians due to ease of language and communication. Three-quarters of the patients have not achieved good control of their diabetes. The study concluded that culturally appropriate education about type 2 diabetes and proper management and treatment options are especially needed in the Vietnamese community (Mull et al., 2001).

Another study among Asian American and Pacific Islander women who delivered babies in a northern California hospital found that 6.1% of Chinese, 6.3% of Filipina, 6.7% of Indian/ Pakistani, 2.2% of Japanese, 4.7% of Korean, 7.2% of Pacific Islander, and 5.7% of Vietnamese mothers had diabetes mellitus. Other studies have shown that women born outside of the United States are significantly more likely to have diabetes during pregnancy (Kiefer, Martin, & Herman, 1999). Since gestational diabetes is an established risk factor for development of type 2 diabetes, additional studies are needed on the manifestations of this disease in immigrant populations such as Vietnamese communities.

Cardiovascular Disease

Cardiovascular disease is a leading cause of death in the United States and in many countries around the world, including Vietnam (Duong, Bohannon, & Ross, 2001). Risk factors for heart disease include low levels of physical activity, low levels of consumption of fruits and vegetables, hypertension, tobacco use, and hyperlipidemia (Grundy, Pasternak, Greenland, Smith, & Fuster, 1999; U.S.

Preventive Services Task Force [USPSTF], 2002). Cardiovascular disease is the leading cause of death among Asian and Pacific Islander women (36% of all deaths) and accounts for 31% of all deaths among Vietnamese women in Vietnam (Hoang, Dao, Wall, Nguyen, & Byass, 2006). Unfortunately, research on cardiovascular disease among Asian American populations, particularly among Vietnamese, is scarce (Coronado et al., 2008).

A few studies have investigated smoking behavior among Vietnamese (Baluja, Park, & Myers, 2003; Bates, Hill, & Barrett-Connor, 1989; Chen, 2001; Ma, Tan, Feeley, & Thomas, 2002), but few have looked at other important risk factors for heart disease, such as level of physical activity, consumption of fruits and vegetables, or frequency of blood pressure and cholesterol checks (Coronado et al., 2008). In a study of 201 Vietnamese in a Gulf Coast community, 44% of participants were hypertensive. Participants said that they believe that hypertension is inherited, has clear symptoms, is caused by lack of daily exercise and by stress, and has no cure. This study demonstrates a need for additional health education regarding hypertension and cardiovascular disease in the Vietnamese American community (Duong et al., 2008).

There is also a need for more preventive education. In a needs assessment survey of 1,523 immigrant Vietnamese American women between the ages of 20 and 79 in Seattle, Washington, researchers examined the relationship between demographic factors and preventive behaviors (Coronado et al., 2008). They found that length of time in the United States is strongly correlated with having received a recent blood pressure check and cholesterol check, but is inversely correlated with level of physical activity and consumption of fruits or vegetables. Having spent 20 years or longer in the United States is also associated with a greater likelihood of smoking. These associations are consistent with previous research showing a correlation between the adoption of more high-risk behaviors and acculturation as well as an increase in access to health care for established immigrants compared to more recent arrivals (Kim, Ziedonis, & Chen, 2007). These findings confirm the need for continued development and implementation of targeted educational campaigns to reduce the risk of cardiovascular disease among Vietnamese Americans. Encouraging the maintenance of protective health practices, such as eating fruits and vegetables and not smoking, may be especially impactful for recent immigrants who have traditionally healthy diets. Additionally, expanding access to preventive health care services, such as cholesterol and blood pressure testing, might reduce the prevalence of cardiovascular disease and mortality among Vietnamese Americans (Coronado et al., 2008).

Obesity

Obesity is a growing health problem in the United States, including for Vietnamese Americans. While rates of obesity and being overweight are lower among Asian American adults than among the general population of adults, evidence is mounting that the risk of being even mildly overweight may be greater for Asian Americans, including Vietnamese Americans, than for other ethnic groups (Harrison et al., 2005). Likewise, the prevalence of being overweight in younger generations has increased dramatically over the last few decades (Ogden, Flegal, Carroll, & Johnson, 2002), doubling since 1980 for children and tripling for adolescents (Hedley et al., 2004). In fact, Asian Americans and Pacific Islanders have the fastest-growing rate of overweight and obese children. Unfortunately, studies and data on Vietnamese American communities are very limited. One study that examined survey results from the National Latino and Asian American Survey, a nationally-representative health population survey with 2,554 Latinos and 2,095 Asian Americans (of which 516 were Vietnamese) from 2002 to 2003, found statistically significant increases in Body Mass Index (BMI) and obesity for the Chinese and "other Asian" subgroups. In contrast, among Vietnamese, there was a statistically significant decrease in BMI and obesity between the first and second generation, but data were insufficient to generate

estimates for the third generation (Bates, Acevedo-Garcia, Alegria, & Krieger, 2008).

In another study survey with 2,816 Vietnamese, white, African American, and Hispanic adolescents in Worcester, Massachusetts, Vietnamese students had a 35.5% and 15.3% greater intake of fruits and vegetables, respectively, but had a 44.6% lower intake of dairy foods than white students. The study authors noted that this behavior may be culturally shaped, since the native Vietnamese diet is low in animal products and high in fruits and vegetables. However, although their diet is *relatively* high in fruits and vegetables, Vietnamese students still do not consume at least five servings per day (Wiecha, Fink, Wiecha, & Hebert, 2001). These findings are consistent with results from other studies and points to the need for more education and interventions that promote healthy eating (Harrison et al., 2005; McGarvey et al., 2006). The 2005 *Report of the U.S. Dietary Guidelines Advisory Committee* concluded that greater consumption of fruits and vegetables is associated with better weight management and reduced risk of type 2 diabetes, cancer, stroke, and perhaps other cardiovascular diseases (DHHS/USDA, 2005). It is therefore crucial to promote these healthy eating practices in Vietnamese American communities.

Tuberculosis

Health beliefs and misconceptions of illness may hinder recognition of the early symptoms or warning signs and delay access to medical treatment for certain diseases. This is especially true for infectious diseases such as tuberculosis (TB). For instance, focus groups conducted in Vietnam found that four types of tuberculosis are recognized (Long, Johansson, Diwan, & Winkist, 1999): (1) *Lao truyen* or inherited TB that is passed down from older generations to younger through family blood; (2) *Lao luc* or physical TB that is caused by hard work, which is believed to affect more men than women; (3) *Lao tam* or mental TB that is caused by too much worrying, which is believed to affect more women than men; and (4) *Lao phoi* or lung TB that is caused by transmission of TB germs through the respiratory system, which is believed to affect more men than women.

In the United States, one study found that newly arrived Vietnamese immigrants in New York feel that tuberculosis is an infectious lung disease, with symptoms such as coughing, weakness, and weight loss (Carey et al., 1997). Some believe that hard manual labor, smoking, alcohol consumption, and poor nutrition are risk factors. Nearly all respondents in this study said that having TB would adversely affect their work, family relationships, and community activities. However, many Vietnamese respondents incorrectly said that it is not possible to have asymptomatic latent TB infection and that TB infection always leads to disease. These beliefs may contribute to delays in TB diagnosis and treatment as well as possible social stigma and social isolation due to incorrect beliefs about transmission routes. As such, more education is needed on infectious diseases such as TB so that immigrant communities who are at high risk, like the Vietnamese, can reduce the prevalence of and mortality from these diseases.

Hepatitis B

Southeast Asians, including Vietnamese Americans, have higher rates of liver cancer than any other racial or ethnic group in the United States. In fact, Vietnamese American men are over ten times more likely to be diagnosed with liver cancer than white men (in California they are seven times more likely). This disparity is attributable to high rates of hepatitis B virus (HBV) infection. A population-based in-person survey conducted in Seattle in 2002 with 345 men and 370 women found that 81% of the respondents had heard of hepatitis B and 67% had been tested for HBV. A majority of participants said that HBV can be transmitted during sexual intercourse, by sharing toothbrushes, and by sharing razors. Less than half said that hepatitis B is not spread by eating food prepared by an infected person or by coughing. One-third did not recall being tested for HBV (Taylor et al., 2005). Low levels of HBV testing remain a

problem in many Vietnamese American subgroups. The study researchers concluded that health education about HBV transmission could encourage patients to seek testing. They recommended targeting intervention programs specifically to Vietnamese immigrant communities who lack a regular source of health care and to physicians who serve Vietnamese communities (Taylor et al., 2004; Taylor et al., 2005).

Cancer

Cancer is one of the leading causes of death for Vietnamese men and women in the United States (Hoyert & Kung, 1997; Shinagawa et al., 1999). High smoking rates and exposure to second-hand smoke contribute to high cancer rates. According to Surveillance, Epidemiology, and End Results data (Miller et al., 1996), rates of nasopharynx, liver, and stomach cancers are high among Vietnamese men. The same study indicated high rates of death for Vietnamese women from cervical, stomach, and thyroid cancers.

A more recent study in California found that Vietnamese have among the highest incidence of and death rates from liver, lung, and cervical cancer (McCracken et al., 2007). In California Vietnamese men have the highest incidence of and death rates from liver cancer of all Asian ethnic groups (54.3 and 35.5 per 100,000, respectively); the incidence rate is more than seven times higher for Vietnamese men than for non-Hispanic white men. Stomach and lung cancer rates are also high for Vietnamese in California, with Vietnamese males having the second highest incidence and the third highest death rate from stomach cancer compared to other Asian ethnic groups. Both Vietnamese men and women have the highest lung cancer incidence rates, even though Vietnamese women have the lowest prevalence of smoking compared to all other Asian groups. Vietnamese women have the highest incidence of and mortality from cervical cancer compared to other Asian ethnic groups. These data mirror national statistics, which show that Vietnamese women suffer from cervical cancer at five times the rate of white women. Much of this can be explained by the lack of Pap testing. For instance, Vietnamese women in California have one of the lowest prevalence of Pap testing within the past 3 years (69.8% compared to 83.8% for Non-Hispanic white women) (McCracken et al., 2007).

Schulmeister and Lifsey (1999) found that Vietnamese American women generally believe that their risk of cervical cancer is low. Some barriers to screening include not having a regular doctor or a gynecologist, cost, and fear of the test. Significant barriers for breast and cervical cancer screening among Vietnamese women include embarrassment and shyness during the physical examination due to cultural taboos regarding private body parts and structural issues such as lack of insurance (Nguyen, Kagawa-Singer, Tanjasiri, & Foo, 2003). Other studies have shown that promising interventions, such as increasing education and access to cancer screening and care have involved media campaigns that address cultural stigmas and beliefs and the use of lay health workers or community-based navigators (Mock, Nguyen, Nguyen, Bui-Tong, & McPhee, 2006; Nguyen, Tran, Kagawa-Singer, & Foo, 2011; Nguyen, Vo, Doan, & McPhee, 2006; Nguyen, Vo, McPhee, & Jenkins, 2001).

Elderly and End-of-Life Care

Cultural issues significantly influence health care and end-of-life decision-making. According to Braun, Pietsch, and Blanchette (2000), culture influences a wide variety of attitudes and medical decisions about death and dying. For example, some Buddhists may believe that those who die in hospitals may have lost souls that wreak havoc on the living, so they avoid hospitals when sick and subsequently delay medical care.

Another issue related to end-of-life care is organ donation. Some Vietnamese are not willing to be organ donors because they believe that donors will be reborn without all of their vital organs in the next life. Some believe that decisions by family members to donate the organs of their dying elders are a sign of disrespect and lack of filial piety (Nakasone, 2000). Despite these cultural barriers, the willingness of Vietnamese to

be organ donors may be increasing. According to Hai et al., (1999), Vietnamese would be more willing to donate organs and tissue if they were doing so for close relatives or friends, if medical care was provided to the donor's family, or if monetary rewards were given for such donations.

The issue of advanced directives among Southeast Asians, including Vietnamese elders, is another area that needs to be examined further. Vaughn, Kiyasu, and McCormick (2000) found that nursing home residents were often listed as "no code" on their resident charts because they had not specified what was to be done in case of a terminal prognosis. Some Vietnamese regard life-saving medical interventions, such as organ transplants or cardiac resuscitation, as disturbing the natural flow of life and as signaling a "bad death," while others view stopping life support as causing or speeding a loved one's death. Palliative care, with its comforting, peaceful, and family-supportive dimensions, may be more acceptable to certain Vietnamese. Many Vietnamese are influenced by Catholic, Taoist, and Buddhist beliefs regarding life and death (Ta & Chung, 1990). Some Vietnamese may not want the dying person to be told that he or she is dying because doing so will bring bad luck (Calhoun, 1985), others may feel that doing so will cause the person to lose hope, some may not want to upset the loved one, and some may think that the information will bring death sooner or feel that discussions about dying show a lack of respect for the soon-to-be departed (Crow, Matheson, & Steed, 2000).

Mental Health

As outlined at the beginning of this chapter, Vietnamese immigrants and refugees have had to endure many traumas resulting from their exodus from Vietnam. More than 35 years after the war, many Vietnamese are still suffering from the effects of wartime experiences and their aftermath, including post-traumatic stress, culture shock, the loss of loved ones, adaptation and discrimination challenges, and economic hardship. These traumatic experiences create substantial mental health needs for Vietnamese communities

(Gold, 1992). Despite these needs, Vietnamese Americans drastically underutilize mental health services (Leong, 1986; Nguyen, 1999) and are prone to stop treatment prematurely (Leong & Lau, 2001). This is consistent with the patterns for Asian Americans in general, who are seen as the "model minority," having few social and mental health problems (Sue & Morishima, 1982; Sue & Sue, 1999). However, research over the last three decades has shown that Asian Americans suffer disproportionately from a range of mental health problems that defy the stereotype of the "model minority."

In addition, studies looking at intergroup heterogeneity among persons receiving mental health services demonstrate poorer functioning in Southeast Asian groups, like the Vietnamese, compared to East Asian groups. These differences are undoubtedly linked to their refugee experiences and the subsequent hardships in obtaining services. For example, Vietnamese "re-education camp" survivors have a higher prevalence of psychiatric disorders compared to the general population and to other groups of Vietnamese refugees (Hinton et al., 1993). They have a 90% prevalence rate for post-traumatic stress disorder and a 49% prevalence rate for major depression (Mollica et al., 1998). Utilization rates are much lower and premature termination rates are much higher among Vietnamese than among other ethnic groups (Zane, Hatanaka, Park, & Akutsu, 1994). When they do receive mental health services, Southeast Asian groups, including Vietnamese, show less improvement than other Asian groups (Ying & Hu, 1994). These findings point to the importance of understanding immigration-related factors, as well as place of birth and age/generation group, in explaining the use of mental health services among Vietnamese communities (Abe-Kim et al., 2007). The effect of perceived discrimination and language proficiency on service use also indicates a need for more bilingual services and greater collaboration between formal service systems and community resources (Spencer, Chen, Gee, Fabian, & Takeuchi, 2010).

Recent studies have also highlighted addictive behaviors such as gambling and substance abuse as increasing problems for the Vietnamese American community, especially in places such as California, where Vietnamese populations are larger and gambling casinos are more readily accessible (Glionna, 2006). Studies have indicated that binge drinking is twice as common among Vietnamese men when compared to the general population of the United States (Makimoto, 1998). Among the Asian immigrant populations, Vietnamese have higher levels of alcohol consumption than Japanese, Chinese, Koreans, and Filipinos (Caetano, Clark, & Tam, 1998). Additional research is needed in these areas because of the important implications for health and mental health concerns in the Vietnamese community.

Domestic Violence

Until recently, domestic violence in Asian American immigrant communities, including Vietnamese communities, has been largely ignored by social scientists and policy makers (Kim-Goh & Baello, 2008). This lack of attention is due, in part, to the enduring myth of the "model minority," which perpetuates the notion that all Asian American families are highly educated, physically and emotionally healthy, and financially successful (Leong & Lau, 2001). Another factor contributing to the lack of awareness and research on domestic violence in these communities is that relatively few individuals report incidents of domestic violence to the authorities (Ho, 1990). Research indicates that racial or ethnic minority women may cope with spousal abuse differently than other women (Bauer, Rodriguez, Quiroga, & Flores-Ortiz, 2000; Gondolf, 1997; Huisman, 1996). For example, Asian American women are less likely than women from other racial or ethnic groups to report abuse to the police, or they only report abuse when it is critically severe (Huisman, 1996; Rimonte, 1989). In addition, Asian American women often do not use formal services, such as women's shelters, hospitals, victim service agencies, or lawyers (Bauer et al., 2000; Rimonte, 1989).

Despite the low levels of reporting of domestic violence, domestic violence is a significant issue in Vietnamese communities (Nguyen, 2005).

In one study, 78% of Vietnamese women interviewed indicated that they had experienced physical or verbal abuse within the past year (Tran, 1997).

There appears to be a link between traditional Asian values and domestic violence. In particular, Baba and Murray (2003) identified three major variables that affect violence in relationships among Vietnamese immigrants in the United States: cultural adaptation and traditional gender roles, decision-making power, and marital conflict. With regard to culture and gender roles, the authors found that men who adhere strictly to traditional Vietnamese cultural perspectives are more likely to abuse their partner.

A qualitative study of Vietnamese American immigrants' attitudes toward marital violence found that husbands' patriarchal beliefs and dominant role in the family cause conflicts regarding changing norms and values and that these conflicts are related to domestic abuse (Bui & Morash, 1999). Another study that involved in-depth interviews with 34 abused Vietnamese American women selected from four Vietnamese communities in the United States (Orange County, California; Houston, Texas; Boston, Massachusetts; and Lansing, Michigan) and 11 Vietnamese Americans who had contacts with Vietnamese American victims of domestic violence through their jobs examined help-seeking behavior among abused Vietnamese Americans. This study found that abused Vietnamese American women often seek help from their personal networks as a first resort. However, this sometimes backfires because the advice of family and friends is not always constructive or helpful. Many victims are told to "wait for their spouse to change" or to "avoid making their spouse angry" in order to preserve familial honor or to "save face." When confiding in their support networks does not help, Vietnamese women may turn to the criminal justice system and various victim service agencies; however, the decisions of Vietnamese American women to reach out are complex and shaped by a mix of structural, cultural, and organizational factors. Acculturation on the part of both abused women and victim services could facilitate the efforts of Vietnamese women to seek help outside their personal networks (Bui, 2003). This finding is consistent with other studies that have looked at acculturation and its effects on attitudes toward domestic violence (Kim-Goh & Baello, 2008).

Nail Salons and Occupational Hazards

In 1987 there were 3,900 licensed Vietnamese nail salon workers in the United States; by 2002 this number had increased to 39,600, a tenfold increase in 15 years. The nail salon industry attracts so many Vietnamese workers that Vietnamese is one of the primary foreign-language options for the license examinations in California (California State Board of Barbering and Cosmetology [BBC], 2006). In California, an estimated 59–80% of all manicurists are Vietnamese and 95% are female (Federman, Harrington, & Krynski, 2006; NAILS, 2006).

Vietnamese nail salon workers tend to work long hours in poorly ventilated environments. They are exposed disproportionately to products that contain toxic and potentially hazardous chemicals, including solvents, plasticizers, resins, and acids (Roelofs, Azaroff, Holcroft, Nguyen, & Doan, 2008). Despite these hazards, few studies have examined the chronic health effects of these chemicals on workers.

In a recent survey of 71 Vietnamese nail technicians in Boston, workers reported having experiencing work-related musculoskeletal disorders, headaches, and skin and respiratory problems, and these problems were significantly associated with the degree of exposure, such as poor air quality. The study found that when the workers were away from work for a day or two, the symptoms improved. The absence of skin disorders was associated with the use of gloves, and the presence of musculoskeletal symptoms was associated with the number of years working as a nail technician (Roelofs et al., 2008).

A pilot project of Vietnamese nail salon workers in Alameda County, California (Quach et al., 2008) produced similar findings. In order to inform future health interventions and reduce occupational exposures, researchers conducted face-to-face surveys with a sample of 201 Vietnamese nail salon workers at 74 salons.

A majority of those surveyed (80%) reported that they are concerned about their health. A large proportion (62%) reported having experienced some health problem after they began working in the industry, especially acute health problems that may be associated with exposure to solvents (for example, skin, eye, and throat irritations, breathing difficulties, numbness, and headaches). The study findings also highlighted a critical need to investigate the breast cancer risks of nail salon workers due to their routine use of carcinogenic and endocrine-disrupting chemicals. It is crucial that more research studies be conducted and health interventions be developed for this target community (Quach et al., 2008).

Recommendations and Conclusion

Cultural and social factors play a pivotal role in the health status of Vietnamese Americans. Since a majority of Vietnamese Americans are foreign born, language and cultural barriers remain a major issue in accessing health information and services. For effective communication, health care documentation should be translated to Vietnamese and should be written in easily understood language and presented with visual aids.

The National Assessment of Adult Literacy (NAAL) reported that only 12% of adults nationally have proficient health literacy (Office of Disease Prevention and Health Promotion, n.d.). Nationally, the groups most likely to have low health literacy are the elderly, racial and ethnic populations, immigrants, low-income communities, and individuals with chronic mental and physical conditions (Kutner, Greenberg, & Paulsen 2006). For Vietnamese Americans, data on health literacy are lacking entirely (Dang, 2011). As presented earlier in this chapter, a significant number of Vietnamese Americans have lack of knowledge or misconceptions about certain diseases. These need to be addressed if Vietnamese Americans are to seek out and receive adequate health care. It is also important to improve patient-provider communication. Many recent Vietnamese immigrants and first generation Vietnamese Americans often do not express their health care concerns or

criticism to their health care providers because they fear negative reactions or reprisal by their providers and subsequently do not get good care (Ngo-Metzger et al., 2003). Some Vietnamese Americans feel that they are not respected and are discriminated against due to language and cultural barriers (Dang, 2011; Spencer et al., 2010).

Although research on the health of Vietnamese Americans has been increasing in recent years, significant gaps remain in health data on this population. More comprehensive health research is needed in areas such as diabetes, hypertension, cardiovascular disease, tuberculosis, Hepatitis B, obesity, mental health, gambling, domestic violence, and environmental and occupational hazards. There is a need for more national surveys exploring Vietnamese Americans and health. Research should also explore comparative analysis by age/generation group, socioeconomic and educational backgrounds, acculturation levels, geographical regions, and gender. National data sets should disaggregate data by ethnic group and geography in order to illuminate the diversity of Asian Americans, particularly Vietnamese Americans, so that better health outcomes can be achieved.

References

Abe-Kim, J., Takeuchi, D. T., Hong, S., Zane, N., Sue, S., Spencer, M. S., et al. (2007). Use of mental health – Related services among immigrant and US-born Asian Americans: Results from the National Latino and Asian American study. *American Journal of Public Health, 97*(1), 91–98.

American Community Survey. (2009). Retrieved http://www.census.gov/acs/www/.

Baba, Y., & Murray, S. B. (2003). Spousal abuse, Vietnamese children's reports of parental violence. *Journal of Sociology and Social Welfare, 30,* 97–122.

Baker, S. B., Calvert, R., Dols, J., Payne, L., & Reyes, A. (2000). Asian American diabetes prevalence and awareness: Telephone survey results. *Diabetes Care, 49*(Suppl. 1), A16.

Baluja, K. F., Park, J., & Myers, D. (2003). Inclusion of immigrant status in smoking prevalence statistics. *American Journal of Public Health, 93,* 642–646.

Bates, L. M., Acevedo-Garcia, D., Alegria, M., & Krieger, N. (2008). Immigration and generational trends in body mass index and obesity in the United States: Results of the National Latino and Asian American Survey, 2002–2003. *American Journal of Public Health, 98*(1), 70–77.

Bates, S. R., Hill, L., & Barrett-Connor, E. (1989). Cardiovascular disease risk factors in an Indochinese population. *American Journal of Preventive Medicine, 5*, 15–20.

Bauer, H., Rodriguez, M., Quiroga, S., & Flores-Ortiz, Y. (2000). Barriers to health care for abused Latina and Asian immigrant women. *Journal of Health Care for the Poor and Underserved, 11*, 33–44.

Braun, K. L., Pietsch, J. H., & Blanchette, P. L. (2000). *Cultural issues in end-of-life decision making.* Thousand Oaks, CA: Sage.

Bui, H. N. (2003). Help-seeking behavior among abused immigrant women: A case of Vietnamese American women. *Violence Against Women, 9*, 207–238.

Bui, H. N., & Morash, M. (1999). Domestic violence in the Vietnamese immigrant community: An exploratory study. *Violence Against Women, 5*(7), 769–795.

Caetano, R., Clark, C. L., & Tam, T. (1998). Alcohol consumption among racial/ethnic minorities: Theory and research. *Alcohol Health and Research World, 22*, 233–238.

Calhoun, M. A. (1985). The Vietnamese woman: Health/illness attitudes and behaviors. *Health Care for Women, 6*, 61–72.

California State Board of Barbering and Cosmetology (BBC). (2006). *Application for examination.* Sacramento, CA: Author.

Carey, J. W., Oxtoby, M. J., Nguyen, L. P., Huynh, V., Morgan, M., & Jeffrey, M. (1997). Tuberculosis beliefs among recent Vietnamese Refugees in New York state. *Public Health Reports, 112*, 66–72.

Carter, J. S., Pugh, J. A., & Monterrosa, A. (1996). Non-insulin-dependent diabetes mellitus in minorities in the United States. *Annals of Internal Medicine, 125*, 221–232.

Chen, M. S., Jr. (2001). The status of tobacco cessation research for Asian Americans and Pacific Islanders. *Asian American and Pacific Islander Journal of Health, 9*, 61–65.

Coronado, G., Woodall, E. D., Do, H., Li, L., Yasui, Y., & Taylor, V. (2008). Heart disease prevention practices among immigrant Vietnamese women. *Journal of Women's Health, 17*(8), 1293–1300.

Crow, K., Matheson, L., & Steed, A. (2000). Informed consent and truth-telling: Cultural directions for healthcare providers. *Journal of Nursing Administration, 30*, 148–152.

Dang, J. K. (2011). Vietnamese Americans and health literacy. *Vietnam Talking Points.* Retrieved http://talk.onevietnam.org/vietnamese-americans-and-health-literacy-ready/.

Dao, T. V., & Bankston, C. L., III. (2010). Vietnamese in the USA. In K. Potowski (Ed.), *Language diversity in the USA* (pp. 128–145). New York: Cambridge University Press.

DHHS/USDA. (2005). *Nutrition and your health: Dietary guidelines for Americans. 2005 dietary guidelines advisory committee report.* Retrieved http:www.health.gov/dietaryguidelines/dga2005/report/.

Duong, D. A., Bohannon, A. S., & Ross, M. C. (2008). A descriptive study of hypertension in Vietnamese Americans. *Journal of Community Health Nursing, 18*, 1–11.

Federman, M. N., Harrington, D. E., & Krynski, K. J. (2006). Vietnamese manicurists: Are immigrants displacing natives or finding new nails to polish? *Industrial & Labor Relations Review, 59*, 302–318.

Fujimoto, W. Y. (1995). Diabetes in Asian and Pacific Islander Americans. In *Diabetes in America* (2nd ed., pp. 661–677). Bethesda, MD: National Institutes of Health/National Institute of Diabetes and Digestive and Kidney Diseases, NIH publication 95-1468.

Glionna, J. M. (2006). Gambling, addiction, and Asian culture. *Asian-Nation: The Landscape of Asian America.* Retrieved: http://www.asiannation.org/gambling.shtml/.

Gold, S. J. (1992). Cross-cultural medicine a decade later: Mental health and illness in Vietnamese Refugees. *The Western Journal of Medicine, 157*, 290–294.

Gondolf, E. (1997). Batterer programs: What we know and need to know. *Journal of Interpersonal Violence, 12*, 83–98.

Gordon, S., Bernadett, M., Evans, D., Shapiro, NB., & Dang, L. (2009). Vietnamese culture: Influences and implications for health care. *Molina Health Care.* Retrieved http://www.molinahealthcare.com/medicaid/providers/common/pdf/vietnamese%20culture%20-%20influences%20and%20implications%20for%20health%20care_material%20and%20test.pdf?E=true.

Grundy, S. M., Pasternak, R., Greenland, P., Jr Smith, S., & Fuster, V. (1999). Assessment of cardiovascular risk by use of multiple-risk-factor assessment equations: A statement for healthcare professionals from the American Heart Association and the American College of Cardiology. *Circulation, 100*, 1481–1492.

Hai, T. B., Eastlund, T., Chien, L. A., Duc, P. T., Giang, T. H., Hoa, N. T., et al. (1999). Willingness to donate organs & tissues in Vietnam. *Journal of Transplantation Coordination, 9*, 57–63.

Harrison, G., Kagawa-Singer, M., Foerster, S., Lee, H., Kim, L. P., Nguyen, T.-U., et al. (2005). Seizing the moment: California's opportunity to prevent nutrition-related health disparities in low-income Asian American populations. *Cancer, 104*(Suppl. 12), 1293–1300.

Hedley, A. A., Ogden, C. L., Johnson, C. L., Carroll, M. D., Curtin, L. R., & Flegal, K. M. (2004). Prevalence of overweight and obesity among US Children, adolescents, and adults, 1999–2002. *Journal of the American Medical Association, 291*, 2847–2850.

Hinton, W. L., Chen, Y.-c. J., Du, N., Tran, C. G., Giaouyen, M. A., Lu, F., et al. (1993). DSM-III—R disorders in Vietnamese refugees: Prevalence and correlates. *The Journal of Nervous and Mental Disease, 181*(2), 113–122.

Ho, C. (1990). An analysis of domestic violence in Asian American communities: A multicultural approach to counseling. *Women and Therapy, 9*(12), 129–150.

Hoang, V. M., Dao, L. H., Wall, S., Nguyen, T. K., & Byass, P. (2006). Cardiovascular disease mortality and its association with socioeconomic status: Findings from a population-based cohort study in rural Vietnam, 1999–2003. *Preventing Chronic Disease, 3*(A89), 1–11.

Hoyert, D. L., & Kung, H. (1997). Asian or Pacific Islander mortality, selected states, 1992. *Monthly Vital Statistics Report, 46*(Suppl. 1), 1–63.

Huisman, K. (1996). Wife battering in Asian American communities: Identifying the service needs of an overlooked segment of the U.S. population. *Violence Against Women, 2*, 260–283.

Kiefer, E., Martin, J., & Herman, W. H. (1999). Impact of maternal nativity on the prevalence of diabetes during pregnancy among U.S. Ethnic Groups. *Diabetes Care, 22*(5), 729–735.

Kim, S. S., Ziedonis, D., & Chen, K. W. (2007). Tobacco use and dependence in Asian Americans: A review of the literature. *Nicotine & Tobacco Research, 9*, 169–184.

Kim-Goh, M., & Baello, J. (2008). Attitudes toward domestic violence in Korean and Vietnamese immigrant communities: Implications for human services. *Journal of Family Violence, 23*, 647–654.

Kutner, M., Greenberg, E., Jin, Y., & Paulsen, C. (2006). *The health literacy of America's adults: Results from the 2003 National Assessment of Adult Literacy*. Washington, DC: U.S. National Center for Education Statistics.

Leong, F. T. L. (1986). Counseling and psychotherapy with Asian Americans: Review of the literature. *Journal of Counseling Psychology, 33*, 196–206.

Leong, F. T. L., & Lau, A. S. L. (2001). Barriers to providing effective mental health services to Asian Americans. *Mental Health Services Research, 3*(4), 201–214.

Long, N. H., Johansson, E., Diwan, V. K., & Winkist, A. (1999). Different tuberculosis in men and women: Beliefs from focus groups in Vietnam. *Social Science and Medicine, 49*, 815–822.

Ma, G., Tan, Y., Feeley, R. M., & Thomas, P. (2002). Perceived risks of certain types of cancer and heart disease among Asian American smokers and non-smokers. *Journal of Community Health, 27*, 233–246.

Makimoto, K. (1998). Drinking patterns and drinking problems among Asian-Americans and Pacific Islanders. *Alcohol Health and Research World, 22*(4), 270–275.

McCracken, M., Olsen, M., Chen, M. S., Jemal, A., Thun, M., Cokkinides, V., et al. (2007). Cancer incidence, mortality, and associated risk factors among Asian Americans of Chinese, Filipino, Vietnamese, Korean, and Japanese ethnicities. *CA: a Cancer Journal for Clinicians, 57*, 190–205.

McGarvey, E. L., Collie, K. R., Fraser, G., Shufflebarger, C., Lloyd, B., & Norman Oliver, M. (2006). Using focus group results to inform preschool childhood obesity prevention programming. *Ethnicity and Health, 11*(3), 265–285.

McNeely, M., & Boyko, E. J. (2004). Type 2 diabetes prevalence in Asian Americans. *Diabetes Care, 27*(1), 66–69.

Miller, B. A., Kolonel, L. N., Berstein, L., Young, J. L., Jr., Swanson, G. M., West, D., et al. (Eds.). (1996). *Racial/ethnic patterns of cancer in the United States 1988–1992*. Bethesda: National Cancer Institute, (NIH Pub. No. 96-4104).

Mock, J., Nguyen, T., Nguyen, K. H., Bui-Tong, N., & McPhee, S. J. (2006). Processes and capacity-building benefits of lay health worker outreach focused on preventing cervical cancer among Vietnamese. *Health Promotion Practice, 7*, 223S–232S.

Mollica, R. F., McInnes, K., Pham, T., Fawzi, M. C. S., Murphy, E., & Lin, L. (1998). The dose-effect relationships between torture and psychiatric symptoms in Vietnamese ex-political detainees and a comparison group. *Journal of Nervous Mental Disorder, 186*, 543–553.

Montero, D. (1979). Vietnamese refugees in America: Toward a theory of spontaneous international migration. *International Migration Review*. Retrieved http://www.jstor.org/pss/2545179.

Mull, D. S., Nguyen, N., & Mull, J. D. (2001). Vietnamese diabetic patients and their physicians: What ethnography can teach us. *The Western Journal of Medicine, 175*, 307–311.

NAILS. (2006). 2006 nail technician demographics. In *Nails magazine 2005–2006 big book*. Torrance, CA: Author.

Nakasone, R. Y. (2000). Buddhist issues in end-of-life decision making. In K. L. Braun, J. H. Pietsch, & P. L. Blanchette (Eds.), *Cultural issues in end-of-life decision making* (pp. 213–230). Thousand Oaks, CA: Sage.

Nelson, K. R., Bui, H., & Samet, J. H. (1997). Screening in special populations: A "case study" of recent Vietnamese immigrants. *American Journal of Medicine, 102*, 435–440.

Ngo-Metzger, Q., Massagli, M. P., Clarridge, B. R., Manocchia, M., Davis, R. B., Iezzoni, L. I., & Phillips, R. S. (2003). Linguistic and cultural barriers to care: Perspectives of Chinese and Vietnamese immigrants. *Journal of General Internal Medicine, 18*(1), 44–52.

Nguyen, Q. X. (1999). *Vietnamese individuals' attitudes toward seeking mental health services: Influence of cultural variables*. Ann Arbor, MI: Bell & Howell, UMI No. 9967270.

Nguyen, T. D. (2005). *Domestic violence in Asian American communities: A cultural overview*. Lanham, MD: Lexington Books.

Nguyen, T.-U., Kagawa-Singer, M., Tanjasiri, S. P., & Foo, M. A. (2003). Vietnamese American women's health: A community perspective and report. *Amerasia Journal, 29*(1), 183–197.

Nguyen, T.-U., Tran, J. H., Kagawa-Singer, M., & Foo, M. A. (2011). A qualitative assessment of community-based breast health navigator services for Southeast Asian women in Southern California: Recommendations for developing a navigator training curriculum. *American Journal of Public Health, 101*(1), 87–93.

Nguyen, B. H., Vo, P. H., Doan, H. T., & McPhee, S. J. (2006). Using focus groups to develop interventions to promote colorectal cancer screening among Vietnamese Americans. *Journal of Cancer Education, 21*, 80–83.

Nguyen, T., Vo, P. H., McPhee, S. J., & Jenkins, C. N. (2001). Promoting early detection of breast cancer among Vietnamese-American women. Results of a controlled trial. *Cancer, 92,* 267–273.

Office of Disease Prevention and Health. (n.d.). *Quick guide to health literacy.* U.S. Department of Health and Human Services. Retrieved http://www.health.gov/communication/literacy/quickguide/factsbasic.htm.

Ogden, C. L., Flegal, K. M., Carroll, M. D., & Johnson, C. L. (2002). Prevalence and trends in overweight among US children and adolescents, 1999–2000. *Journal of the American Medical Association, 288,* 1728–1732.

Pham, T. M., Rosenthal, M. P., & Diamond, J. J. (1999). Hypertension, cardiovascular disease, & health care dilemmas in the Philadelphia Vietnamese community. *Family Medicine, 31,* 647–651.

Quach, T., Nguyen, K.-D., Doan-Billings, P.-A., Okahara, L., Fan, C., & Reynolds, P. (2008). A preliminary survey of Vietnamese nail Salon workers in Alameda County, California. *Journal of Community Health, 33,* 336–343.

Rimonte, N. (1989). Domestic violence among Pacific Asians. In Asian Women United of California (Ed.), *Making waves: An anthology of writings by and about Asian American Women* (pp. 327–337). Boston: Beacon.

Roelofs, C., Azaroff, L. S., Holcroft, C., Nguyen, H., & Doan, T. (2008). Results from a community-based occupational health survey of Vietnamese-American nail salon workers. *Journal of Immigrant and Minority Health, 10,* 353–361.

Rumbaut, R. (1995). Vietanmese, Laotian, and Cambodian Americans. In P. G. Min (Ed.), *Asian Americans: Contemporary trends and issues* (pp. 232–266). Thousand Oaks, CA: Sage.

Rutledge, P. J. (1992). *The Vietnamese experience.* Bloomington/Indianapolis: Indiana University Press.

Schulmeister, L., & Lifsey, D. S. (1999). Cervical cancer screening knowledge, behaviors, and beliefs of Vietnamese women. *Oncology Nursing Forum, 26,* 879–887.

Shinagawa, S., Kagawa-Singer, M., Chen, M., Tsark, J., Palafox, N., & Mackura, G. (1999). Cancer registries and data for Asian Americans and native Hawaiians and Pacific Islanders: What registrars need to know. *Journal of Registry Management, 26,* 128–141.

Siganga, W. W., & Huynh, T. C. (1997). Barriers to the use of pharmacy services: The case of ethnic populations. *Journal of the American Pharmacy Association, NS37,* 335–340.

Spencer, M. S., Chen, J., Gee, G. C., Fabian, C. G., & Takeuchi, D. T. (2010). Discrimination and mental health-related service use in a national study of Asian Americans. *American Journal of Public Health, 100*(12), 2410–2417.

Sue, S., & Morishima, J. K. (1982). *The mental health of Asian-Americans.* San Francisco: Jossey-Bass.

Sue, D. W., & Sue, D. (1999). *Counseling the culturally different* (3rd ed.). New York: Wiley.

Ta, M., & Chung, C. (1990). Death and dying: A Vietnamese cultural perspective. In J. K. Parry (Ed.), *Social work practice with the terminally III: A transcultural perspective* (pp. 191–204). Springfield, IL: Charles C. Thomas.

Tanjasiri, S. P., Kagawa-Singer, M., Nguyen, T. N., & Foo, M. A. (2002). Collaborative research as an essential component for addressing cancer disparities among Southeast Asian and Pacific Islander women. *Health Promotion Practice, 3*(2), 144–154.

Taylor, V. M., Choe, J. H., Yasui, Y., Li, L., Burke, N., & Jackson, C. (2005). Hepatitis B awareness, testing, and knowledge among Vietnamese American men and women. *Journal of Community Health, 30*(6), 477–490.

Taylor, V. M., Yasui, Y., Burke, N., Nguyen, T., Chen, A., Acorda, E., et al. (2004). Hepatitis B testing among Vietnamese American men. *Cancer Detection and Prevention, 28*(3), 170–177.

Tran, C. G. (1997). *Domestic violence among Vietnamese Refugeee women: Prevalence, abuse characteristics, psychiatric symptoms, and psychological factors.* Doctoral dissertation, Boston University, Boston

Trinh, T. N. L. (2002). *Vietnamese traditional family values.* Retrieved http://www.vietspring.org/values/traditionalval.html.

Tung, T. M. (1980). *Indochinese patients.* Washington, DC: Action for South East Asians.

U.S. Preventive Services Task Force (USPSTF). (2002). *Guide to clinical preventive services: Screening for breast cancer.* Baltimore: Wiliams & Wilkins.

Vaughn, G., Kiyasu, E., & McCormick, W. C. (2000). Advance directives preferences among subpopulations of Asian nursing home residents in the Pacific Northwest. *Journal of the American Geriatrics Society, 48,* 554–557.

Wiecha, J. M., Fink, A. K., Wiecha, J., & Hebert, J. (2001). Differences in dietary patterns of Vietnamese, White, African-American, and Hispanic adolescents in Worcester, Mass. *Journal of the American Dietetic Association, 101*(2), 248–251.

Yee, B. W. K. (1999). Influence of traditional and cultural health practices among Asian women. In *Agenda for research on women's health for the 21st century. Report of the task force on the NIH women's health research Agenda for the 21st Century* (Differences among populations of women, Vol. 6, pp. 150–165). Santa Fe, NM: Office of Research on Women's Health, National Institutes of Health, July 1997.

Yee, B. W. K. (2004). *Health and health care of Southeast Asian American elders: Vietnamese, Cambodian, Hmong and Laotian elders.* Standford University. Retrieved: http://www.stanford.edu/group/ethnoger/southeastasian.html.

Ying, Y. W., & Hu, L. T. (1994). Public outpatient mental health services: Use and outcome among Asian Americans. *The American Journal of Orthopsychiatry, 64*(3), 448–455.

Zane, N., Hatanaka, H., Park, S. S., & Akutsu, P. (1994). Ethnic specific mental health services: Evaluation of the parallel approach for Asian-American clients. *Journal of Community Psychology, 22,* 68–81.

Emerging South Asian Americans and Health

8

Shilpa Patel and Nadia Islam

Introduction

South Asian Americans, comprised of individuals from the countries of India, Bangladesh, Pakistan, Sri Lanka, Nepal, and Bhutan, encompass a wide group that varies in terms of ethnicity, language and health. However, this rich diversity is generally masked in health research as all of these groups are often lumped into the Asian American group. Further, when the Asian American literature disaggregates into the South Asian group, much of this research focuses on the Asian Indians and does not consider the other groups in the South Asian population. This lack of research on within-group differences among this diverse group is needed as they could explain many of the racial and ethnic health disparities that this group faces (Bulatao & Anderson, 2004).

Two growing South Asian populations with distinctive characteristics that should be studied more are Bangladeshis and Pakistanis in America. These groups, relatively new to the South Asian American community but experiencing tremendous population growth, share both commonalities and differences with Asian Americans. Bangladeshis and Pakistanis have varied socioeconomic backgrounds, unique cultural factors, and face various environmental factors compared to other ethnic groups in the United States. All of these factors combine to affect the health status of Pakistanis and Bangladeshis and thus a more detailed understanding of these factors, separate and in combination, is needed in order to mitigate the barriers and health conditions these groups deal with.

Immigration Patterns

The immigration experience of Bangladeshis and Pakistanis is quite different from other South Asian Americans. A large influx of Asian Indians came into the United States in the 1960s and 1970s. Most of these immigrants were well-educated young professionals that came to the country for work (Bateman, Abesamis, & Ho-Asjoe, 2009). However, most of the Bangladeshis and Pakistanis immigrated to the United States in the 1980s, after the Asian Indians had already settled into the country. These groups were often less educated, had a lower income level, and had higher unemployment rates compared to the previous South Asian immigrants (Trinh-Shevrin, Islam, & Rey, 2009). This lack of educational and financial resources is an added layer of vulnerability that these two groups must also deal with as they begin their life in the United States.

S. Patel (✉)
NYU School of Medicine,
NYU Prevention Research Center, NYU Center for the Study of Asian American Health, New York, USA
e-mail: Shilpa.Patel@nyumc.org

N. Islam
Department of Medicine, NYU Prevention Research Center, NYU Center for the Study of Asian American Health, New York University School of Medicine, New York, NY
e-mail: nadia.islam@nyumc.org

G.J. Yoo et al. (eds.), *Handbook of Asian American Health*,
DOI 10.1007/978-1-4614-2227-3_8, © Springer Science+Business Media, LLC 2013

Both of these populations have recently experienced dramatic growth. The 2009 American Community Survey reported the Bangladeshi population grew to 102, 983 individuals, a dramatic 149% increase from the 2000 Census (US Census, 2000). Certain areas have seen even larger population growth of Bangladeshis. From 1990 to 2000, the Bangladeshi population in New York City increased by 471% (CSAAH, 2007). The Pakistani population in the United States also saw a similar increase. The American Community Survey lists the population at 333,064 individuals in 2009, which corresponds to a population increase of 117% in 9 years (US Census, 2000). From 1990 to 2000, the Pakistani group grew by 154% in the country (CSAAH, 2007).

Bangladeshi Americans

In 2000, there were almost 12 million people who reported being either Asian alone or in combination with other races. Of this group, 57,412 individuals identified themselves as Bangladeshi only or in some combination in 2000. Of the Bangladeshi population that is 25 years and over, about half (45%) had a bachelors degree or higher. Most of this population (83%) was foreign-born, with 86% speaking a language other than English at home. The median household income of Bangladeshi-Americans in 2000 was slightly lower than the national median income at $37,074 compared to national median income of $41,994. However, the Bangladeshi per capita income of $13,532 was substantially lower than the national average of $21,587. Similarly, a large number of Bangladeshis faced financial difficulty as over 20% of the population lived under the poverty level in 2000 (Table 8.1) (US Census, 2000).

Demographic data is quite different for the Bangladeshi population when disaggregated by gender. Eighteen percent of Bangladeshi men over 25 years in the 2000 Census had less than a high school education, yet about half (51%) had a bachelor's degree or higher. Thirty-two percent of Bangladeshi women reported that they had less than a high school education and only 36% had a bachelor's degree or higher. Both groups

Table 8.1 Characteristics of Bangladeshis from 2000 U.S. census

General characteristics	Bangladesh	Total population
Total population	57,412	281,421,906
Male	33,403	138,053,563
Female	24,009	143,368,343
Median age	29	35
Under 5 years	5,691	19,175,798
18 years and over	40,575	209,128,094
Population 25 years and over	34,669	182,211,639
High school graduate or higher	26,631	146,496,014
Bachelors degree or higher	15,715	44,462,605
Foreign born	47,740	31,107,889
Speak a language other than English at home	49,354	46,951,595
Median household income in 1999 (dollars)	$37,074	$41,994
Per capita income in 1999 (dollars)	$13,532	$21,587
Individuals below poverty level	12,953	33,899,812

are linguistically isolated. Almost a third of Bangladeshi men and women reported that they had no one over the age of 14 that spoke English well at home (Trinh-Shevrin et al., 2009).

Pakistani Americans

There were 204,309 individuals who reported being either Pakistani only or Pakistani in combination with another race living in the United States. Of the population that is 25 years and over, about half (51%) had a bachelors degree or higher. Seventy-five percent of the population group was foreign-born and 83% spoke a language other than English at home. The median household income level of Pakistanis in the United States at $45,576 was higher than the national average of $41,994 but like the Bangladeshi group, the per capita income for Pakistanis at $17,685 was lower than the national average at $21,587. Another similarity to the

Table 8.2 Characteristics of Pakistani Americans, US Census (2000)

General characteristics	Bangladeshi	Total population
Total population	204,309	281,421,906
Male	115,016	138,053,563
Female	89,293	143,368,343
Median age	28	35
Under 5 years	20,617	19,175,798
18 years and over	137,004	209,128,094
Population 25 years and over	116,623	182,211,639
High school graduate or higher	94,573	146,496,014
Bachelors degree or higher	60,027	44,462,605
Foreign born	154,300	31,107,889
Speak a language other than English at home	170,308	46,951,595
Median household income in 1999 (dollars)	$45,576	$41,994
Per capita income in 1999 (dollars)	$17,685	$21,587
Individuals below poverty level	36,598	33,899,812

Bangladeshis is many of the Pakistanis living in the United States were experiencing financial distress, as about 18% lived under the poverty level in 2000 (US Census, 2000) (Table 8.2).

There are other similarities between Bangladeshi and Pakistani Americans. Important gender differences among the Pakistani American population, especially in terms of educational attainment are noted. Only 14% of the Pakistani male population in the United States had less than a high school education in 2000, while over half had a bachelor's degree or higher. On the other hand, a quarter of the Pakistani female population had less than a high school education but 44% had a bachelor's degree or higher. Although not as high as the Bangladeshi population, Pakistani men and women also reported a high degree of linguistic isolation, with rates in both groups at about 15% (Trinh-Shevrin et al., 2009).

Health Issues Facing the Bangladeshi and Pakistani Populations

Asian Americans have often been grouped as one demographic in medical research, mostly due to the limited sample size of this population in studies. One of the results of this grouping is that this group is often labeled the "model minority," where Asian Americans are generally thought to be in better health than the general population because of their higher socioeconomic status and better health status compared to other groups in the country (APIAHF, 2006). In general, Asians Americans have a lower prevalence and, as a result, lower cause-specific death rates, for almost all of the leading causes of death compared to all other ethnic groups in the United States (Bateman et al., 2009).

Some studies do evaluate South Asians as an aggregated separate group, yet even this distinction conceals some important details about Pakistanis and Bangladeshis as well as other characteristics of this diverse group (Islam, Kwon, Senie, & Kathuria, 2006). To reiterate, not all South Asian Americans are uniformly wealthy and/or healthy. Further, when the South Asian group is actually disaggregated, most authors focus on Asian Indians and often do not consider Bangladeshis or Pakistanis separately.

Diabetes

One disease prevalent among Asians in general and South Asians in particular is diabetes mellitus. Diabetes is now the fifth leading cause of death for the Asian American and Pacific Islander population (The Office of Minority Health, 2007). Using data from the National Health Interview Survey from 1997 to 2008, Lee, Brancati, and Yeh, (2011) found that even though Asian Americans had lower rates of several risk factors for diabetes, including higher education and less smoking, they still were 30% more likely to have Type 2 diabetes compared to Whites (Lee et al.). The South Asian community is especially vulnerable to the disease, with an incidence rate that is two to seven times higher than the rates of non-Hispanic Whites in the country (Bhopal et al., 1999; Rajpathak et al., 2010).

Perhaps more alarming, when the data on diabetes is disaggregated, it is apparent that Pakistanis and Bangladeshis are especially vulnerable to the disease. Bangladeshis in their native country already have high rates of the disease. In 2000, the World Health Organization reported that Bangladesh had 3,196,000 diabetics, which is projected to increase to 11,140,000 by 2030. Though some research has found a higher prevalence of diabetes in urban populations (8.1%) compared with rural populations (2.3%) in Bangladesh (Hussain, Rahim, Azad Khan, Ali, & Vaaler, 2005), other research has shown that diabetes is on the increase even in rural populations in Bangladesh (Rahim et al., 2007).

Consequently, the disease is also prevalent among Bangladeshi immigrants living abroad. In the United Kingdom, the source of many studies on the Bangladeshi immigrant population, Bangladeshis have a higher prevalence of diabetes compared to any other ethnic group (Choudhury, Brophy, & Williams, 2009), though screening rates for diabetes among these groups are also low. In the United States, results from a community health and resource needs assessment among South Asians in New York City found that two-thirds of the respondents had ever been screened for diabetes, with 17% of those respondents were told by health professionals that they had diabetes (CSAAH, 2007).

Gestational diabetes, linked to adverse infant health outcomes including childhood obesity as well as later maternal development of Type 2 diabetes, is also higher among Bangladeshis and Pakistanis. Thorpe et al. (2005) analyzed 1.5 million New York City birth records between 1990 and 2001. The authors discovered that South and Central Asian women had the highest prevalence of gestational diabetes in New York City (11.1%) compared to other racial and ethnic groups in New York City (4.2%). Women of these populations also had one of the highest increases for gestational diabetes, specifically a 95% increase since 1990, compared to other women in NYC.

When this group is further disaggregated, Bangladeshis and Pakistanis are found to be even more vulnerable to gestational diabetes. In an analysis of NYC births between 1995 and 2003, Savitz et al. found that among the high rates of gestational diabetes for South Central Asians, the greatest risks were for women from Bangladesh (RR = 7.1) and Pakistan (RR = 4.6), and their risk seemed to be rising over time (Savitz, Janevic, Engel, Kaufman, & Herring, 2008).

Cardiovascular Disease

Similar to diabetes, rates of cardiovascular disease (CVD) are prevalent among South Asians. In this population, the leading cause of mortality among Asian Indians in the United States is due to CVD (Chang, Fernando, de Abrew, & Sheriff, 1998), while first generation Asian Indians have a higher prevalence of CVD compared with other Asians and non-Hispanic Whites (Enas et al., 1996).

In another parallel to diabetes, Bangladeshis and Pakistanis are particularly vulnerable to CVD among South Asians. The two groups have an increased risk of dying from coronary heart disease (CHD) compared to Whites (Williams, Stamatakis, Chandola, & Mark Hamer, 2010), with Pakistani women in particular at a higher risk for cardiovascular disease compared to American women, possibly due to the higher risk of developing dyslipidemia in this group (Periyakoil, Mendez, & Buttar, 2010). Bhopal et al. (1999) also reported that among Indian, Pakistani, Bangladeshi and European individuals, Bangladeshi men and women had the highest risk profiles for 9 of the 15 coronary heart disease risk factors (Bhopal et al., 1999). Additionally, in a study of Asian Americans in Northern California, South Asians were 3.7 times more likely to have ischemic heart disease compared to other Asian ethnic groups (Klatsky, Tekawa, Armstrong, & Sidney, 1994).

The risk of CHD for these two groups seems to be increasing with acculturation. Harding, Rosato and Teyhan, (2008) found that the risk for coronary mortality increased with time for Bangladeshis and Pakistanis in Wales and England (Harding et al.). The authors posit several reasons for this finding, including positive selection of more recent migrants to Wales and England, environmental factors in the country of origin and country of immigration that could affect risk of getting the disease later in life, and artefactual factors including the limited sample size.

Bangladeshis also have higher rates of metabolic syndrome, which increases the risk of heart disease. Metabolic syndrome is a combination of risk factors such as elevated blood pressure, dyslipidemia, and elevated glucose levels (Grundy et al., 2005). A recent study of 91 Bangladeshi immigrant men in Texas found that 38% had this syndrome. Significant risk factors for metabolic syndrome for this sample included poor self-rated health status, younger age and increased weight (Rianon & Rasu, 2010).

Cancer

Some diseases have become more prevalent among South Asians as they have immigrated to other parts of the world. One such disease is cancer. As South Asians immigrate to the US and the UK and adopt a more Western lifestyle, rates of cancer increase compared to those still residing in the native country (Deapen, Liu, Perkins, Bernstein, & Ross, 2002; Harding, 2003; Winter et al., 1999). In effect, incidence rates for common cancers such as colon and breast cancer – while decreasing for the general population – are actually increasing for South Asian immigrants in the US over time (Jain, Mills, & Parikh-Patel, 2005). Rates for lung cancer among South Asian men in Britain are also increasing (Smith, Peake, & Botha, 2003).

Although much research has not been conducted among Bangladeshis in the US in terms of cancer, recent studies combining Indian and Pakistani together as one group have shown greater cancer morbidity compared to other South Asians. By using Surveillance, Epidemiology, and End Results (SEER) data, Kakarala found that Asian Indians/Pakistani women younger than 40 years are being diagnosed with breast cancer at a disproportionately higher rate compared to Caucasian women (Kakarala, Rozek,

Cote, Liyanage, & Brenner, 2010). Similarly, by using SEER data from 17 regions, Ooi et al. found that compared to non-Hispanic White women, Asian Indian/Pakistani women had higher odds of being diagnosed with a more advanced stage of breast cancer (Stage III or Stage IV), but had lower odds of dying from the disease (Ooi, Martinez, & Li, 2010).

Men also experience cancer incidence and prevalence changes associated with emigration from their native country. Prostate cancer, which is not prevalent in most Asian countries, is now a significant health risk for Asian American men. Moreover, prostate cancer is now the most commonly diagnosed cancer for Asian Indian/Pakistani men (Bateman et al., 2009; Hossain, Sehbai, Abraham, & Abraham, 2008).

One of the reasons for the increased cancer morbidity and mortality is low rates of cancer screening. By utilizing SEER data from five regions, Hedeen et al. found that Asian American women, and in particular Indian/Pakistani women who immigrated to the United States, were not receiving timely mammograms. As a result, more women in these groups were found to have a greater proportion of tumors that were larger than 1 cm, compared to white females with breast cancer. Of note, this was not observed among Indian/Pakistani women who were born in America, which suggests that immigrants in particular are affected by the increase in breast cancer morbidity (Hedeen, White, & Taylor, 1999).

Smaller community based studies have also found low rates of cancer screening for South Asian women. Using a community sample of South Asians in New York City, Islam et al. (2006) reported 70% of South Asian women over the age of 40 had ever had a mammogram, while 67% of women had ever had a Pap test, far from an ideal number (Islam et al., 2006). Data from a Community Health Needs Assessment of South Asians in New York City found that only 32% of South Asian respondents over 50 years had received a colonoscopy, 59% of women had ever had a Pap smear and 78% of women over age 40 had ever had a mammogram (CSAAH, 2007).

Glenn conducted a study of South Asian subgroups in California. Concurring with previous studies, screening rates for South Asians in California were low, with just over half of respondents (57%) reporting getting a Pap test in the past 3 years and only 25% of eligible patients receiving a screening for colorectal cancer (Glenn, Chawla, Surani, & Bastani, 2009a). However, important subgroup differences were seen in receiving different types of cancer screening. For instance, only 4% of eligible Bangladeshis had received a colon cancer screening, yet Pakistanis – who were significantly less likely to get a mammogram – were more likely to get a screening for cervical or colorectal cancer. The authors observed the most significant factor affecting cancer screening was insurance status (Glenn et al.).

Domestic Violence

South Asian women in the United States are at high risk for encountering domestic violence in their lives, with one survey of immigrant South Asian women finding that one in four reported domestic violence in her home (Ayyub, 2000). Other studies have documented an even higher prevalence. A survey of South Asian immigrant women in the Boston area found that 40.8% of the respondents reported intimate partner violence or needing medical care because of intimate partner violence from current male partners in their lifetime. Further, 37% of the sample reported having encountered intimate partner violence in the past year (Raj & Silverman, 2002). The effects of domestic violence are detrimental and can include a loss of self-esteem and identity, depression, anxiety, post traumatic stress syndrome (PTSD), and suicidal ideation (Hurwitz, Gupta, Liu, Silverman, & Raj, 2006; Midlarsky, Venkataramani-Kothari, & Plante, 2006).

However, these women are not seeking care for services related to domestic violence. In the aforementioned study conducted in Boston, only 11% of the women who had reported intimate partner violence actually received any counseling related to the abuse (Raj & Silverman, 2002).

Rianon and Shelton recruited a total of 29 married Bangladeshi immigrant women from Houston, Texas. The authors found that almost all (91%)

said that domestic violence existed in the Bangladeshi community. Most of the respondents (84%) reported that husbands and/or their in-laws were responsible for the abuse. Although most women recognized that domestic violence existed in their community, only two reported actual abuse from their partner (Rianon & Shelton, 2003).

Past literature has suggested that certain characteristics of the general Asian community, including gender roles, the stigma of divorce, and the lack of support systems for some immigrant women, may actually increase the occurrence and tolerance of domestic violence in this community (Midlarsky et al., 2006). In addition, these same factors also prevent women from seeking help for domestic violence. Other factors that may prevent South Asian women from seeking help are often tied to immigration. Besides losing the social support and network from their home country, Asian women also face cultural barriers like limited English skills that make these women financially, emotionally, and legally dependent on their abusive partners (Lee & Hadeed, 2009). The social isolation felt by these women are particularly important to experiencing domestic violence as research has shown an association between social isolation and an increased likelihood of experiencing severe intimate partner violence. Raj found that women who reported having no local family members (other than spouse and children) were three times more likely than those with family in the United States to have been physically abused by their partner (Raj & Silverman, 2003).

Mental Health

South Asians, particularly Pakistanis, are currently experiencing high rates of common mental disorders, anxiety, and depression, even after accounting for measures of socioeconomic status such as employment and social class. In a cross-sectional study conducted in England, the prevalence of common mental disorders was statistically higher for Pakistani men aged 35–54 years and for older Indian and Pakistani women (aged 55–74 years) compared to White respondents of the same age and gender (Weich et al., 2004).

Similarly, Gater et al. (2009) reported that Pakistani women had a higher prevalence of depression compared to White women in England (Gater et al.).

Conversely, the differences between these two groups were no longer significant after the authors adjusted for factors like social support or social difficulties, suggesting that such factors play an important role in Pakistani women and the incidence of depression (Gater et al., 2009). Similarly, a qualitative study of British Pakistani women being treated for depression by Gask, Aseem, Waquas, and Waheed, (2011) found that themes including feeling isolated and feeling "stuck" regarding difficulties with family and martial conflicts were most often cited by these women (Gask et al.). A smaller study of Pakistanis in the UK exploring the social origins of depression found that significant factors included marital, health and housing issues (Husain, Creed, & Tomenson, 1997).

Adolescent Pakistanis have also experienced mental health issues. In a school based survey of nine different ethnic groups, Pakistani youths were at high risk for suicidal behaviors. Compared to White students, this group had a higher rate of suicide attempts and a higher prevalence of suicidal thoughts. The effect persisted even after adjusting for factors such as age, gender, and socioeconomic status (Roberts, Chen, & Roberts, 1997).

The Influence of Social and Cultural Practices on Health and Illness

Numerous sociocultural traditions and practices are associated with the Pakistani and Bangladeshi population that can affect their health and illness. Most of the population from Bangladesh and Pakistan are of the Muslim faith (US Dept of State, 2010). Accordingly, their religious practices and beliefs can have an impact on the health status and behaviors among community members. Muslim women may have reservations regarding engaging in physical activity in public due to prescriptions regarding modest dress in the Muslim tradition. Similarly, Muslim women may be reluctant to seek care from male physicians, particularly regarding sexual health.

At the same time, given the important role of faith in these populations, faith-based strategies may be useful means of health promotion and prevention. For example, Muslim Bangladeshi and Pakistani families often attend weekly Friday prayer services at mosques, which may serve as an opportunity to disseminate health messages and programs. The acculturative process among Pakistani and Bangladeshi immigrants living abroad, whereby they adopt a more "Western lifestyle," may also impact health. As these groups adopt a Western lifestyle, some protective cultural practices they may have had in their native country decrease (Trinh-Shevrin et al., 2009). The effect of these acquired lifestyle habits are further exacerbated by difficulties in accessing healthcare services, as well as linguistic, cultural, economic, and social barriers that these groups may face (Trinh-Shevrin et al.).

Alcohol and Substance Use

Because the Muslim faith bans the use of alcohol and other substances like drugs, rates of alcohol and substance use among these groups are extremely low. Rates of substance use are especially low for women because of their Muslim faith. However, as these groups become more Westernized, rates of alcohol and substance use may rise.

Diet

Diets in the South Asian culture, including the Pakistani and Bangladeshi communities, are often high in saturated fats. For instance, (Kamath et al., 1999) found that compared to American women, Indian and Pakistani women had a higher fat intake (Kamath et al.). In turn, such dietary choices may affect rates of nutritionally-linked diseases like diabetes and CVD by influencing relevant clinical outcomes. In a cross-sectional survey of European, African-Caribbean, and Pakistani individuals in Manchester, England, Vyas et al. found that the highest overall BMI and the highest female waist-to-hip ratio were measured in the female

Pakistani group. Pakistani men and women also had the greatest percentage of energy derived from fat in their diets (Vyas et al., 2003). The dietary habits of these groups may also worsen with greater acculturation (Lauderdale & Rathouz, 2000; Raj, Ganganna, & Bowering, 1999). These observations correlate with other studies, stating as South Asians immigrate to other countries and adopt their diet, they change the frequency of how often they eat traditional food and increasingly consume Western foods (McKeigue et al., 1988).

Smoking

South Asians often use smokeless tobacco in addition to the cigarettes that are more popular in America. Smokeless tobacco encompasses many types of products but for Pakistanis and Bangladeshis, the most common form are *paan*, *paan masala*, *zarda*, and *gutka*. These products are comprised of tobacco, betel nut (also known as areca nut), and other spices and fruits. Both the tobacco and the areca nut in these products are carcinogenic leading to an increase of certain cancers like oral cancers among South Asians (Glenn, Surani, Chawla, & Bastani, 2009b).

Compared to the general population of the U.S., both Pakistani and Bangladeshi men have a higher prevalence of smoking and using these smokeless products (Bhopal et al., 1999; Periyakoil et al., 2010). Smoking in these two groups is very gender specific, as Pakistani and Bangladeshi women have very low smoking rates, though this may change with increasing acculturation (Bush, White, Kai, Rankin, & Bhopal, 2003).

There are consistent reports that smoking and use of tobacco products by Pakistani and Bangladeshi men in particular is frequent. In comparing risk factors for coronary heart disease in Indian, Pakistani, Bangladeshi and European individuals, Bhopal et al. (1999) found that Bangladeshis had the highest prevalence of smoking of all of the groups studied (Bhopal et al., 1999). The high prevalence of smoking among Bangladeshis and Pakistanis is also seen in the United States. Glenn et al. (2009b) reported Bangladeshis living in California were signifi-

cantly more likely to use smokeless tobacco products and Pakistanis were significantly more likely to be daily smokers, when compared to Asian Indians (Glenn et al.).

In a qualitative study conducted by Bush et al., (2003) in the United Kingdom, the authors found that smoking in Bangladeshi men may be more of a culturally specific social phenomenon. In examining the reasons why they smoked, the authors theorized that smoking contributed to group cohesion and identity more among Bangladeshi men than their Pakistani counterparts (Bush et al.).

Exercise

Physical activity among South Asians is generally low, even after taking into account differences in age, sex and subgrouping (Rajpathak et al., 2010; Williams et al., 2010). In particular, Pakistanis and Bangladeshis are more likely to have a sedentary lifestyle compared to other South Asian groups, as well as other ethnic groups in general (Bhopal et al., 1999; Periyakoil et al., 2010). In a longitudinal study of the UK South Asian population, Williams et al. (2010) found that a substantial proportion of the excess mortality in CHD in a South Asian sample could be explained by differences in leisure time physical activity. Likewise, Hayes et al. (2002) reported that South Asians residing in Newcastle, England – and in particular Pakistanis and Bangladeshis – are less physically active than other Europeans. Asian Indian and Pakistani women had lower energy expenditure compared to American females (Kamath et al., 1999). The sedentary lifestyle may contribute to the excess risk of diabetes and CHD morbidity and mortality in these two groups (Hayes et al., 2002; Williams et al., 2010).

The lack of exercise is also observed in younger South Asians. Fischbacher, Hunt, and Alexander (2004) reviewed numerous studies of physical activity and fitness among South Asians living in the United States. The authors reviewed 12 studies of adults and five involving children. All but one study among adolescents found that South

Asian groups had much lower levels (~50–75%) of physical activity compared to the general U.S. population. Among the four studies that looked at different subgroups of South Asians, the Bangladeshi population had the lowest levels of physical activity.

Knowledge of Disease

Knowledge of diseases like diabetes and cardiovascular disease, and how to prevent or manage them, is generally low among South Asians. In a cross-sectional study of South Asians adults in Illinois, Kandula et al. (2010) found that 89% knew little or nothing about coronary heart disease. Knowledge on how to control the disease was especially low. Few respondents knew that controlling blood pressure, cholesterol and diabetes could affect coronary heart disease, with 53% of respondents believing that heart attacks were not preventable.

Disaggregating data into different groups of South Asians reveals various distinctions. Choudhary et al. (2009) found that Bangladeshi individuals residing in the UK did not understand what caused or how to prevent diabetes. Correspondingly, Rankin and Bhopal (2001) found that, among different groups of South Asians in the UK, Bangladeshis had the lowest levels of knowledge about heart disease and diabetes. A study of Bangladeshis in New York City found that over 80% of the sample did not know the meaning of Hemoglobin (Hb) A1c, which is an indicator of diabetes control (Islam et al., 2011).

Language

Over 90% of both the Bangladeshi and Pakistani population speak a language other than English at home and over half of the Bangladeshi population have limited English proficiency, a potential barrier to accessing health services. Bangladeshis experience some of the highest levels of linguistic isolation – having no one 14 years or older in the home that speaks English well – among all AAPI groups (Trinh-Shevrin et al., 2009).

Needed Future Directions in Research for this Group

Given the rich diversity the South Asian American group encompasses, much more study is needed to understand the complexity of this population. Specifically, disaggregated data on members of the South Asian group is necessary to understand the relevant differences among the different sub-populations. However, there are relatively few sources that collect enough data on the general Asian American population to produce meaningful results. Data that allows the disaggregation of the Asian American group, or the disaggregation of the South Asian group, is even rarer. As such, more research is needed that collects enough information that allows the disaggregation of the South Asian American population so these within-group differences are shown.

Focused research is especially needed for Pakistani and Bangladeshi Americans as this population continues to increase, particularly via immigration, to the United States. Not only do these two groups face unique health issues compared to other South Asian groups, they also have numerous financial and social stressors not experienced by South Asian immigrant groups. Pakistani and Bangladeshi Americans have lower socioeconomic status and are more linguistically isolated compared to other South Asians. As such, more information is desirable to understand how this combination of environmental and personal factors affects the health of Pakistanis and Bangladeshis.

Studies focusing on educating these groups on the prevention and management of prevalent diseases are imperative as many investigations demonstrate that Bangladeshis in particular do not know the cause of diabetes and other diseases, let alone what can be done preventatively. A potential resource in educating Pakistanis and Bangladeshis in America may be primary care providers. As such, general information about diseases like diabetes and cancer screenings that is delivered in a culturally appropriate manner from providers could help to ameliorate knowledge gaps in these groups.

Cultural sources such as ethnic language media and local ethnic organizations should also be included as health resources. By delivering health education in the ethnic language, it makes such information more accessible than traditional sources. Previous studies have already found that ethnic media is an effective way to reach the Asian American population (Jenkins et al., 1997, 1999).

Additionally, there are a number of community organizations that are already helping the Pakistani and Bangladeshi population with health-related issues. Examples include the community-based organization Andolan, helping South Asian workers deal with abusive employers (Andolan, 2010). Sakhi is another community-based organization in New York City dedicated to ending violence against women of South Asian origin (Sakhi, 2010). These same resources can be utilized to help educate Pakistanis and Bangladeshis about health.

The various social and economic factors that Pakistanis and Bangladeshis face after immigrating to the United States make the use of the community-based participatory research (CBPR) framework, set forth by Tandon and Kwon, potentially more constructive in garnering needed data. As Pakistanis and Bangladeshis in the United States are not as proficient in English and are more likely to be recent immigrants compared to other ethnic groups, these groups might be wary of a more traditional top-down research paradigm that collects personal information. These two populations have significant health needs, yet traditional research has not captured the health disparities that Pakistanis and Bangladeshis face. CBPR may be useful in collecting information on the health needs of these two groups more accurately. Also, the CBPR approach would allow for a more tailored and culturally appropriate study design. Finally, the use of CBPR with these groups would empower Pakistanis and Bangladeshis as individuals, as they can become agents of change within this framework rather than passive research participants (Trinh-Shevrin et al., 2009).

One such project currently focusing on Bangladeshi Americans is the Diabetes Research, Education and Action for Minorities (DREAM) at New York University. The DREAM project is a 5-year community based participatory research study based in the Center for the Study of Asian American Health at the NYU Langone Medical Center. The goal of the project is to develop, implement, and test a Community Health Worker (CHW) Program designed to improve diabetes control and diabetes-related health complications for the Bangladeshi community in New York City. The community health workers in the DREAM project are community leaders within the Bangladeshi community and as such, the delivery of diabetes education by these leaders may be more effective in educating this group about diabetes than a traditional educational intervention. Results from the pilot study found both a number of facilitators and barriers to diabetes care for this population. Facilitators for managing and preventing diabetes for NYC Bangladeshis included low stigma surrounding the disease and the Bangladeshi media, whereas diabetes-related barriers included language and the widespread availability of high fat food. The results from the pilot study also suggested that CHWs could help the population effectively manage and prevent diabetes and improve behaviors surrounding the disease, including nutrition and exercise (Islam et al., 2011).

More studies that focus on these two groups are needed to improve the health of Bangladeshi and Pakistanis in the United States. These emerging South Asian groups face many barriers that impede health care access in the United States. Efforts must be made to help mitigate the problems that these groups face. Their unique social and cultural factors make efforts to reach this population a vital goal for health care resources and providers.

References

Andolan. (2010). From http://www.andolan.net/index.htm

APIAHF. (2006). Health brief: South Asians in the United States 2010. Retrieved http://www.apiahf.org/resources/resources-database/south-asians-united-states.

Ayyub, R. (2000). Domestic violence in the South Asian Muslim immigrant population in the United States.

Journal of Social Distress and the Homeless, 9, 237–248.

Bateman, W. B., Abesamis, N. F., & Ho-Asjoe, H. (2009). *Praeger handbook of Asian American health: Taking notice and taking action.* Santa Barbara, CA: Praeger.

Bhopal, R., Unwin, N., White, M., Yallop, J., Walker, L., Alberti, K. G. M. M., et al. (1999). Heterogeneity of coronary heart disease risk factors in Indian, Pakistani, Bangladeshi, and European origin populations: Cross sectional study. *British Medical Journal, 319*(7204), 215–220.

Bulatao, R. A., & Anderson, N. B. (2004). *Understanding racial and ethnic differences in health in late life: A research agenda.* Washington, DC: The National Academies Press.

Bush, J., White, M., Kai, J., Rankin, J., & Bhopal, R. (2003). Understanding influences on smoking in Bangladeshi and Pakistani adults: Community based, qualitative study. *British Medical Journal, 326*(7396), 962.

Chang, A. A., Fernando, D. J., de Abrew, K., & Sheriff, M. H. (1998). Teaching and learning about diabetes mellitus: A clarification. *The Ceylon Medical Journal, 43*(2), 115.

Choudhury, S. M., Brophy, S., & Williams, R. (2009). Understanding and beliefs of diabetes in the UK Bangladeshi population. *Diabetic Medicine, 26*(6), 636–640.

CSAAH. (2007). *Community health needs and resource assessment: An exploratory study of South Asians in NYC.* New York: NYU Center for the Study of Asian American Health.

Deapen, D., Liu, L., Perkins, C., Bernstein, L., & Ross, R. K. (2002). Rapidly rising breast cancer incidence rates among Asian-American women. *International Journal of Cancer, 99*(5), 747–750.

Enas, E. A., Garg, A., Davidson, M. A., Nair, V. M., Huet, B. A., & Yusuf, S. (1996). Coronary heart disease and its risk factors in first-generation immigrant Asian Indians to the United States of America. *Indian Heart Journal, 48*(4), 343–353.

Fischbacher, C. M., Hunt, S., & Alexander, L. (2004). How physically active are South Asians in the United Kingdom? A literature review. *Journal of Public Health (Oxford), 26*(3), 250–258.

Gask, L., Aseem, S., Waquas, A., & Waheed, W. (2011). Isolation, feeling 'stuck' and loss of control: Understanding persistence of depression in British Pakistani women. *Journal of Affective Disorders, 128*(1–2), 49–55.

Gater, R., Tomenson, B., Percival, C., Chaudhry, N., Waheed, W., Dunn, G., et al. (2009). Persistent depressive disorders and social stress in people of Pakistani origin and white Europeans in UK. *Social Psychiatry and Psychiatric Epidemiology, 44*(3), 198–207.

Glenn, B. A., Chawla, N., Surani, Z., & Bastani, R. (2009a). Rates and sociodemographic correlates of cancer screening among South Asians. *Journal of Community Health, 34*(2), 113–121.

Glenn, B. A., Surani, Z., Chawla, N., & Bastani, R. R. (2009b). Tobacco use among South Asians: Results of a community-university collaborative study. *Ethnicity and Health, 14*(2), 131–145.

Grundy, S. M., Cleeman, J. I., Daniels, S. R., Donato, K. A., Eckel, R. H., Franklin, B. A., et al. (2005). Diagnosis and management of the metabolic syndrome: An American Heart Association/National Heart, Lung and Blood Institute Scientific Statement. *Circulation, 112*(17), 2735–2752.

Harding, S. (2003). Mortality of migrants from the Indian subcontinent to England and Wales: Effect of duration of residence. *Epidemiology, 14*(3), 287–292.

Harding, S., Rosato, M., & Teyhan, A. (2008). Trends for coronary heart disease and stroke mortality among migrants in England and Wales, 1979–2003: Slow declines notable for some groups. *Heart, 94*(4), 463–470.

Hayes, L., White, M., Unwin, N., Bhopal, R., Fischbacher, C., Harland, J., et al. (2002). Patterns of physical activity and relationship with risk markers for cardiovascular disease and diabetes in Indian, Pakistani, Bangladeshi and European adults in a UK population. *Journal of Public Health Medicine, 24*(3), 170–178.

Hedeen, A. N., White, E., & Taylor, V. (1999). Ethnicity and birthplace in relation to tumor size and stage in Asian American women with breast cancer. *American Journal of Public Health, 89*(8), 1248–1252.

Hossain, A., Sehbai, A., Abraham, R., & Abraham, J. (2008). Cancer health disparities among Indian and Pakistani immigrants in the United States: A surveillance, epidemiology, and end results-based study from 1988 to 2003. *Cancer, 113*(6), 1423–1430.

Hurwitz, E. J., Gupta, J., Liu, R., Silverman, J. G., & Raj, A. (2006). Intimate partner violence associated with poor health outcomes in U.S. South Asian women. *Journal of Immigrant and Minority Health, 8*(3), 251–261.

Husain, N., Creed, F., & Tomenson, B. (1997). Adverse social circumstances and depression in people of Pakistani origin in the UK. *The British Journal of Psychiatry, 171*, 434–438.

Hussain, A., Rahim, M. A., Azad Khan, A. K., Ali, S. M., & Vaaler, S. (2005). Type 2 diabetes in rural and urban population: Diverse prevalence and associated risk factors in Bangladesh. *Diabetic Medicine, 22*(7), 931–936.

Islam, N., Kwon, S. C., Senie, R., & Kathuria, N. (2006). Breast and cervical cancer screening among South Asian women in New York city. *Journal of Immigrant and Minority Health, 8*(3), 211–221.

Islam, N., Tandon, D., Mukherju, R., Tanner, M., Ghosh, K., Alam, G., et al. (2011). Understanding barriers and facilitators to diabetes control and prevention in the New York city Bangladeshi community: A mixed-methods approach to inform the development of a community health worker intervention. *The American Journal Public Health*, [In press].

Jain, R. V., Mills, P. K., & Parikh-Patel, A. (2005). Cancer incidence in the south Asian population of California, 1988–2000. *Journal of Carcinogenesis, 4*, 21.

Jenkins, C. N., McPhee, S. J., Le, A., Pham, G. Q., Ha, N. T., & Stewart, S. (1997). The effectiveness of a media-led intervention to reduce smoking among Vietnamese-American men. *American Journal of Public Health, 87*(6), 1031–1034.

Jenkins, C. N., McPhee, S. J., Bird, J. A., Pham, G. Q., Nguyen, B. H., Nguyen, T., et al. (1999). Effect of a media-led education campaign on breast and cervical cancer screening among Vietnamese-American women. *Preventive Medicine, 28*(4), 395–406.

Kakarala, M., Rozek, L., Cote, M., Liyanage, S., & Brenner, D. E. (2010). Breast cancer histology and receptor status characterization in Asian Indian and Pakistani women in the U.S. – a SEER analysis. *BMC Cancer, 10*, 191.

Kamath, S. K., Hussain, E. A., Amin, D., Mortillaro, E., West, B., Peterson, C. T., et al. (1999). Cardiovascular disease risk factors in 2 distinct ethnic groups: Indian and Pakistani compared with American premenopausal women. *American Journal of Clinical Nutrition, 69*(4), 621–631.

Kandula, N. R., Tirodkar, M. A., Lauderdale, D. S., Khurana, N. R., Makoul, G., & Baker, D. W. (2010). Knowledge gaps and misconceptions about coronary heart disease among U.S. South Asians. *American Journal of Preventive Medicine, 38*(4), 439–442.

Klatsky, A. L., Tekawa, I., Armstrong, M. A., & Sidney, S. (1994). The risk of hospitalization for ischemic heart disease among Asian Americans in northern California. *American Journal of Public Health, 84*(10), 1672–1675.

Lauderdale, D. S., & Rathouz, P. J. (2000). Body mass index in a US national sample of Asian Americans: Effects of nativity, years since immigration and socioeconomic status. *International Journal of Obesity and Related Metabolic Disorders, 24*(9), 1188–1194.

Lee, Y.-S., & Hadeed, L. (2009). Intimate partner violence among Asian immigrant communities: Health/mental health consequences, help-seeking behaviors, and service utilization. *Trauma, Violence & Abuse, 10*(2), 143–170.

Lee, J. W., Brancati, F. L., & Yeh, H. C. (2011). Trends in the prevalence of type 2 diabetes in Asians versus whites: Results from the United States National Health Interview Survey, 1997–2008. *Diabetes Care, 34*(2), 353–357.

McKeigue, P. M., Marmot, M. G., Syndercombe Court, Y. D., Cottier, D. E., Rahman, S., & Riemersma, R. A. (1988). Diabetes, hyperinsulinaemia, and coronary risk factors in Bangladeshis in east London. *British Heart Journal, 60*(5), 390–396.

Midlarsky, E., Venkataramani-Kothari, A., & Plante, M. (2006). Domestic violence in the Chinese and South Asian immigrant communities. *Annals of the New York Academy of Sciences, 1087*, 279–300.

Ooi, S. L., Martinez, M. E., & Li, C. I. (2010). Disparities in breast cancer characteristics and outcomes by race/ethnicity. *Breast Cancer Research and Treatment*.

Periyakoil, V., Mendez, J., & Buttar, A. B. (2010). Health and health care for Pakistani American elders.

Retrieved http://www.stanford.edu/group/ethnoger/pakistani.html.

Rahim, M. A., Hussain, A., Azad Khan, A. K., Sayeed, M. A., Keramat Ali, S. M., & Vaaler, S. (2007). Rising prevalence of type 2 diabetes in rural Bangladesh: A population based study. *Diabetes Research and Clinical Practice, 77*(2), 300–305.

Raj, A., & Silverman, J. G. (2002). Intimate partner violence against South Asian women in greater Boston. *Journal of the American Medical Women's Association, 57*(2), 111–114.

Raj, A., & Silverman, J. G. (2003). Immigrant South Asian women at greater risk for injury from intimate partner violence. *American Journal of Public Health, 93*(3), 435–437.

Raj, S., Ganganna, P., & Bowering, J. (1999). Dietary habits of Asian Indians in relation to length of residence in the United States. *Journal of the American Dietetic Association, 99*(9), 1106–1108.

Rajpathak, S. N., Gupta, L. S., Waddell, E. N., Upadhyay, U. D., Wildman, R. P., Kaplan, R., et al. (2010). Elevated risk of type 2 diabetes and metabolic syndrome among Asians and south Asians: Results from the 2004 New York City HANES. *Ethnicity & Disease, 20*(3), 225–230.

Rankin, J., & Bhopal, R. (2001). Understanding of heart disease and diabetes in a South Asian community: Cross-sectional study testing the 'snowball' sample method. *Public Health, 115*(4), 253–260.

Rianon, N. J., & Rasu, R. S. (2010). Metabolic syndrome and its risk factors in Bangladeshi immigrant men in the USA. *Journal of Immigrant Health, 12*(5), 781–787.

Rianon, N. J., & Shelton, A. J. (2003). Perception of spousal abuse expressed by married Bangladeshi immigrant women in Houston, Texas, U.S.A. *Journal of Immigrant Health, 5*(1), 37–44.

Roberts, R. E., Chen, Y. R., & Roberts, C. R. (1997). Ethnocultural differences in prevalence of adolescent suicidal behaviors. *Suicide & Life-Threatening Behavior, 27*(2), 208–217.

Sakhi. (2010). About sakhi for South Asian women. Retrieved http://www.sakhi.org/about/index.php.

Savitz, D. A., Janevic, T. M., Engel, S. A. M., Kaufman, J. S., & Herring, A. H. (2008). Ethnicity and gestational diabetes in New York City, 1995–2003. *BJOG: An International Journal of Obstetrics and Gynaecology, 115*(8), 969–978.

Smith, L. K., Peake, M. D., & Botha, J. L. (2003). Recent changes in lung cancer incidence for south Asians: A population based register study. *British Medical Journal, 326*(7380), 81–82.

The Office of Minority Health. (2007). *HHS fact sheet: Minority health disparities at a glance*. US Department of Health and Human Services.

Thorpe, L. E., Berger, D., Ellis, J. A., Bettegowda, V. R., Brown, G., Matte, T., et al. (2005). Trends and racial/ethnic disparities in gestational diabetes among pregnant women in New York City, 1990–2001. *American Journal of Public Health, 95*(9), 1536–1539.

Trinh-Shevrin, C., Islam, N. S., & Rey, M. J. (2009). *Asian American communities and health.* San Francisco: Wiley.

US Census. (2000). Retrieved http://www.census.gov/.

US Dept of State. (2010). *Background 2010.* Retrieved http://www.state.gov/r/pa/ei/bgn/3452.htm.

Vyas, A., Greenhalgh, A., Cade, J., Sanghera, B., Riste, L., Sharma, S., et al. (2003). Nutrient intakes of an adult Pakistani, European and African-Caribbean community in inner city Britain. *Journal of Human Nutrition and Dietetics, 16*(5), 327–337.

Weich, S., Nazroo, J. Y., Sproston, K., McManus, S., Blanchard, M., Erens, B., et al. (2004). Common mental disorders and ethnicity in England: The EMPIRIC study. *Psychological Medicine, 34*(8), 1543–1551.

Williams, E. D., Stamatakis, E., Chandola, T., & Mark Hamer, M. (2010). Physical activity behaviour and coronary heart disease mortality among South Asian people in the UK: An observational longitudinal study. *Heart.* doi:10.1136/hrt.2010.201012.

Winter, H., Cheng, K. K., Cummins, C., Maric, R., Silcocks, P., & Varghese, C. (1999). Cancer incidence in the south Asian population of England (1990–92). *British Journal of Cancer, 79*(3–4), 645–654.

Southeast Asian American Health: Socio-Historical and Cultural Perspectives

Khatharya Um

Whenever I think about all that happened in Cambodia, my chest gets tight. It is so painful to recall. I don't want to think about it because I get a headache.

Cambodian woman survivor-Oakland, California

Introduction

Understanding of the state and conditions of new Asian American communities must begin with recognition of the multiplicity, diversity and disparity within and among the groups. Health conditions and concerns reflect an individual's and a group's experiences before, during, and after migration, which makes it difficult to generalize. Factors such as access to healthcare in the home country, migration related trauma, and socio-economic status both in the home country and in the U.S. all impact health and mental well-being of communities.

Though Southeast Asia, as a region, covers ten countries, this article focuses on communities in the U.S. that are often referred to simply as "Southeast Asian refugees," and more specifically on the smaller Cambodian and Laotian (including Hmong) American populations. Vietnamese Americans, which comprise a much larger community, will be discussed in a separate chapter. While in more recent years, other countries in the region such as Burma (Myanmar) have produced refugees, the term remains principally associated with the earlier communities that,

K. Um (✉)
Asian American and Asian Diaspora studies Program, Department of Ethnic Studies, University of California, Berkeley, CA, USA
e-mail: umk@berkeley.edu

despite their distinct histories, cultures, traditions, and migration experiences, are bound by their shared experience as political refugees of the wars in Southeast Asia, otherwise known as the "Vietnam War".

Southeast Asian Americans: History, Migration and Community Formation

Following the Communist takeover of Vietnam, Laos and Cambodia in 1975, nearly 3 million refugees left their homelands. An estimated 2 million of them were permanently resettled in third countries principally in Western democracies, the majority in the U.S. Unlike economic immigrants, these were refugees who were forcibly displaced by the sudden collapse of the pro-American governments in Vietnam, Cambodia, and Laos, and by the fear of Communist persecution. Many were evacuated with the Americans; others made their way out on their own recourse. Though a small group of the less educated, including fishermen, farmers, and rank-and-file soldiers, also managed to escape, most of those who were resettled in the United States in 1975–1976 were individuals associated with American foreign missions, military and civilian elites, diplomats, professionals, and their families.

The exodus in 1975 was followed by renewed refugee conditions in Southeast Asia in the late 1970s and early 1980s. In all three countries-Vietnam, Laos and Cambodia - socialist revolution adversely affected many groups. In Cambodia, state-sponsored terror, inhumane labor camps, mass starvation and death from diseases, deprivation, and execution became key features of life under the Khmer Rouge. Though less extremist, developments in Vietnam and Laos also involved persecution of certain classes and groups, including ethnic minorities. The Laotian highland ethnic minority communities, particularly the Hmong, but also Thai Dam, and Mien, were persecuted by the Pathet Lao regime for their affiliation with the Americans and continued anti-communist resistance. As in Cambodia, many civilians, commercial elites and military personnel were sent to re-education camps, also referred to as "seminar" in Laos.

As a result of these developments, the late 1970s to early 1980s saw yet another spike in refugee exodus from Cambodia and Laos. The overthrow of the Khmer Rouge regime in 1979 engendered cross-border flight into Thailand of close to 800,000 Cambodians. In response to, and in anticipation of continued persecution, lowland and highland Laotians also escaped Laos at an unprecedented number. Hmong, Mien, Khmu, Thai Dam, fled from their upland dwellings, eluding captivity by pursuing soldiers, and crossed the Mekong into Thailand.

As compared to the earlier cohort, the majority of the later arrivals were less educated and urbane. Most endured many more challenges prior to and during flight. The journey to the Thai border camps across minefields and treacherous mountain ranges and waters of the Mekong resulted in more deaths and separation. Many never reached Thai soil. The majority of those who successfully reached Thailand had to endure protracted stay in the refugee camps before their final resettlement. In the early 2000, some 15,000 Hmong were resettled in the U.S. after decades of living illegally in Thailand. In all, some 1,146,650 Southeast Asian refugees were resettled in the United States from 1975 to 2002. Though refugees are spread out throughout the US, California, Massachusetts, Minnesota, Iowa, Texas and Washington State became home to a sizeable Cambodian community and to large and diverse Laotian community (Southeast Asian Resource Action Center, 2004).

	Less than HS education (%)	Lack of eng. competency (%)
Cambodian	38.1	43.7
Hmong	42.4	45.2
Laotian	35.7	43.8

Source: U.S. Census, American Community Survey, 2005–2007 3-year estimates

	Per capita income	Below poverty (%)	Cash assistance (%)	No insurance (%)
Cambodian	$13,624	21	14.3	21.1
Hmong	$8,470	31.7	27.1	15.9
Laotian	$13,914	13.4	8.9	18.5

Source: Winston Tseng and Khatharya Um, presentation at Hmong Health Conference, University of Merced, 2010

Social, Political and Cultural Experiences Affecting Health

As with many emerging communities, the state of Southeast Asian health and mental health is informed by a number of factors, namely pre-migration experiences with modern healthcare system, historical political experiences including flight and long term stay in refugee camps, and post-resettlement challenges such as poverty. Access to modern health care in Laos and Cambodia was essentially limited to urban dwellers, and affordable to an even smaller subset of the population. The majority of those living in rural communities relied on traditional healing practices, ceremonies, and rituals for their well-being. Given the high representation of rural dwellers, many first generation Southeast Asian refugees in the U.S. have limited experience with modern healthcare systems prior to migration. Most continue to resort to traditional healing practices even after resettlement in the U.S. (Buchwald, Panwala, & Hooton, 1992). The high cost of modern healthcare in Southeast Asia also meant that the notion of preventive care is not an ingrained idea in many older Southeast Asian Americans. These factors bear significantly on the way that Southeast Asian refugees think about health issues and priorities.

Whether urban or rural, most Southeast Asians nevertheless harbor some traditional notions about health and well-being. Health is viewed systemically, based on the concepts of interconnections and equilibrium. The interconnection between mind and body also extends to desired balance in terms of essence (yin/yang), the Ayurvedic elements of water, fire, earth, and wind, and between the physical and the metaphysical realms, namely of body, spirits and "soul." The Mien, for instance, attribute certain illnesses to the loss of one of the 12 souls, a notion shared by other Southeast Asian cultural communities. Similarly, Southeast Asians also believe that ancestral spirits are important to the overall well-being of their posterity (Fadiman, 1997); they can either help or harm, and must be pacified with the appropriate rituals. For some ailments, it may involve placating the spirits with offerings of food, flowers, music, or through holy ablution. Physiological equilibrium can also be restored through therapeutic intervention such as coining and cupping aimed at "unblocking the wind."

Above all Southeast Asian health and mental health conditions were most adversely affected by their recent historical experiences. During the Vietnam War, Cambodia was one of the most heavily bombed countries in the world. Tragically, the end of the war did not produce peace but mass atrocities committed by one of the most brutal regimes of the twentieth century against its own people. In less than four years under the Khmer Rouge, over 1 million Cambodians out of a population of 7 million perished from starvation, hard labor, torture and execution. These compounding experiences with acute deprivations and depravity left enduring health effects on the Cambodian refugee population. Postwar situations in Laos were also challenging. Many who were sent to re-education camps, including the royal family, perished in detention. The survivors bore long-term health consequences from chronic exposure to malnutrition, diseases and torture.

The plight of many refugees did not end with exit from their countries. Many had to endure protracted stay in the border camps where undernourishment, overcrowding, unsanitary conditions and violence continued to negatively impact their physical and mental well-being. Even more acute than the diseases, was the violence that was bred in the toxic environment of over-density,

fear, uncertainty and hopelessness, and in the culture of impunity that prevailed in the conflict-fraught borderland through which many refugees journeyed. This was allowed to perpetuate by the absence of protective mechanisms in non-UN monitored camps. Fear of jeopardizing the family's resettlement prospect compelled many refugees, especially women and the elderly, to hide their health conditions, including late-term pregnancies, thereby denying themselves of pre-natal and other critical care. In some instances, pregnant women may resort instead to traditional forms of intervention and care that may have unintended long-term effects on them and their babies.

Post Resettlement Experiences and Health Implications

While resettlement may yield physical security, it also presented, for many Southeast Asian refugees, different and additional challenges. The majority of the Cambodian refugee population were survivors of the Khmer Rouge genocidal regime and, like most of the highland Laotian, have little or no formal education, and limited English language competency. Lacking much of the social capital to function effectively in America's post-industrial society, Cambodian, Hmong and Laotian Americans are highly represented in low -wage, low skill and often-hazardous occupational sectors. For the highland Laotian refugees, such as the Hmong, Mien, and Thai-Dam, negotiating a world that is fundamentally different from upland Laos can be a daunting process. Many Hmong families attempted to re-engage farming, especially in Central California, the state's agricultural valley. After years of struggle, successful Hmong farms began to emerge in California and the East Coast. In the Tri-State areas, the Lee poultry farm was one of the success stories in agro-farming. Most refugee families, however, continue to face economic challenges.

The rate of poverty is high in the Cambodian and Laotian communities, and is especially acute among female-headed household. A study of the community in Rhode Island reveals that

Southeast Asians are four times as likely to live in poverty. Economic marginalization is also tied to challenging living conditions, diet and lifestyles that have wide ranging health effect. Significantly, most of the medically underserved areas in California are located in the regions of Northern and Central California with high concentrations of Southeast Asians (University of California Multi Campus Policy Research Initiative, 2010).

Because of the affordability of housing, most Southeast Asian refugees were resettled in America's inner cities where crime and economic blight are prominent features, and where reception by pre-existing communities is, in many instances, tepid or even outrightly hostile. Many stayed, less by choice than by circumstances. As the economy contracts, anti-immigrant sentiments implicate all forms of different-ness. Violence, real and symbolic, pursued refugees into exile. As new communities, ones which are living reminders of an unpopular war, they are vulnerable targets. These incorporation and acculturation challenges constitute new and compounding stressors for the refugee populations, with significant and adverse bearing on their health.

State and Conditions of Southeast Asian Health Issues

In fundamental ways, Southeast Asian Americans embody their historical experiences. Especially for survivors of the Khmer Rouge genocidal regime, effects of hard labor, starvation, and chronic fear leave long lasting and deep imprints on their physical and mental health. Experiences with acute malnutrition and outright starvation were common, and may be linked to the cirrhosis of the liver that is found among surviving refugees. Hard labor and deprivation resulted in the overuse of muscles and bones and overall physical stress on the body that induce signs of premature aging and reduce resistance to disease. Because of overcrowding and protracted exposure to open sewage, smoke filled evenings of burning garbage, and in the case of the Hmong

refugees from Wat Tham Krabok, airborne particles from the nearby stone quarry, many refugees were afflicted with respiratory problems, gastrointestinal and airborne diseases, especially tuberculosis, as well as other diseases induced by the unsanitary conditions in the camps. Gastrointestinal disorder could also be persisting with parasites found in their system 10 years after resettlement.

In addition to the pre-existing conditions, acculturation stressors and other factors associated with migration and resettlement are also shown to have significant correlation to failing health. Among Southeast Asians, hypertension, high cholesterol, heart disease, obesity, smoking related conditions and diabetes are leading health concerns; one study notes that over 61% of Southeast Asians are at moderate to high risk in at least one category (Bates, Hill, & Barrett-Conner, 1989).

High Cholesterol and Diabetes

National data on Southeast Asians underscore the health concerns: 6% of Southeast Asians have diabetes, and 30% have cholesterol (CAPI, 2010). In two community-based studies, 13–42% of Hmong adults were found to be diabetic (CAPI, 2010). In Long Beach California, 23% of Cambodians surveyed reported having diabetes (National Cambodian American Health Initiative [NCAHI], 2007).

Hypertension, Cardiovascular and Cerebrovascular Diseases

Exposure to extreme conditions- starvation, punishing labor, torture and fear- also stresses the heart and vascular system. The hyper-alert state induced by these conditions, combined with migration and acculturation related stress, generate high cortisol levels that contribute to cardiovascular and cerebrovascular diseases, and cancer (Peeke & Chrousos, 1995; Schneiderman, Antoni, Saab, & Ironson, 2001). Nationwide statistics indicate that 21% of Southeast Asian Americans have hypertension (CAPI, 2010). In California, one of the few states in the nation that maintain disaggregated health statistics, analysis of the Health Indicators For California's Minority Populations revealed that Cambodians have four times the death rate from stroke compared to the White population. Though there is little scholarly attention paid to it, there may be some correlation between the sudden death syndrome that affected some Hmong men and heart arrhythmias. Trauma is also known to engender metabolic disorder, including abnormal thyroid functions that afflict many Southeast Asian refugees.

Cancer

Along with cardiovascular diseases, cancer is another leading cause of death among Southeast Asian Americans. The rate of liver cancer among Cambodians is 6.3 times greater than Whites (NCAHI, 2007). Conditions that involve chronic inflammation and that injure or stress the liver are linked to liver cancer (CAPI, 2010). In addition to smoking and other contributors, many refugees were exposed in the border refugee camps to tuberculosis and hepatitis B and C, which are linked to liver cancer. Among Southeast Asian refugees, the rates of chronic hepatitis B infection are 25–75 times that of the national average (CAPI, 2010).

Other forms of cancer are also prevalent in Cambodian and Laotian refugee populations. Among Hmong women, the rate of cervical cancer is more than three times that of other Asian/Pacific Islander groups, which already have much higher rates than Whites (Mills, Yang, & Riordan, 2005). The rate of lung cancer is also high and can be attributed to the prevalence of smoking, particularly among Southeast Asian men (35–42%), and exposure to secondary smoke. For older Cambodian and Lao women, in particular, the popular practice of chewing lime-coated betel nuts, which is also a mild stimulant, exposes them to the risk of oral squamous cell cancer that is prevalent throughout Southeast Asia, though virtually no research has been done regarding its prevalence among Southeast Asians in the United States. In addition, the rate of nasopharyngeal cancer is also high among Southeast Asians, at 13.9 times that of Whites for Cambodian Americans, and 35 times that of Whites for Hmong (Mills et al., 2005; CAPI, 2010). Studies have associated certain carcinogenic substance found in salty fish and vegetable preserves that are common in Southeast Asian diets with nasopharyngeal cancer. Stomach cancer is also common among Southeast Asian Americans; for Cambodians, the rate is 2.5 times greater than those in the general population (NCAHI, 2007).

Environmentally Related Health Issues

Inserted into impoverished communities and challenging working conditions, Southeast Asian refugees also find themselves in substandard housing and schools with asbestos and lead-based paints, and in working conditions that are injurious to their health; in some instances, these factors exacerbate the health conditions that they had prior to resettlement. Those engaged in agriculture are exposed to pesticide, while those in service sectors such as nail salons and dry cleaning are subjected to chemicals that have long-term hazardous effects. Along with other environmentally induced health issues, asthma is highly prevalent among Southeast Asian Americans. Nationally, 16% of Southeast Asian Americans have asthma (CAPI, 2010) though the rate is likely to be higher among children, and in certain geographical communities. Additionally, the repetitive work associated with assembly line work in various industries such as meatpacking and textile factories, and in high tech sectors extracts a physical toll and aggravates conditions that many refugees already have because of their prior subjugation to forced labor.

For economic reasons and for taste, many refugees also supplement their food supply by fishing and catching shellfish in local waters that are polluted. In a study of the Southeast Asian community in Rhode Island, over 50% of the respondents indicated that they fish in the local waters and consume their catch; another 48% indicated that they had received local catches from their friends. Southeast Asians, in general, not only consume greater amount of fish than what is recommended by the Food and Drugs Administration but also tend to leave no parts untouched, including those areas where toxins and mercury are heavily concentrated.

Resettlement Related Health Concerns

Research on Hmong refugees in California has shown that some health conditions appear to exacerbate with the length of stay in the United States (Kunstadter et al., 2000). Hmong in Fresno, California for instance register three times the rate of hypertension found in Hmong in Thailand. Similarly, the prevalence of diabetes among Hmong in California is 17 times that of Thai Hmong (CAPI, 2010). Studies have linked some of these emerging health concerns, namely diabetes and high cholesterol, to changes in lifestyle and diet, including increased consumption of meat, fast foods and sodas by Southeast Asian children. In addition, traditionally consumed fruits and vegetables that may help counter some of the adverse effects of traditional diets consisting, for many communities, of white rice and salty fish products, are unavailable in the United States. Furthermore, as compared to their counterparts in Asia, Southeast Asians in the United States are much more sedentary as disengagement from the farming lifestyle, cold weather and neighborhood safety issues undercut their ability to walk to places and to be more active. Linguistic isolation also means physical isolation, especially for elderly Southeast Asians.

Arguably, many of these lifestyle changes occurred even prior to resettlement. Surveys of Hmong recent arrivals from Wat Tham Krabok, who had been confined to this camp city for over a decade, reveal that 13.7% of those between the ages of 0–20 and 33.4% of those over 20 years of age were overweight, and 14.8% were obese upon arrival. If left unattended and potentially exacerbated by post-resettlement conditions, obesity could lead to diabetes. Excess weight, however, is not the only cause. Presence of insulin resistance had been found among Vietnamese Americans

who were not overweight (Minh et al., 1997), though no data is available for Cambodians and Laotians.

The emergence of certain health issues such as diabetes, hypertension, high cholesterol, cardiovascular disease and obesity among Southeast Asians after resettlement in the United States have led some researchers to refer to these conditions as "New World Syndrome" (Weiss, Ferrel, & Hanis, 1984). Despite this disposition, ethnic specific data is scarce. We also know little about the health conditions of young American-born and raised Southeast Asians as most of the existing scholarship deal largely with the heath and mental health concerns of first generation adult refugees. We have virtually no information on the developmental impact of camp conditions on children conceived or born in the refugee camps and who are now in their adulthood. In the same vein, practices such as bottle feeding and early weaning have been widely adopted by Southeast Asian American mothers but there is virtually no information regarding the impact that these shifts may have on children's development. Nor is there much attention paid to the health, including sexual health, implications of the changing lifestyle and habits of Southeast Asian American youths. The little that we do know points to some concerns. A study of the Hmong community in the Midwest, for instance, reveals a high teen pregnancy rate, while a study of Southeast Asian children in Minnesota, the overwhelming majority of whom were likely to be American born, indicated above average blood pressure among Cambodian girls, which may indicate future problem with hypertension. More information and pro-active community education are also needed about genetic disorders such as Thalassimia that affected an estimated 3.6% Southeast Asian Americans, especially those of Chinese ancestry.

Mortality Rate

As with stroke and hypertension, mortality rate from diabetes for Southeast Asians, especially Cambodians, is very high, almost six times that of the general population. With some of the conditions, especially cervical cancer, high mortality rate, in large part, is due to delayed detection (CAPI, 2010).

Mental Health

Physical and mental health cannot be easily separated as many physical health conditions are linked to anxieties and disorders, while the physical duress of torture, for instance, engenders multifaceted and long term consequences (NCAHI, 2007). In effect, the historical traumas that Southeast Asian refugees experienced not only left physiological damage but also enduring psychological scars (Kinzie et al., 1998). Evidence shows that Cambodians who had lived through the Vietnam War and the Khmer Rouge genocidal regime and who were admitted to the United States in the mid 1970s through the mid -1980s encountered some 8–16 major trauma experiences (Kinzie et al., 1984; Mollica, Lavelle, & Khoun, 1986; Realmuto, Ann, Hubbard, Groteluschen, & Chhun, 1992) that correspond with those described in the literature on survivors of the Nazi concentration camps and on prisoners of war. As a result, anxiety disorders, of varying degree of acuteness, are prevalent in the community. Many of the manifestations of the Concentration Camp Syndrome are registered in the Cambodian survivors in the United States. Lassitude, failing memory and inability to concentrate, sleeplessness, sense of insufficiency, headaches, depression and social adjustment problems impaired their ability to function optimally. A 2005 Rand study of Cambodians in Long Beach revealed that 62% of adults over age 32 have post-traumatic stress disorder (PTSD), and 51% manifest symptoms of depression, as compared to 4% and 6.7% of the general population respectively. Children and the elderly are especially vulnerable. A study of Cambodians in San Jose found that "sadness from obsessive thinking" about losses and traumatic events were root causes of common illnesses in elderly populations who have few coping mechanisms (Handelman & Yeo, 1996). Many are

linguistically isolated, and have difficulty reconciling with the disorienting changes in their lives, not the least of which are changes within the family and home. The recent murder-suicide of a Cambodian grandmother in Seattle is a shrill reminder of the latent threat of trauma.

For Southeast Asians, mental health as a concept is relatively new; one is either crazy or not. In fact, the term mental health has no direct and precise equivalent in many Southeast Asian languages. In some instances, the term has been used interchangeably with "mental illness." Given the cultural stigma associated with mental impairment, Southeast Asians are reluctant to seek help. They also have difficulty sharing their intimate feelings with strangers, which makes therapy sessions that rely on talking a culturally alien experience. Moreover, many Southeast Asians understand these conditions in cultural terms. Given the traditional beliefs that health and well-being rest on the equilibrium between the internal and external environment, between the physical and the metaphysical, many look upon recurrent nightmares and "hearing voices" as visits by ancestral spirits and restless souls demanding acknowledgement and pacification. As such, instead of, or in addition to, relying on Western interventions, many Southeast Asians seek solace through traditional healing in chants, rituals and ceremonies that are considered to be important intercessions to redress the imbalance in one's life.

With limited expression and outlet, trauma is often internalized and manifested in other forms. Many refugees turn to and, in many instances, excessively rely upon, suppressive substance such as alcohol, sleeping pills, and prescription drugs in the efforts to alleviate insomnia and obsessive thinking. It is significant to note that in a 1987 United Nations Border Relief Organization report, intoxication was listed as one of the leading causes of death in women. In the highland Laotian communities where opium was commonly used in ceremonies and for medicinal purpose, addiction remains a problem among the older generation even after resettlement. Other self-destructive activities such as gambling addiction are also on the rise. A 2003 study of Southeast Asians in Connecticut concluded that the rate of pathological gambling is 10 to 25 times as high as that of the general population, even higher than those of high-risk groups. Trauma also feeds the cycle of violence that destabilizes families and communities. Homicide is one of the leading causes of death among young Southeast Asian males. Statistics from the Department of Corrections in California show that 40% of the 64 Cambodians serving sentences in prison are there for killing some one. Another 11% are there for assault. In many instances, these crimes were gang related. They reflect the persistence and prevalence of violence in Southeast Asian American lives. In other instances, violence turns inwardly in the form of domestic violence.

Similar to the physiological disorders, we know little about the potential for trans-generational transmission of trauma in Southeast Asian families, though it has been suggested in studies of other historical instances. Reports from community-based programs seem to indicate that the shadow of trauma remains unlifted for subsequent generations and that mental health needs are significant among Southeast Asian youths (CAPI, 2010). What we do know anecdotally is that language loss and corresponding limited communication within the family impede the ability of young Southeast Asians to make sense of their histories and of their families' experiences. Alienation from family, community and society, in turn, is among the root causes of delinquency among many Southeast Asian youth, and a prime motivator for gang participation.

Structural Barriers to Healthcare Access

For many Southeast Asians, limited education not only means economic marginality and challenging living and working conditions but also impeded access to quality care. According to the U.S. Census (2009), an estimated 21% Cambodian, 19% Laotian and 16% Hmong Americans have no health insurance coverage. Because of the nature of their employment and the absence of

effective coverage, many feel that they cannot afford to take time off to go to the doctor, or are not inclined to make preventive care a priority. Additionally, the healthcare system in the United States can involve lengthy and confusing bureaucracy particularly for people with limited education and English proficiency. Southeast Asians often complain about having to first see their primary physicians before being allowed to see a specialist, with the former doing little other than providing them with a referral. As such, even those with health benefits may be deterred by the opportunity cost of taking time off to see a doctor, and are reluctant to do so except in dire conditions. Among other reasons, the reluctance to see a doctor or to comply with the need for return visits lead many Southeast Asian patients to resort to self-diagnosis and self-medication, including manipulating dosage and cutting pills in half, and to share prescriptions, all with grave medical implications. In the same vein, many Southeast Asians also simultaneously seek both Western and Eastern care, in some instances with counter-interactive effects. Nursing mothers who had just given birth may resort to alcohol-soaked herbal medicine to "strengthen the nerves."

Lack of English language proficiency and linguistic support in the healthcare system for Southeast Asian language speakers also impede access to quality care. The Rhode Island Office of Minority Health noted that 84% of Asians over age five speak a language at home other than English. Nationally, over 41% of Cambodians and Hmong, and over 38% of Laotians have limited English proficiency (American Community Survey, 2009). Moreover, because of their limited access to Western medical care, many Southeast Asians either do not know their family medical history or only know them in terms of traditional health concepts and are unable to translate them into English and into Western scientific concepts. While more materials are now available in Southeast Asian languages, many Southeast Asians, particularly women, are functionally illiterate. Similarly, despite increases in the number of bilingual and bi-cultural staff, the level of representation of Cambodian, Hmong and Mien Americans in healthcare professions remains insufficient to meet the needs of these growing communities. In California, there are only 142 Khmer speaking licensed physicians to serve approximately over 68,000 Cambodians, though this census number is most likely to be an undercount. For Hmong, the ratio is 194 for over 67,000 (University of California Multi Campus Policy Research Initiative, 2010). Given that not many Southeast Asian languages are taught in schools and colleges, truly bilingual and bicultural staff is not easy to find, as young Southeast Asian Americans may have mastery over the English language but not necessarily the same level of fluency in their native languages. Additionally, many of the scientific concepts and medical terminology such as PTSD or stress do not have a Southeast Asian equivalent. For instance, there is no Hmong word for cancer; in some instances, the term that is used is "death" (CAPI, 2010). Continued scarcity of fully bilingual staff, particularly in the smaller Southeast Asian linguistic groups, means persisting problems with information access, questionable translation quality, and inappropriate use of translators. Language barrier also makes it difficult for Southeast Asian patients to obtain the necessary information about complicated procedures, a situation that is exacerbated by the rapid pace in which patients are processed through office visits. Lack of sufficient explanation may lead Southeast Asian patients not to comply with drug regiments and/or to stop taking medications when the symptoms had disappeared or to lessen the dosage either to economize or to lessen the effects because of the notion that Western medicine is "too strong" for Asian constitution (CAPI, 2010). In the worst case scenarios, patients may find themselves unwittingly consenting to medical procedures that they may not otherwise agree to do had there been sufficient explanations. In one instance, an elderly Cambodian gentleman who only had his young daughter as a translator did not fully understand that his state insurance would cover only full dentures and not the partials that he had wanted until all his teeth had been pulled out.

For some Southeast Asian groups, community-based organizations are able to provide supplemental support in the generation of translated materials and the provision of interpreters. For Cambodian, Lao, and Mien in particularly, these internal resources are scarce. At present, there are only 35 Cambodian mutual assistance agencies to serve close to 300, 000 Cambodians in the U.S., an actual decline from the over 200 such organizations a decade prior. While culturally informed and community tailored programs, including those involving community health navigators, have been found to be effective in providing critical support to Cambodian and Laotian communities (Nguyen, Tanjasiri, Kagawa-Singer, Tran, & Foo, 2008), more resources need to be invested in the proliferation of such programs to many more locales, and in the delivery of quality staff training.

Culture, Gender and Health

As referenced earlier, culture impacts how Southeast Asians view their health condition and priorities and how effectively they access care (CAPI, 2010; Kramer, Kwong, Lee, & Chung, 2002; Uba, 1992). Cultural beliefs and misconceptions about illnesses may lead Southeast Asian to delay seeking medical help. The erroneously held notion about cervical cancer as being caused by promiscuity, for instance, may prevent Southeast Asian women from seeking diagnosis and treatment out of shame, as well as give others in monogamous relationships a false sense of immunity. Many Cambodian and Laotian women are also deterred by their sense of modesty and cultural understanding of virginity from submitting to Pap smear screening, which prevents early detection of cervical cancer.

Given the cultural emphasis on modesty, age and gender matter when pairing patients with healthcare providers and interpreters. Southeast Asian elders, in particular, feel tremendous reluctance to discuss their intimate health history with younger doctors and translators, particularly of a different sex. It is culturally difficult for older Southeast Asian women to discuss reproductive and intimate health issues with younger, especially male translators and healthcare professionals. The heavy reliance on children, relatives and untrained individuals for translation, all of which are considered poor practices by the industry's standards but are widely prevalent, raises separate but equally grave concerns (Yee, n.d.).

Culturally informed notions of loyalty and respect for authority figures as well as the emphasis on non-confrontation also make it difficult for many Southeast Asian patients to question their doctors, or even to seek clarification or a second opinion, for fear of appearing disrespectful. Southeast Asian patients may be reluctant to change doctors, even if the latter are uncaring or ineffectual, because they don't want to offend them or to appear disloyal. By extension, notions of filial duty, respect for elders and self sacrifice may also interfere with the need for self-protection on the part of caregivers when attending to family members with infectious diseases. In the same vein, the cultural emphasis on stoicism and general sense of fatalism may also deter elderly Southeast Asians from speaking up and seeking help before their conditions had become serious (Uba, 1992). Though it varies according to cultural communities, there may also be general anxieties, especially among highland Laotians, about certain procedures such as biopsies and transplants that are perceived to be unnatural interventions, which may prevent Southeast Asians from seeking that recourse.

Gendered notions about acceptable social behaviors also have health implications. Cambodian cultural aphorisms such as "men are like gold nuggets and women worsted cotton" may foster a feeling of immunity and a degree of acceptance of high-risk behaviors of Cambodian men. Though they are challenged by diseases such as HIV/AIDS, the notions that certain behaviors are natural and, above all, expungeable continue to prevail.

Conclusion: The Importance of Knowing

Despite the size of the populations, length of residency, and the fact that they constitute the fastest growing Asian American populations, we still know relatively little about Southeast Asian American health. In part, this is the result of the comparatively recent formation of the communities and, for many of the Southeast Asian groups, their statistically small size. In part, and as a result of the latter, it is because of the virtual absence of disaggregate data and ethnic specific studies. Studies that are nation-wide or multi-local, longitudinal, and sufficiently disaggregated along ethnic lines are particularly scarce.

Of the research that has been done on this highly diverse population, comparatively more is available on Vietnamese Americans and, to a lesser extent, on Hmong Americans than on Cambodian and other Laotian groups. More research, in general, is needed on the relationship between the effects of acculturation and other forms of stress and physical health. While new scholarship on health and health disparities has begun to address the intersectionality of race, gender, and culture, much more research is also needed on the ways that ethnic, cultural and gender factors inform Southeast Asian health issues, including how ethnicity may potentially affect differential response to drug efficacy. Similarly, how gender and culture may inform the way that Southeast Asian men and women manifest and cope with anxiety and depression is an important question that remains insufficiently addressed. Data on Asian American women reveals that they have twice the rate of serious psychological distress than Asian American men, though similar data is not available for the different Southeast Asian groups. There are also disconcertingly few systematic studies on the health and mental health conditions of those who came to the U.S. in their pre-adolescence, i.e. the second-generation cohorts, or who are American-born. As such, in addition to a more robust understanding of the general health conditions of Southeast Asian Americans, what is needed are national datasets that can be disaggregated on multiple dimensions particularly ethnicity, gender and geography. Additionally, more national longitudinal studies are necessary for our understanding of these complex health issues, including the trans-generational transmission of trauma.

For research and information to have a meaningful impact on healthcare access and delivery, it must be widely shared with the numerous stakeholders, including policy makers and community advocates, and must inform our critical approach to continuous improvement and reform. Given cultural and structural barriers to equitable access to care, greater resources must be dedicated to the training and development of bilingual and bicultural staff and health navigators, to the enhancement of community education and outreach programs, and to the overall capacity building of community based organizations that work intimately with these under-served populations. Along with research, there has to be more societal investment in the development of linguistic and cultural competencies among American healthcare providers, and in the cultivation of more Southeast Asian American health practitioners.

References

American Community Survey. (2009). Retrieved http://www.census.gov/acs/www/.

Bates, S. R., Hill, L., & Barrett-Conner, E. (1989). Cardiovascular disease risk factors in an Indochinese population. *American Journal of Preventive Medicine, 5*, 15–20.

Buchwald, D., Panwala, S., & Hooton, T. (1992). The use of traditional health practices by Southeast Asian refugees in a primary care clinic. *Western Journal of Medicine, 156*, 507–511.

Center for Eliminating Health Disparities. *Chronic disease and pain management*. University of Minnesota.

Fadiman, A. (1997). *The spirit catches you and you fall down*. Union Square West, New York: Farrar, Straus and Giroux.

Handelman, L., & Yeo, G. (1996). Using explanatory models to understand chronic symptoms of Cambodian refugees. *Family Medicine, 28*, 271–276.

Kinzie, J. D., Denney, D., Riley, C., Boehnlein, J., McFarland, B., & Leung, P. (1998). A cross-cultural study of reactivation of posttraumatic stress disorder symptoms: American and Cambodian psychophysiological response to viewing traumatic video scenes. *Journal of Nervous Mental Disorder, 186*, 670–676.

Kinzie, D., Fredrickson, R., & Ben, R. (1984). Posttraumatic Stress Disorder among survivors of Cambodian Concentration Camps. *American Journal of Psychology, 141*, 645–650.

Kramer, E. J., Kwong, K., Lee, E., & Chung, H. (2002). Cultural factors influencing the mental health of Asian Americans. *Western Journal of Medicine, 176*(4), 227–231.

Kunstadter, P., Wong, C., Lee, S., Xiong, G., Vang, V., & Comerford, M. (2000, November 15). *Blood pressure increases with length of stay in the U.S. among Hmong refugees in California*. Presented at the 128th annual meeting of APHA.

Mills, P. K., Yang, R. C., & Riordan, D. (2005). Cancer incidence in the Hmong in California, 1988–2000. *Cancer, 104*(Suppl. 12), 2969–2974.

Mollica, R. F., Lavelle, J., and Khoun, F. (1986). *Khmer Widows: At highest risk*, presented at the American Friends Service Committee Conference on Cambodian Mental Health, New York, May 24, 1986.

National Cambodian American Health Initiative. (2007). *Health Emergency*. Report 2007.

Nguyen, T.-U. N., Tanjasiri, S. P., Kagawa-Singer, M., Tran, J. H., & Foo, M. A. (2008). Community health navigators for breast and cervical cancer screening among Cambodian and Laotian women: Intervention strategies and relationship building processes. *Society for Public Health Education, 9*(4), 356–367.

Peeke, P. M., & Chrousos, G. P. (1995). Hypercortisolism and obesity. *Annals of the New York Academy of Sciences, 771*, 665–676.

Pierce, A. (2010). *Health disparities among Southeast Asian and African refugee communities*. CAPI Report.

Realmuto, G. M. M., Ann, C., Hubbard, J., Groteluschen, A., & Chhun, B., (1992). Adolescent survivors of massive childhood trauma in Cambodia: life events and current symptoms. *Journal of Traumatic Stress, 5*.

Schneiderman, N., Antoni, M. H., Saab, P. G., & Ironson, G. (2001). Health psychology: Psychosocial and biobehavioral aspects of chronic disease management. *Annual Review of Psychology, 51*, 555–580.

Southeast Asian Resource Action Center, " Southeast Asian Statistical Profile 2004", Washington DC. 2004

Uba, L. (1992). Cultural barriers to healthcare for Southeast Asian refugees. *Public Health Reports, 107*, 544–548.

University of California Multi Campus Policy Research Initiative. (2010). Ethnic health assessment for Asian Americans and Pacific Islander Americans.

Van Minh, H., Thanh, L. C., Thi, B. N., Trinh, T. D., Tho, T. D., & Valensi, P. (1997). Insulinaemia and slight overweight: The case of Vietnamese hypertensives. *International Journal of Obesity Related Metabolic Disorders, 21*, 897–902.

Weiss, K. M., Ferrel, R. F., & Hanis, C. L. (1984). A new world syndrome of metabolic diseases with a genetic and evolutionary basis. *Yearbook of Physical Anthropology, 27*, 153–178.

Yee, B. W. K. (n.d.). *Health and Health Care of Southeast Asian American elders:Vietnamese, Cambodian, Hmong and Laotian elders*. Consortium of Geriatric Education Centers [undated].

Mixed Asian Americans and Health: Navigating Uncharted Waters

Cathy J. Tashiro

Introduction

What are the health implications of being a mixed Asian American? Very little is known about this diverse and rapidly expanding population. The little we do know is complicated by the collision between biological concepts of "race" and the social process of racial categorization. Asian America includes such diverse populations that it's difficult to make biological generalizations about them. Yet there are some well-established differences between *certain* Asian groups and the majority population that have important health implications. Two examples will be discussed in this chapter. For people of mixed Asian ancestry who may also have ancestral roots in Europe, Africa, and/or the Americas, the complexities of possible combinations and their implications are daunting. But there is an urgent need to tease apart the social and biological meanings of being a mixed Asian American. Researchers whose studies are discussed in this chapter are beginning to do this important work. Hopefully, in the near future, a mixed Asian American confronted with health risks by race who asks "But what does this mean for me?" will find real answers.

C.J. Tashiro (✉)
Nursing Program, University of Washington Tacoma,
Tacoma, WA, USA
e-mail: ctashiro@u.washington.edu

Demographics

According to the U.S. Census Bureau (2011), the population of the two or more race category grew by almost 32% between 2000 and 2010. The number of multiracial children increased by close to 50% in this period (The New York Times, 2011). Over 2.6 million people identified with two or more races and claimed "Asian" as one of their ancestries in 2010, about 15% of a total of over 17 million claiming "Asian alone or in combination" as their race(s). Clearly people of mixed heritage are a significant part of Asian America. Over 70% of mixed Asian Americans of two races claim "White" as their non-Asian race.

Asian intermarriage rates vary widely by gender and generational status, with women and the native-born generally much more likely to marry outside of their racial or ethnic group. In their analysis based on data from the 2000 U.S. census, Lee and Boyd (2008) found Japanese and Filipinos most likely to marry outside of their ethnic groups, while Asian Indians and Chinese were least likely to do so. Southeast Asians also had low rates of intermarriage relative to other Asian ethnic groups. These patterns may change as native-born children of more recent immigrants become adults. Authors Hidalgo and Bankston (2010) examined Asian American outmarriage trends from 1980 to 2005. Across this period, about a fifth of married Asian Americans were married to non-Asian spouses, predominantly Whites. The proportion of mixed marriages of couples of child-rearing ages was even higher during this period, resulting in rapid growth of the younger mixed Asian American population. Research indicates that individuals of mixed race and mixed race households tend to live in more multiethnic neighborhoods than their single-race counterparts (Clark & Mass, 2009). Some have wondered if mixed race Asians, particularly those with one White parent, are fulfilling the classic assimilationist model articulated by sociologist Milton Gordon (1964). However, the emerging picture of mixed Asian America is diverse socioeconomically and generationally, and includes all of the Asian subgroups, plus ancestors from all the world's continents. One size does not fit all.

Health and Mixed Race

Historically, there has been little research on the health of mixed race people. This will change as the multiracial population grows and the practice of allowing survey respondents to self-identify with more than one race becomes the norm. Early mixed race health research focused on the birth outcomes of mixed Black/White infants. For example, Collins and David (1993) compared birth weights of mixed Black/White infants based on the race of the father and mother, with single race White and Black infants. Low birth weight puts infants at risk and is much more common for African American babies. Collins and David found a gradient of risk, with infants born to mixed couples when the mother was Black, close to the level of risk experienced by infants born to two Black parents, intermediate risks with Black father/White mother, and the least risk for infants born to two White parents. Collins and David suggested that the physiological effects of the stress of racism on Black mothers, and thereby on their infants in utero, accounted for the poorer outcomes to Black mothers, regardless of the race of the father. For mixed Asians of this age group, bilirubin levels in mixed Asian/White infants were found to be intermediate between those of East Asians (typically higher) and White infants in one study (Setia, Villaveces, Dhillon, &

Mueller, 2002). A few studies of health issues affecting mixed race Asians have shown higher self-reported diabetes and cardiovascular disease (Gomez, Kelsey, Glaser, Lee, & Sidney, 2004), higher rates of being overweight or obesity than their respective parent racial groups (Albright, Steffen, Wilkens, Henderson, & Kolonel, 2008), and relatively high rates of hypertension for multiracials in general (Ochner, Ayala, & Jiles, 2006). However, the literature is sparse, and none of these studies broke out their mixed Asian populations by Asian ethnic group. Much more research needs to be done before these findings can be considered definitive.

Social and Psychological Health

While the research on physical health outcomes of mixed Asian Americans is limited, there is a growing body of research that seems to indicate increased risk for behavioral problems. In their landmark study based on analysis of the National Longitudinal Study of Adolescent Health, Udry, Lim, and Hendrickson-Smith (2003) found greater behavioral risk behaviors for youth who self-identify with more than one race when compared with their monoracial counterparts. Though not broken down by subgroups, the mixed Asian American youth were significantly more likely than their monoracial Asian counterparts to report somatic symptoms and fair/poor health, suicidal ideation, substance use, school problems, and having had sex. Since then, additional studies have found indications of increased behavioral risks for mixed Asian Americans (Choi, Harachi, Gillmore, & Catalano, 2006).

Sense of attachment to social groups and institutions is an important factor in youth substance abuse. Supportive schools and communities can play a positive role in prevention (Mayberry, Espelage, & Koenig, 2009). Mixed race students may be less attached to their schools (Jackson, & LeCroy, 2009), though the level of attachment can be related to factors like the racial composition of the school and the particular racial mix of the mixed race individual. For example, Cheng and Klugman (2010) found that Asian/White students were less affected by the racial composition of their schools, whereas Asian/Black students felt a greater sense of attachment the larger the percentage of Black students in their schools, and the converse for the White percentage. The authors hypothesize that the asset of part White ancestry enabled the Asian/White students to socialize more comfortably in predominantly White environments.

Increased substance abuse among mixed Asian Americans and Pacific Islanders has been identified through analysis of several large data sets by Price, Risk, Wong, and Klingle (2002). Their analysis of data from the Add Health survey showed particularly high rates of substance use for mixed Chinese and mixed Vietnamese youth relative to their monoracial Asian counterparts. Relatively high rates of DUIs have been found for mixed race adults (Caetano & McGrath, 2005), though the particular "mixes" were not broken out in this study. High rates of smoking among mixed race Asian American adults in comparison to monoracial Asian subgroups have been found (Gomez, Kelsey, Glaser, Lee, & Sidney, 2004).

In an analysis of 1999–2002 data from the National Survey on Drug Use and Health (NSDUH) Sakai, Wang, and Price (2010) examined substance use and abuse for mixed Asian Americans and Pacific Islanders by ethnic subgroups, comparing them with their monoracial API counterparts and Caucasians. Lifetime use of alcohol by mixed race Asians was greater than that of Asians and less than that of Caucasians, which the authors suggest indicates a possible genetic component since most mixed Asians have Caucasian ancestry. Yet rates of actual dependency on alcohol were higher than Caucasians for the mixed race groups in the study, suggesting a social etiology. Regarding drug use, multiracial Native Hawaiians, Filipinos, and Koreans described significantly higher lifetime use than their monoracial counterparts. The rates of drug use and dependence for other mixed Asian American ethnic groups also exceeded their monoracial Asian counterparts, though establishing statistical significance could have been hampered by small sample sizes. Mixed race Filipinos may be particularly at risk for substance use.

Though much more research is needed to definitively establish elevated behavioral risks for mixed Asian Americans, it is important to consider why this trend might be real. In a society in which race is still one of the most powerful identifiers, people of mixed race can experience a profound sense of not quite belonging (Tashiro, 2011). There are unique stressors faced by people of mixed race in a society that is still highly racialized. At least one study found that some issues related to discrimination and identity may be more acute for mixed race adolescents than monoracial minority youth (Choi, Harachi, Gillmore, & Catalano, 2006). Mixed Asian Americans may feel a sense of exclusion from either parent's racial or ethnic group (Hall, 2004; AhnAllen, Suyemoto, & Carter, 2006; Shih, Bonam, Sanchez, & Peck, 2007). Physical appearance, familiarity with the Asian culture of ancestry, last name, and language fluency are some of the important factors that can influence perceptions of a mixed Asian American's "authenticity" as an Asian American. Reflected appraisals, that is, how one imagines how others see oneself, based on appearance and cultural familiarity with the Asian heritage, can strongly influence identity (Khanna, 2004). Conversely, being identified as Asian, or non-white can lead to race-based exclusion by whites, which may be more acute for "minority-mixed" Asian Americans. Because mixed race Asian Americans are most commonly half White, their issues have been studied more. There is a need for more research on the particular issues faced by mixed Asian Americans with other minority group ancestries.

How one identifies may be related to how being mixed is experienced. Identifying as non-White may play a protective role. In a study of the impact of stress on biracial girls, those who identified with their non-White ancestry (Hispanic, Asian, or Black) experienced significantly higher self-esteem than those who identified as White (Phillips, 2004). In this study, girls of mixed Asian/White ancestry were significantly more likely to experience physical symptoms and substance use than their non-mixed Asian counterparts. Believing that race is intrinsically biological may be associated with a lower sense of psychological well-being (Sanchez & Garcia, 2009). Understanding that race is a social construction may soften the impact of racial stereotypes (Shih, Bonam, Sanchez, & Peck, 2007).

What About Genetics?

Perhaps the biggest health risk to mixed race Asian Americans is health care provider assumptions about their race and presumed genetic tendencies based on superficial characteristics like appearance and surname (Tashiro, 2001, 2003). For example, in a conversation with an acquaintance of mixed Japanese/White ancestry who recently had orthopedic surgery, he mentioned that the dose of Warfarin he was taking to prevent blood clots "wasn't working" and had to be increased. Warfarin, also known by the brand name Coumadin, is an anticoagulant commonly prescribed to people after orthopedic surgery to lower their risk of potentially fatal blood clots. When I asked him what his original dose was, it was the standard starting dose for Asians. Clearly, whoever prescribed the Coumadin presumed he was Asian only. It is well established that populations throughout the world differ in their response to Coumadin, and East Asians typically need lower doses than Caucasians to get the desired therapeutic effect (Ross et al., 2010). The risks of too high a Coumadin dose are potentially fatal, and excess bleeding is one of the most common medication-induced serious side effects. In 2006, the U.S. Food and Drug Administration (FDA) required Bristol-Meyers Squibb Company, the manufacturer of Coumadin, to include a warning for bleeding risk in their product insert, which also includes the probable need for lower starting doses for Asians. However, the risk of too low a dose, such as that prescribed for my acquaintance, is that it will be ineffective, hence failing to prevent blood clots. To add to the complexity of the pharmacogenetics involved, different populations within Asia have different configurations of the genetic factors associated with response to Coumadin. For example, while the optimal dose for people of East Asian ancestry is the lowest of the ethnoracial groups, the effective dose for

South Asians is significantly higher (Chan et al., 2011). Thus, in this case, reliance on our socially constructed category of "Asian American" has little utility for patient care. Add the complexity of mixed ancestry from Europe, Africa, and/or the Americas, and the predictability of response to medications based on race becomes virtually impossible, indeed potentially dangerous. Though populations may show some genetic variations, these are not based on "race," which is a social means of categorizing people devoid of biological meaning. The existence of people of mixed race highlights the contradictions of our common beliefs about race. The growth of pharmacogenetics and genomics may eventually make it possible to target individual therapies when there is a documented genetic component, but we are still a long way from this being realistic and accessible to most people. In the meantime, health care providers need to be educated about the growing mixed race population and to not make race-based assumptions about their patients.

Another arena involving genetics for mixed Asian Americans is the ability to tolerate alcohol. Many East Asians, (predominantly Chinese, Japanese, and Koreans) lack the aldehyde dehydrogenase isozyme, which makes them unable to fully metabolize alcohol, giving rise to a variety of unpleasant symptoms, such as flushing, rapid heart rate, and in extreme cases, fainting. A look at my own mixed race Japanese/White family's ability to tolerate alcohol shows the difficulty of predicting how the genes will be expressed. My Nissei father was so intolerant of alcohol that even minute quantities of alcohol in food would make him extremely ill. My mother, of northern European ancestry, has no trouble with alcohol. My sister, like my father, has been known to faint after just one drink. My brother tolerates alcohol well. I can drink a few sips. It has been assumed that this difficulty metabolizing alcohol explains the generally lower rates of alcohol abuse amongst Asian Americans relative to other groups. But the question of whether the relatively high rates of alcohol use among some mixed Asian American groups is due to genetic admixture or to the unique psychosocial issues associated with being mixed needs much more exploration (Sakai, Wang, & Price, 2010).

Unanswered Questions and Future Research

There now exists a robust amount of well-crafted research connecting experiences of racism and discrimination with health outcomes like hypertension and other health issues, such as the birth weight study of mixed race infants by Collins and David (1993) discussed previously. We need more research on the unique ways that mixed Asian Americans experience the contradictions of race, exclusion, and difference, and how these experiences might "get in the body." We need more research on mixed Asian Americans with African American, Latino, and Native American ancestry. In particular, we need research that looks at the long-term effects of the unique racial position of mixed Asian Americans on the mind and body, as well as the meaning of identity over the life course. We know from the literature on adverse childhood events (ACES) that youth trauma can manifest itself in poorer health in adulthood (Anda et al., 2006). Are there similar complex biosocial pathways through which experiences of difference manifest themselves over time? At the same time, for the many healthy mixed Asian Americans, what family and community factors facilitate positive development and health? Hopefully, the future will bring solid answers to these questions, as well as a decline in the belief in the mutual exclusivity of the "races" that so plagues people of mixed ancestry. This will bring greater health in its fullest meaning to our entire society.

References

AhnAllen, J. M., Suyemoto, K. L., & Carter, A. S. (2006). Relationship between physical appearance, sense of belonging and exclusion, and racial/ethnic self-identification among multiracial Japanese European Americans. *Cultural Diversity & Ethnic Minority Psychology, 12*(4), 673–686. doi:10.1037/1099-9809.12.4.673.

Albright, C. L., Steffen, A., Wilkens, L. R., Henderson, B. E., & Kolonel, L. N. (2008). The prevalence of obesity in ethnic admixture adults. *Obesity, 16*(5), 1138–1143.

Anda, R. F., Felitti, V. J., Bremner, J. D., Walker, J. D., Whitfield, C., Perry, B. D., et al. (2006). The enduring effects of abuse and related adverse experiences in childhood: A convergence of evidence from neurobiology and epidemiology. *European Archives of Psychiatry and Clinical Neuroscience, 256*, 174–186.

Caetano, R., & McGrath, C. (2005). Driving under the influence (DUI) among U.S. ethnic groups. *Accident Analysis and Prevention, 37*, 217–224.

Chan, S. L., Suo, C., Lee, S. C., Goh, B. C., Chia, K. S., & Teo, Y. Y. (2011). Translational aspects of genetic factors in the prediction of drug response variability: A case study of warfarin pharmacogenomics in a multiethnic cohort from Asia. *The Pharmacogenomics Journal*, 1–7.

Cheng, S., & Klugman, J. (2010). School racial composition and biracial adolescents' school attachment. *The Sociological Quarterly, 51*(1), 150–178. doi:10.1111/j.1533-8525.2009.01166.x.

Choi, Y., Harachi, T. W., Gillmore, M. R., & Catalano, R. F. (2006). Are multiracial adolescents at greater risk? Comparisons of rates, patterns, and correlates of substance use and violence between monoracial and multiracial adolescents. *The American Journal of Orthopsychiatry, 76*(1), 86–97. doi:10.1037/0002-9432.76.1.86.

Clark, W. A. V., & Maas, R. (2009). The geography of a mixed-race society. *Growth and Change, 40*(4), 565–593.

Collins, J. W., & David, R. J. (1993). Race and birthweight in biracial infants. *American Journal of Public Health, 83*(8), 1125–1129.

Gomez, S. L., Kelsey, J. L., Glaser, S. L., Lee, M. M., & Sidney, S. (2004). Immigration and acculturation in relation to health and health-related risk factors among specific Asian subgroups in a health maintenance organization. *American Journal of Public Health, 94*(11), 1977–1984.

Gordon, M. (1964). *Assimilation in American life*. New York: Oxford University Press.

Hall, C. C. I. (2004). Mixed-race women: One more mountain to climb. *Women & Therapy, 27*(1/2), 237–246.

Hidalgo, D. A., & Bankston, C. L. (2010). Blurring racial and ethnic boundaries in Asian American families: Asian American family patterns, 1980-2005. *Journal of Family Issues, 31*(3), 280–300.

Jackson, K. F., & LeCroy, C. W. (2009). The influence of race and ethnicity on substance use and negative activity involvement among monoracial and multiracial adolescents of the Southwest. *Journal of Drug Education, 39*(2), 195–210.

Khanna, N. (2004). The role of reflected appraisals in racial identity: The case of multiracial Asians. *Social Psychology Quarterly, 67*(2), 115–131. doi:10.1177/019027250406700201.

Lee, S. M., & Boyd, M. (2008). Marrying out: Comparing the marital and social integration of Asians in the U.S. and Canada. *Social Science Research, 37*, 311–329.

Mayberry, M. L., Espelage, D. L., & Koenig, B. (2009). Multilevel modeling of direct effects and interactions of peers, parents, school, and community influences on adolescent substance use. *Journal of Youth and Adolescence, 38*(8), 1038–1049.

Ochner, M., Ayala, C., & Jiles, R. (2006). Effect of race category redefinition on hypertension and hypercholesterolemia prevalence in the behavioral risk factor surveillance system, 1999 and 2001. *Ethnicity & Disease, 16*(1), 152–158.

Phillips, L. (2004). Fitting in and feeling good: Patterns of self-evaluation and psychological stress among biracial adolescent girls. *Women & Therapy, 27*(1), 217–236.

Price, R. K., Risk, N. A., Wong, M. M., & Klingle, R. S. (2002). Substance use and abuse by Asian Americans and Pacific Islanders: Preliminary results from four national epidemiologic studies. *Public Health Reports, 117*(Suppl. 1), S39–S50.

Ross, K. A., Bigham, A. W., Edwards, M., Gozdzik, A., Suarez-Kurtz, G., & Parra, E. J. (2010). Worldwide allele frequency distribution of four polymorphisms associated with warfarin dose requirements. *Journal of Human Genetics, 55*, 582–589.

Sakai, J. T., Wang, C., & Price, R. K. (2010). Substance use and dependence among native Hawaiians, other Pacific Islanders, and Asian ethnic groups in the united states: Contrasting multiple-race and single-race prevalence rates from a national survey. *Journal of Ethnicity in Substance Abuse, 9*(3), 173–185.

Sanchez, D. T., & Garcia, J. A. (2009). When race matters: Racially stigmatized others and perceiving race as a biological construction affect biracial people's daily well-being. *Personality and Social Psychological Bulletin, 35*(9), 1154–1164.

Saulny, S. (2011, March 25). Census data presents rise in multiracial population of youths. *The New York Times*, p. A3.

Setia, S., Villaveces, A., Dhillon, P., & Mueller, B. A. (2002). Neonatal jaundice in Asian, white, and mixed-race infants. *Archives of Pediatric Adolescent Medicine, 156*, 276–279.

Shih, M., Bonam, C., Sanchez, D., & Peck, C. (2007). The social construction of race: Biracial identity and vulnerability to stereotypes. *Cultural Diversity & Ethnic Minority Psychology, 13*(2), 125–133. doi:10.1037/1099-9809.13.2.125.

Tashiro, C. J. (2001). Mixed but not matched: Multiracial people and the organization of health knowledge. In C. Nakashima & T. Williams (Eds.), *The sum of our parts: Mixed heritage Asian Americans* (pp. 173–182). Philadelphia: Temple University Press.

Tashiro, C. J. (2003). Health issues facing mixed race people. In M. Kelley & M. P. P. Root (Eds.), *Multiracial child resource book* (pp. 26–31). Seattle, WA: The Mavin Foundation.

Tashiro, C. J. (2011). *Standing on both feet: Voices of older mixed race Americans*. Boulder, CO: Paradigm.

U.S. Census Bureau. (2011). Profile of general population and housing characteristics 2010: 2010 demographic profile data. Retrieved May 29, 2011, from http://factfinder2.census.gov/faces/tableservices/jsf/pages/productview.xhtml?src=bkmk.

Udry, J. R., Lim, R. M., & Hendrickson-Smith, J. (2003). Health and behavior risks of adolescents with mixed-race identity. *American Journal of Public Health, 93*(11), 1865–1870.

Acculturation and Culture: A Critical Factor for Asian Americans' Health

11

Yijie Wang and Su Yeong Kim

Ting is a 24-year-old who immigrated to the U.S. from China when she was 8 years old. Two months ago, she was diagnosed with bipolar disorder at the only bilingual mental health center in her city. Her parents communicated with staff members in Chinese, explaining that Ting had suffered from severe mood swings since college. She had barely managed to graduate, and had not held a job ever since. Although they knew that something was wrong with her, Ting's parents never talked about her problem with anyone outside their own family. They were ashamed that Ting was unemployed and sometimes manic; they also did not know where to ask for help. It was not until Ting went a whole week with only 10 hours of sleep that her parents finally took her to a local hospital and asked for treatment. At the hospital, they experienced great difficulty trying to communicate with the hospital staff in English. Finally, Ting was referred the local bilingual mental health center. However, even with professional help, Ting's parents have not accepted the idea that Ting needs medication to control her condition, and are insisting that acupuncture is a better choice.

The example of Ting and her family illustrates many of the cultural and acculturative factors that are typically associated with Asian American health problems. First of all, Ting's family did

Y. Wang (✉) • S.Y. Kim
Department of Human Development and Family
Sciences, University of Texas at Austin,
Austin, TX, USA
e-mail: yiwang@prc.utexas.edu;
suyeongkim@mail.utexas.edu

not seek professional help until after Ting had already been suffering from bipolar disorder for several years. Asian Americans are less likely than other Americans to utilize mental health services or communicate about their problems with people outside their families (Zhang, Snowden, & Sue, 1998). One reason is that a mental health problem is considered a sign of weakness in traditional Asian cultures, and families do not want to be stigmatized (Kim, Atkinson, & Umemoto, 2001). Interestingly, when Ting's family finally sought professional help, they focused on her insomnia rather than her mood swings. Even after Ting was diagnosed with a mood disorder, they preferred traditional Chinese treatment over medication. Asian cultures tend to hold a holistic view of mind–body relationships, which may explain why Asian Americans with mental health problems are likely to report somatic symptoms and prefer traditional treatments that target both mind and body (Chun, Enomoto, & Sue, 1996). Finally, Ting's family experienced a lot of difficulties communicating with the staff members at the hospital, where there were no bilingual services available for them. The lack of multicultural expertise in the mainstream U.S. culture is another reason for Asian Americans' underutilization of health services. To address this issue, much needs to be done to increase multicultural competency in health services (Hwang, 2006).

In this chapter, we highlight aspects of the acculturation process that are important in gaining a better understanding of Asian Americans' mental and physical health. We will first discuss the concept of acculturation, including a review of various acculturation strategies, dimensions, and measures. Then, we will examine cultural forms of expressing distress, and discuss the relationship between acculturation and health, both mental and physical. After summarizing the current research findings on acculturation and heath, we will discuss future directions for research.

Conceptualizing Acculturation

Concept of Acculturation

A classic definition of acculturation was proposed by Redfield, Linton, and Herskovits (1936): "Acculturation comprehends those phenomena which result when groups of individuals having different cultures come into continuous first-hand contact with subsequent changes in the original culture patterns of either or both groups" (p. 149). Although this definition suggests possible changes in both groups, it is often the minority group who is expected to change and adapt to the mainstream culture in order to survive and succeed, as opposed to the other way around (Yoon, Langrehr, & Ong, 2011). Therefore, in the literature on minority adjustment in the U.S., "acculturation" is mainly used to describe the changes taking place within ethnic minority groups, even though some changes may also occur in the mainstream group.

For immigrants, there are two aspects to the process of acculturation: participating in the mainstream culture and retaining the heritage culture. These two aspects used to be considered as two extremes on a continuum. In this view, becoming oriented to the mainstream culture means simultaneously relinquishing the heritage culture. This unilinear framework appears often in the sociological literature, which uses the term "assimilation" to describe the process through which immigrants, their children, and their children's children gradually lose their culture of origin and become an indistinguishable part of the mainstream society. In contrast, a bilinear model, which appears more often in the recent psychological literature, conceptualizes acculturation as two separate processes. In this view, an individual who is highly oriented towards the mainstream culture may also be highly oriented towards his/her heritage culture.

Empirical studies that directly compare the two models suggest that it is important to consider immigrant generational status in providing support for each of the two models. For example, Tsai, Ying, and Lee (2000) compared the relationship between the meanings of "being Chinese" and "being American" in a sample of 122 U.S.-born Chinese, 119 immigrant Chinese who arrived in the U.S. before age 12, and 112 immigrant Chinese who arrived in the U.S. after age 12. They found that "being Chinese" was unrelated to "being American" among U.S.-born Chinese, whereas "being Chinese" was negatively related to "being American" among immigrant Chinese, whether they had arrived before or after age 12 (Tsai et al., 2000). These findings suggest that for U.S.-born Chinese, how they feel about "being Chinese" develops separately from how they feel about "being American." For foreign-born immigrants, however, feeling more American goes hand-in-hand with feeling less Chinese. In other words, Tsai and colleagues' research suggests that a unilinear framework may best explain the acculturation process for foreign-born immigrants, whereas the bilinear framework is a more accurate explanation of the acculturation process for U.S.-born Asian Americans.

We have chosen to adopt the bilinear model of acculturation in this chapter, which discusses the effects of both participating in the mainstream culture and retaining the heritage culture on Asian Americans' health. Not only does the bilinear model better capture the complexity of the acculturation process, but it can also accommodate the linear perspective within the bilinear model. This inclusiveness is helpful, since some studies referenced in the current chapter still use a unilinear model.

Acculturation Strategies and Adjustment

Berry (1980) proposed four different acculturation strategies, based on various levels of orientation towards the mainstream and heritage cultures: integration, assimilation, separation and marginalization. Each strategy is related to a specific adjustment outcome. Immigrants who choose the strategy of integration are highly oriented towards both the mainstream and the heritage culture. Integrated individuals usually exhibit a high level of participation and proficiency in the mainstream culture; at the same time, they maintain the heritage culture to a great degree. Such individuals are considered to be well adjusted, and their health status generally supports this view. It is likely that they experience better health because they are more flexible in personality, have more social support, and experience mutual acceptance from peers in two different cultures, both mainstream and heritage (Berry, 1997).

Those who choose the strategy of assimilation are oriented towards the mainstream culture rather than towards the heritage culture. Assimilated individuals participate fully in the mainstream culture, and refuse to maintain their heritage culture. However, as Asian Americans are often perceived as "perpetual foreigners," they may not be able to participate fully in the mainstream culture (Kim, 2009).

Separation is the strategy of maintaining a high orientation towards one's heritage culture at the cost of orienting towards the mainstream culture. Separated individuals do not have contact with the mainstream culture, choosing instead to focus on their heritage culture. They may experience rejection from the mainstream group, yet they often benefit from social support within their close-knit heritage group.

Marginalization happens when immigrants have low orientations towards both cultures. Marginalized individuals do not participate in the mainstream culture, yet they also lose connection with their heritage culture. Such individuals are considered to be at highest risk for adjustment problems. This is probably because they are likely to experience both rejection from the mainstream group and loss of social support from the heritage group (Berry, 1997).

In sum, among the four acculturation strategies, integration represents the most adaptive strategy, marginalization represents the least adaptive strategy, with assimilation and separation being intermediate (Berry, 1997).

Measures of Acculturation

Acculturation encompasses a broad spectrum of changes in the lives of ethnic minorities. Accordingly, there are various approaches to measuring acculturation. In the sociological literature, indirect measures such as generational status, age of arrival and length of residency in the U.S. are frequently used as proxies of acculturation. Sociological theories of immigrant assimilation hypothesize that a longer exposure to the mainstream culture results in a higher level of acculturation. Individuals who have been in the U.S. for a longer period of time are considered more acculturated than those who have recently immigrated; another assumption is that each successive generation will naturally become more acculturated (Gordon, 1964). However, some scholars have questioned the use of generational status as a measurement of acculturation among Asian Americans. Waters and Jimenez (2005) noted that for early European immigrants, the hiatus of immigration during the Great Depression caused some cultural distance between generations, such that being in a later generation was usually synonymous with being more acculturated. For post-1965 Asian immigrants, on the other hand, immigration has been more or less constant, which means that belonging to a later generation does not guarantee distance from, or higher levels of acculturation than, first generation Asian immigrants.

Instead of the proximal measures of acculturation that commonly appear in the sociological literature, the psychological literature gives greater emphasis to an individual's behavioral and psychological dimensions of acculturation. Kim and Abreu (2001) reviewed the content of acculturation measures currently being used, and summarized four basic dimensions: cultural behavior, cultural values, cultural knowledge, and cultural identity. Cultural behavior includes "friendship choice, preferences for television programs and reading materials, participation in cultural activities, contact with the heritage culture, language use, food choice and music preference." The cultural values dimension includes "attitudes and beliefs about social relations, cultural customs, cultural traditions, gender roles, and health and illness". Cultural knowledge includes "culturally specific information such as names of historical leaders in the heritage and mainstream cultures, and the significance given to culturally specific activities." Cultural identity refers to "attitudes towards one's cultural identity, attitudes toward mainstream and heritage groups, and level of comfort towards people from mainstream and heritage groups."

Different dimensions of acculturation tend to develop at different rates (Kim & Abreu, 2001). For example, behavioral acculturation may proceed faster than value acculturation, as individuals may feel compelled to adopt certain behaviors, but not values, in order to survive in the mainstream society (Szapocznik & Kurtines, 1980; Szapocznik, Scopetta, Kurtines, & Arandale, 1978). In a similar vein, Kim, Atkinson, and Yang (1999) found that the increase in mainstream cultural behaviors proceeded faster than the decline in heritage culture values. Even within each dimension, different sub-dimensions might change at various rates. For example, the acquisition of language proceeded faster than the increase in mainstream social interactions (Lee, Goldstein, Brown, & Ballard-Barbash, 2010). These findings suggest that it is important to examine the acculturation process by looking separately at each dimension, along with its sub-dimensions, in addition to developing more effective ways to measure overall levels of acculturation.

A single measure of a specific dimension may not provide a complete picture of the acculturation process. It is important to recognize this point, as some studies have assessed acculturation with a single indicator, such as language use, which is considered a proximal measure of acculturation by some scholars but not others (Chun, Organista, & Gerardo, 2003). Kim and Abreu (2001) state that language use is in fact an indicator of behavioral acculturation rather than a proxy measure for acculturation in general. For our purposes, language use alone will be considered as a proxy measure only if it is the sole measure of acculturation in a given study. This is because that a single indicator such as language use cannot fully capture the range of psychological experience associated with the complex process of acculturation.

The following review of the literature on acculturation and health will examine various dimensions of acculturation. It is important to note that although many theories of acculturation posit behavioral and psychological dimensions of the process, many of the studies we review employ a proximal measure, such as generational status, length of residency or language use, as the sole measure of acculturation.

Acculturation, Culture and Mental Health

Acculturation and Psychological Well-being

Most research on the relationship between acculturation and psychological well-being has focused on a specific mental health problem, such as depression and anxiety, or on a global index of various mental health symptoms referred to as "psychological distress." When indices of psychological well-being are examined in the same study, they are often shown to be related to acculturation in similar ways. However, researchers do not agree on whether acculturation enhances or detracts from psychological well-being. This debate is especially apparent in epidemiological studies, which usually employ standardized clinical diagnostic interviews and evaluate them alongside proxy measures of acculturation, such as generational status, age of immigration and length of stay in the United States (Hwang, Chun, Takeuchi, Myers, & Siddarth, 2005; Takeuchi et al., 1998, 2007). Although such studies generally take the perspective that immigrants are at greater risk for negative outcomes as they acculturate and live in United States into later generations (Takeuchi et al., 2007), research findings are not always consistent with this perspective. Study findings can contradict each other, depending on the measure of acculturation used.

Using a large-scale sample of 1,747 Chinese Americans between the ages of 18 and 65 living in the Los Angeles area (the Chinese American Psychiatric Epidemiological Study, or CAPES), Hwang and colleagues (2005) found that individuals who immigrated at younger ages were more likely to experience depression than those who immigrated at older ages. However, the likelihood of experiencing a first onset of depression decreased as the length of time an individual stayed in the U.S. increased. Using the same CAPES dataset, Takeuchi and colleagues (1998) found that among highly acculturated individuals (as indicated by language use, ethnicity of the workplace and food choices), women were twice as likely as men to experience depression, whereas among less acculturated individuals, there was no gender difference in depression. Using a nationally representative sample of Asian Americans from the National Latino and Asian American Study (NLAAS), Takeuchi et al. (2007) found that U.S.-born Asian American women experienced higher rates of lifetime depression and anxiety disorders than did foreign-born Asian American women, and that Asian American men who were more fluent in English experienced lower rates of depression and anxiety disorders during both a particular 12-month period and over the course of their life. In other words, although current research findings indicate possible gender and generational differences in the relationship between acculturation and psychological wellbeing, the direction of such relationships is not yet clear. While the CAPES and NLAAS datasets suggest that some proxy measures of acculturation (younger age at immigration, being in the U.S.-born second generation) are risk factors for clinically significant levels of depression, other proxy measures (English language fluency, when it is the only indicator of acculturation in a study) may protect individuals from experiencing clinically significant mental health problems.

In comparison, smaller-scale studies have yielded more consistent results using depressive symptoms scales and psychological measures of acculturation, such as behaviors, values and identities. Such studies suggest that a high level of acculturation is related to a lower risk of developing mental health problems. For example, using a sample of 107 Asian American college students, Hwang and Ting (2008) measured behavioral and value dimensions of acculturation and explored their relationships to mental health. Results showed that individuals who identified with American culture to a greater degree reported lower levels of psychological distress and depressive symptoms, whereas identification with the heritage culture was not significantly related to psychological wellbeing. Similarly, in a study of 104 Chinese international graduate and undergraduate students in the United States, Wang and Mallinckrodt (2006) found that higher behavioral and value acculturation towards American culture, as opposed to behavioral and value acculturation towards the heritage culture, was related to experiencing lower levels of psychological distress.

Stress that is related to the process of adapting to a new environment, or acculturative stress, is considered to be a primary risk factor for decreased psychological wellbeing (Berry, Kim, Minde, & Mok, 1987). Acculturative stress can be the result of a wide range of difficulties, such as those presented by the language barrier, challenges in new jobs, discrimination, or disruptions in family functions (Hwang & Ting, 2008). A lower level of acculturation to the mainstream culture is related to increased acculturative stress. For example, in a sample of 118 Korean Americans, Shim and Schwartz (2007) found that individuals who had lived in the U.S. for less time were less oriented towards the mainstream culture and adhered more strongly to the heritage culture; these individuals were also more likely to experience cultural adjustment difficulties, or in other words, acculturative stress. Unfortunately, a higher level of acculturative stress is related to poorer psychological wellbeing. In a sample of 319 Chinese, Japanese and Korean immigrant adolescents, Yeh (2003) found that those with lower cultural adjustment difficulties, or low acculturative stress, reported fewer problems with their mental health. Finally, Hwang and Ting (2008) directly tested the potential mediating effect of acculturative stress in the relationship between acculturation and psychological wellbeing. They found that a low level of acculturation was related to more acculturative stress, which in turn was associated with more psychological distress and a higher incidence of clinical depression.

Based on the above findings for Asian American adults, orientation towards the mainstream culture seems more important than orientation towards the heritage culture for psychological wellbeing. However, the pattern for adolescents seems to be the opposite: for them, orientation towards the heritage culture seems to be more important for psychological well-being. Kim, Gonzales, Stroh and Wang (2006) examined the relationship between behavioral and value dimensions of acculturation and depressive symptoms in a sample of Korean American, Chinese American, and Japanese American parents and adolescents. Results showed that adolescents with a lower orientation towards Asian culture reported more depressive symptoms, and parents with a lower orientation towards American culture reported more depressive symptoms. Using a sample of Chinese Canadian families, Costigan and Dokis (2006) found that only the difference between parents' and adolescents' orientations toward Chinese culture (and not the difference in their mainstream orientations) was related to adolescents' depressive symptoms. Specifically, when their parents were strongly oriented towards Chinese culture, adolescents with a low level of Chinese orientation reported more depressive symptoms.

Although the different effects of acculturation on individuals of various ages is a topic that needs further research, it is possible that there are age-specific acculturative stressors. To illustrate, a major stressor for adults in immigrant families is learning how to participate in the mainstream culture, as adults need to succeed in a career that most likely puts them in daily contact with the mainstream culture. In comparison, a major stressor for adolescents in immigrant families may be discrepant acculturation levels between them and their parents, since a gap between them and their parents can lead to disrupted family functioning and poorer adolescent mental health (Crane,

Ngai, Larson, & Hafen, 2005). A low level of orientation towards the heritage culture may be especially problematic for adolescents, as this can cause their parents to feel dismayed or even betrayed (Ying, 1999). At the same time, immigrant parents usually want their children to be oriented to the mainstream culture, believing that this is necessary in order to succeed in mainstream society (Costigan & Dokis, 2006).

In short, the current literature has reached no consensus on the relationship between acculturation and psychological well-being. Sociological studies using proximal measures of acculturation usually argue that Asian Americans who immigrated at a younger age or who belong to a later generation (and who are thus presumably more acculturated to the mainstream culture) are at increased risk for maladjustment, while psychological studies using behavioral and value measures of acculturation usually find that individuals with a low level of acculturation are at increased risk for maladjustment, possibly due to increased acculturative stress. To further complicate matters, the relative importance of mainstream versus heritage cultural orientation may not be the same for children and adults, given that some acculturative stressors seem to be age-specific.

Culture and Somatic Symptoms

When considering the relationship between culture and mental health among Asian Americans, it is important to address the mental health problems that are rooted in Asian cultures. One example of this kind of culturally distinctive problem is somatization. Somatization refers to the tendency to experience, communicate and seek medical help for physical distress due to psychological stress (Lipowski, 1988). Somatic distress may include "headaches, stomach pains, inability to concentrate, chronic fatigue, sleep difficulties, or loss of sensory functioning" (Chun et al., 1996, p. 348).

Although somatic symptoms seem to be co-morbid with affective disorders across cultures (Gureje, Simon, Ustun, & Goldberg, 1997), Asians are more likely than Westerners to experience, or at least to communicate, somatic symptoms (Lin & Cheung, 1999). For example, in an initial attempt to examine cross-culture differences in somatization, Kleinman (1977) found that 88% of 25 Taiwanese patients with depressive symptoms initially reported somatic symptoms without dysphoric affect, whereas only 20% of 25 western patients reported somatic symptoms. Similarly, in a sample of 85 Chinese American and 85 European American patients referred for psychiatric consultation, Hsu and Folstein (1997) found that 28.6% of Chinese American patients and 9.5% of European American patients reported somatic suffering, persisting in attributing their problems to physical causes even when no such cause was found. Waza, Graham, Zyzanski, and Inoue (1999) compared the medical records of 104 patients in Japan and 85 patients in the U.S. with a diagnosis of depression, and found more somatic complaints in Japanese patients' records. In a study of anxiety disorder in Nepal and the U.S., Hoge and colleagues (2006) found that although patients from the two countries had similar overall anxiety scores, Nepali patients scored higher on the somatic subscale, whereas American patients scored higher on the psychological subscale. High rates of somatic symptoms among Asians and Asian Americans appear to be consistently supported by the literature.

Scholars have proposed several explanations for the high levels of somatization observed in the Asian population. One explanation is related to the fact that distress is often presented in culturally specific ways. In other words, every culture has its "idiom of distress" (Nichter, 1981). Specifically, individuals in Asian culture prefer to communicate physical discomfort rather than emotional pain when they discuss their psychological distress, even though they are fully aware that emotional stressors may be responsible for triggering their somatic symptoms (Cheung & Lau, 1982). In a longitudinal study on Vietnamese refugees in the U.S., Lin and colleagues found that although most of the participants reported only somatic symptoms in the initial interview, they reported both psychological and somatic symptoms when they were asked specifically about their psychological symptoms in later

interviews (Lin, Masuda, & Tazuma, 1982; Lin, Tazuma, & Masuda, 1979; Masuda, Lin, & Tazuma, 1980). In a study comparing 175 Chinese and 107 Canadian outpatients with depressive symptoms, Ryder and colleagues (2008) found that the Chinese reported more somatic symptoms, whereas the European Canadians reported more psychological symptoms; they suggest that the tendency among Chinese outpatients to report more somatic symptoms was due to the devaluation of emotional expression in this group.

Kirmayer (2001) further proposed that, since psychopathology is associated with social stigma in Asian culture, communicating psychological distress in a somatic form is a culturally appropriate way of expressing psychological distress, as it enables individuals in Asian culture to seek professional help without being stigmatized. Several studies support this notion, which seems especially salient when it comes to individuals who have already reached clinically significant levels of psychological distress. For example, in a sample of 224 outpatients with depressive symptoms and individuals without any history of mental health problems in China, Yen, Robins, and Lin (2000) found that after controlling for depression levels, Chinese outpatients were more likely to report somatic symptoms than were Chinese individuals without any history of mental health problems. Similarly, Weiss, Tram, Weisz, Rescorla, and Achenbach (2009) compared somatic and psychological symptoms of depression between children in the U.S. and Thailand. They found that in the clinic-referred sample, Thai children reported higher levels of somatic versus depressive symptoms compared to U.S. children. Collectively, these findings suggest that the Asian preference for expressing psychological distress in somatic terms may be more operative when individuals are experiencing severe mental health problems, or among those who have already sought out professional help to deal with their psychological distress.

There may, however, be a more fundamental reason why Asians and Asian Americans are more likely than their Western counterparts to report somatic symptoms. Somatization represents not just a culturally specific way of expressing psychological distress, but also a way of conceptualizing it. Rather than making a distinction between psychological and physical experience, as Western culture tends to do, most Asian cultures hold a holistic view of the relationship between mind and body (Tseng, 1975). Traditional Chinese medicine emphasizes that both mental and physical health depend on the balance of two energy forces, *yin* and *yang*, and that when this balance is disrupted, the imbalance should be treated in both the mind and body (Chun et al., 1996). In this view, it follows that manifestations of psychological distress in Asian individuals would include not only psychological symptoms but also somatic symptoms.

Studies on culture-bound syndromes provide evidence for the holistic view of mind and body common among Asian cultures. For example, ethnic Koreans who are seeking professional help often report that they suffer from *hwa-byung*, a culture-bound syndrome that includes both psychological and physical symptoms (Lin, 1983). *Hwa-byung* means, literally, "fire sickness," which includes "a multitude of somatic and psychological symptoms, including constricted, oppressed, or 'pushed-up' sensations in the chest, palpitations, 'heat sensation,' flushing, headache, 'epigastric mass (lump in epigastrium),' dysphoria, anxiety, irritability, and difficulty in concentration" (Lin et al., 1992, p. 386). Individuals suffering from *hwa-byung* believe that their problems are caused by "chronic unresolved anger that led to the imbalance of the body by the excessive accumulation of the fire element, as conceptualized in Oriental medicine theories" (Lin & Cheung, 1999, p. 777). In a community sample of 109 Korean Americans, Lin and colleagues (1992) found that individuals who reported suffering from *hwa-byung* were more likely to be diagnosed with Diagnostic and Statistical Manual of Mental Disorders-III (DSM-III) major depression, to have had a history of depression diagnosis, or to report more depressive symptoms, which suggests that *hwa-byung* may be a culture-bound form of depression. More recently, in a sample of 1,352 individuals in Korea, Ketterer and colleagues (2010) found

that *hwa-byung* is characterized by general health problems, gastrointestinal symptoms, hopelessness, and anger, which suggests that *hwa-byung* may not have an exact counterpart in Western culture.

Another example of a culture-bound syndrome is neurasthenia, *shenjing shuairuo*, in Chinese culture. It is "an ailment with vague, protean signs and symptoms due to weakness of the nervous system, the brain and the body generally," accompanied by "bodily weakness, fatigue, tiredness, headaches, dizziness, and a range of gastrointestinal and other complaints" (Kleinman, 1982, p. 122). In a sample of 100 patients diagnosed with neurasthenia in China, Kleinman (1982) found that 83% of them could also be diagnosed with major depression. More recently, in a community sample of 1,610 Chinese Americans, Takeuchi, Chun, Gong, and Shen (2002) found that life stressors (e.g., financial stress) were related to neurasthenia but not to depressive symptoms. This evidence suggests neurasthenia may be a better indicator than depression for psychological distress in Asian Americans (Chun, Moos, & Cronkite, 2006).

To summarize, the literature shows that Asian Americans are more likely than European Americans to express their psychological problems in physical terms. A good explanation for this phenomenon may be the fact that Asian cultures emphasize the connection between mind and body. This culturally specific view of health may also contribute to culture-bound syndromes such as *hwa-byung* and *shenjing shuairuo*, which encompass both psychological and physical forms of discomfort.

Acculturation, Culture and Counseling

Asian Americans tend to underutilize mental health services compared to European Americans. In a randomly selected sample of 161 Asian Americans and 1,332 European Americans in the Los Angeles area (Epidemiologic Catchment Area study, ECA), Zhang and colleagues (1998) found that Asian Americans were less likely than European Americans to disclose their mental health problems to others, including friends or relatives, religious figures, psychiatrists or mental health specialists, and physicians. In addition, Asian Americans were less likely to use mental health facilities, including mental health centers, psychiatric outpatient clinics at a general hospital or university hospital, hospital emergency rooms, crisis centers or hotline programs, self-help groups, spiritualists, herbalists or natural therapists. Perhaps a more serious problem is that, although Asian Americans tend to underutilize counseling services, they may be more likely than European Americans to experience severe disturbances in their mental health. In a sample of 3,729 Asian American and 3,553 European American outpatients, Durvasula and Sue (1996) found that compared to European American outpatients, Asian American outpatients tended to receive more severe diagnoses, function more poorly and display more psychotic symptoms.

Scholars have proposed several reasons for Asian Americans' underutilization of counseling services. One is that Asian cultures hold a negative view of counseling, which may discourage Asian Americans from seeking professional help (Kim et al., 2001). Asian cultures also value self-control and restraint over emotional expressiveness and expect individuals to solve psychological problems by themselves. Disclosing personal problems to, or seeking help from, people other than one's family members is considered a sign of weakness that brings disgrace to the family (Kim et al., 2001).

From this perspective, a high level of adherence to Asian cultural values is likely to be related to a lower likelihood of seeking professional psychological help. Kim (2007) examined the effects of orientation towards the mainstream and heritage cultures on 146 Asian American college students' professional help-seeking attitudes. The study reported that individuals with a higher orientation towards the heritage culture were less likely to recognize the need for psychological help and were less tolerant of stigma; additionally, they were less open to, and less confident about, consulting mental health professionals. However, higher acculturation towards the mainstream culture was not

significantly related to attitudes about seeking professional psychological help. Using a sample of 242 Asian American college students, Kim and Omizo (2003) found additional support for the idea that individuals with a higher adherence to Asian values hold more negative attitudes toward seeking professional help and are therefore less willing to see a counselor.

Another reason for Asian Americans' underutilization of counseling is that mainstream counseling is often lacking in multicultural sensitivity and competency, which discourages Asian Americans from consulting mental health professionals about their psychological problems (Hwang, 2006). Sue and Sue (1999) proposed three strategies to improve multicultural counseling effectiveness: counselors need to be aware of their own cultural values and potential biases, counselors need to understand their clients' cultural values and potential differences between the counselors' and clients' cultural values, and counselors need to use culturally appropriate interventions. Supporting Sue and Sue's recommendation, in a sample of 146 Asian American college students, Kim, Ng, and Ahn (2005) found that Asian American students perceived greater alliance and empathy from their counselors when counselors expressed agreement with students' opinions on the cause of their problems. Further, in a sample of 116 Asian American college students, Li and colleagues (2007) found that when counselors did express culturally inconsistent statements during the counseling process, students perceived these counselors to be more competent if they acknowledged potential inconsistencies and encouraged clients to express their own opinions.

In sum, the literature shows that although Asian Americans tend to underutilize counseling services, they may actually be more likely than European Americans to experience severe mental health problems. Asian Americans may be reluctant to use counseling services due to culturally specific attitudes that discourage individuals from seeking professional help, or because there is a lack of competent multicultural counseling services currently available.

Acculturation, Culture and Physical Health

Acculturation, Culture and Smoking Behavior

Smoking is the single leading cause of preventable death in the United States; even exposure to secondhand smoke can cause serious disease, including lung cancer and heart disease (Centers for Disease Control and Prevention [CDCP], 2011c). In national surveys covering the period from 2006 to 2008, the prevalence of smoking among the Asian American population was 21.2% for male adults, 8.8% for female adults, 5.2% for male youth and 2.9% for female youth, rates that are lower than those found among other ethnic groups (CDCP, 2011a). In comparison, the smoking rate in Asian Americans' native countries is usually much higher for men and lower for women. In a recent global report, the current smoking rate is 57.4% for men and 2.6% for women in China, 52.8% for men and 5.8% for women in Korea, 57.0% for men and 10.8% for women in India, 39.9% for men and 10.0% for women in Japan, 40.3% for men and 7.1% for women in the Philippines, 36.6% for men and 1.6% for women in Thailand, and 34.8% for men and 1.8% for women in Vietnam (World Health Organization [WHO], 2009). The data show that Asian American men are less likely to smoke than their ethnic counterparts living in Asia, whereas Asian American women are more likely to smoke than their ethnic counterparts living in Asia.

The difference between smoking rates in the Asian American population and the rates in their native countries may be related to the different views of smoking held by the mainstream American and Asian cultures. Asian cultures have a more positive view of smoking in men but a more negative view of smoking in women. For example, in Korean culture, smoking is a medium for social interaction among males: it is usual for men to initiate a conversation by offering cigarettes to others; when offered a cigarette, men are expected to accept such an offer, as turning it

down is interpreted as impolite. In addition, since adult men comprise the group with the highest social status in Korean culture, and since smoking is socially approved only for this group, smoking can become a way for Korean youths to identify themselves with adult men by appearing more mature and masculine. In comparison, smoking is considered to be inappropriate for women in most Asian cultures, due to traditional gender roles. For example, female smokers are perceived as unfit mothers and wives in Korean culture (Kim, Son, et al., 2005). For this reason, even though smoking is considered less acceptable in American culture than it is in Asian cultures, smoking in women is more likely to be tolerated in American culture than it is in Asian cultures (An, Cochran, Mays, & McCarthy, 2008).

As American and Asian cultures hold different views of smoking in men and women, it is possible that acculturation plays an important role in Asian Americans' smoking behavior. In fact, a number of studies have found that a higher level of acculturation is associated with lower smoking rates in Asian American male adults but with higher smoking rates in Asian American female adults (for a review, see Kim et al., 2005; Zhang & Wang, 2008). Almost all the available studies on this topic have used concurrent data and a single proximal measure of acculturation, such as length of stay in the U.S., generational status, or language proficiency. Generally, the smoking rate in Asian American men is lower if they were born in the U.S. (Maxwell, Bernaards, & McCarthy, 2005), have lived longer in U.S. (Juon, Kim, Han, Ryu, & Han, 2003), or are more fluent in English (Tang, Shimizu, & Chen, 2005). These associations are reversed for Asian American women (Ma et al., 2004; Maxwell et al., 2005). A recent meta-analysis of 21 studies published between 1994 and 2005 confirmed that acculturation to the mainstream society is a protective factor for Asian American men but a risk factor for Asian American women in terms of their smoking behaviors (Choi, Rankin, Stewart, & Oka, 2008). The reliance on proxy measures of acculturation in past studies means that more research is needed to examine the relationship between smoking behavior and additional domains of acculturation, including the behavioral, cultural values, attitudes and identification domains of acculturation.

However, it seems clear that social support for smoking is implicated in the relationship between acculturation and Asian American smoking behaviors. In Kim et al., (2005) interview with 22 Korean American men about their experiences of smoking in Korea and the U.S., many current smokers reported that they felt "timid" smoking in public places in the U.S., where smoking around people is perceived to be socially unacceptable, and where they were sometimes clearly asked not to smoke, or to stop smoking in public. Hofstetter and colleagues (2007) examined the effect of social support on smoking behavior in a sample of 2,830 Korean Americans. They found that both men and women were more likely to start smoking when they experienced more social support for smoking, and that persistent smokers reported having more social reinforcers than did smokers who quit (Hofstetter et al., 2007).

The possible effect of social support on the relationship between acculturation and smoking behavior seems particularly evident among Asian American youth. Studies have found that acculturation is a risk factor for smoking in Asian American youth (Chen et al., 2009; Chen, Unger, Cruz, & Johnson, 1999). It is possible that when Asian American youth are more acculturated into the mainstream culture, they are more likely to interact with peers who smoke, as there is a higher incidence of smoking in the mainstream culture than among Asian Americans (CDCP, 2011a). Several studies have directly tested the effect of peer group smoking on the smoking behaviors of Asian American youth. In a sample of 3,268 Asian American adolescents from various ethnic backgrounds, Weiss and Garbanati (2006) found that adolescents of both genders and from all ethnic backgrounds were more likely to smoke when they perceived more acceptance of smoking in their peer groups. Moreover, in a sample of 1,248 Asian American adolescents of various ethnicities, Thai, Connell, and Tebes (2010) found a significant mediating effect of peer smoking

behavior in the relationship between acculturation and adolescents' smoking behavior. In other words, adolescents who were more acculturated had more friends who were currently smoking, which in turn was related to more smoking behavior among Asian American adolescents.

To summarize, a high orientation towards the mainstream culture tends to decrease the likelihood of smoking in men, but it increases the likelihood of smoking in women and adolescents. This is probably due to the different cultural views of smoking in Asian and American cultures for men, women and adolescents. Special attention needs to be paid to adolescent smokers, as they are greatly influenced by their social environment, especially their peer group.

Acculturation, Culture and Chronic Diseases

Chronic diseases, such as heart disease, cancer and diabetes, are the leading causes of death and disability in the U.S. (Kung, Hoyert, Xu, & Murphy, 2008). Generally, the rate of chronic diseases in the Asian American population is lower than, or similar to, that found in other groups. For example, in a recent national health survey, Asian American adults were less likely to be diagnosed with cancer or any type of heart disease than were European American adults (Sondik, Madans, & Gentleman, 2010). The rate of diagnosed diabetes is 8.4% among Asian American adults, compared to 7.1% in non-Hispanic whites, 11.8% in Hispanics, and 12.6% in non-Hispanic blacks (CDCP, 2011b).

Although the rate of chronic diseases in Asian Americans is relatively low, Asian Americans are more likely than those in their native countries to experience chronic disease (Cook, Goldoft, Schwartz, & Weiss, 1999; Flood et al., 2000; Stanford, Herrinton, Schwartz, & Weiss, 1995; Ueshima et al., 2007). This discrepancy suggests a possible effect of acculturation on chronic diseases. Generally, Asian Americans with higher levels of acculturation are more likely to have a chronic disease. For example, Huang and colleagues (1996) examined the relationship between acculturation and the prevalence of diabetes in a sample of 8,006 Japanese American men in Hawaii. They found that Japanese Americans who were born in the U.S. and those who had stayed in the U.S. for a longer period were more likely to have diabetes (Huang et al., 1996). In another sample of 3,809 Japanese Americans in California, Marmot and Syme (1976) measured the behavior and value dimensions of acculturation and examined their relationships to the prevalence of coronary heart diseases. They found that Japanese Americans who were more acculturated were more likely to have coronary heart disease compared to those who were less acculturated.

Diet habits often change during the process of acculturation, which may explain some of these research findings on chronic disease in the Asian American population. A number of studies have demonstrated that Asian Americans' diet decreases in quality as they acculturate into the mainstream culture. For example, in a sample 486 Korean Americans, Kim and Chan (2004) examined the relationship between the behavioral and attitude dimensions of acculturation and dietary habits. They found that less acculturated Korean Americans tended to consume more traditional Korean food, such as rice, *chigae* (stew) and *kimchi*, whereas more acculturated Korean Americans tended to consume more Western food, such as bread, spaghetti, ham, chocolate, candies and diet soft drinks. In addition, more acculturated Korean Americans tended to take in more sweets and total fat, both of which have been implicated in the development of chronic diseases (Kim & Chan, 2004). In another sample of 243 Chinese Americans in the Philadelphia region, Liu and colleagues (2010) measured acculturation, using English proficiency and social interactions with the mainstream culture as measures, and examined its relationship with diet quality, including dietary variety, adequacy of nutrients, moderation of intake (total fat, saturated fat, cholesterol, sodium, and empty calorie foods), and overall dietary balance. They found that although more acculturated Chinese Americans had diets with more variety and nutritional adequacy,

their diets also tended away from moderation (in other words, this group consumed more total fat and calories), which is a risk factor for chronic diseases (Liu et al., 2010).

To summarize, it appears that adopting unhealthy dietary habits, and thus increasing the risk of developing chronic diseases, is currently part of the process of acculturation to mainstream American culture. Many studies cited here used a proximal measure of acculturation, such as generational status and length of residency. Although we did review studies using behavioral measures of acculturation, such as social interaction in the mainstream culture, more research is needed to understand the ways in which additional domains of acculturation relate to chronic diseases.

Acculturation, Health Prevention, Management, and Health Care Utilization

Not only do Asian Americans underutilize mental health services, but they are also less likely to use other health care services. A nationally representative survey on health care quality indicated that compared to the overall American population, Asian Americans are less likely to receive counseling services for smoking cessation (79% of overall U.S. smokers vs. 68% Asian American smokers), healthy diet and weight (49% of overall U.S. population vs. 35% of Asian Americans), and exercise (19% of overall U.S. population vs. 14% of Asian Americans) (Hughes, 2002).

Scholars have proposed several reasons for the underutilization of health care services in the Asian American population. One reason is that Asian Americans might prefer more traditional forms of treatment, such as acupuncture, and are therefore likely to consult traditional healers rather than seeking out Western health care services. A national health care quality survey showed that Asian Americans were two to three times as likely as the overall U.S. population to use the services of traditional healers and acupuncturists (Collins et al., 2002). Among those who used alternative care, 27% of Asian

Americans reported using alternative care because of cultural or religious beliefs, as compared to 8% of the overall U.S. population (Collins et al., 2002). From this perspective, a higher level of orientation towards the heritage culture may be related to a tendency to seek traditional Asian treatment. However, studies on this issue have used proximal measures of acculturation, such as generational status and length of residency in the U.S. Using a nationally representative sample, Lee and colleagues (2010) examined the relationship between acculturation and the use of complementary and alternative medicine. They found that Asian Americans who had been in the U.S. for a shorter time were more likely to use the services of acupuncturists and traditional Chinese medicine practitioners.

Another possible reason why Asian Americans underutilize health services may have to do with their limited expertise in the mainstream culture. For example, Asian Americans who are not fluent in English may experience difficulties in accessing health care information, which hinders their utilization of health services. In addition, Asian Americans who lack knowledge about mainstream health practices may also underutilize health care services. From this perspective, a lower level of language fluency and a lack of knowledge about the mainstream society may be related to lower use of health care services. In a sample of 380 Cambodian, Chinese, Indonesian, Korean, and Vietnamese American women, Nguyen, Leader, and Hung (2009) found that individuals with lower level of English proficiency were less likely to acknowledge the availability of a cancer vaccine, but more likely to acknowledge, mistakenly, the availability of a vaccine for non-vaccine-preventable cancers. In addition, in a sample of 315 Asian Indian, Chinese, Filipino, Korean, and Taiwanese American women, Wu and Ronis (2009) found that individuals who held inaccurate beliefs and lacked knowledge about mammography screening, as promoted in the mainstream culture, were less likely to have been regularly and recently screened for breast cancer. Relevant knowledge in this case included the recommended intervals for breast exam and mammography, which conditions increase the chances of getting breast cancer, and the recommended frequency for mammograms for women with different backgrounds (Wu & Ronis, 2009). Similarly, in a sample of 1,181 Korean American families, Chen and colleagues (2009) found that parents who received a variety of information on health insurance and assistance on their insurance application were more likely to apply for health insurance for their children, as compared to parents who did not receive any information or assistance in applying for available insurance.

What we know about the effect of acculturation on Asian Americans' health care utilization suggests that it is important to promote culturally competent health care services. Unfortunately, the mainstream health care services currently available may not be ideal for the Asian American population. In a national survey, Ngo-Metzger, Legedza, and Phillips (2004) found that Asian Americans were more likely than European Americans to be unsatisfied with their health care. Compared to European Americans, Asian Americans were more likely to report that their regular doctors were not of the same ethnicity and did not understand Asian Americans' background and values, and that their doctors "did not listen to everything patients had to say," "spend as much time as patients wanted," or "involve patients in decisions about care as much as patients wanted" (Ngo-Metzger et al., 2004). In a qualitative study of type 2 diabetes management experiences among 40 Chinese patients and their spouses, Chun and colleagues (2004) found that culturally competent health care can help improve diabetes management among patients who are dealing with a language barrier. Participants reported that bilingual Chinese medical staff members' knowledge of Chinese diet and food practices and their ability to provide emotional support, in addition to the availability of Chinese-language health education materials, on-site translator services and ethnically-matched health care providers, directly enhanced their diabetes management practices.

In all, the current literature suggests that when providing health care services for Asian Americans, it is important to take into consideration their traditional cultural beliefs and treatment practices, and to develop more culturally competent mainstream health care services by removing language barriers, promoting health management education, and providing emotional support.

Future Directions

In this chapter we have reviewed both the sociological and psychological literature on acculturation and its effect on Asian Americans' mental and physical health. Although much has been accomplished in understanding the link between acculturation and the mental/physical health of Asian Americans, a variety of topics still need further research. It is particularly important to gather more information on the effect of acculturation on health for various dimensions of acculturation, including cultural behaviors, values, knowledge and identity. Most current studies rely on a single proximal measure of acculturation, such as generational status or English language fluency. Such studies sometimes yield inconsistent findings, as we saw in the research on acculturation/assimilation and psychological wellbeing. Different dimensions of acculturation proceed at different rates, which means that they may also have different effects on those who are in the process of acculturating. In addition, some dimensions of acculturation may be more closely related to a specific type of health status or health behavior. Access to health information and knowledge about health insurance are both of great relevance to Asian Americans' cancer management and prevention behaviors, and heritage cultural orientation may play a central role in Asian Americans' utilization of Asian culture-specific services. It is important to examine specific dimensions of acculturation, in addition to measuring the overall level of acculturation, in order to gain a more comprehensive view of Asian Americans' health outcomes.

Research on this topic would also be improved if more studies adopted the bilinear model of acculturation. As we discussed, mainstream and heritage cultural orientations may affect different aspects of Asian Americans' well-being in various ways. It is important to distinguish between the two orientations and to examine both orientations together in future studies. According to Berry's theory of acculturation strategies, each strategy results in a distinctive pattern of adjustment. For this reason, it may also be beneficial to include Berry's acculturation strategies as part of the bilinear model of acculturation.

Another direction for future studies would be to examine the effect of acculturation on health among different age groups. The majority of the current literature focuses on college students and adults, giving less attention to children and elders. There are a few topics, such as alcohol use and risky sexual behaviors that are studied mainly in adolescents. The effects of acculturation on health may be different for people in different developmental stages, as they are faced with distinct acculturative stressors. For children and elders in Asian American families, one crucial task is to handle cultural discrepancies between them and the adults in the family: children tend to be more oriented towards American culture than their parents are (Portes & Rumbaut, 1996), and elders tend to be more oriented towards their heritage culture than their adult children are (Trinh & Ahmed, 2009). In contrast, the most important task for Asian American adults, especially immigrant adults, may be to attain proficiency in the mainstream culture in order to survive and succeed in their career. Therefore, future studies need to explore specific acculturation stressors for diverse age groups in order to gain a more nuanced understanding of the relationship between acculturation and health.

It would also be beneficial to examine different ethnic groups within the Asian American population. Although some epidemiological studies include comparisons of groups from various countries of origin, most of the current literature focuses on East Asians, such as Chinese, Japanese and Koreans. As a group, East Asians enjoy higher socioeconomic status than some other Asian subgroups, such as the Hmong, who are far more likely to experience poverty (Reeves & Bennett, 2004). It is important to examine Asian American subpopulations like the Hmong, as they may be more likely than East Asian subgroups to have risk factors for health problems.

Finally, future studies need to examine the underlying mechanisms of the relationship between acculturation and health. As more and more evidence demonstrates that there is a significant link between acculturation and health, it makes sense to investigate the reasons for such a link. The current literature has indicated that acculturative stressors may be a key factor linking acculturation and health outcomes together. More studies are needed to explore specific processes related to various acculturative stressors. For example, discrepant acculturation levels between parents and children in Asian American families may compromise family functioning, leading to poor health outcomes in both children and adults. Similarly, a low orientation towards both the heritage culture and the mainstream culture may weaken marginalized individuals' social networks and diminish their social support, placing their mental and physical health at risk. It is critical to explore these kinds of mediating processes, because having a better understanding of potential mediators between acculturation and health will enable researchers to provide valuable suggestions for interventions aimed at improving the lives of Asian Americans.

References

An, N., Cochran, S. D., Mays, V. M., & McCarthy, W. J. (2008). Influence of American acculturation on cigarette smoking behaviors among Asian American subpopulations in California. *Nicotine & Tobacco Research, 10*, 579–587.

Berry, J. W. (1980). Social and cultural change. In H. C. Triandis & R. Brislin (Eds.), *Handbook of cross-cultural psychology* (Social psychology, Vol. 5, pp. 211–279). Boston: Allyn & Bacon.

Berry, J. W. (1997). Immigration, acculturation, and adaptation. *Applied Psychology, 46*, 5–34.

Berry, J. W., Kim, U., Minde, T., & Mok, D. (1987). Comparative studies of acculturative stress. *International Migration Review, 11*, 491–510.

Centers for Disease Control and Prevention. (2011a). CDC health disparities and inequalities report – United States, 2011. *Morbidity and Mortality Weekly Report, 60*, 1–113.

Centers for Disease Control and Prevention. (2011b). *National diabetes fact sheet: National estimates and general information on diabetes and prediabetes in the United States, 2011*. Atlanta, GA: U.S. Department of Health and Human Services, Centers for Disease Control and Prevention.

Centers for Disease Control and Prevention. (2011c). *Tobacco use: Targeting the nation's leading cause of death. At a glance 2011*. Atlanta, GA: U.S. Department of Health and Human Services, Centers for Disease Control and Prevention.

Chen, J. Y., Swonger, S., Kominski, G., Liu, H., Lee, J. E., & Diamant, A. (2009). Cost-effectiveness of insuring the uninsured: The case of Korean American children. *Medical Decision Making, 29*, 51–60.

Chen, X., Unger, J. B., Cruz, T. B., & Johnson, C. A. (1999). Smoking patterns of Asian-American youth in California and their relationship with acculturation. *Journal of Adolescent Health, 24*, 321–328.

Cheung, F. M., & Lau, B. W. K. (1982). Situational variations of help-seeking behavior among Chinese patients. *Comprehensive Psychiatry, 23*, 252–262.

Choi, S., Rankin, S., Stewart, A., & Oka, R. (2008). Effects of acculturation on smoking behavior in Asian Americans: A meta-analysis. *Journal of Cardiovascular Nursing, 23*, 67–73.

Chun, K. M., Chesla, C. A., & Kwan, C. M. L. (2004). So we adapt step by step: Acculturation experiences affecting diabetes management and perceived health for Chinese American immigrants. *Social Science & Medicine, 72*, 256–264.

Chun, C.-A., Enomoto, K., & Sue, S. (1996). Health care issues among Asian Americans: Implications of somatization. In T. Mann (Ed.), *Handbook of diversity issues in health psychology* (pp. 347–365). New York: Plenum Press.

Chun, C.-A., Moos, R. H., & Cronkite, R. C. (2006). Culture: A fundamental context for the stress and coping paradigm. In P. T. P. Wong & L. C. J. Wong (Eds.), *Handbook of multicultural perspectives on stress and coping* (pp. 29–53). Dallas, TX: Spring Publications.

Chun, K. M., Organista, P. B., & Gerardo, M. (2003). *Acculturation: Advances in theory, measurement, and applied research*. Washington, DC: American Psychological Association.

Collins, K. S., Hughes, D. L., Doty, M. M., Ives, B. L., Edwards, J. N., & Tenney, K. (2002). *Diverse communities, common concerns: Assessing health care quality for minority Americans*. New York: The Commonwealth Fund.

Cook, L. S., Goldoft, M., Schwartz, S. M., & Weiss, N. S. (1999). Incidence of adenocarcinoma of the prostate in Asian immigrants to the United States and their descendants. *Journal of Urology, 161*, 152–155.

Costigan, C. L., & Dokis, D. P. (2006). Relations between parent-child acculturation differences and adjustment within immigrant Chinese families. *Child Development, 77*, 1252–1267.

Crane, D. R., Ngai, S. W, Larson, J. H., & Hafen, M., Jr. (2005). The influence of family functioning and parent-adolescent acculturation on North American Chinese adolescent outcomes. *Family Relations, 54*, 400–410.

Durvasula, R., & Sue, S. (1996). Severity of disturbance among Asian American outpatients. *Cultural Diversity and Mental Health, 2*, 43–51.

Flood, D. M., Weiss, N. S., Cook, L. S., Emerson, J. C., Schwartz, S. M., & Potter, J. D. (2000). Colorectal cancer incidence in Asian migrants to the United States and their descendants. *Cancer Causes & Control, 11*, 403–411.

Gordon, M. M. (1964). *Assimilation in American life: The role of race, religion, and national origins*. New York: Oxford University Press.

Gureje, O., Simon, G. E., Ustun, T. B., & Goldberg, D. P. (1997). Somatization in cross-cultural perspective: A World Health Organization study in primary care. *The American Journal of Psychiatry, 154*, 989–995.

Hofstetter, C. R., Hovell, M. F., Jung, K.-R., Raman, R., Irvin, V., & Ni, R. (2007). The first puff: Forces in smoking initiation among Californians of Korean descent. *Nicotine & Tobacco Research, 9*, 1277–1286.

Hoge, E. A., Tamrakar, S. M., Christian, K. M., Mahara, N., Nepal, M. K., Pollack, M. H., et al. (2006). Cross-cultural differences in somatic presentation in patients with generalized anxiety disorder. *The Journal of Nervous and Mental Disease, 194*, 962–966.

Hsu, L. K. G., & Folstein, M. F. (1997). Somatoform disorders in Caucasian and Chinese Americans. *The Journal of Nervous and Mental Disease, 185*, 382–387.

Huang, B., Rodriguez, B. L., Burchfiel, C. M., Chyou, P.-H., Curb, J. D., & Yano, K. (1996). Acculturation and prevalence of diabetes among Japanese-American men in Hawaii. *American Journal of Epidemiology, 144*, 674–681.

Hughes, D. L. (2002). *Quality of health care for Asian Americans: Findings from the Commonwealth Fund 2001 Health Care Quality Survey*. New York: The Commonwealth Fund.

Hwang, W.-C. (2006). The psychotherapy adaptation and modification framework: Application to Asian Americans. *American Psychologist, 61*, 702–715.

Hwang, W.-C., Chun, C.-A., Takeuchi, D. T., Myers, H. F., & Siddarth, P. (2005). Age of first onset major depression in Chinese Americans. *Cultural Diversity and Ethnic Minority Psychology, 11*, 16–27.

Hwang, W.-C., & Ting, J. Y. (2008). Disaggregating the effects of acculturation and acculturative stress on the mental health of Asian Americans. *Cultural Diversity and Ethnic Minority Psychology, 14*, 147–154.

Juon, H.-S., Kim, M., Han, H., Ryu, J. P., & Han, W. (2003). Acculturation and cigarette smoking among Korean American men. *Yonsei Medical Journal, 4*, 875–882.

Ketterer, H., Han, K., & Weed, N. C. (2010). Validation of a Korean MMPI-2 Hwa-Byung scale using a Korean normative sample. *Cultural Diversity and Ethnic Minority Psychology, 16*, 379–385.

Kim, B. S. K. (2007). Adherence to Asian and European American cultural values and attitudes toward seeking professional psychological help among Asian American college students. *Journal of Counseling Psychology, 54*, 474–480.

Kim, B. S. K. (2009). Acculturation and enculturation of Asian Americans: A primer. In N. Tewari & A. Alvarez (Eds.), *Asian American psychology: Current perspectives* (pp. 97–112). Mahwah, NJ: Erlbaum.

Kim, B. S. K., & Abreu, J. M. (2001). Acculturation measurement: Theory, current instruments, and future directions. In J. G. Ponterotto, J. M. Casas, L. A. Suzuki, & C. M. Alexander (Eds.), *Handbook of multicultural counseling* (pp. 394–424). Thousand Oaks, CA: Sage.

Kim, B. S. K., Atkinson, D. R., & Umemoto, D. (2001). Asian cultural values and the counseling process: Current knowledge and directions for future research. *The Counseling Psychologist, 29*, 570–603.

Kim, B. S. K., Atkinson, D. R., & Yang, P. H. (1999). The Asian Values Scale: Development, factor analysis, validation, and reliability. *Journal of Counseling Psychology, 46*, 342–352.

Kim, J., & Chan, M. M. (2004). Acculturation and dietary habits of Korean Americans. *British Journal of Nutrition, 91*, 469–478.

Kim, S. Y., Gonzales, N. A., Stroh, K., & Wang, J. J.-L. (2006). Parent-child cultural marginalization and depressive symptoms in Asian American family members. *Journal of Community Psychology, 34*, 167–182.

Kim, B. S. K., Ng, G. F., & Ahn, A. J. (2005). Effects of client expectation for counseling success, client-counselor worldview match, and client adherence to Asian and European American cultural values on counseling process with Asian Americans. *Journal of Counseling Psychology, 52*, 67–76.

Kim, B. S. K., & Omizo, M. M. (2003). Asian cultural values, attitudes toward seeking professional psychological help, and willingness to see a counselor. *The Counseling Psychologist, 31*, 343–361.

Kim, S. S., Son, H., & Nam, K. A. (2005). The sociocultural context of Korean American men's smoking behavior. *Western Journal of Nursing Research, 27*, 604–623.

Kim, S. S., Ziedonis, D., & Chen, K. W. (2007). Tobacco use and dependence in Asian Americans: A review of the literature. *Nicotine & Tobacco Research, 9*, 169–184.

Kirmayer, L. J. (2001). Cultural variations in the clinical presentation of depression and anxiety: Implications for diagnosis and treatment. *The Journal of Clinical Psychiatry, 62*, 22–28.

Kleinman, A. M. (1977). Depression, somatization, and the new cross-cultural psychiatry. *Social Sciences and Medicine, 11*, 3–10.

Kleinman, A. M. (1982). Neurasthenia and depression: a study of somatization and culture in China. *Culture, Medicine and Psychiatry, 6*, 117–190.

Kung, H.-C., Hoyert, D. L., Xu, J., & Murphy, S. L. (2008). Deaths: final data for 2005. *National Vital Statistics Reports, 56*, 1–124.

Lee, J. H., Goldstein, M. S., Brown, E. R., & Ballard-Barbash, R. (2010). How does acculturation affect the use of complementary and alternative medicine providers among Mexican- and Asian-Americans? *Journal of Immigrant and Minority Health, 12*, 302–309.

Li, L. C., Kim, B. S. K, & O'Brien, K. M. (2007). An analogue study of the effects of Asian cultural values and counselor multicultural competence on counseling process. *Psychotherapy Theory Research Practice Training, 44*, 90–95.

Lin, K.-M. (1983). Hwa-byung: a Korean culture-bound syndrome? *The American Journal of Psychiatry, 140*, 105–107.

Lin, K.-M., & Cheung, F. (1999). Mental health issues for Asian Americans. *Psychiatric Services, 50*, 774–780.

Lin, K.-M., Lau, J. K. C., Yamamoto, J., Zheng, Y.-P., Kim, H.-S., Cho, K.-H., et al. (1992). Hwa-byung: a community study of Korean Americans. *The Journal of Nervous and Mental Disease, 180*, 386–391.

Lin, K.-M., Masuda, M., & Tazuma, L. (1982). Adaptational problems of Vietnamese refugees: Part III. Case studies in clinic and field: Adaptive and maladaptive. *Psychiatric Journal of the University of Ottawa, 7*, 173–183.

Lin, K.-M., Tazuma, L., & Masuda, M. (1979). Adaptational problems of Vietnamese refugees: Part I. Health and mental health status. *Archives of General Psychiatry, 36*, 955–961.

Lipowski, Z. J. (1988). Somatization: The concept and its clinical application. *The American Journal of Psychiatry, 145*, 1358–1368.

Liu, A., Berhane, Z., & Tseng, M. (2010). Improved dietary variety and adequacy but lower dietary moderation with acculturation in Chinese women in the United States. *Journal of the American Dietetic Association, 110*, 457–462.

Ma, G. X., Tan, Y., Toubbeh, J. I., Su, X., Shive, S. E., & Lan, Y. (2004). Acculturation and smoking behavior in Asian-American populations. *Health Education Research, 19*, 615–625.

Marmot, M. G., & Syme, S. L. (1976). Acculturation and coronary heart disease in Japanese-Americans. *Journal of Epidemiology, 104*, 225–247.

Masuda, M., Lin, K.-M., & Tazuma, L. (1980). Adaptational problems of Vietnamese refugees: Part II. Life changes and perception of life events. *Archives of General Psychiatry, 37*, 447–450.

Maxwell, A. E., Bernaards, C. A., & McCarthy, W. J. (2005). Smoking prevalence and correlates among Chinese- and Filipino-American adults: Findings from the 2001 California Health Interview Survey. *Preventive Medicine, 41*, 693–699.

Ngo-Metzger, Q., Legedza, A. T. R., & Phillips, R. S. (2004). Asian Americans' reports of their health care experiences: Results of a national survey. *Journal of General Internal Medicine, 19*, 111–119.

Nguyen, G. T., Leader, A. E., & Hung, W. L. (2009). Awareness of anti-cancer vaccines among Asian American women with limited English proficiency: An opportunity for improved public health communication. *Journal of Cancer Education, 24*, 280–283.

Nichter, M. (1981). Idioms of distress: Alternatives in the expression of psychosocial distress: A case study from South India. *Culture, Medicine and Psychiatry, 5*, 379–408.

Portes, A., & Rumbaut, R. G. (1996). *Immigrant America: A portrait*. Berkeley, CA: University of California Press.

Redfield, R., Linton, R., & Herskovits, M. J. (1936). Memorandum on the study of acculturation. *American Anthropologist, 56*, 149–152.

Reeves, T. J., & Bennett, C. E. (2004). *We the People: Asians in the United States, Census 2000 Special Reports*. Washington, DC: United States Census Bureau.

Ryder, A. G., Yang, J., Zhu, X., Yao, S., Yi, J., Heine, S. J., & Bagby, R. M. (2008). The cultural shaping of depression: Somatic symptoms in China, psychological symptoms in North America? *Journal of Abnormal Psychology, 117*, 300–313.

Shim, Y. R., & Schwartz, R. C. (2007). The relationship between degree of acculturation and adjustment difficulties among Korean immigrants living in a Western society. *British Journal of Guidance and Counselling, 35*, 409–426.

Sondik, E. J., Madans, J. H., & Gentleman, J. F. (2010). Summary Health Statistics for U.S. Adults: National Health Interview Survey, 2009. *Vital and Health Statistics, 249*, 1–86.

Stanford, J. L., Herrinton, L. J., Schwartz, S. M., & Weiss, N. S. (1995). Breast cancer incidence in Asian migrants to the United States and their descendants. *Epidemiology, 6*, 181–183.

Sue, D. W. & Sue, D. (1999). *Counseling the culturally diverse: Theory and practice*. New York: Wiley.

Szapocznik, J., & Kurtines, W. (1980). Acculturation, biculturalism, and adjustment among Cuban Americans. In A. M. Padilla (Ed.), *Psychological dimensions on the acculturation process: Theory, models, and some new findings* (pp. 139–159). Boulder, CO: Westview.

Szapocznik, J., Scopetta, M. A., Kurtines, W., & Arandale, M. D. (1978). Theory and measurement of acculturation. *Interamerican Journal of Psychology, 12*, 113–120.

Takeuchi, D. T., Chun, C.-A., Gong, F., & Shen, H. (2002). Cultural expressions of distress. *Health, 6*, 221–236.

Takeuchi, D. T., Chung, R. C.-Y., Lin, K.-M., Shen, H., Kurasaki, K., Chun, C.-A., et al. (1998). Lifetime and twelve-month prevalence rates of major depressive episodes and dysthymia among Chinese Americans in Los Angeles. *The American Journal of Psychiatry, 155*, 1407–1414.

Takeuchi, D. T., Zane, N., Hong, S., Chae, D. H., Gong, F., Gee, G. C., et al. (2007). Immigration-related factors and mental disorders among Asian Americans. *American Journal of Public Health, 97*, 84–90.

Tang, H., Shimizu, R., & Chen, M. S., Jr. (2005). English language proficiency and smoking prevalence among California's Asian Americans. *Cancer, 104*, 2982–2988.

Thai, N. D., Connell, C. M., & Tebes, J. K. (2010). Substance use among Asian American adolescents:

Influence of race, ethnicity, and acculturation in the context of key risk and protective factors. *Asian American Journal of Psychology, 1*, 261–274.

Trinh, N.-H., & Ahmed, Iqbal. (2009). Acculturation and Asian American elderly. In N.-H. Trinh, Y. C. Rho, F. G. Lu, & K. M. Sanders (Eds.), *Handbook of mental health and acculturation in Asian American families* (pp. 167–178). Totowa, NJ: Humana Press.

Tsai, J. L., Ying, Y.-W., & Lee, P. A. (2000). The meaning of "being Chinese" and "being American": Variation among Chinese American young adults. *Journal of Cross-Cultural Psychology, 31*, 302–332.

Tseng, W-s. (1975). The nature of somatic complaints among psychiatric patients: The Chinese case. *Comprehensive Psychiatry, 16*, 237–245.

Ueshima, H., Okayama, A., Saitoh, S., Nakagawa, H., Rodriguez, B. L., Sakata, K., et al. (2007). Differences in cardiovascular disease risk factors between Japanese in Japan and Japanese-Americans in Hawaii: the INTERLIPID study. *Journal of Human Hypertension, 17*, 631–639.

Wang, C.-C. D. C., & Mallinckrodt, B. (2006). Acculturation, attachment, and psychosocial adjustment of Chinese/Taiwanese international students. *Journal of Counseling Psychology, 53*, 422–433.

Waters, M. C., & Jimenez, T. R. (2005). Assessing immigrant assimilation: New empirical and theoretical challenges. *Annual Review of Sociology, 31*, 105–125.

Waza, K., Graham, A. V., Zyzanski, S. J., & Inoue, K. (1999). Comparison of symptoms in Japanese and American depressed primary care patients. *Family Practice, 16*, 528–533.

Weiss, J. W., & Garbanati, J. A. (2006). Effects of acculturation and social norms on adolescent smoking among Asian-American subgroups. *Journal of Ethnicity in Substance Abuse, 5*, 75–90.

Weiss, B., Tram, J. M., Weisz, J. R., Rescorla, L., & Achenbach, T. M. (2009). Differential symptom expression and somatization in Thai versus U.S. children. *Journal of Consulting and Clinical Psychology, 77*, 987–992.

World Health Organization. (2009). *WHO report on the global tobacco epidemic, 2009: Implementing smoke-free environments*. Geneva: World Health Organization.

Wu, T.-Y., & Ronis, D. (2009). Correlates of recent and regular mammography screening among Asian-American women. *Journal of Advanced Nursing, 65*, 2434–2446.

Yeh, C. J. (2003). Age, acculturation, cultural adjustment, and mental health symptoms of Chinese, Korean, and Japanese immigrant youths. *Cultural Diversity and Ethnic Minority Psychology, 9*, 34–48.

Yen, S., Robins, C. J., & Lin, N. (2000). A cross-cultural comparison of depressive symptom manifestation: China and the United States. *Journal of Consulting and Clinical Psychology, 68*, 993–999.

Ying, Y.-W. (1999). Strengthening Intergenerational/Intercultural Ties In Migrant Families: A New Intervention For Parents. *Journal of Community Psychology, 27*, 89–96.

Yoon, E., Langrehr, K., & Ong, L. Z. (2011). Content analysis of acculturation research in counseling and counseling psychology: A 22-year review. *Journal of Counseling Psychology, 58*, 83–96.

Zhang, A. Y., Snowden, L. R., & Sue, S. (1998). Differences between Asian and White Americans' help seeking and utilization patterns in the Los Angeles area. *Journal of Community Psychology, 26*, 317–326.

Zhang, J., & Wang, Z. (2008). Factors associated with smoking in Asian American adults: A systematic review. *Nicotine & Tobacco Research, 10*, 791–801.

Asian Americans and Racism: Mental Health and Health Consequences

12

Alvin N. Alvarez and Jaeyoun Shin

Imagine you and your entire family – grandparents, parents, aunts, uncles, siblings, cousins, and even babies – had to leave your home whether you liked it or not. You can only take two suitcases so this means you need to sell your home and all your possessions – cars, furniture, clothes, pets, everything – for a fraction of their cost. By the way, you may only have two days to do this. Strangers have been nosing around your house constantly looking to profit from the bargains they can get off you and your family. Then you're herded to live in horse stables where you wait to be sent to yet another site that's hundreds if not thousands of miles away from everything you know. There you'll be living in communal barracks with hundreds of people in the desert or the mountains with little space and no privacy. No one can tell you how long you and your family will have to endure this. There's no police, no lawyer, no judge, no government official who can or will protect you since this is actually being enforced by the government, the legal authorities, and the military. You and your family haven't done anything wrong nor is there any evidence that you have, there are no warrants, no due process, no trials. Regardless of whether or not you are a citizen of the United States, your main offense is that you are a member of a particular racial ethnic group. Imagine that for a moment and think of the impact this would have on you and your family – in terms of your finances, your education, your jobs, your physical health, your psychological health, your family functioning. Imagine what you would do and how you would react.

While this may be an imaginary scenario for many people, for nearly 120,000 Japanese Americans living on the West Coast in the spring of 1942, this scenario was an all too real nightmare that came to be recognized as one of the most powerful examples of institutional racism against Asian Americans in the history of the United States. While experiences of racial discrimination – of which the internment is an extreme example – have been a facet of life for many Asian Americans, the pressing question for scholars in disciplines such as psychology, public health, sociology, and nursing revolves around the impact of racism on one's psychological and physical well being. Questions such as: Does racial trauma like the internment affect your psychological well-being? How do people cope with racial discrimination? Does racial discrimination have a long term impact across generations? While these are clearly questions of both empirical and clinical relevance, in all likelihood, these may also be questions of personal relevance for those of us or our families who have experienced some form of racial discrimination. Although many of us may not have

A.N. Alvarez (✉)
College of Health and Human Services, Department of
Counseling, San Francisco State University,
San Francisco, CA
e-mail: aalvarez@sfsu.edu

J. Shin
Pyramid Alternatives, Inc., Pacifica California, CA, USA

G.J. Yoo et al. (eds.), *Handbook of Asian American Health*,
DOI 10.1007/978-1-4614-2227-3_12, © Springer Science+Business Media, LLC 2013

directly experienced racism to the degree that the Japanese American internees faced, Asian Americans continue to experience racial discrimination in one form or another. Consequently, given the clinical, intellectual and perhaps personal significance of racism, the current chapter provides an overview of the research on Asian Americans' experiences with racism and its impact on health and mental health. To provide a conceptual foundation for the literature on racism, the chapter begins with key definitions and conceptual frameworks about racism followed by a discussion of how the topic of racism targeted at Asian Americans has been examined. The chapter then examines the impact of racism on the mental health, health and behaviors of Asian Americans as well as the factors that influence this experience such as protective factors and within-group differences. Lastly, the chapter concludes by examining the implications and future directions of the research on Asian Americans' experiences with racism.

Conceptual Foundations

The image of racism elicits powerful images for those of us in the United States, from entire families being herded onto trains during the Japanese American internment to police attacking civil rights demonstrators in Birmingham to Klansmen in hoods burning crosses. Yet, what is racism, racial discrimination and prejudice? How are these different? Is racism always this overt? Is racism an action or a belief? Is racism something that happens between individuals? Can it be racial discrimination if it's not intentional? In order to provide a foundation for this chapter, it may be helpful to review an operational definition of racism. While various scholars have wrestled with the definition of racism, the current chapter will use Jones' (1997) conceptualization since it highlights key dimensions of racism that distinguish it from concepts such as racial prejudice and discrimination. According to Jones, "racism results from the transformation of race prejudice and/or ethnocentrism through the exercise of power against a racial group

defined as inferior, by individuals and institutions with the intentional and unintentional support of the entire culture" (Jones, 1997, p. 172). In this definition, it is important to note that racism is rooted in racial prejudice – an attitude that classifies individuals and groups as being inferior based on race. However, whereas prejudice is attitudinal, the key distinction between racism and racial prejudice is that racism is behavioral and an act of discrimination or differential treatment by individuals and institutions that is legitimized by the larger society. While many people may be racially prejudiced as individuals, racism occurs when power is granted to individuals, institutions and the larger culture to create and perpetuate a system of beliefs and actions that is supported as being normative by society as a whole. In turn, the support of the larger society gives racism its legitimacy and the power to dominate another racial group. Thus, a key feature of racism is reflected in the power that one group has to act upon their racially prejudiced attitudes and to use both individuals and institutional systems to enforce those attitudes.

Building upon this foundation, Jones argued that racism can be classified into three broad types: (a) individual, (b) institutional, and (c) cultural. Individual racism occurs when individuals act upon their racial prejudice and engage in behaviors that reflect their beliefs in their own racial superiority. Individual racism can range from teasing and verbal harassment to treating others rudely based on race to physical assaults and even homicides based on race. In contrast, institutional racism occurs when social institutions such as schools, governments, banks, businesses, law enforcement, judicial courts and so forth create and enforce laws, policies and regulations that serve to restrict a racial group's life choices and deny their access to social resources. Examples of institutional racism can be found in housing policies, disparities in health care access, university admissions, judicial sentencing, immigration legislation and so forth. Lastly, cultural racism occurs when the values, worldviews, traditions, norms and cultural products of one racial group are denigrated. Thus, cultural racism may be operating when aspects of one's life such as one's appearance, patterns of communications, family structure, ways of dress, traditional holidays, as well as the art and history of a minority racial group are devalued and regarded as inferior by the dominant racial group.

Racism and Asian Americans

Racism in its various forms has been a persistent challenge for Asian Americans beginning with the large scale immigration of Chinese laborers in the 1840s (Chan, 1991). Although Asian laborers were intentionally recruited to work on plantations, canneries and railroads, individual racism remained deeply rooted in the belief that Asians were an inferior group of "heathens" and "barbarians." As Asian laborers became perceived as economic competition, individual racism against Asians was often manifested in vandalism, destruction of property, physical assaults, lynchings, murders and mass expulsions out of ethnic enclaves. Chan writes that 15 Chinese were hung during the Los Angeles Chinese Massacre of 1871, five Chinese were set on fire in Chico in 1877, and 28 Chinese miners were killed in Rock Springs, Wyoming in 1885. Similar to the Chinese, other Asian ethnic communities encountered similar forms of individual racism such as the robbery and expulsion of Asian Indians farm workers in Live Oak in 1908, the armed expulsion of Japanese laborers in Turlock in 1921, and the attacks on Filipino workers by a mob of 400 White workers in Watsonville in 1930. Indeed, it is important to note that although different Asian ethnic groups immigrated at various points in time, the experience of anti-Asian violence was a strikingly consistent thread in the experiences of different Asian ethnic communities.

To further reinforce acts of individual racism, institutional racism against Asian Americans was also manifested in municipal, state and federal legislation designed to restrict their opportunities and deny access to resources at a systemic level. At the state and municipal level, anti-miscegenation laws were enforced to restrict interracial marriages, alien land laws were passed to prevent Asian Americans from owning property, taxes were imposed that specifically targeted Asian businesses, and educational codes were enforced to maintain segregated schools (Ancheta, 1998). At the federal level, glaring examples of institutional racism can be found in anti-Asian exclusion laws that sought to limit the immigration of specific Asian ethnic groups, beginning with the Page Law of 1875, which despite being aimed at prostitutes, effectively barred all Chinese women since they were all labeled as prostitutes, followed by the Chinese Exclusion Act of 1882 barring all Chinese immigration, the Gentlemen's Agreement of 1907 which excluded Japanese immigration, the Immigration Act of 1917 which excluded other potential Asian immigrants who were not already targeted in prior legislation, and the Tydings-McDuffie Act of 1934 which effectively reduced Filipino immigration to 50 persons per year (Ancheta, 1998). Yet, the most glaring instance of institutional racism against Asian Americans was the forced incarceration of Japanese Americans – most of whom were American citizens – that was depicted in the beginning of this chapter.

Although history provides ample evidence of racism against Asian Americans, racism continues to be a contemporary challenge in the lives of Asian Americans. A particularly insidious racial stereotype of Asian Americans can be found in the model minority myth. First emerging in a 1966 *New York Times Magazine* article and popularized in subsequent accounts in the media, the model minority myth portrays Asian Americans as being academically, economically and educationally successful (Lee, 1996). In short, the image suggests that Asian Americans have overcome the racial barriers that face other minority groups and implicitly suggests that racial discrimination, in particular, is no longer a barrier for this community. While numerous scholars (Lee, 1996; Lee, Nga-Wing, & Alvarez, 2009) have presented cogent critiques of this myth (e.g., aggregating the data on Asian Americans hides existing inequities and obscures important ethnic group differences), the stereotype continues to persist. For instance, a 2009 poll sponsored by the Committee of 100 – a Chinese American advocacy group – found that 57% of the general population continue to regard Asian Americans as more successful than other Americans (Committee of 100, 2009). The same poll also found evidence that Asian Americans continue to be stereotyped as perpetual foreigners – a group that despite numerous generations in this country are still regarded as "unassimilable" and "not American." The poll found that 45% of the general population (up from 37% in 2001) believed that Asian Americans are more loyal to their country of origin than the United States. The fact that nearly half of the participants were suspicious about the loyalty of Asian Americans is particularly troubling given that this underlying attitude was precisely the belief system that fueled the internment of Japanese Americans in World War II despite the fact that 62% of the internees were American citizens (Chan, 1991).

At an institutional level, racism continues to fuel regulations, policies and practices that continue to target and adversely affect Asian Americans. Ancheta (1998) observed that English-only initiatives have targeted both Asian and Latino Americans by attempting to eliminate bilingual ballots, bilingual government forms, and access to bilingual government services such as public safety, healthcare, social welfare and court translations. On a similar note, Asian Americans have been the targets of language and accent discrimination in the workplace such that workers have been penalized, reprimanded or fired for having accents and/or not speaking English at work. Similarly, Asian Americans have also faced glass ceiling effects in the workplace that have limited their ability to advance on the career ladder. According to a report by the United States Equal Employment Opportunity Commission (EEOC), factors such as perceived lack of leadership skills, low social skills, passivity, and being perceived as foreigners "have become the framework of barriers establishing glass or bamboo ceilings which prevent Asian American Pacific Islanders (AAPIs) from moving into the upper tiers of an organization" (Ancheta, 2008, p. 2). Indeed, in a Gallup survey (2005), 31% of Asian Americans report having been the target of workplace discrimination, the highest rate of any racial ethnic group. Interestingly, despite having the highest rates of workplace discrimination, the EEOC has found that Asian Americans generally have the lowest rates of reporting such incidents (Equal Employment Opportunity Commission [EEOC], 2008). Lastly, since the 1980s, there has been an ongoing debate about the use of implicit quotas or differential standards of admissions at elite public and private universities that have resulted in lower admission rates of qualified Asian American students, a phenomenon Kang (1996) has referred to as "negative action." According to Kang, negative action occurs when an institution rejects Asian Americans who would otherwise had been admitted if they were White.

Given these instances of contemporary racism and racial discrimination, it is not surprising that Asian Americans continue to report that they encounter racial discrimination. For instance, in the National Latino and Asian American Study – the first nationwide study of its kind – 74% of Asian American reported some form of unfair treatment in their lifetime (Chae et al., 2008). Similarly, 58% of Chinese Americans in the Committee of 100 poll reported that they faced unfair treatment, primarily in the form of verbal harassment and disrespectful or differential service (Committee of 100, 2009). Yet, beyond unfair treatment, racism has also fueled acts of vandalism, harassment, assaults, and at its most extreme, homicide. Indeed, the murder of Vincent Chin in 1982, when disgruntled factory workers chased and beat a Chinese American man with bats, has been a powerful catalyst for reminding Asian Americans about the lethal potential of racism. Yet, since Vincent Chin, there has been ample evidence of the violence that racism can instigate. According to the National Asian Pacific American Legal Consortium (2003), the number of incidents of anti-Asian violence ranged from 275 to 507 incidents from 1991 to 2001, figures which have generally been regarded as an underreport of the phenomenon. Thus, from racial stereotypes to institutional racism to anti-Asian violence, racism has been and continues to be a challenge in the lives of Asian Americans.

Studies on Racism and Asian Americans

Despite the clear historical and contemporary evidence of racial discrimination against Asian Americans, research into racism's impact on the psychological and physical well being of Asian Americans – or any other community of color for that matter – has only recently emerged. Indeed, in reviews of the empirical literature on studies of racism, Paradies (2006) found that out of a total of 138 studies across all racial groups, only six studies were conducted prior to 1990. Similarly, Gee, Ro, Shariff-Marco, and Chae (2009) found that out of 62 studies of racism against Asian Americans specifically, only three were conducted prior to 2000. Of these studies, the bulk of the research has focused on what has been referred to as microaggressions or everyday racism, a form of individual racism that involves verbal and behavioral insults or differential treatment that are racially derogatory. It is not surprising that Young and Takeuchi lamented as recently as 1998 that "more is known about the details of racism against Asian Americans within the socio-historical context of the United States… than about the psychological impact of racism on Asian American individuals" (Young & Takeuchi, 1998, p. 428). Nevertheless, since 2000, the research on the physical and psychological impact of racism has been a rapidly emerging body of literature for Asian Americans as well as other communities of color.

Yet before we can examine what has been found in the literature on racial discrimination, it may be helpful to provide a conceptual model for understanding the relationship between racial discrimination and its psychological and physical outcomes. The most common conceptual framework for understanding the impact of racism has been a stress-coping model (Clark, Anderson, Clark, & Williams, 1999). In other words, racial discrimination is a stress-inducing phenomenon. To illustrate this framework, a review of Clark et al.'s (1999) biopsychosocial model of the impact of racism may be helpful in highlighting the conceptual linkages between racism and its

outcomes (See Fig. 12.1). According to this model, when an experience is perceived to be racist, this results in psychological and physiological stress responses that over time may adversely impact one's health. The linkage between racial discrimination and its physical and psychological outcomes is influenced by a number of factors: (a) constitutional, (b) sociodemographic, (c) psychological and behavioral, and (d) coping responses. Constitutional factors refer to within-individual characteristics such as physical appearance, skin tone, or family's health history, that may influence the experience of racial discrimination and/or its impact on health outcomes. For instance, individuals who come from families with a history of mental illness such as depression or anxiety may be particularly vulnerable to experience these outcomes when encountering racism than individuals who come from families without such a history. Sociodemographic factors refer to social status variables such as age, gender, socioeconomic status, educational level, and so forth that may shape the frequency with which one encounters racial discrimination, the ability to cope with such experiences, as well as the resources for doing so. Psychological and behavioral factors refer to intrapsychic and overt patterns of action and reaction that influence how one perceives and responds to racism. This may include factors such as self-esteem, ethnic identity, anger expression, hostility, and perceived control. Lastly, coping refers to cognitive and behavioral efforts designed to reduce the stress associated with an experience. These may include coping strategies such as avoidance, denial, problem-solving, and seeking emotional support or advice. Model, constitutional, sociodemographic, psychological and behavioral factors influence whether an individual perceives an event to be racially discriminatory as well as the manner in which one copes with such events. When an event is perceived to be racially motivated, a number of acute psychological and physiological stress responses may be elicited. Psychological stress responses may include anxiety, helplessness, and frustration and physiological stress responses may include impairments to immune and cardiovascular systems. Lastly, insofar as these acute

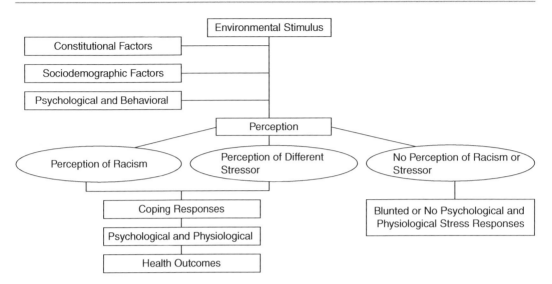

Fig. 12.1 Biopsychosocial Effects of Perceived Racism Clark et al., (1999)

stress responses persist over time, then Clark et al. argued that health outcomes such as depression, high blood pressure, and psychological distress may be adversely impacted.

Racial Discrimination and Mental Health

The study of Asian Americans' experiences of racial discrimination has primarily focused on the effects of racial discrimination on Asian Americans' mental health. In Gee et al.'s (2009) review of this literature, 40 studies or 64% of the published literature in this area has focused on mental health outcomes. These mental health outcomes include depression, psychological distress, anxiety, post-traumatic stress disorder (PTSD), negative self-image and identity, and low self-esteem (see Table 12.1). Among these psychological difficulties, depression and psychological distress are the most common symptoms found in studies. As we reflect back on the internment scenario depicted at the beginning of the chapter, an immediate question that comes to mind is: "Do people experience any psychological difficulty when they encounter racial discrimination?" With 92% of studies demonstrating a positive linkage between racial discrimination

and adverse psychological outcomes, the consistent answer to date appears to be "Yes."

Gee et al. (2009) reported that about 45% of studies found a positive relationship between Asian Americans' experiences with racial discrimination and depressive symptoms and general psychological distress. In other words, people tend to feel more depressed and their general psychological functioning is detrimentally affected as they encounter more episodes of racial discrimination. Noh, Kaspar, Hou, Rummens, and Beiser (1999) found that perceived discrimination had a significant and positive relationship with depression among Southeast Asian refugees in Canada. Those who had experienced racial discrimination reported higher depression scores compared to their counterparts who had no experiences of racism. Yip, Gee, and Takeuchi (2008) studied the relationship between racism and psychological distress. In order to assess psychological distress, they measured the prevalence of negative feelings participants experienced in the past 30 days. The authors stated that experiences of racism were positively associated with psychological distress. In addition, the existing although limited literature suggests that racial discrimination can have a long term and adverse impact on developmental outcomes among adolescents, including increased depression and

Table 12.1 Summary of findings of the impact of Racism on mental health, health and behavioral outcomes

Independent variables	Dependent variables (outcomes)	Association
Racism	Mental health outcomes	
	Psychological distress	(+)
	Depression	(+)
	Anxiety	(+)
	PTSD	(+)
	Self-image	(−)
	Self-esteem	(−)
	Identity	(+), (−)
	Physical health	
	Physical functioning, chronic health conditions	(−), Poorer health
	Body mass index	(+), Increased BMI, obesity
	Cardiovascular disease	(+)
	Cholesterol levels	(+)
	Diabetes symptoms	(+)
	Respiratory conditions	(−)
	Pain conditions	(+)
	Self-rated health	(−)
	Behavioral concerns	
	Alcohol/drug abuse, dependence	(+)
	Suicide ideation and suicide attempts	(+)
	Unprotected sexual activity among Asian American gay men	(+)

Note: (+) indicates positive association, (−) indicates negative association between racism and health outcomes

alienation, and declined school engagement and academic grades. In one of the few longitudinal studies on the topic, Benner and Kim (2009) found that seventh and eighth grade middle-school adolescents, who experienced chronic daily discrimination, were more likely to struggle with socioemotional challenges and academic functioning even later in their eleventh or twelfth grade in high school.

Anxiety coupled with depressive symptoms is also a relatively common outcome for Asian Americans who have faced situations of racial discrimination. Male participants in a study by Cassidy, O'Connor, Howe, and Warden (2004) showed an inverse relationship between frequency of racial discrimination and personal and ethnic self-esteem. As participants experienced more racial discrimination, they reported lower personal and ethnic self-esteem, which eventually led to increased depression and anxiety. Another study examining Asian American college students

found that minority college students were at greater risk for trait anxiety, which are "individual differences in enduring anxiety and predisposition to respond anxiously to stressful situations" (Hwang & Goto, 2008, p. 329), as they experienced more discrimination in social and professional settings. More strikingly, racial discrimination has been linked to the experience of post-traumatic stress disorder (PTSD) in a limited series of studies. Loo et al. (2001) found that among Asian American veterans in Vietnam, the experience of looking like the enemy, identifying with Vietnamese culture, and being treated with hostility and prejudice by other soldiers were significant racial stressors. Loo, Fairbank, and Chemtob (2005) found a positive association between symptoms of PTSD and "adverse race-related events" in a sample of Asian American Vietnam veterans. Indeed, Loo and her colleagues found that the relationship between these race-related stressors and PTSD was *significantly* above and beyond the stress associated with combat exposure.

Over time, perceived racial discrimination also shapes or influences one's self-image and self-esteem in an unhealthy manner. It is especially true for children and adolescents who may be particularly vulnerable since they are still in the developmental stage of forming their identity and establishing their self-esteem. In regard to this concern, a number of researchers have conducted studies that have substantiated hypothesized associations between experiences of racism and unhealthy self-image, identity, and low self-esteem. For example, in one of the few qualitative studies in the area, South Asian women recalled that as they were initially encountering racism as children and adolescents, they were prone to develop low self-esteem, as evidenced by feelings of insecurity and being unattractive (Beharry & Crozier, 2008). This may have been associated with the internalization of the perception that the dominant White culture was the normative standard. As one of the participants reported, "I think when I was in elementary, junior high, I was more 'oh how I wish I could be blonde like my friends.'" (Beharry & Cozier, 2008, p. 268). This finding is particularly salient since Asian American children and adolescents generally report a higher level of racial discrimination from their peers than other youth of color (Greene, Way, & Pahl, 2006; Rosenbloom & Way, 2004). Strikingly, Greene et al. found that depressive symptoms and decreased self-esteem were accelerated over time for adolescents who reported more experiences of racial discrimination relative to those with fewer experiences of discrimination. The available evidence suggest that experiences of racial discrimination tend to affect Asian Americans' self-esteem in a negative manner. However, there may be mitigating factors in the impact of racism for adolescents. The self-esteem of adolescents with a strong sense of belonging to one's ethnic group appeared to be less affected by experiences of discrimination (Greene et al., 2006). This finding was consistent with another study done with Chinese American youth. Rivas-Drake, Hughes, and Way (2008) reported that participants with positive regard toward their Chinese ethnic group presented higher self-esteem in situations of peer discrimination.

Racial Discrimination and Physical Health

Although not many studies have focused on the relationships between racial discrimination and physical health, the existing studies in this area have consistently indicated that Asian Americans experience negative physical health outcomes because of perceived discrimination. Gee et al. (2009) reported that 26% of the published studies focused on the relationship between physical health outcomes and discrimination against Asian Americans, with the majority focusing on overall indicators of physical health. These negative physical health outcomes include global physical functioning, cardiovascular disease, cholesterol levels, diabetes symptoms, body mass index, and chronic health conditions.

So how is it that discrimination can cause such serious physical illnesses? After all, these incidents of discrimination seem somewhat trivial, being treated differently, being ignored, being treated with less respect. According to Clark et al.'s (1999) biopsychosocial model, the experience of discrimination can contribute to allostatic load, the physiological impact of being exposed to chronic stress. In other words, the accumulated stress that results from one's experiences with perceived discrimination can also result in adverse consequences for one's physical well-being over the long term. While each individual incident of discrimination may appear "trivial," it may be the accumulated and repeated exposure to discrimination that may have a long-term impact on one's overall physical wellness. In support of this theoretical proposition, Gee, Spencer, Chen, and Takeuchi (2007) found that everyday discrimination was positively associated with measures of chronic health conditions as well as specific health conditions such as chronic pain, cardiovascular disease, and respiratory disease. The findings are even more noteworthy when one accounts for the fact that Gee and his colleagues found this association even after accounting for multiple demographic factors such as age, gender, income, education and marital status, which suggests that the relationship between discrimination and physical health occurs across gender, age, income, etc. Moreover, it is important to note that Gee and his colleagues focused on the impact of microaggressions in this current study, a seemingly innocuous form of discrimination, thereby suggesting that despite it's seemingly trivial nature, microaggressions can have a significant impact on one's physical well-being (Gee et al., 2007).

Although the majority of studies have focused on global indicators of physical health, the results of a limited number of disease-specific studies have also corroborated the linkage between perceived discrimination and various health conditions. Iyer and Haslam (2003) examined the relationship between racial teasing (i.e., name-calling, behavior related teasing, appearance related teasing, and social exclusion) and body image and eating disturbance among South Asian women. The results indicated that racial teasing was positively associated with disturbed eating behavior and body image dissatisfaction. Iyer and Haslam speculated that "being teased on account of visible signs of their ethnic difference might lead some girls to be dissatisfied with their appearance and to resort to disturbed eating patterns in an attempt to reshape it (p. 146)." and that this form of discrimination may reinforce a sense of marginalization that may be manifested pathologically. On a related note, there is evidence to suggest that an association exists between racial discrimination and body weight (Gee, Ro, Gavin, & Takeuchi, 2008). Gee et al. found that racial discrimination was associated with increased body mass index (BMI) and obesity, an association that was strengthened with the time spent in the United States. This finding was consistent even after controlling other possible factors, such as weight discrimination and social desirability bias. In other words, racial discrimination is a contributing factor for being overweight and obese among Asian Americans. Knowing that an increasing number of people are struggling with obesity, it is imperative to pay close attention to this association.

Other health concerns are also closely associated with racial discrimination, including cardiovascular disease, respiratory conditions, diabetes symptoms, pain conditions, chronic health conditions, and self-rated health, physical functioning (Harris et al., 2006; Piette, Bibbins-Domingo, & Schillinger, 2006; Yoo, Gee, & Takeuchi, 2009). Piette et al., (2006) found that people of color with diabetes who experienced health care discrimination reported lower levels of glycemic control and higher levels of cholesterol. Regarding physical functioning, Harris et al. (2006) utilized the SF-36 physical functioning scale to measure participants' self-rated physical functioning, i.e., a person's physical activities from vigorous activities like running and lifting heavy objects to walking more than a mile to bathing or dressing during a typical day. The findings revealed that across age and gender, people with more exposure to racial discrimination reported lower physical functioning compared to those with no exposure. In addition, racial discrimination has been associated with increased chronic health conditions defined as diagnosed medical conditions such as "high blood pressure, heart attack or any other heart disease, cancer, diabetes or sugar diabetes, anxiety or depression, obesity, and asthma" in the past 5 years (Yoo et al., 2009). In a longitudinal study with ethnic minority women – including Asian Americans – Brown, Matthews, Bromberger, and Chang (2006) examined the relationship between unfair treatment and blood pressure. Although Chinese American and Japanese American women did report they experience unfair treatment, the authors found no significant association between blood pressure and perceived unfair treatment, which is inconsistent with studies of other ethnic minority groups, such as African Americans and Latinos. More empirical studies on Asian Americans may be needed to examine racial discrimination and its impact on the cardiovascular system and blood pressure.

Although the majority of studies have focused on racial microaggressions, there is limited evidence that other forms of racism may also have an impact on one's physical health. De Castro, Gee, and Takeuchi (2008) studied Filipino

Americans and the association between racial discrimination in the workplace and general health conditions. In their study, de Castro et al. defined workplace discrimination as the expectation that Filipinos had to work harder than others and that they were less likely to get promotions or raises. The results indicated that workplace discrimination was positively correlated with overall deterioration in physical health among Filipino American participants even after controlling for the experience of everyday discrimination and overall job concerns. In effect, these findings indicate that workplace discrimination – above and beyond everyday racial microaggressions – is a unique form of racism that can be a significant stressor in the lives of Asian Americans that merits further investigation.

Racial Discrimination and Health-Related Behaviors

Just as racial discrimination has negatively influenced Asian Americans' mental and physical health, the existing evidence suggests that racial discrimination also has an adverse impact on health-related behaviors. To date, studies have examined racial discrimination's impact on substance abuse or dependence, unprotected sexual intercourse, help-seeking and utilization and even suicidality. Asian Americans who reported high levels of racial discrimination are at greater odds of having a history of alcohol abuse or dependence, drinking heavily, or being a current smoker compared to their counterparts (Chae et al., 2008; Yen, Ragland, Greiner, & Fisher, 1999). Indeed, Chae et al. (2008) found that Asian Americans who reported high levels of racial discrimination had more than three times the odds of being a smoker than individuals who did not report experiencing discrimination. Likewise, Yen, Ragland Greiner, and Fisher (1999) found that those who reported high levels of discrimination were more likely to be dependent on alcohol and be heavy drinkers than those who reported no experiences of discrimination; in fact, participants who faced high levels of discrimination drank an average of 13 drinks more per month than those who did not

experience discrimination. Extending the evidence that racial discrimination is associated with self-destructive health behaviors, one study has found that high levels of racial discrimination are also associated with suicidal ideation and suicidal attempts. Specifically, Cheng et al. (2012) found that high levels perceived discrimination was associated with 1.5 times increase in the odds of having suicidal ideation as well as 1.4 times increase in the odds of actually attempting suicide.

While the majority of studies in this area have focused on Asian Americans in general, the pattern of associations between racial discrimination and self-injurious behavior has also been found within the Asian American gay community. In particular, Yoshikawa, Wilson, Chae, and Cheng (2004) found that racism against Asian American gay men is a significant factor that is associated with increased depressive symptoms as well as higher rates of unprotected anal intercourse with a secondary partner. Moreover, Wilson and Yoshikawa (2004) found that Asian American gay men who responded to discrimination with self-blame or self-attribution were more likely to engage in sexual behaviors that placed them at greater risk for HIV. The authors speculated that "the interview data suggested that in stigmatizing themselves, some respondents placed themselves at risk in an effort to be more attractive to sexual partners" (Wilson & Yoshikawa, 2004, p. 77). In support of this proposition, Han (2008) has argued that in gay communities dominated largely by White men, the idealization of White men and the marginalization of Asian American gay men may lead Asian American gay men to engage in high risk sexual behavior in an effort to win the "favor" of White men. As one of Han's participants poignantly states, "If I want to get laid, I had to fit what they want me to be. If I wanted to be myself, I don't get laid very often" (p. 834).

Given the clear damage that racial discrimination can cause both psychologically and physically, it is even more troubling that racial discrimination can also influence whether or not Asian Americans seek help as well as their perceptions of the quality of that help. Burgess, Ding, Hargreaves, van Ryn, and Phelan (2008) found that moderate to high levels of everyday discrimination were associated with underutilization of both medical and mental health care. In effect, the impact of racial discrimination on Asian Americans' physical and psychological well-being may be compounded by the likelihood that discrimination itself may inhibit Asian Americans from seeking the help they need. Moreover, once they do seek health care, Asian Americans also reported facing discrimination from their health care providers (Lee, Ayers, & Kronenfeld, 2009). Providing us with some insights into what happens in the doctor-patient interaction, Ngo-Metzger, Legedza, and Phillips (2004) found that Asian Americans were more likely than White patients to report that physicians did not spend much time with them, did not listen to them, and did not involve them in health care decisions. Likewise, Asian Americans perceived that their doctors were less likely to know about their culture or background and were less likely to discuss lifestyle or mental health concerns. As a result, it is not surprising that the perceived quality of health care for Asian Americans is negatively associated with the experience of discrimination and differential treatment (Ngo-Metzger et al., 2004; Sorkin, Ngo-Metzger, & De Alba, 2010). Taken together, (Lee, Ayers et al., 2009a) found that the poorer health status of Asian Americans – as well as other people of color – was associated with both provider discrimination and the delay in seeking treatment. Consequently, in addition to the direct effect of racial discrimination on health and mental health, Asian Americans' health may be further exacerbated by the hesitation to seek help and the lower quality of health care services they receive.

Contributing Factors

In the previous section, we looked at the empirical evidence of racial discrimination on overall health among Asian Americans and found that racial discrimination generally has a negative impact on health and mental health. Although this emerging literature has been critical in documenting the outcomes of racial discrimination, important

questions remain about the factors that mitigate these outcomes. What factors exacerbate or worsen these outcomes? What factors ameliorate the negative impact of racial discrimination on mental health and health? Although less numerous than the outcomes-focused research on racism, emerging studies on both coping strategies and ethnic identity have yielded findings that merit further investigation.

To understand this line of research, it may be helpful to have a clearer understanding of the roles of moderators and mediators. Frazier, Tix, and Barron (2004) define a moderator as "a variable that alters the direction or strength of the relation between a predictor and an outcome" while a mediator is "a variable that explains the relation between a predictor and an outcome" (p. 116). Moreover, Frazier et al. (2004) note that a causal relationship between variables exists in mediation models, but not in moderation models. Nevertheless, it is important to note that what defines a moderator or mediator is dependent on the theory underlying your hypotheses; it is possible that a variable can be mediator in one theory and a moderator in another. Let us take a look at examples of moderators and mediators for a better understanding of how they are examined in studies of racial discrimination among Asian Americans.

Although questions about coping with discrimination would seem to be a logical area of investigation, only a limited number of studies have been conducted in this area (Alvarez & Juang, 2010; Wei, Ku, Russell, Mallinckrodt, & Liao, 2008). In our search of the literature, there have only been eight studies on the relationship between racial discrimination and coping among Asian Americans. In a study of the moderating effects of three coping strategies (reflective, suppressive, and reactive coping strategies) on racial discrimination and depressive symptoms, Wei et al. (2008) found that suppressive coping (i.e., avoidance and denial) enhanced the relationship between racial discrimination and depressive symptoms for Asian international students. Similarly in their study of Filipino Americans, Alvarez and Juang (2010) found that the use of avoidance coping was associated with higher levels of psychological distress and lower levels of self-esteem. Avoiding or denying racial discrimination – particularly when it is a chronic and ongoing experience – can become psychologically challenging. In contrast, Noh et al. (1999) found that in a sample of Southeast Asian Canadian refugees, the use of forbearance or avoidant strategies were actually effective in coping with racial discrimination. Thus, various authors (Alvarez & Juang, 2010; Noh & Kaspar, 2003) have cautioned that coping may be highly contextual and the effectiveness of a specific coping strategy may vary depending on variables such as socioeconomic resources, educational capital, and acculturation to the dominant society.

In terms of coping as a protective factor, the research is mixed. A few studies have examined the role of support-seeking in responding to racism (Alvarez & Juang, 2010; Yoshikawa et al., 2004). In their study of Asian American gay men, Yoshikawa et al. (2004) found that conversations with friends and family about one's experiences with discrimination were associated with lower levels of high risk sexual behaviors. Conversely, the authors found that in the face of high levels of racial discrimination, individuals who were less likely to seek social support were significantly more likely to engage in high risk sexual behaviors. In contrast, Alvarez and Juang (2010) have found that the use of social support as a coping strategy was associated with higher levels of psychological distress. Alvarez and Juang have speculated that seeking the support of others and talking about one's experiences with racism may be emotionally provocative and distressing and that the effect of support seeking may depend on the type of support that one receives. On a related note, Wei et al. (2008) found that when Asian students utilized lower levels of reactive coping – such as responding emotionally and impulsively to presenting problems – the relationship between racial discrimination and depressive symptoms became non-significant. Although clearly speculative, these results may be pointing to the importance of helping Asian Americans manage the emotional reactions to racial discrimination. Lastly, there has been limited evidence to indicate that an active style of coping – such as being proactive and developing a plan – can be an adaptive form of coping for some individuals (Alvarez & Juang, 2010; Noh & Kaspar, 2003). In their study of Korean Canadians, Noh and Kaspar found that a problem focused style of coping mitigated the depressive symptoms associated with racial discrimination. Similarly, Alvarez and Juang (2010) found that active coping in the face of racism was associated with lower psychological distress and higher self-esteem. As Alvarez and Juang observed, active coping "may elicit a sense of self-efficacy or empowerment that mitigates one's psychological distress and perhaps the sense of helplessness and victimization associated with the experience" (p. 75). In short, the limited evidence in this area suggests that coping strategies can play an important factor in one's experiences with racial discrimination; however, determining what is an adaptive or maladaptive style of coping remains an issue in need of further investigation.

Another line of investigation has focused on the role of ethnic identity as a factor that influences the relationship between racial discrimination and its outcomes. Ethnic identity refers to one's sense of pride in and identification with one's ethnic group and the values, traditions, worldviews, and beliefs of that group. Various scholars have theorized that ethnic identity can serves as a buffer that reduces the adverse effects of racism by instilling a sense of pride in one's ethnic group and providing a sense of belonging with one's community, a proposition that has found support in the literature (Greene et al., 2006). Mossakowski (2003) stated that ethnic identity was found to reduce the depressive symptoms associated with both lifetime and everyday experiences of racism among Filipino American subjects. However, additional findings have suggested that the influence of ethnic identity is far more complex than what was initially believed. Although Yip et al. (2008) found that ethnic identity was a protective factor for U.S. born Asian Americans between 41 and 50 years old, they also found that a strong ethnic identity exacerbated the relationship between discrimination and psychological distress among U.S. born individuals between 31 and 40 years old as well as those between 51 and 75 years old. In addressing these seemingly contradictory findings, Yip et al. argue that one's ethnic identity is a dynamic and continually evolving phenomenon and therefore its role as a protective or exacerbating factor may also shift throughout the lifespan. Further detail is offered by Yoo and Lee (2008), who stated that a strong ethnic identity exacerbated the relationship between racial discrimination and situational well-being when faced with multiple experiences of racial discrimination. According to the authors, when individuals are faced with extensive experiences of discrimination that denigrate an aspect of their identity that is highly valued by an individual (i.e., a strong ethnic identity), then that individual may be more vulnerable to experiencing adverse outcomes, a phenomenon referred to as rejection sensitivity. Despite the variability in these emerging findings, what we can draw from these results is that there is a critical need to continue examining the complexities of how ethnic identity and coping influence the linkages between racial discrimination and health outcomes.

Within Group Differences

Although much of the focus of the literature has been on Asian Americans as a racial group, numerous scholars have long pointed to the importance of addressing the diversity in this community along dimensions such as ethnicity, generational status, socioeconomic status, and so forth (Lee et al., 2009a, 2009b). By extension, it is natural to ask if there are within group differences in the racial experiences of Asian Americans. Do Asian American ethnic groups experience racism differently? Are there differences according to gender? How do immigrants and U.S. born Asian Americans differ in their encounters with racism? While the answers to such relevant questions are still emerging, the existing literature does point to important within group differences in how Asian Americans experience and respond to racial discrimination. In terms of experiences with discrimination by ethnic group, researchers have found some intriguing differences. Gee and Ponce (2010) using statewide data from the California Health

Interview Survey found that Filipino Americans reported the highest levels of racial discrimination (33%), followed by Japanese (28%), Chinese (28%), Korean (25%), and with South Asians (23%) and Vietnamese Americans (23%) reporting the lowest percentage of racial discrimination. Similarly, in the National Latino and Asian American Study, Gee et al. (2007) found that Filipino Americans reported the highest levels of perceived discrimination followed by Chinese Americans and then Vietnamese Americans. Why are there such ethnic group differences in reporting racial discrimination? Although more research is needed to answer this question, Alvarez and Juang (2010) have speculated that the histories of the various ethnic groups may be a contributing factor. Given that the Philippines had a relatively long history of colonization – almost 350 years of colonization by Spain and followed by 47 years of colonization by the U.S – it is possible that Filipinos may be more sensitive to experiences of racial discrimination. Likewise, phenotype may also be a factor given the differences in the physical appearance, hair, and skin color of Asian Americans (Gee et al., 2009). It is possible that Asian Americans with a darker skin tone, such as many Filipinos, may be the targets of more racial discrimination than Asian Americans with a lighter skin tone.

Gender has also emerged as another notable within-group factor to consider when examining Asian Americans' perceptions of and coping with racial discrimination. Using data from the National Latino and Asian American Study, Hahm, Ozonoff, Gaumond, and Sue (2010) reported that men were more likely to report medium to high levels of perceived discrimination than women (56% vs. 48%). Similarly, a number of studies using convenience samples have also found that men reported more experiences of racial discrimination than women (Alvarez & Juang, 2010; Cassidy et al., 2004; Kuo, 1995; Liang, Alvarez, Juang, & Liang, 2007). In the few studies conducted on coping and racial discrimination, gender differences have also been found. In a sample of Asian American college students, Liang et al. (2007) found that in responding to racial discrimination, men were more likely to use active coping whereas women were more likely to use support-seeking coping. Similarly, in a sample of Filipino Americans, Alvarez and Juang (2010) found that women reported more use of support-seeking coping strategies than men did and that men were more likely to use avoidance coping than women. Lastly, there has also been evidence that women and men may experience different outcomes in the face of racism. For instance, Cassidy et al. (2004) found that personal and collective self-esteem mediated the impact of racism on depression and anxiety for men but not women. Additionally, Hahm et al. (2010) found that although women and men experienced the same outcomes as a result of racism, the threshold for experiencing these symptoms differed by gender. Specifically, a greater proportion of women (32–50%) than men (25%) who reported medium to high levels of discrimination experienced physical and mental health concerns such as suicidal ideation, chronic headaches and depression. Lower levels of discrimination may be needed to precipitate adverse health outcomes for women – a finding referred to as differential gender vulnerability. While various authors have speculated that these gender differences may reflect factors such as gender role socialization, differential exposure to additional forms of discrimination such as sexism, and so forth, further research is clearly needed in this area to clarify why such differences exist.

Generational status is also an important factor in understanding the relationship between racial discrimination and health outcomes. Studies have indicated that Asian American immigrants with different generational statuses report different levels of racial discrimination. Kuo (1995), found that American-born Asian American participants (second-generation or beyond) reported more experiences of discrimination compared to their first-generation counterparts, who were born outside of the U.S. However, Yip et al. (2008) and Ying, Lee, and Tsai (2000) reported a contradictory finding that foreign-born first-generation immigrants indicated more racial discrimination than those born in the U.S. However, it is important to note that there were no differences in the effects of racism across generational status (Yip et al., 2008). There are

competing potential explanations for these findings. One possible explanation is that U.S. born Asian Americans, who are raised in this country's educational and social systems, may be more sensitive to and aware of racial discrimination. In other words, U.S. born Asian Americans may have had more exposure to racism. Alternatively, Asian immigrants to this country may be the targets of more racism since they may be less acculturated, less proficient with English, and therefore perceived as "outsiders." As with other aspects of within group differences, further research in this area is clearly needed to better understand the role of generational status and nativity on Asian Americans' experiences with racism.

Future Directions in Research

As mentioned earlier, research on Asian Americans and their experiences with racial discrimination has had a relatively short history. While there are clear trends in the data, there are also important limitations in these studies that can point to improvements in future research.

First, most studies are based primarily on self-report, retrospective, and aggregate experiences rather than specific and current incidents of racism. In short, these studies rely on participants' subjective, past memories of their overall experiences with racial discrimination rather than their actual experiences with specific instances of racial discrimination. By relying on retrospective memories, it is possible that Asian Americans may be distorting – both underreporting or overreporting – their experiences with racism. Their experiences of racial discrimination can be exaggerated out of emotional distress, fear, or anger. In other cases, people may minimize their experiences with racial discrimination in order to 'not make a big deal out of it'. Moreover, by relying on scales that aggregate participant's responses, the data is based essentially on the "average" experience of racism; thereby obscuring our ability to understand how individuals respond to specific incidents of racism. Aggregating participants' experiences with racism, neglects the fact that the manner in which Asian

Americans respond and cope with racial teasing is most likely quite different than how they deal with the loss of a job or how they deal with witnessing racial stereotypes in a movie. Given that each instance of racial discrimination can be idiosyncratic (Alvarez & Juang, 2010), there is a need for greater specificity in the type of racism that is being investigated and how one copes with and responds to those specific incidents.

On a related issue, it is important to note that studies have focused primarily on microaggressions or everyday racial discrimination. Although these studies have excelled in confirming that people experience subtle forms of racism on a daily basis, it is still possible that people experience other types of racism, on which we are less clear. In contrast to the emphasis on individual racism such as microaggressions, there has been a limited amount of research conducted on the experience of institutional racism and the effects of discriminatory policies and legislation. Similarly, the majority of studies of racial discrimination have been largely acontextual with limited attention to how people are treated in specific settings such as their workplace, schools, and health settings. One possible strategy for future studies is to use qualitative methods – interviews, focus groups, diary reports – that allow individuals to address specific and perhaps a broader range of incidents of racial discrimination. Given that the vast majority of studies have utilized quantitative methods, the use of qualitative methodologies may also help to broaden our exploration of the actual experiences of Asian Americans.

Parallel to the need for more specificity in understanding the various types of racial discrimination, more studies on different Asian ethnic groups are needed. As discussed earlier, Asian Americans are heterogeneous in terms of culture, history, language, educational attainment, socioeconomic status and religion. Moreover, each ethnic group has varied experiences of immigration to the U.S. For instance, Vietnamese Americans came to the U.S. largely as political refugees while Korean Americans primarily immigrated here voluntarily. It is possible that their perceptions of the United States, their access to economic as well as educational resources may also shape how they experience racial discrimination. In addition, different phenotypes – from South Asians to East Asians to Southeast Asian American – may influence the severity and frequency of racial discrimination. Indeed, the National Asian Pacific American Legal Consortium (2003) has noted that since the terrorist attacks on September 11, 2011, South Asian Americans have been subjected to more racial profiling that has resulted in a notable spike in their experiences with anti-Asian harassment and violence. Unfortunately, the majority of studies have focused on a select group of Asian Americans, such as Chinese and Filipino Americans. Therefore, it is crucial to attend to Asian ethnic groups that have been relatively understudied such as Southeast Asians and Asian Indians.

Lastly, although the large majority of studies have clearly documented how racial discrimination affects Asian Americans' psychological and physical health, we are less clear about the protective factors that mitigate these outcomes. Given that much of this research has been quite limited and often yielding contradictory findings, definitive answers about the role of factors such as self-esteem, ethnic identity, coping and social support have been elusive. We now know that racial discrimination happens and has a negative impact on Asian Americans. It is imperative to direct our attention to examining the protective and possibly preventive factors that have a direct bearing on the interventions that health care practitioners can use in working with Asian Americans.

References

Alvarez, A. N., & Juang, L. P. (2010). Filipino Americans and racism: A multiple mediation model of coping. *Journal of Counseling Psychology, 57*(2), 167–178. doi:10.1037/a0019091.

Ancheta, A. N. (1998). *Race, rights and the Asian American experience*. New Brunswick, NJ: Rutgers University Press.

Beharry, P., & Crozier, S. (2008). Using phenomenology to understand experiences of racism for second-generation south Asian women. *Canadian Journal of Counseling, 42*(4), 262–277.

Benner, A. D., & Kim, S. Y. (2009). Experiences of discrimination among Chinese American adolescents and the consequences for socioemotional and academic development. *Developmental Psychology, 45*(6), 1682–1694. doi:10.1037/a0016119.

Brown, C., Matthews, K. A., Bromberger, J. T., & Chang, Y. (2006). The relation between perceived unfair treatment and blood pressure in a racially/ethnically diverse sample of women. *American Journal of Epidemiology, 164*(3), 257–262. doi:10.1093/aje/kwj196.

Burgess, D. J., Ding, Y., Hargreaves, M., van Ryn, M., & Phelan, S. (2008). The association between perceived discrimination and underutilization of needed medical and mental health care in a multi-ethnic community sample. *Journal of Health Care for the Poor and Underserved, 19*(3), 894–911. doi:10.1353/hpu.0.0063.

Cassidy, C., O'Connor, R. C., Howe, C., & Warden, D. (2004). Perceived discrimination and psychological distress: The role of personal and ethnic self-esteem. *Journal of Counseling Psychology, 51*(3), 329–339. doi:10.1037/0022-0167.51.3.329.

Chae, D. H., Takeuchi, D. T., Barbeau, E. M., Bennett, G. G., Lindsey, J., & Krieger, N. (2008). Unfair treatment, racial/ethnic discrimination, ethnic identification, and smoking among Asian Americans in the national Latino and Asian American study. *American Journal of Public Health, 98*(3), 485–492.

Chan, S. (1991). *Asian Americans: An interpretive history*. Boston: Twayne.

Cheng, J. K. Y., Fancher, T. L., Ratanasen, M., Conner, K. R., Duberstein, P. R., Sue, S., & Takeuchi, D. (2012). Lifetime suicidal ideation and suicide attempts in Asian Americans. *Asian American Journal of Psychology, 1*(1), 18–30.

Clark, R., Anderson, N., Clark, V., & Williams, D. (1999). Racism as a stressor for African Americans: A biopsychosocial model. *The American Psychologist, 54*, 805–816. doi:10.1037/0003-066X.54.10.805.

Committee of 100. (2009). *Still the other: Public attitudes towards Chinese and Asian Americans*. New York: Author.

de Castro, A. B., Gee, G. C., & Takeuchi, D. T. (2008). Workplace discrimination and health among Filipinos in the United States. *American Journal of Public Health, 98*(3), 520–526. doi:10.2105/AJPH.2007.110163.

Equal Employment Opportunity Commission. (2008). *Asian American and Pacific Islander group report to the chair of the equal employment opportunity commission*. Washington, DC: Author.

Frazier, P. A., Tix, A. P., & Barron, K. E. (2004). Testing moderator and mediator effects in counseling psychology research. *Journal of Counseling Psychology, 51*(1), 115–134. doi:10.1037/0022-0167.51.1.115.

Gallup. (2005). *Employee discrimination in the workplace*. Washington, DC: Author.

Gee, G. C., & Ponce, N. (2010). Associations between racial discrimination, limited English proficiency, and health-related quality of life among 6 Asian ethnic groups in California. *American Journal of Public Health, 100*(5), 888–895. doi:10.2105/AJPH.2009.178012.

Gee, G. C., Spencer, M. S., Chen, J., & Takeuchi, D. T. (2007). A nationwide study of discrimination and chronic health conditions among Asian Americans. *American Journal of Public Health, 97*(7), 1275–1282. doi:10.2105/AJPH.2006.091827.

Gee, G. C., Ro, A., Gavin, A., & Takeuchi, D. T. (2008). Disentangling the effects of racial and weight discrimination on body mass index and obesity among Asian Americans. *American Journal of Public Health, 98*(3), 493–500. doi:10.2105/AJPH.2007.114025.

Gee, G. C., Ro, A., Shariff-Marco, S., & Chae, D. (2009). Racial discrimination and health among Asian Americans: Evidence, assessment, and directions for future research. *Epidemiologic Reviews, 31*, 130–151. doi:10.1093/epirev/mxp009.

Greene, M. L., Way, N., & Pahl, K. (2006). Trajectories of perceived adult and peer discrimination among Black, Latino, and Asian American adolescents: Patterns and psychological correlates. *Developmental Psychology, 42*(2), 218–238. doi:10.1037/0012-1649.42.2.218.

Hahm, H. C., Ozonoff, A., Gaumond, J., & Sue, S. (2010). Perceived discrimination and health outcomes: A gender comparison among Asian-Americans nationwide. *Women's Health Issues, 20*(5), 350–358. doi:10.1016/j.whi.2010.05.002.

Han, C-s. (2008). A qualitative exploration of the relationship between racism and unsafe sex among Asian Pacific Islander Gay Men. *Archives of Sexual Behavior, 37*(5), 827–837. doi:10.1007/s10508-007-9308-7.

Harris, R., Tobias, M., Jeffreys, M., Waldegrave, K., Karlsen, S., & Nazroo, J. (2006). Racism and health: The relationship between experience of racial discrimination and health in New Zealand. *Social Science & Medicine, 63*(6), 1428–1441.

Hwang, W.-C., & Goto, S. (2008). The impact of perceived racial discrimination on the mental health of Asian American and Latino college students. *Cultural Diversity and Ethnic Minority Psychology, 14*(4), 326–335. doi:10.1037/1099-9809.14.4.326.

Iyer, D. S., & Haslam, N. (2003). Body image and eating disturbance among South Asian-American women: The role of racial teasing. *International Journal of Eating Disorders, 34*(1), 142–147. doi:10.1002/eat.10170.

Jones, J. M. (1997). *Prejudice and racism* (2nd ed.). New York: McGraw Hill.

Kang, J. (1996). Negative action against Asian Americans: The internal instability of Dworkin's defense of affirmative action. *Harvard Civil Rights-Civil Liberties Review, 31*, 1–47.

Kuo, W. H. (1995). Coping with racial discrimination: The case of Asian Americans. *Ethnic and Racial Studies, 18*, 109–127.

Lee, S. (1996). *Unraveling the "model minority" stereotype: Listening to Asian American youth*. New York: Teachers College Press.

Lee, R. M. (2005). Resilience against discrimination: Ethnic identity and other-group orientation as protective factors for Korean Americans. *Journal of Counseling Psychology, 52*(1), 36–44. doi:10.1037/0022-0167.52.1.36.

Lee, C., Ayers, S. L., & Kronenfeld, J. J. (2009a). The association between perceived provider discrimination, health care utilization, and health status in racial and ethnic minorities. *Ethnicity & Disease, 19*(3), 330–337.

Lee, S. J., Nga-Wing, A. W., & Alvarez, A. N. (2009b). The model minority and perpetual foreigner: Stereotypes of Asian Americans. In N. Tewari & A. N. Alvarez (Eds.), *Asian American psychology: Current perspectives* (pp. 69–84). New York: Psychology Press.

Liang, C. T. H., Alvarez, A. N., Juang, L. P., & Liang, M. X. (2007). The role of coping in the relationship between perceived racism and racism-related stress for Asian Americans: Gender differences. *Journal of Counseling Psychology, 54*(2), 132–141. doi:10.1037/0022-0167.54.2.132.

Loo, C. M., Fairbank, J. A., Scurfield, R. M., Ruch, L. O., King, D. W., Adams, L. J., et al. (2001). Measuring exposure to racism: Development and validation of a race-related stressor scale (RRSS) for Asian American Vietnam veterans. *Psychological Assessment, 13*(4), 503–520. doi:10.1037/1040-3590.13.4.503.

Loo, C. M., Fairbank, J. A., & Chemtob, C. M. (2005). Adverse race-related events as a risk factor for post-traumatic stress disorder in Asian American Vietnam veterans. *The Journal of Nervous and Mental Disease, 193*(7), 455–463. doi:10.1097/01.nmd.0000168239. 51714.e6.

Mossakowski, K. N. (2003). Coping with perceived discrimination: Does ethnic identity protect mental health? *Journal of Health and Social Behavior, 44*(3), 318–333. doi:10.2307/1519782.

National Asian Pacific American Legal Consortium. (2003). *Remembering: A ten year retrospective.* Washington, DC: Author.

Ngo-Metzger, Q., Legedza, A. T. R., & Phillips, R. S. (2004). Asian Americans' Reports of Their Health Care Experiences: Results of a National Survey. *Journal of General Internal Medicine, 19*(2), 111–119. doi:10.1111/j.1525-1497.2004.30143.x.

Noh, S., & Kaspar, V. (2003). Perceived discrimination and depression: Moderating effects of coping, acculturation, and ethnic support. *American Journal of Public Health, 93*(2), 232–238. doi:10.2105/AJPH.93.2.232.

Noh, S., Kaspar, V., Hou, F., Rummens, J., & Beiser, M. (1999). Perceived racial discrimination, depression, and coping: A study of Southeast Asian refugees in Canada. *Journal of Health and Social Behavior, 40*(3), 193–207. doi:10.2307/2676348.

Paradies, Y. C. (2006). A systematic review of empirical research on self-reported racism and health. *International Journal of Epidemiology, 35*, 888–901. doi:10.1093/ije/dyl056.

Piette, J. D., Bibbins-Domingo, K., & Schillinger, D. (2006). Health care discrimination, processes of care, and diabetes patients' health status. *Patient Education and Counseling, 60*(1), 41–48. doi:10.1016/j.pec.2004.12.001.

Rivas-Drake, D., Hughes, D., & Way, N. (2008). A closer look at peer discrimination, ethnic identity, and psychological well-being among urban Chinese American sixth graders. *Journal of Youth and Adolescence, 37*(1), 12–21. doi:10.1007/s10964-007-9227-x.

Rosenbloom, S. R., & Way, N. (2004). Experiences of discrimination among African American, Asian American, and Latino adolescents in an urban high school. *Youth & Society, 35*(4), 420–451. doi:10.1177/0044118X03261479.

Sorkin, D. H., Ngo-Metzger, Q., & De Alba, I. (2010). Racial/ethnic discrimination in health care: Impact on perceived quality of care. *Journal of General Internal Medicine, 25*(5), 390–396. doi:10.1007/s11606-010-1257-5.

Wei, M., Ku, T.-Y., Russell, D. W., Mallinckrodt, B., & Liao, K. Y.-H. (2008). Moderating effects of three coping strategies and self-esteem on perceived discrimination and depressive symptoms: A minority stress model for Asian international students. *Journal of Counseling Psychology, 55*(4), 451–462. doi:10.1037/a0012511.

Wilson, P. A., & Yoshikawa, H. (2004). Experiences of and responses to social discrimination among Asian and Pacific Islander Gay Men: Their relationship to HIV risk. *AIDS Education and Prevention, 16*(1), 68–83. doi:10.1521/aeap. 16.1.68.27724.

Yen, I. H., Ragland, D. R., Greiner, B. A., & Fisher, J. M. (1999). Racial discrimination and alcohol-related behavior in urban transit operators: Findings from the San Francisco Muni health and safety study. *Public Health Reports, 114*, 448–458.

Ying, Y.-W., Lee, P. A., & Tsai, J. L. (2000). Cultural orientation and racial discrimination: Predictors of coherence in Chinese American young adults. *Journal of Community Psychology, 28*(4), 427–442. doi:10.1002/1520-6629(200007)28:4.

Yip, T., Gee, G. C., & Takeuchi, D. T. (2008). Racial discrimination and psychological distress: The impact of ethnic identity and age among immigrant and United States-born Asian adults. *Developmental Psychology, 44*(3), 787–800. doi:10.1037/0012-1649.44.3.787.

Yoo, H. C., & Lee, R. M. (2005). Ethnic identity and approach-type coping as moderators of the racial discrimination/well-being relation in Asian Americans. *Journal of Counseling Psychology, 52*(4), 497–506. doi:10.1037/0022-0167.52.4.497.

Yoo, H. C., & Lee, R. M. (2008). Does ethnic identity buffer or exacerbate the effects of frequent racial discrimination on situational well-being of Asian Americans? *Journal of Counseling Psychology, 55*(1), 63–74. doi:10.1037/0022-0167.55.1.63.

Yoo, H. C., Gee, G. C., & Takeuchi, D. (2009). Discrimination and health among Asian American immigrants: Disentangling racial from language discrimination. *Social Science & Medicine, 68*(4), 726–732.

Yoshikawa, H., Wilson, P. A.-D., Chae, D. H., & Cheng, J.-F. (2004). Do family and friendship networks protect against the influence of discrimination on mental health and HIV risk among Asian and Pacific Islander Gay Men? *AIDS Education and Prevention, 16*(1), 84–100. doi:10.1521/aeap. 16.1.84.27719.

Young, K., & Takeuchi, D. T. (1998). Racism. In L. C. Lee & N. S. Zane (Eds.), *Handbook of Asian American psychology* (pp. 401–432). Thousand Oaks, CA: Sage.

Asian Americans, Socio-Economic Status and Health: Current Findings and Future Concerns

Wei Zhang

Introduction

Mrs. Yeh decided to immigrate to the United States at the beginning of the twenty-first century with her husband, who was accepted by the Ph.D. program in Computer Sciences. This was a tough decision for Mrs. Yeh because she was a successful doctor in Hangzhou, one of the most developed cities in China. Migrating to the U.S. means that she had to give up her career and adjust herself to a completely new cultural environment.

The first couple of months after she arrived in the U.S., she was actually very happy. Relaxing from her previous heavy workload, she initially very much enjoyed her new environment. But as time went by, she increasingly felt lonely, anxious, and stressful. She started to miss her family, colleagues, and friends in China. In addition, though she can read and write English well, Mrs. Yeh did not have sufficient English-speaking skills to communicate with others in the still unfamiliar culture. A major blow to her was she was not able to continue working as a doctor because her degree and license of medicine earned in China were not recognized in the United States. To get back to the profession she loved, Mrs. Yeh would have no choice but to start all over again.

Ahead of her was preparing for English exams and applying for medical schools. Then it would require Mrs. Yeh to successfully complete her studies and find an internship at a hospital somewhere before she could restart and establish her own practice. The entire process might take about a decade. Therefore, she asked herself, as a woman in her early thirties, do I even want to give it a try?

Mrs. Yeh had a high socioeconomic status (SES) in China. Her past success and her education should allow her to have higher levels of self-esteem and sense of personal control to help address many new challenges in a new country. Nevertheless, a high SES in China is not easily transferable in the United States. The loss of social status due to immigration may adversely affect general health and well-being. Should Mrs. Yeh decide to re-establish her previous personal socioeconomic status and occupation in the United States, she faces a potentially time consuming as well as stressful process, which in turn, could take an additional toll on her already declining mental and physical health.

The story of Mrs. Yeh reveals how SES is an important factor in the study of Asian American health. Moreover, given that the majority of Asian Americans are immigrants, the relationship between SES and health should be examined within larger contexts, including immigration. Family support, education, nativity, English proficiency, and personal appraisal of SES are just a few of the factors related to immigration and SES. The present review will include an introduction of studies documenting the parallels

W. Zhang, Ph.D. (✉)
College of Social Sciences, Sociology Department, University of Hawaii at Manoa, Honolulu, HI, USA
e-mail: weizhang@hawaii.edu

G.J. Yoo et al. (eds.), *Handbook of Asian American Health*,
DOI 10.1007/978-1-4614-2227-3_13, © Springer Science+Business Media, LLC 2013

between SES and health using the first nationally representative sample of Asian Americans, the National Latino and Asian American Study (NLAAS). Another important dynamic is the correlation between neighborhoods and poverty, two important explanatory mechanisms that could underlie the link between SES and health for Asian Americans. Alternative measures of SES better suited for this racial group will be introduced. Lastly, suggestions for future research in this topic will be presented via a comprehensive conceptual model that summarizes relationships among several key concepts.

Connecting SES and Health

Asian Americans represent one of the fastest growing racial minorities in the United States, with the majority being immigrants (Barnes & Bennett, 2002). Based on the most recent Census data, The Asian American population will triple in growth and represent an approximate 8% of the entire American population in 2050. Given their equivalent and even better socioeconomic and health profile as a group compared to non-Hispanic whites, Asian Americans are often portrayed as the "model minority" (Peterson, 1966, p. 180). Yet are they really the model minority? A closer look at this population segment provides a definitely "no" answer to this question.

Despite the U.S. government's tendency to combine individuals with origins in "any of the original people of the Far East Southeast Asia, or the Indian subcontinent" (Reeves & Bennett, 2004) and to create a larger category of "Asian Americans" for planning and demographic purposes, this group is extremely diverse with respect to country of origin, languages and dialects, religions, immigration history, socioeconomic status, and other factors that might affect their health (McCracken et al., 2007). Socioeconomic status (SES) is an example of a variable with substantial within-group distinctions. Specific data from the 2000 U.S. Census reports the median family income for all Asian Americans was approximately $59,324, yet this masks the wide range within subgroups. For example, the average

income of $32,284 for Hmong is vastly different from the $70,849 for Japanese. Poverty rates vary from 6.3% for Filipino to 29.3% for Cambodian and 37.8% for Hmong. Though 44% of the overall Asian American population had a college level education, less than 10% of Cambodians, Hmong, and Laotians had a bachelor's degree.

Socioeconomic status is associated with a wide range of health problems such as low birth weight, cardiovascular diseases, hypertension, arthritis, diabetes, and cancer (Alder & Newman, 2002). Link and Phelan (1995) assert the most fundamental cause of health disparity is socioeconomic disparities. Sociologists traditionally assess SES by indicators of education, income, and occupation. Of these three indicators of SES, the educational gradient in health is regarded as one of the more robust associations in social science research (Lynch, 2003) because education generally precedes and shapes other aspects of SES such as income and occupation (Mirowsky & Ross, 2003).

How does SES impact health for Asian Americans? In reviewing the first ever nationally representative sample of Asian Americans, the aforementioned 2002–2003 National Latino and Asian American Study (NLAAS) discloses several interesting patterns. First, there is significant diversity in SES, immigration-related factors, and self-rated health (SRH) across four major Asian American groups in the data (Table 13.1). South Asians, Japanese, and Koreans (Gee, Ro, Gavin, & Takeuchi, 2008), exceeded the Chinese, Filipinos and Vietnamese in college-level education. The Filipinos reported the highest household income and were most likely to be employed among the four listed groupings. Consistent with previous literature (e.g., Frisbie, Cho, & Hummer, 2001), Vietnamese were the most disadvantaged with respect to almost every indicator of SES, reporting the lowest educational attainment and household income, but the second highest unemployment rate. Gender make-up and age distribution were found to be almost equivalent across the four listed ethnic groups. Divorce/separation/ widowhood rate ranged from 6.6% for Vietnamese to slightly over 10% for Chinese. In terms of migration status, the proportion of U.S.-born

Table 13.1 Distributions of demographics, socioeconomic status, immigration-related factors, and self-rated physical and mental health of Asian American adults by national origin: U.S. Asian Americans in the national Latino and Asian American study 2002–2003

	Asian whole	Vietnamese	Filipino	Chinese	Other Asians
Demographics					
Sex					
Male	47.4	47.3	47.4	47.2	47.5
Female	52.6	52.7	52.6	52.8	52.5
Age (years)	41.3 (15.6)	41.3 (15.4)	41.8 (16.1)	41.4 (15.4)	41.1 (15.5)
Marital status					
Married	68.8	71.9	68.7	65.8	70.2
Divorced/separated/widowed	8.3	6.6	9.5	10.3	6.7
Never married	22.8	21.5	21.8	23.9	23.0
Socioeconomic status					
Education (years)					
<high school (<12)	14.3	31.8	10.6	17.6	7.8
= high school (12)	17.8	20.8	20.2	16.3	16.5
Some college (13–15)	25.1	23.6	32.2	20.2	25.3
College or more (16)	42.8	23.8	37.1	45.9	50.4
Household income ($)					
<15,000	18.4	25.9	12.9	22.6	15.6
15,000–34,999	12.7	23.0	10.2	13.2	10.0
35,000–74,999	28.5	27.7	29.9	21.3	33.4
75,000	40.5	23.3	46.9	42.9	41.0
Employment status (%)					
Employed	63.9	63.2	66.8	63.4	62.8
Unemployed	6.4	8.5	5.7	5.9	6.4
Not in labor force	29.8	28.2	27.5	30.8	30.8
Immigration-related factors					
Immigration status					
US born	23.8	3.7	31.0	19.1	30.1
0–4 years	13.7	16.4	10.9	14.3	13.8
5–10 years	12.1	26.7	8.0	14.8	7.4
11 years	50.4	53.3	50.1	51.8	48.7
English proficiency					
Good/excellent	62.8	28.0	82.6	48.4	74.6
Poor/fair	37.2	72.0	17.4	51.6	25.4
Self-rated health					
Physical health					
Poor/fair	15.4	21.7	11.6	21.4	10.9
Good/very good/excellent	84.6	78.3	88.4	78.6	89.1
Mental health					
Poor/fair	8.5	11.6	7.0	13.5	4.5
Good/very good/excellent	91.5	88.4	93.0	86.5	95.5
All persons (no.)	2,083	270	449	594	770

Note: Percentages are reported. Except for rounding error, percentages sum to 100.0%. For age, mean and standard deviation (in parenthesis) are reported

Vietnamese was the lowest (3.7%), followed by Chinese (19.1%), other Asians (30.1%), and Filipinos (31.0%). Vietnamese were also the ethnic group with the greatest proportion of very recent immigrants, roughly 16.4% had been in the United States for less than 5 years. For English proficiency, over three-fourths of Filipinos and other Asians reported having English skills either good or excellent, while only 28% of Vietnamese reported sufficient English skills in reading, writing, and speaking. Poorer self-ratings of physical and mental health were found among Vietnamese and Chinese as compared with other Asians and Filipinos.

Second, SES indicators such as educational levels, income levels, and employment status are all significantly related to physical health for Asian Americans (Table 13.2). Education level and fair to poor self-rated physical health were negatively related in a gradient fashion. In other words, every level increase in education is negatively correlated with reports of fair to poor health among respondents. Similar results were found for family income. Individuals reporting an annual family income of at least $35,000 were significantly less likely to report their health was fair or poor than those participants listing a family income of $15,000. Currently employed Asian

Table 13.2 Self-rated poor/fair physical and mental health on socioeconomic status with adjustment for demographics (Model 1 and Model 3) and immigration-related factors (Model 2 and Model 4): U.S. Asians in the National Latino and Asian American study 2002–2003

	Poor/fair physical health		Poor/fair mental health	
Characteristic	Model 1 OR [95% CI]	Model 2 OR [95% CI]	Model 3 OR [95% CI]	Model 4 OR [95% CI]
Education (less than high school[a])				
High school graduate	.91 [.61, 1.33]	1.00 [.67, 1.49]	.54 [.34, .86]**	.62 [.39, .98]*
Some college	.60 [.40, .89]**	.81 [.54, 1.22]	.35 [.22, .57]***	.51 [.31, .84]**
College or more	.50 [.34, .72]*	.75 [.51, 1.12]	.25 [.16, .41]***	.40 [.25, .66]***
Family income (<$15,000[a])				
$15,000–$34,999	.98 [.65, 1.48]	.94 [.62, 1.43]	.82 [.50, 1.36]	.78 [.46, 1.30]
$35,000–$74,000	.58 [.40, .86]**	.59 [.39, .88]**	.53 [.32, .88]*	.53 [.32, .89]*
$75,000	.61 [.42, .89]**	.64 [.43, .95]*	.63 [.39, 1.03]†	.67 [.41, 1.11]
Employment status (unemployed[a])				
Employed	.62 [.37, 1.04]†	.60 [.36, 1.02]†	.86 [.43, 1.72]	.85 [.42, 1.72]
Not in labor force	1.19 [.70, 2.02]	1.27 [.74, 2.17]	1.22 [.60, 2.47]	1.34 [.65, 2.78]
Migration status (U.S. born[a])				
0–4 years		.44 [.26, .77]**		.47 [.22, 1.03]†
5–10 years		.93 [.56, 1.52]		1.34 [.70, 2.59]
11 years		.84 [.58, 1.22]		1.25 [.73, 2.12]
English proficiency (poor/fair[a])				
Good/excellent		.32 [.23, .44]***		.30 [.19, .48]***
National origin (Vietnamese[a])				
Filipino	.60 [.39, .94]*	.97 [.60, 1.55]	.83 [.48, 1.46]	1.39 [.77, 2.51]
Chinese	1.21 [.83, 1.78]	1.32 [.90, 1.95]	1.59 [.99, 2.55]†	1.71 [1.05, 2.76]*
Other Asian	.60 [.40, .90]*	.83 [.54, 1.27]	.61 [.35, 1.04]†	.86 [.49, 1.51]
Gender (male[a])				
Female	1.24 [.96, 1.62]	1.19 [.91, 1.56]	1.25 [.89, 1.75]	1.22 [.87, 1.73]
Age (yr)	1.02 [1.02, 1.03]***	1.02 [1.01, 1.03]**	1.01 [1.00, 1.02]†	1.00 [.99, 1.02]
Marital status (married/cohabiting[a])				
Divorced	.84 [.54, 1.30]	.90 [.57, 1.41]	1.47 [.90, 2.42]	1.64 [.98, 2.73]†
Never married	.89 [.60, 1.33]	.90 [.60, 1.37]	.96 [.57, 1.61]	1.05 [.62, 1.80]

Note: $N = 2,083$

OR odds ratio, *CI* confidence interval

†$p < .1$; *$p < .05$; **$p < .01$; ***$p < .001$

[a]Reference group

Americans showed slightly lower chances of reporting fair or poor physical health. Filipinos and other Asians were less probable to report fair or poor physical health compared to the Vietnamese. The data presented, along with other measures from the NLAAS suggest that the SES and physical health association is quite robust for Asian Americans.

Third, in addition to SES factors, immigration-related factors such as migration status (place of birth and length of residence in the U.S.) and English proficiency (measured by asking respondents how well they spoke, read, and wrote English) were interrelated to self-rankings of physical health. Most recent Asian immigrants were healthier, indicating generally good to excellent health compared to their U.S.-born counterparts. Asian Americans with good to excellent English proficiency were also healthier and significantly less likely to report fair to poor physical health. When self-rated mental health was examined, similar patterns were found: higher levels of education and family income, and better English proficiency are related to a better self-rated mental health.

The NLAAS data presents several important propositions. Comparing results of four Asian ethnic groups with those of Asian Americans as a whole from Table 13.1 confirm that simply focusing on the undifferentiated total Asian group tends to overlook the significant within-group variations in SES, migration status, and health status across Asian ethnic groups. Further, noteworthy SES-related gradients in health, particularly education and income, exist among Asian Americans and should be incorporated in evaluating physical and mental health status, although some other immigration-related factors such as English proficiency also are important.

SES and Health: Explanatory Mechanisms

Why is SES related to individual health? Simply stated, individuals with lower SES are likely to live in poverty. They may not have health insurance at all or have health insurance with limited services, which in combination with other stressors, may put their health at jeopardy. Individuals with lower SES are also likely to live in poor neighborhoods lacking resources. Moreover, they may not have easy access to fresh fruits and vegetables resulting in poorer diet choices. Lack of time, lack of facilities, and safety issues can limit exercise and fitness. Heavy drinking and smoking may temporarily appease stress, yet this adversely affects current and future well-being. The following summary reviews the effects of poverty and impoverished neighborhoods and their implications for the health of Asian Americans.

Poverty and Health

In spite of the aforementioned "model minority" stereotype, Asian Americans are not immune to poverty and its consequences. Poverty often means lack of health insurance, thwarting access to both preventive and therapeutic health care. Medicaid does not always guarantee access to services, since doctors may refuse to participate due to the limited payments offered by the program. Even if doctors accept Medicaid or if health insurance is available, poorer immigrants may encounter language barriers making it difficult to explain symptoms and/or understanding treatment options. Visiting the doctor can mean time off from work, something not easily afforded with low wage employment. Additional expenses, such as transportation costs and child care, can further impede medical care and affect utilization rates among lower SES Asian Americans.

Ghosh (2003) mentioned that, as a group, there are more than two million (17%) Asian Americans and Pacific Islanders (AAPIs) lacking health insurance. The household poverty rate for AAPIs is approximately 14%, compared with only 8% for non-Hispanic whites. A 2008 report pooled data from the 2004 to 2006 Current Population Surveys (CPS), finding that 31% of Koreans and 21% of Vietnamese residing in the United States are currently uninsured, compared to 12% of Japanese and Asian Indians (Kaiser Family Foundation, 2008). Similar results were obtained in a California survey, a state with an AAPI population of around 13%. Over one-third of Koreans and 20% of Vietnamese are uninsured (Brown et al., 2007). Using pooled data from the 2003 to 2005 California Health Interview Surveys, Kao (2010) also disclosed significant ethnic differences in health insurance types and uninsured rates among Asian Americans. The reported differences were at least partially explained by socioeconomic and immigration-related factors. Higher rates of the uninsured among Vietnamese Americans and Chinese Americans are primarily due to their relatively lower levels of income and underemployment. Likewise, Kagawa-Singer and Pourat (2000) reported that the breast and cervical cancer screening rates were below national guidelines for AAPIs, with rates significantly lower for Asian Americans compared to white subjects. Lack of insurance, low income, and lack of primary source of care were all cited as explanations for the low screening participation.

More recently, Yu, Huang, and Singh (2010) analyzed data from the 2003 and 2005 California Health Interview Survey. The findings indicated that Asian Americans have a variety of health care access and utilization patterns, but that lack of health care usage is still a significant problem. For instance, compared with non-Hispanic White children: (1) Korean children are approximately four times more likely to lack health insurance; (2) Filipino children are two times as likely to not have had recent contact with doctor; (3) Chinese, Korean, and Vietnamese children are much more likely to be in fair to poor health status. Family poverty along with other immigration-related factors such as nativity and English proficiency of parents are partially responsible for many of these outcomes.

Taken together, large SES heterogeneity exists within Asian America. Asian ethnicities are overrepresented on both ends of the socioeconomic scale. Many Asian Americans were foreign-born and have limited English proficiency. Because of language barriers, there is considerable unemployment and/or chronic underemployment (temporary, lower-wage jobs), affecting insurance availability. SES, poverty, health insurance, nativity, levels of acculturation are among numerous

factors working together to contribute to a complex portrait of the health and well-being of Asian Americans. Examining Asian American health issues cannot be completed without regard to substantial within-group variations.

Neighborhood and Health

Individual SES commonly determines place of residence, which in turn, can affect individual health. Diez-Roux and Mair (2010) stated there are at least two reasons that account for the increasing scholarly attention on neighborhood contextual factors and individual health. One element is the increasing insufficiency of individual-based explanations on health disparities which ignores group-wide dynamics. Secondly, with the ever-evolving debates about health care and insurance, there is a revitalized interest in understanding the health disparities across different racial and ethnic groups. "Place of residency is strongly patterned by social position and ethnicity" (Diez-Roux & Mair, 2010, p. 125), which necessitates examination of neighborhood characteristics interacting with racial and ethnic differences in health status and care. Using multilevel analyses to link individual level survey data with contextual neighborhood information, recent studies in the U.S. have started to test and identify the independent effect of neighborhood conditions on individual health net of personal characteristics.

Although empirical results remain mixed and inconclusive due to diverse measures of neighborhood attributes, a notable trend within studies suggests the positive association between neighborhood SES and a variety of physical and mental health outcomes. LeClere, Rogers, and Peters (1998) suggested that neighborhood characteristics (as indicated by public assistance, poverty rate, low median income, and female headship rates) predict mortality rates of heart disease in women. Waitzman and Smith (1998) found that residence in a poor area (proportions of low income families, substandard housing, single-parent households, unskilled males in the labor force, adults with low educational attainment) is associated with significantly elevated mortality risk among adults aged 25–54 years. Ross and Mirowsky (2009) disclosed that perceived neighborhood disorder, a more subjective measure of neighborhood perception, is related to higher levels of mental health problems such as depression, anxiety, and anger.

Despite the rapid increase of literature on neighborhood and health in general, it is again noted that very few studies have focused on Asian Americans. The limited information that is available provides mixed findings. Kandula, Wen, Jacobs, and Lauderdale (2009) examined whether neighborhood social and cultural characteristics (e.g., socioeconomics, ethnic composition, and residents' perception of social cohesion) are associated with smoking behavior among Asian Americans in California. Their findings disclose that (1) neighborhood SES (based on Census data on concentrated affluence, concentrated poverty, percentage of college-educated residents, and percentage of home ownership) is not significantly related to smoking behavior among Asian Americans; (2) for women, living in an Asian enclave (a neighborhood with at least 50% Asians) was protective against smoking, whereas (3) for men, higher perceived social cohesion was protective against smoking. The findings underscore that cultural factors may be more important than neighborhood SES in understanding that at least some health behaviors, such as smoking, among Asian Americans. In contrast, Hong (2009) revealed that Asian Americans living in poor neighborhoods and neighborhoods with higher proportions of Asian Americans are more likely to experience poorer mental health. Her findings suggest the importance of neighborhood economic resources and racial heterogeneity in maintaining and promoting better mental health outcomes for Asian Americans.

Zhang et al. (2010) simultaneously examined how individual education levels and neighborhood level of education (i.e., the percentage of the population over the age of 24 with a college degree or higher in the respondent's zip-code area) are related to self-rated health (SRH) in

Hawaii. The authors reported that the health advantages of some Asian Americans (i.e., better self-ratings of general health status) over others in Hawaii are partially explained by their residency concentration in areas with higher percentages of college graduates. Their findings suggest that the presence of more educated people in the community may lead to the possible "spillover" benefits generated by the actions of those with high educational attainment. For instance, well-educated neighbors may effectively mobilize their resources to make their community a better one, providing a safe, convenient, and friendly micro-environment that positively influences health and well-being.

Zhang and Ta (2009) examined the layered social connections (family cohesion, relative and friend support, and neighborhood social cohesion, among others) in relation to self-rated physical and mental health of Asian Americans. The findings revealed that neighborhood social cohesion does have some positive effects on residents' self-rated health. Here, neighborhood social cohesion is defined as whether people in the neighborhood can be trusted, get along with each other, assist in an emergency, and look out for one another. However, the beneficial effects of social cohesion on individual health are again largely explained by individual SES such as education and family income, place of birth, and other types of social connections such as family cohesion and social support from friends and relatives.

Recent Research on SES, Asian Americans and Health

Traditional socioeconomic factors underlie much of the health and illness disparities in American society, yet the SES gradient was found to be attenuated or sometimes even inverted in the data involving Asian Americans and health. Using pooled data from the 1992 to 1995 National Health Interview Survey, Launderdale and Rathouz (2000) found that nativity and ethnicity are stronger predictors of obesity and being overweight than SES among Asian Americans.

The authors reported a weak association between economic status and body mass index for foreign-born Asian American and even a positive association for the foreign-born Asian American men. Likewise, the Filipino American Epidemiological Study (FACES) also showed that education and income were not associated with chronic physical health or psychological distress for Filipino Americans (de Castro, Gee, & Takeuchi, 2008a, 2008b). Walton, Takeuchi, Herting, and Alegria (2009) found that education in their native countries had little positive effect on health among Asian American immigrants, since a foreign education is associated with fewer socioeconomic resources and limited English proficiency. Iceland (1999) reported that foreign-born Asian men have lower earnings relative to native-born non-Hispanic white men, whereas Asian Americans raised in the United States do not show the same disadvantages.

Collectively, the above findings from empirical studies suggest that the traditional indicators of SES such as education, income, and occupation capture some but not all aspects of socioeconomic status of Asian Americans. As previously mentioned, many Asian immigrants educated in their home country may not necessarily find immediate success in the U.S., if ever. The case study of Mrs. Yeh, presented earlier, reflects this observation. Since purchasing power and cost of living varies across the country, reports of average income for different Asian subgroups should be examined in context. Taken together, to study health and well-being of Asian Americans, new indicators of SES more appropriate for Asian Americans may be necessary. Additionally, other dynamics such as nativity, duration of residence, language proficiency should also be assessed, as these immigration-related factors are indicators of social status and success.

de Castro, Gee, & Takeuchi, (2010) proposed some alternative measures of Asian American SES – particularly for immigrants – including financial strain, subjective social status, and economic opportunity. Why is economic opportunity, a subjective evaluation of one's economic chance in the United States, a legitimate indicator of SES? de Castro et al. (2010) argues that the quest to improve one's economic opportunity is particularly important to immigrants. Self-perceived economic opportunity also reflects ones' satisfaction toward current work and attitudes about previous employment experiences. If an individual is optimistic about economic opportunities, better health and well-being is more likely.

Another alternative measure of SES is called *subjective social status*, defined as a specific aspect of SES that reflects one's self-evaluated social standing in the U.S. and in the community where they live. This particular subjective evaluation reflects an individual's reflection of their past experiences as well as current economic conditions. It has been argued that subjective social status was related to health more consistently than other, more objective measures of SES. In general, an increasing number of empirical studies support the concept that this self-perceived measure of social status was strongly related to psychological functioning and a wide range of health related factors among healthy White women (Adler, Epel, Castellazzo, & Ickovics, 2000). This subjective measure served as a better predictor of self-rated health for Chinese American pregnant women, than education and income (Ostrove, Adler, Kuppermann, & Washington, 2000). The measure was negatively related to mood dysfunction among immigrant Asian Americans who arrived in the U.S. after the age of 25 (Leu et al., 2008).

A third alternative measure of SES is financial strain. de Castro et al. (2010) stated that "income and wealth may not necessarily convert into adequate financial resources" (p. 660). Moreover, financial strain – defined as "difficulties in matching fiscal resources (e.g., income) to expenses and demands" (de Castro et al., 2010, p. 660) – should be considered a more important and relevant indicator of economic well-being than income and wealth. Chronic difficulties in paying bills and buying groceries can impact ones' self-esteem and sense of personal control, which in turn erodes psychological well-being and may result in negative physical health outcomes.

Using alternative measures of SES among the Asian sample in the NLAAS and adjusting for the effects for more traditional SES measures, de Castro et al. (2010) found that economic opportunity (followed by financial strain and subjective social status) has strong independent effects on self-rated health (SRH), body mass index (BMI), and smoking behavior. Consider that New York, California, and Hawaii are population hubs for Asian Americans, yet the higher cost of living may amplify insecurities and inadequacies in financial security which can have deleterious effects on well-being. To assess such facets of psychological concerns, both subjective as well as objective measures of SES are vital to obtain a more complete understanding of immigrant and minority populations like Asian Americans, particularly in assessing health and fitness.

Summary and Directions for Future Research

Previous studies demonstrate that SES is still germane in evaluating health outcomes for Asian Americans. Noteworthy is the limitations of traditional measures of SES, indicating the need to incorporate alternative ways of gauging SES. Because the vast majority of Asian Americans were foreign-born, most were educated in their native country and have limited English proficiency. Accordingly, using education as a measure of SES may not lead to the same economic and health returns for Asian Americans. To better assess education, stipulating English competency and foreign education as germane issues would be beneficial. Many Asian Americans reside in costly locales entailing a higher cost of living. The same income level may feel quite satisfactory for Texas residents, yet can be perceived as woefully inadequate for Asian American residents in California or Hawaii.

The limitations of conventional SES measures call for future research, helping develop more alternative SES indicators to better gauge the socioeconomic status of Asian Americans. For instance, subjective measures of SES such as economic opportunity, financial strain and

subjective social status should be considered simultaneously with education, income, and occupation. In addition, neighborhood level characteristics such as neighborhood safety, social cohesion, racial density, unemployment rate and poverty rate should also be examined. Taken together, prospective studies should incorporate both subject and objective measures of SES along with features of the neighborhood.

Immigration-related factors – including nativity, age at immigration, generational status, English proficiency – should also be examined as part of the analysis of SES and health. Disaggregating Asian Americans with respect to specific ethnic groups would improve understanding and subdue the persistent myth of the "model minority." Specific needs can and should be documented and presented for different subgroups.

Suggestions for future studies are summarized in Fig. 13.1. SES should be understood as a multidimensional construct, including aspects of objective SES (i.e. education, income, and occupation), subjective reports, along with other relevant indicators including (but not limited to) nativity, duration of residence in the U.S., and English proficiency. Individual measures of SES should be investigated within the context of neighborhood SES, including both the physical environment (food resources, recreational resources, environmental exposures, quality of housing, healthcare access, etc.) and social environment (safety, social cohesion, social control, neighborhood norms and values, etc.). Although individual SES may shape neighborhood-level SES, both qualities of socioeconomic status will yield independent effects on health, including pathways of poverty, health and fitness-related behaviors, psychological resilience, and social support. In summary, the discussion of SES and its association with health and well-being for Asian Americans would be much more meaningful if we develop a more comprehensive conceptual model and embed our discussions within the contexts of history, culture, ethnicity, and immigration.

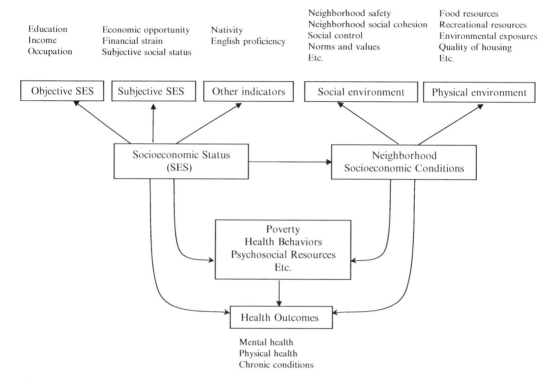

Fig. 13.1 Conceptual models suggesting future studies on SES and health for Asian Americans

References

Adler, N. E., Epel, E. S., Castellazzo, G., & Ickovics, J. R. (2000). Relationship of subjective and objective social status with psychological and physiological functioning: Preliminary data in healthy white women. *Health Psychology, 19*(6), 586–592.

Alder, N. E., & Newman, K. (2002). Socioeconomic disparities in health: Pathways and policies. *Health Affairs, 12*(2), 60–76.

Barnes, J. S., & Bennett, C. E. (2002). *The Asian population of 2000, census 2000 brief.* Washington, DC: US Census Bureau.

Brown, R. E., Lavarreda, S. A., Ponce, N., Yoon, J., Cummings, J., & Rice, T. (2007). *The state of health insurance in California: Findings from the 2005 California health interview survey.* Los Angeles: University of California at Los Angeles, Center for health Policy Research.

de Castro, A. B., Gee, G. C., & Takeuchi, D. T. (2008a). Job-related stress and Chronis health conditions among Filipino immigrants. *Journal of Immigrant and Minority Health, 10*(6), 551–558.

de Castro, A. B., Gee, G. C., & Takeuchi, D. T. (2008b). Relationship between Job dissatisfaction and physical and psychological health among Filipino immigrants. *AAOHN Journal, 56*(1), 33–40.

de Castro, A. B., Gee, G. C., & Takeuchi, D. T. (2010). Examining alternative measures of social disadvantages among Asian Americans: The relevance of economic opportunity, subjective social status, and financial strain for health. *Journal of Immigrant and Minority Health, 12*, 659–671.

Diez-Roux, A. V., & Mair, C. (2010). Neighborhoods and health. *Annals of the New York Academy of Sciences, 1186*, 125–145.

Frisbie, P., Cho, Y., & Hummer, R. (2001). Immigration and the health of Asian and Pacific Islander adults in the Unites States. *American Journal of Epidemiology, 153*(4), 372–380.

Gee, G., Ro, A., Gavin, A., & Takeuchi, D. (2008). Disentangling the effects of racial and weight discrimination on body mass index and obesity among Asian Americans. *American Journal of Public Health, 98*(3), 493–500.

Ghosh, C. (2003). Healthy people 2010 and Asian Americans/Pacific Islanders: Defining a baseline of information. *American Journal of Public Health, 93*(12), 2093–2098.

Hong, S. (2009). *Neighborhood contexts, mental health, and immigration.* PhD. dissertation, School of Social Work, University of Washington, Seattle, WA.

Iceland, J. (1999). Earnings returns to occupational status: Are Asian Americans disadvantaged? *Social Science Research, 28*, 45–65.

Kagawa-Singer, M., & Pourat, N. (2000). Asian American and Pacific Islander breast and cervical carcinoma screening rates and healthy people 2000 objectives. *Cancer, 89*(3), 696–705.

Kaiser Family Foundation & Asian and Pacific Islander American Health Forum. (2008). *Health coverage and access to care among Asian Americans, native Hawaiians and Pacific Islanders (race, ethnicity and health care fact sheet)*. Menlo Park: Kaiser Family Foundations.

Kandula, N. R., Wen, M., Jacobs, E. A., & Lauderdale, D. S. (2009). Association between neighborhood context and smoking prevalence among Asian Americans. *American Journal of Public Health, 99*(5), 885–892.

Kao, D. (2010). Factors associated with ethnic differences in health insurance coverage and type among Asian Americans. *Journal of Community Health, 35*, 142–155.

Launderdale, D. S., & Rathouz, P. J. (2000). Body mass index in a US national sample of Asian Americans: Effects of nativity, years since immigration and socio-economic status. *International Journal of Obesity, 24*, 1188–1194.

LeClere, F. B., Rogers, R. G., & Peters, K. (1998). Neighborhood social context and racial differences in Women's heart disease mortality. *Journal of Health and Social Behavior, 39*, 91–107.

Leu, J., Yen, I. H., Gansky, S. A., Walton, E., Adler, N. E., & Takeuchi, D. T. (2008). The association between subjective social status and mental health among Asian immigrants: Investigating the influence of age at immigration. *Social Science & Medicine, 66*(5), 1152–1164.

Link, B. G., & Phelan, J. (1995). Social conditions as fundamental causes of disease. *Journal of Health and Social Behavior*, (Extra Issue), 80–94.

Lynch, S. M. (2003). Cohort and life-course patterns in the relationship between education and health: A hierarchical approach. *Demography, 40*(2), 309–331.

McCracken, M., Olsen, M., Chen, M. S., Jemal, A., Thun, M., Cokkinides, V., et al. (2007). Cancer incidence, mortality, and associated risk factors among Asian Americans of Chinese, Filipino, Vietnamese, Korean, and Japanese ethnicities. *CA: A Cancer Journal for Clinicians, 57*, 190–205.

Mirowsky, J., & Ross, C. E. (2003). *Education, social status, and health*. New York: Aldine de Gruyter.

Ostrove, J. M., Adler, N. E., Kuppermann, M., & Washington, A. E. (2000). Objective and subjective assessments of socioeconomic status and their relationship to self-rated health in an ethnically diverse sample of pregnant women. *Health Psychology, 19*(6), 613–618.

Peterson, W. (1966, January 9). Success story, Japanese American style. *The New York Times Magazine*, p. 180.

Reeves, T., & Bennett, C. E. (2004). *We the people: Asians in the United States*. Census 2000 Special Reports. Washington, DC: US Census Bureau.

Ross, C., & Mirowsky, J. (2009). Neighborhood disorder, subjective alienation, and distress. *Journal of Health and Social Behavior, 50*, 49–64.

Waitzman, N. J., & Smith, K. R. (1998). Phantom of the area: Poverty-area residence and mortality in the United States. *American Journal of Public Health, 88*(6), 973–976.

Walton, E., Takeuchi, D. T., Herting, J. R., & Alegria, M. (2009). Does place of education matter? Contextualizing the education and health status association among Asian Americans. *Biodemography and Social Biology, 55*(1), 30–51.

Yu, S. M., Huang, Z. J., & Singh, G. K. (2010). Health status and health services access and utilization among Chinese, Filipino, Japanese, Korean, south Asian, and Vietnamese children in California. *American Journal of Public Health, 100*(5), 823–830.

Zhang, W., McCubbin, H., McCubbin, L., Chen, Q., Foley, S., Strom, I., et al. (2010). Education and self-rated health: An individual and neighborhood level analysis of Asian Americans, Hawaiians, and Caucasians in Hawaii. *Social Science & Medicine, 70*, 561–569.

Zhang, W., & Ta, V. M. (2009). Social connections, immigration-related factors, and self-rated physical and mental health among Asian Americans. *Social Science & Medicine, 68*, 2104–2112.

Perceptions and Culturally Responsive Care of Asian Americans with Alzheimer's Disease and Related Dementias

14

Linda A. Gerdner and Gwen Yeo

Introduction

During the summer of 2005, a 67-year old Hmong American man living in Wisconsin was reported missing by family members. He was last seen repairing a fence at the family's home. Family reported that the man was unable to speak any English and had a "minor mental disorder" that involved "short-term memory loss." Family stated that the man had never walked more than three blocks from his home. Three days following his disappearance the authorities launched a "full search." This included a ground search conducted by 40 family members, police, fire fighters, as well as the Canine Emergency Response Team. In addition, the area was searched by airplane. Police even activated a computerized telephone system to alert neighbors that the man was missing. As days passed, the region experienced excessively hot weather, hope began to diminish. After 21 days, the elder was found crawling in tall grass about 2.5 miles from his home. The same $41 dollars was found in his pocket that he had before his disappearance. The man explained to his family that during his absence he had been drinking from a plastic bottle that he filled with

water from a nearby creek. He had not had anything to eat since becoming lost. At night he covered himself with leaves and branches as protection. The man was hospitalized, primarily for treatment of dehydration (Moua, 2005). In this example, dementia was compounded by language and cultural barriers. The survival skills the man had acquired during and following the war, in his homeland of Laos, has been attributed to saving the man's life.

Dementia is a syndrome, or group of symptoms, associated with a progressive loss of memory and other cognitive functions, severe enough to interfere with performing tasks of daily life (American Psychiatric Association, 2000; Green, 2005). The syndrome has a variety of etiologies. Alzheimer's disease is the most common type of dementia. The onset of Alzheimer's disease is gradual and involves continuing cognitive decline. Because of the difficulty in obtaining pathological evidence of Alzheimer's disease, diagnosis is usually determined by ruling out other forms of dementia.

The Alzheimer's Association (2011) estimates that over 5.4 million Americans have a diagnosis of Alzheimer's disease. In a 2010 poll conducted on behalf of the Alzheimer's Association, 70% of family caregivers were white, 15% were African-American, 12% were Hispanic, 1% were Asian-American and 2% were from other ethnic groups.

The majority of research on Alzheimer's disease has focused on large ethnic groups with a long-standing presence in the United States. Gerontologists increasingly recognize the important

L.A. Gerdner (✉) • G. Yeo
Stanford Geriatric Education Center, Center for
Education in Family and Community Medicine,
Stanford University School of Medicine,
Palo Alto, CA, USA
e-mail: lgerdner@gmail.com

G.J. Yoo et al. (eds.), *Handbook of Asian American Health*,
DOI 10.1007/978-1-4614-2227-3_14, © Springer Science+Business Media, LLC 2013

influence that ethnic background has on a person's perception of dementia, caregiving experience and use of formal assistance (Janevic & Connell, 2001; Yeo & Gallagher-Thompson, 2006).

As discussed in other chapters in this volume, the Asian Americans are a very diverse and rapidly growing population whose origins cover most of the countries on the extensive Asian continent. The same is true of the elders in the population, who are those at greatest risk of the various types of dementia. Persons 65 and over years of age who self-identified as Asian, comprise 2.3% of all persons 65 and over years of age in the U.S. in 2000.[1] The percent of those 65 and over comprised 7.7% of all Asian Americans, compared to 12.4% of all older Americans. Significant exceptions among the Asian American subgroups are the 20% of elders in the Japanese American population and the small percent of elders among the newer immigrant groups, especially those from Southeast Asia (Reeves & Bennett, 2004). The size and selected characteristics of the largest older Asian American populations as found in the 2000 census are included in Table 14.1.

With the exception of Japanese Americans, there are no statistics available on the prevalence of Alzheimer's disease in any of the Asian Americans subgroups. However, an analysis of Medicare data from the U.S. Centers for Medicare and Medicaid Services (Porell, 2009) reports that in 2006, 8.1% of Asian-American Medicare beneficiaries aged 65 and older, had a claims-based diagnosis of Alzheimer's disease or related dementia (ADRD). In that same year, the Office of Minority Health and Health Disparities (2009) reported that Alzheimer's disease was the tenth leading cause of death in Asian Americans and Pacific Islanders.

There is wide diversity within the elders in the ethnic subgroups of the Asian American population. Valle (1998) emphasizes the need to consider both the historical and cultural background when working with dementia and their family caregivers

in specific ethnic minority groups, so readers are encouraged to keep the historical background of specific Asian American populations presented in previous chapters in mind as each group is discussed below. This chapter proceeds by discussing the available research on ADRD within some of the largest and most distinctive Asian American subpopulations, Chinese Americans, Filipino Americans, Japanese Americans, Korean Americans, Vietnamese Americans, and Hmong Americans, and the elders in those populations at risk for dementia.

Ethnic Subgroups

Chinese Americans

Demographic Characteristics. Chinese Americans elders are the largest and probably the most diverse ethnic group of Asian American elders. Although there are a large number of second generation Chinese American elders, over 80% are foreign born, and 60% speak little or no English (see Table 14.1). Mandarin and Cantonese are the most common languages spoken by Chinese American elders, although there are several other Chinese languages used as well.

Prevalence of Dementia. A study of elders in Shanghai found that the prevalence of dementia was 4.6% of the population (Zhang et al., 1990), but there are no statistics on the prevalence of ADRD among Chinese Americans. This may be attributed to the negative stigma that many Chinese Americans associate with the disease. This stigma has served as an impediment for the participation of Chinese Americans in studies of ADRD and has led to delays in seeking medical care until the advanced stages of the disease (Zhan, 2004). For example, Huang et al. (2003) used minimum data sets plus sociodemographic characteristics and health status of older Chinese in a study of those who were newly admitted to a nursing home. Three-fourths of these residents had cognitive impairment that was underdiagnosed on admission.

---

[1] At the time of this writing, the 2010 census data were not available.

Table 14.1 Selected demographic characteristics of older Americans by ethnicity, aged 65 and over (U.S. Census 2000)

Population	Number ≥65	Percent ≥65 in population (%)	In poverty (%)	With disability (%)	Living alone (%)	Education (%)		Foreign born*	Speak little or no English (%)
						<9 yrs.	≥College		
Total Americans	34,991,753	12.4	9.9	41.9	27.8	16.7	33.5	N/A	4.0
Asian Americans	800,795	7.7	11.9	40.8	12.9	30.9	34.0	N/A	41.0
Chinese	235,995	9.6	15.7	36.8	14.0	38.0	33.3	84.2%	59.8
Filipino	164,768	8.7	8.2	47.1	6.7	29.4	42.3	90.5%	22.6
Japanese	161,288	20.4	5.6	33.0	21.9	11.3	33.5	20.0%	10.7
Korean	68,505	6.2	20.9	40.0	19.0	31.7	32.1	90.2%	63.9
Vietnamese	58,241	5.0	15.0	54.2	7.0	47.3	17.2	92.1%	73.5
Hmong	4,698	2.6	27.4	59.2	5.1	91.6	3.0	92.61%	83.8
Asian Indian	66,834	3.8	8.3	42.1	6.0	31.6	40.0	88.9%	35.4
Cambodian	6,570	3.8	22.7	62.3	4.4	73.7	9.5	100.0%	79.7
Laotian	6,106	3.4	18.0	54.9	3.8	72.9	7.3	–	79.2
Pakistani	4,804	3.0	12.7	45.2	2.6	30.7	38.9	96.7%	39.8

Notes: Developed by Gwen Yeo, Wendy King, and Linda Gerdner from File Nos. 1, 2, 3, and 4 of the 2000 Census and from Reeves and Bennett, 2004.
*Adapted 2000 Census Data provided to author (GY) by A. Locsin, National Asian Pacific Center on Aging, Seattle, WA.

Perceptions of Dementia and Other Cultural Issues Affecting Dementia Care. There are no terms in the Chinese language that equate to the diagnostic term for Alzheimer's disease. Words that have been used by the lay community to describe the associated symptoms are *chi dai. Chi* is translated as "confused or stupid" and *dai* means "losing one's mind or catatonic" (Zhan, 2004, p. 20). This term reflects a negative stigma associated with the disease that may cause shame to the family, resulting in social isolation of the elder.

Studies have shown that Chinese American family caregivers often attribute dementia to a natural part of the aging process (Braun, Jeanette, Sheila, Sasaki, & Meininger, 1995; Levkoff, Levy, & Weitzman, 1999; Mahoney, Cloutterbuck, Neary, & Zhan, 2005; Zhan, 2004). This belief is reflected in the term, *hu tu*, used by some to describe the symptoms associated with ADRD. The term means "forgetful in old age" (Mahoney et al., 2005, p. 787).

The accompanying symptoms of dementia have also been attributed to the negative energies resulting from "bad feng shui" (Mahoney et al., 2005; Zhan, 2004) and past psychological trauma (e.g., traumatic experiences during China's Cultural Revolution) (Levkoff et al., 1999).

Assessment. There are a number of assessment tools that are culturally and linguistically appropriate for the assessment of cognitive impairment in the Chinese population. For example the Mini-Mental State Exam originally developed by Folstein, Folstein, and McHugh (1975) has been adapted and translated into Cantonese (Chiu, Lee, Chung, & Kwong, 1994). In addition, several versions of the MMSE have been adapted and translated into Mandarin. These include the Chinese Mini Mental Status (CMMS) (Katzman et al., 1988) and the Chinese-adapted MMSE (CAMSE) (Xu et al., 2003).

Alternative instruments include the Mini Cog (Borson, Scanlan, Brush, Vitaliano, & Dokmak, 2000), Cognitive Abilities Screening Instrument (Teng et al., 1994), and the Mattis Dementia Rating Scale (Chan, Chol, Chiu, & Lam, 2003). Refer to a detailed discussion of assessing cognitive status in Asian Americans, including Chinese Americans by Dick, Dick-Muehlke, and Teng (2006).

Family Caregiving. Filial piety as embraced by the philosophies of Confucianism, Buddhism, and Daoism has become an integral aspect of traditional Chinese culture (Wang et al., 2006). Filial piety is the virtue of love, honor and respect for one's elders and would thus influence the caregiving role. In addition, based on beliefs of Confucianism, the eldest son has the primary responsibility for decisions in the care of his parents. All Chinese American family caregivers of elders with ADRD, in a study conducted by Levkoff et al. (1999), were found to adhere to this norm. However, informants questioned whether this norm should be maintained in the U.S. Similarly, another study conducted by Mahoney et al. (2005) found that although the eldest son held the primary responsibility for the care of his parent, there was a tendency for other family members to withdraw their support. This was attributed to the negative stigma associated with the disease (Mahoney et al., 2005; Zhan, 2004).

Levkoff et al. (1999) found that all the Chinese American caregivers in their study used services and/or long-term care provided by Chinese-affiliated organizations. Informants discussed language barriers and lack of cultural preferences such as food, in "mainstream" community services. In contrast, participants in Zhan's (2004) study reported that following medical diagnosis there was lack of community resources to support the caregiver, this included an overall lack of linguistically and cultural appropriate information on ADRD.

Gallagher-Thompson et al. (2003) developed a culturally and linguistically appropriate training program for Chinese American caregivers regarding the behavioral management of elders with ADRD. This experimental in-home program was found to be more effective in reducing caregiver related stress and symptoms compared to telephone support (Gallagher-Thompson et al., 2007). The psycho-educational intervention was adapted to be more efficient by delivering content through a series of videos (skill training). Findings of a preliminary study indicated promising results when compared to a commercial DVD (Gallagher-Thompson et al., 2010). The video and accompanying workbook are available at http://sgec.stanford.edu/resources/.

Filipino Americans

Demographic Characteristics. In 2000, there were nearly 165,000 older persons of Filipino heritage living in the U.S., making them the second largest older Asian American sub group (Yeo, 2009). As noted in Table 14.1, almost 80% of older Filipino Americans do speak English (and usually Tagalog and other Filipino languages as well) even though 90% were foreign born. This is attributed to English being taught in schools in the Philippines and used widely in business.

Prevalence of Dementia. There are no data on the prevalence of ADRD in Filipino Americans. However, the Philippine Neurological Association collaborated with the National Nutrition survey and determined the prevalence of ADRD in the Philippines to be approximately 11.5% in persons 60–69 years of age and 15.6% for persons 70 and older (Marasigan, 2008).

Perceptions of Dementia and Other Cultural Issues Affecting Dementia Care. The signs and symptoms associated with dementia are often attributed to a natural part of the aging process in the traditional Filipino culture (Braun et al., 1995; McBride, 2006).

Assessment. The literature does not report any screening tools that have been culturally and linguistically adapted for Filipinos or Filipino Americans. However, Marasigan (2008) does report that dementia screening tools and neuropsychological assessment have been translated and validated for use by clinicians practicing in the Philippines.

Family Caregiving. Filipino Americans participated in a series of focus groups conducted by Braun et al. (1995) in Hawaii for the purpose of exploring the perception and care of elders with ADRD. Findings emphasized that elders are traditionally viewed with great respect. Caregiving is viewed as a family responsibility and a means of reciprocity. Traditionally, it is often the first-born adult child, regardless of sex, who is responsible for making decisions regarding the elder's care (McBride, 2006). There is often a reluctance to seek assistance outside of the extended family (Braun et al., 1995).

It is estimated that 85% of Filipino Americans are of the Catholic faith (Sanchez & Gaw, 2007). Religiosity often serves as a "vital force" for coping with stressors and "accepting suffering as a spiritual offering" (McBride, 2006, p. 198). This perception is consistent with focus group participants who used descriptors such as, "it is God's will, we just have to accept it," and "God does not give you jobs that you cannot handle" (Braun et al., 1995, p. 123). Many Filipino Americans turn to the Catholic community for spiritual, emotional, and moral support (McBride, 2006). Sanchez and Gaw (2007) also emphasize the important role of prayer and spiritual counseling when Filipino Americans are confronted with mental health issues.

As previously stated there is a tendency to avoid seeking medical care for the symptoms associated with ADRD. Chow, Ross, Fox, Cummings, and Lin (2000) analyzed data from the Minimum Uniform Dataset that was collected at nine California Alzheimer's Disease and Diagnosis and Treatment Centers. Of the total 9451 cases, only 0.8 percent were Filipino Americans. These findings represents a low proportion of service use, compared to the 2.5% of Filipino Americans among older Californians (Yeo, 2007).

There is need for educational programs on ADRD that are culturally and linguistically appropriate to the Filipino American community. Braun et al. (1995) developed and tested educational outreach materials with a convenience sample of 26 Filipino Americans (ages 28–82 years) who were recruited through churches in Hawaii. The majority (75%) of participants were female, had a high school education, and had lived in the U.S. an average of 10 years. A pre-test was used to determine the participants overall knowledge regarding ADRD. This was followed by the presentation of a video and brochures that were culturally tailored for Filipino Americans and presented in the Ilocano language. Post-test scores revealed significant improvement in knowledge compared to pre-test scores. For example, following the presentation of educational materials, participants were familiar with the term Alzheimer's disease, were able to recognize symptoms and behaviors associated with the disease and identified the importance of consulting a physician when these symptoms were noted. Following the presentation, a greater proportion of participants were also able to identify a community agency, such as the Alzheimer's Association, where they could seek assistance.

Japanese Americans

Demographic Characteristics. Older Japanese Americans who are at risk for dementia and/or caregiving for spouses with dementia are, as a group, the most acculturated of all the populations of Asian American elders. As indicated by Table 14.1, Japanese Americans 65 years of age and older are generally well-educated and most, but not all, speak English. The current older cohort is primarily *Nisei*, or second generation American, children of the original immigrants, the *Issei*. Many of their children, the *Sansei*, who are even more diverse and acculturated are or will be the family caregivers of their parents with dementia.

In spite of their familiarity with the U.S. society, however, there are unique historical events that have influenced Japanese American elders and their response to dementia. After enduring decades of discrimination since their arrival in the U.S., during WWII, all individuals of Japanese descent living on the West Coast, most of whom were U.S. citizens, were forced to leave their homes and property on a few days' notice, and were interned in barren, harsh conditions in isolated areas. Most of the *Nisei* outside of Hawaii experienced this internment and the continuing discrimination following their return home. Many of the young men were part of the units of Japanese American volunteers who fought in the European front and were the most decorated military units in WWII. These experiences have been a unifying thread for the Japanese American elders and their families (Hikoyeda, Mukoyama, Liou, & Masterson, 2006).

Prevalence of Dementia. Japanese Americans are the only Asian American population in which reliable data are available on the prevalence of dementia. A longitudinal study of Japanese

Table 14.2 Rates of dementia among Japanese Americans

	Hawaii (men only)	Washington
Alzheimer's disease	4.7%	4.46%
Vascular dementia	3.8%	1.85%
Ages	≥71, age standardized	≥Age 65
Source	White et al. (1996)	Graves et al. (1996)

American men in Hawaii (White et al., 1996) and a study of Japanese American men and women in King County (Seattle), Washington (Graves et al., 1996), both found rates of Alzheimer's disease comparable to those found with older non-Latino white populations in the U.S. In Hawaii, however, there were higher rates of vascular dementia, which is similar to earlier studies of elders in Japan (Larson & Imai, 1996). In the Hawaiian study, depression was found to be a major risk factor for dementia among the Japanese American men (Irie et al., 2008), and among the Washington sample those with a higher body mass index had a lower risk of dementia (Hughes, Borenstein, Schofield, Wu, & Larson, 2009) (Table 14.2).

Perceptions of Dementia and Other Cultural Issues Affecting Dementia Care. As is the case with other Asian populations, symptoms of dementia are frequently seen as part of normal aging. In the Hawaiian study, either family members did not recognize the problem or there were no assessment performed in 60 percent of the cases of identified dementia (Ross et al., 1997). Dementia was sometimes attributed to genes, bad karma, or family upbringing. Other studies indicate that some Japanese Hawaiians believed people with dementia were insane (Braun & Browne, 1998; Hikoyeda, 2010; Hikoyeda et al., 2006), and describe the influence on common responses to dementia of traditional Japanese values originating in the *Meiji* era in Japan from Buddhist, Shinto, and Confucian teachings brought by the *Issei* immigrants. A feeling of fatalism, acceptance, or "nothing can be done" (*shikataganai*) may influence a family who does not take a parent with memory problems for assessment. Duty to care for parents and grandparents is a strong obligation in filial piety (*oyakoko*), which traditionally falls to the oldest son, even though in reality most of the everyday responsibility falls on the daughter-in-law. Refusal of needed services may be related to the value of *enryo*, which encourages initial refusal of food or help so as not to appear greedy; *gaman*, which mandates stoicism in adverse situations; or *haji*, a sense of shame that reflects on the family if dementia is perceived as a stigma.

Assessment. Because most of the current cohort of older Japanese Americans speak English and are fairly well acculturated, there is less need for translated assessment instruments than with other Asian elders. However, there are a few elders who were educated in Japan or are more recent immigrants, so the availability of a comprehensive battery of cognitive measures in Japanese translated by the Kame project (Graves et al., 1996) in Seattle is important. Of particular note is the Japanese translation of the Cognitive Abilities Screening Instrument (CASI) which was specifically designed for easy cross cultural adaptation and has been used successfully with Japanese American elders in Hawaii and Washington state and in Japan (Dick et al., 2006).

Family caregiving. Adams, Aranda, Kemp, and Takagi (2002) studied stress and coping in family caregivers of persons with dementia from four ethnic backgrounds. Findings indicated that female Japanese American caregivers were similar to the other groups in most aspects. However, they were found to score higher on pessimistic appraisal due to *shikatanagai*, and were second only to Mexican Americans in depression. In a few cities, primarily on the West Coast, Japanese specific services and residential programs have been developed, as an extension of family caregiving, for elders who are more comfortable in an environment that reflects the Japanese culture and language. However, with the increasing acculturation of *Nisei* and *Sansei* and the changing roles of women, there is more acceptance and preference for blended services that serve all elders (Hikoyeda et al., 2006; Young, McCormick, & Vitaliano, 2002).

Vietnamese Americans

Demographics Characteristics. Older Americans from Vietnamese backgrounds are almost all refugees or immigrants who came to the U.S. as adults in one of several waves beginning with the traumatic sudden evacuation from Saigon in the chaos at the end of the Vietnam War in 1975. As a result of the diversity of backgrounds and experiences, there is a wide range of acculturation in the Vietnamese elders in the U.S. (Tran, Tran, & Hinton, 2006). As indicated in Table 14.1, almost half of Vietnamese American elders had less than a ninth grade education, and almost three-fourths spoke little or no English in 2000.

Prevalence of Dementia. There are no known studies of the prevalence of dementia among Vietnamese Americans or adults in Vietnam.

Perceptions of Dementia and Other Cultural Factors Affecting Dementia Care. Like many other Asian cultures, Vietnamese culture is family oriented, and sees the responsibility of care for older adults to be the family's alone.

It is common for individuals from a Vietnamese background to describe dementia symptoms with terms that emphasize confusion and to attribute those symptoms to aging (Tran et al., 2006). Other contributions to the understanding of dementia among the population come from the traditional Eastern medicine concepts of the integration of mind and body such as *Qi*, the vital life force, and the theory of the need for balance between *yin* and *yang*, frequently translated as "hot" and "cold." To sustain good health, it is important to maintain the flow of *Qi* through the body, which can be depleted by excesses of an indulgent life style. Imbalance of *yin* and *yang* and its consequent disease can be prevented by regulating emotions, thoughts, and behavior, as well as balancing diet and medications (Tran et al., 2006). Examples of the application of these concepts were found when dementia was attributed to "thinking too much," "worrying too much," being stressed, and too much "heat" among Vietnamese American caregivers of family members with dementia (Hinton, Franz, Yeo, & Levkoff, 2005; Yeo, Tran, Hikoyeda, & Hinton, 2001).

Spiritual influences are also connected to the understanding of, and response to, dementia through the diverse Vietnamese backgrounds of Buddhism, Taoism, Confucianism, and Catholicism, which may be combined in individuals' belief systems (Tran et al., 2006). One caregiver believed his wife was possessed by a spirit which caused her dementia and "bizarre" behavior. Others considered it fate or karma, and responded to it with perseverance and endurance, even in the face of extreme burden, feeling that as children there was no other choice but to care for their parent (Yeo et al., 2001). The stigma on the family was a theme expressed by 78 percent of Vietnamese American family caregivers of persons with dementia in a small qualitative study (Liu, Hinton, Tran, Hinton, & Barker, 2008).

Assessment. There are no known documented dementia assessment tools specifically for the Vietnamese population. However, a memory measure using pictures developed especially for low literacy populations from various backgrounds was tested on Vietnamese elders as well as other ethnic groups and found to differentiate elders with dementia from those without dementia better than the ten other neuropsychological tests in the study (Kempler, Teng, Taussig, & Dick, 2010).

The stigma on the family of having a member with dementia and the belief that it is normal in old age, have been identified as barriers to having an assessment performed. Recommendations for the assessment include being careful to show the elder utmost respect because of the prestige traditionally reserved for older adults in Vietnamese society. These include using honorific titles, greeting the elder first, avoiding eye contact, and using both hands to give something to the elder. Recent immigrants may be unfamiliar with shaking hands. A challenge for clinicians may be to identify the ability of an elder to perform tasks independently because of the Vietnamese pattern of dependency of elders on family members as part of showing respect (Tran et al., 2006).

Family Caregiving. Family based care is expected in the traditional Vietnamese culture. If adult children cannot care for an elder, other relatives may be brought in. In cases of extreme burden, some adult children make extensive sacrifices to fulfill the obligation of filial piety because they feel it is never acceptable not to care for their parents. When family care is not possible and formal services have to be used, extreme guilt can result (Tran et al., 2006; Yeo et al., 2001).

Korean Americans

Demographic Characteristics. Most older Korean Americans came to the U.S. after 1965 when the Immigration and Naturalization Act was passed. By 2000, 90 percent of Korean American elders were foreign born and almost two-thirds spoke little or no English (Moon, 2006; Yeo, 2009). The majority are Protestant Christian (Kwon, 2003). Many elders from Korea continue to immigrate to the U.S. following retirement or widowhood to be with their adult children (followers of children). As a result, there will continue to be a sizable proportion of older Korean immigrants in the United States, individuals who are foreign born and less acculturated to American culture.

Prevalence of Dementia. There is no known data on prevalence of dementia among Korean Americans. In rural areas of Korea the prevalence was between 9.5% and 10.8% of the population. By comparison, in Seoul, the age standardized rate was 8.2% (5.4% Alzheimer's disease (AD) and 2.0% vascular dementia (VD) (Lee, Lee, Ju, et al., 2002). In Busan, Korea's second largest city, Busan, the age and sex standardized rate was 7.0% (Kim, Jeong, Chun, & Lee, 2003). An interesting finding in both the Seoul and Busan studies was the large gender difference in prevalence. In Seoul 4.5% males were found to be in the dementia range (2.4% AD and 0.9% VD) compared to 10.4% (7.2% AD and 2.6% VD) for females. After controlling for age and education, however, the gender differences were not significant (Lee, Lee, Ju, et al., 2002). In Busan, 2.4% of males and 10.5% of females had dementia, and education was highly correlated with dementia scores; the 34% of the study population with zero years of schooling had a prevalence rate of 13.5%, while there were no cases in the 26% of elders with middle school through college level of education (Kim et al., 2003).

Perceptions of Dementia and Other Cultural Issues Affecting Dementia Care. Similar to other Asian cultures, the traditional Korean values emphasize filial piety (*hyo*) and the strong importance of family and kinship. Sang Lee and her colleagues (Lee, Diwan, & Yeo, 2010; Lee, Lee, & Diwan, 2010) found several beliefs about mental illness. Specifically, it was common for Korean immigrants to believe that memory loss and dementia are a normal part of aging; dementia is a form of insanity which leads to stigmatization of the family; living alone, and/or being physically, mentally, or socially inactive causes dementia; introverted or passive personalities lead to dementia. Many immigrants consider stress and brain chemistry contributing to dementia, but also attribute suppressed emotions such as anger and frustration from unresolved family or personal conflicts, a lifetime of hardships, or issues that cannot be shared with others as also contributing factors to the disease. Slightly less than half of those surveyed believed that environmental stress due to immigration, while about a quarter of respondents attribute an imbalance between *yin* and *yang* as factors in dementia.

Assessment. Because of the research that has been done on dementia in Korea, there are a number of cognitive assessment instruments that have been translated into the Korean language and used successfully with older Koreans in Korea. There are no known reports of their use in the U.S. with Korean Americans, but because almost all older Korean Americans speak Korean at home, the availability of these instruments is a very important resource for cognitive assessment. One of the most important resources is the Korean adaptation of the screening instrument, the Mini-Mental State Examination, the MMSE-K (Kwon & Park, 1989). It was translated and validated for use with low literacy Korean elders which included changing some items to be culturally appropriate. The battery of assessment instruments

in the Consortium to Establish a Registry for Alzheimer's Disease Assessment Packet (CERAD) has also been translated into Korean (CERAD-K), found to be reliable and valid with older Koreans (Lee, Lee, Lee, et al., 2002), and was used in the Seoul study (Lee, Lee, Ju, et al., 2002). A large number of other cognitive assessment instruments have been developed or translated into Korean, including behavior rating scales, staging measures, informant interviews, and assessments of advanced stages of dementia.

Family caregiving. Korean American family caregivers provide care in the context of the strong traditional values of *hyo*, or filial piety, which specifies that older parents should be cared for by the oldest son. Many families continue those traditions, although the real responsibility usually falls on the daughter-in-law. However, both elders and their children in the U.S. are gradually moving away from the strict adherence to those norms (Han, Choi, Kim, Lee, & Kim, 2008; Moon, 2006). Han et al. found a continuum of filial piety among Korean American caregivers, with some feeling it was inhumane not to care for parents with dementia, and at the other end, some seeing nursing homes as positive options. Most found caregiving very physically and psychologically demanding, especially with the pressure of employment or running small businesses. Often caregivers felt unappreciated by other family members. Using services in the U.S. health care system was difficult and unsatisfying because of language and food differences. Lee and Casado (2011) found generally positive attitudes toward using formal non-family care programs for elders with dementia in a sample of non caregiving Korean American adults. The belief that dementia is a normal part of aging and the cultural stigma it brings are barriers to using community support services among Korean American families (Lee, Lee, et al., 2010).

Hmong Americans

Demographic Characteristics. The Hmong, while living in Laos, served America during the Vietnam

War. Hmong immigration to the U.S. started in 1975. As indicated in Table 14.1, older adults comprise a smaller percentage of the Hmong population than in any other Asian American group. The Hmong elders are also the least educated and most poverty stricken of all the Asian American elders, and only 16 percent speak English well. A very small percentage of the Hmong elders live alone.

Prevalence and Assessment of Dementia. There are no statistics on the prevalence of dementia within the Hmong American community. This may be attributed to two primary reasons. First, the overall use of medical care by Hmong American elders is generally limited to emergency situations. Secondly, there is a lack of available linguistically and culturally appropriate tools for the assessment of dementia in Hmong elders (Gerdner, Xiong, & Yang, 2006).

Perceptions of Dementia and Other Cultural Issues Affecting Dementia Care. There are no words in the Hmong language for the diagnostic term of Alzheimer's disease, but the concept is not unfamiliar to the Hmong people. The Hmong term *tem toob* has no direct English translations, but is used to describe an elder with so many thoughts that the person is prone to forgetfulness. This term has been incorporated into a long-standing Hmong proverb, *Ntoo laus ntoo khoob, neeg laus neeg tem toob*, comparing an elder with memory impairment to that of a tree that has been hollowed with age (Gerdner, Xiong, & Cha, 2006).

The traditional spiritual beliefs of the Hmong people include a form of animism and ancestor worship. It is believed that approximately 70 percent of Hmong Americans have retained these traditional beliefs (Pfeifer & Lee, 2005). Within this belief system each person has multiple souls. These souls must remain in harmony to sustain health and well-being. Illness occurs when one or more of these souls separate from the body. Consistent with this belief system, the Hmong have traditionally attributed chronic confusion and memory impairment to soul loss (Gerdner, Xiong, & Cha, 2006). As a result, a shaman may be consulted for spiritual intervention. Refer to Gerdner, Xiong, and Cha (2006) for a detailed discussion.

Traditionally the Hmong also acknowledge that some conditions have a physical cause, requiring the need for a variety of traditional folk remedies including herbal preparations and other organic substances (i.e., dried animal parts) (Bliatout, 1991). For a detailed discussion of some of the remedies traditionally used for chronic confusion and memory impairment, refer to Gerdner, Xiong, and Cha (2006).

Family Caregiving. Gerdner, Tripp-Reimer, and Yang (2008) conducted the first focused ethnographic study to explore the perception, care, and preferred treatment of Hmong American elders with symptoms of dementia (i.e. chronic confusion, memory impairment). The study included in-depth interviews with 15 Hmong American family caregivers.

The majority of families maintained the traditional norm that the eldest son has the primary responsibility for his aging parents, with his wife providing the actual care. However, conflicts with the norm are emerging among the Hmong living in America. All viewed caregiving as reciprocal for the love and care given by the elder generation and a model of traditional values for the younger generation. Overall, female caregivers were pleased to devote their time and attention to the caregiving role and took enormous pride in this endeavor. It was, however, more difficult for those women who were forced to juggle a career outside of the home along with the traditional role of wife and mother. Overall, informants were opposed to nursing homes and viewed the care of elders as a family responsibility.

The majority of caregivers attributed the elders' symptoms to "soul loss" or a natural part of the aging process. Regardless of the personal beliefs of the family caregiver, a shaman was consulted when the elder retained beliefs of animism and ancestor worship.

Treatment from a physician was not generally sought, unless accompanied by a health crisis (e.g. cerebral vascular accident). Even when the elder was given a formal diagnosis of dementia there was often a lack of understanding or a misunderstanding of medical terminology.

Overall, findings revealed that dementia in the Hmong American community was an important but often overlooked issue. A critical need was identified for the development of culturally and linguistically appropriate educational materials. Elders often lived in a multi-generation home with grandchildren who had an especially difficult time understanding the progressive memory and behavioral changes associated with the disease. As a beginning effort, a bilingual (Hmong/English) picture book entitled, *Grandfather's Story Cloth* (Gerdner & Langford, 2008) was developed to address this issue. Themes from the life experiences of family caregivers were used to create a culturally meaningful storyline, see Gerdner (2008).

Community Resources

In many cities with large populations of elders from Asian backgrounds, ethnic specific senior organization are available that provide dementia related services, and sometimes residential services. Local Area Agencies on Aging Information and Assistance programs offer information on these services. Some examples are Kin On in Seattle (http://www.kinon.org/), Yu Ai Kai in San Jose (http://www.yuaikai.org/), Asian Community Center and Homes in Sacramento (http://www.accsv.org/) and South Cove Manor in Boston (http://www.southcovemanor.com).

On Lok Lifeways

Another example of a community resource is On Lok Lifeways, the first PACE (Program for All Inclusive Care for the Elderly) program. On Lok began in the Chinatown area of San Francisco in the 1970s and has grown to include many diverse communities in their multiple centers.

On Lok implements a variety of culturally responsive activity programs for their Asian American clients, such as Chinese Americans. The majority of these programs are conducted in the Cantonese dialect, with some conducted in Toishanese and Mandarin. An activity for Chinese American elders with mild dementia involves a rendition of the traditional "wishing tree" during the Chinese lunar New Year. This ritual involves writing personal wishes on a piece of red paper or cloth and throwing them onto a tree branch, with the belief that the wishes will come true. To adapt as an indoor activity, a large plant serves as the "wishing tree." This activity stimulates conversations among elders on advance care planning and what they hope for at this stage of their lives.

Supervised ethnic cooking activities have been a successful reminiscence activity for individual groups of Korean Americans, Vietnamese Americans, and Chinese Americans. Plans are underway to expand this program with other Asian American subpopulations.

To serve the needs of family caregivers, On Lok provides a series of ten educational workshops presented in Cantonese. For example, during one workshop a physician addresses treatment for dementia from the perspectives of both Western and Eastern medicine. Following formal presentations, attendees are divided into small groups for the opportunity to share their experiences with other caregivers.

Alzheimer's Association

The National Alzheimer's Association website has an Asian web portal that offers disease related information online in Chinese, Korean and Vietnamese (refer to http://www.alz.org/asian/chinese.asp). Local chapters of the Alzheimer's Association are tailored to the communities they serve. For example, the Northern California and Northern Nevada Chapter serves a large ethnic population, including Asian Americans. This chapter provides culturally specific programs implemented to address cultural barriers in this assigned region. Support groups are offered to Asian American caregivers in multiple languages such as, Cantonese, Mandarin, Japanese, Vietnamese, and English.

In addition, the Bridge to Healthy Families is an Asian Pacific Islander Dementia Care Network that supports families caring for a family member with ADRD in Sacramento. This program is a collaboration of the Asian Community Center, Alzheimer's Association, and University of California at Davis Alzheimer's Disease Center. A care advocate and community nurse serve as access points for the Asian Pacific Island community. Responsibilities include educating family caregivers and health care professionals about dementia and directing them to available resources.

The Chinese Alzheimer's Forum is an annual educational program offered to the general public on Alzheimer's related research and caregiver issues and presented entirely in Mandarin.

Stanford Geriatric Education Center

The Stanford Geriatric Education Center (SGEC) is a consortium of the Stanford University of School of Medicine, San Jose State University, and Community Health Partnership. The Center provides multidisciplinary education programs on ethnogeriatrics (health care of elders from diverse ethnic populations). Dementia in diverse communities is a major part of the SGEC's ongoing training programs, including a webinar series in 2009–2010 on assessment of dementia and family caregiving on the following Asian American subpopulations: Chinese, Japanese, Korean, Vietnamese, Hmong, and Filipino. The 2011 series included a presentation entitled "Dementia Assessment and Family Caregiving: Chinese American and Other Asian Americans." Recordings and handouts of these webinars are all available at no cost on the SGEC website (http://sgec.stanford.edu/). Another resource is the book *Ethnicity and Dementias* (2nd edition), edited by Drs. Gwen Yeo and Dolores Gallagher-Thompson. The book includes chapters on prevalence, assessment and seven chapters on working with families in different Asian American populations. Further a special issue of *Hallym International Journal of Aging* showcased research focusing on dementia within the Asian American community.

Future Research Needs

The National Alzheimer's Project Act (Public Law 111–375) was passed unanimously by both houses of Congress and signed into law by President Obama on January 4, 2011. This law has important implications for ADRD as it affects the different subpopulations of Asian America. For example, Section 2.5 of this law addresses the need for ethnic and racial populations who are at higher risk for Alzheimer's disease or who are least likely to receive care, to be included in clinical, service and research efforts as a means of decreasing health disparities. Section 2.6 calls for coordination with international bodies to integrate and inform the fight against Alzheimer's disease globally.

There is a critical need for research to establish the prevalence and risk factors for dementia among all of the rapidly growing older Asian American subpopulations to supplement the work that has already been done with Japanese Americans. Although this type of research in small populations is very difficult and expensive to do, it is critical in establishing the ethnic specific profiles and needs for culturally appropriate services. The amount of dementia related research conducted with the Asian American population varies by subgroup. The individual subgroups presented here have been the focus of the majority of research, with Chinese Americans and Japanese Americans having the strongest foundation of work. There is need to develop educational outreach materials that are linguistically and culturally appropriate to alleviate the overall stigma that is often associated with ADRD within many of the Asian American subpopulations. Adaptation and translation of cognitive screening tools are needed for subgroups such as Filipino Americans, Vietnamese Americans, and Hmong Americans. It is recommended that researchers collaborate with trusted community organizations for development and testing of family based educational programs related to ADRD. There is also need for the development of intervention studies for the management of dysfunctional behaviors.

References

Adams, B., Aranda, M., Kemp, B., & Takagi, K. (2002). Ethnic and gender differences in distress among Anglo American, African American, Japanese American, and Mexican American spousal caregivers of persons with dementia. *Journal of Clinical Geropsychology, 8*, 279–301.

Alzheimer's Association. (2011). Alzheimer's disease facts and figures. Retrieved May 21, 2011, from http://www.alz.org/downloads/Facts_Figures_2011.pdf.

American Psychiatric Association. (2000). *Diagnostic and statistical manual of mental disorders* (4th ed., text rev.). Washington, DC: Author

Bliatout, B. T. (1991). Hmong healing practitioners. *Healing Forum, 2*, 58–66.

Borson, S., Scanlan, J., Brush, M., Vitaliano, P., & Dokmak, A. (2000). The mini-cog: A cognitive 'vital signs' measure for dementia screening in multi-lingual elderly. *International Journal of Geriatric Psychiatry, 15*(11), 1021–1027.

Braun, K. L., & Browne, C. V. (1998). Perceptions of dementia, caregiving and help seeking among Asian and Pacific Islander Americans. *Health and Social Work, 23*, 262–274.

Braun, K. L., Jeanette, C. T., Sheila, M. F., Sasaki, P. A., & Meininger, L. (1995). Developing and testing outreach materials on Alzheimer's disease for Asian and Pacific Islander Americans. *The Gerontologist, 25*(1), 122–126.

Chan, A. S., Chol, A., Chiu, H., & Lam, L. (2003). Clinical validity of the Chinese version of mattis dementia rating scale in differentiating dementia of Alzheimer's type in Hong Kong. *Journal of the International Neuropsychological Society, 9*, 45–55.

Chiu, H., F. K., Lee, H. C., Chung, W. S., & Kwong, P. K. (1994). Reliability and validity of the Cantonese version of the Mini-Mental State Examination – A preliminary study. *Hong Kong Journal of Psychiatry* 4(Suppl. 2):25–28.

Chow, T. W., Ross, L., Fox, P., Cummings, J. L., & Lin, K.-M. (2000). Utilization of Alzheimer's disease community resources by Asian-Americans in California. *International Journal of Geriatric Psychiatry, 15*, 838–847.

Dick, M., Dick-Muehlke, C., & Teng, E. L. (2006). Assessment of cognitive status in Asians. In G. Yeo & D. Gallagher-Thompson (Eds.), *Ethnicity and the dementias* (2nd ed., pp. 55–69). New York: Taylor & Francis/Routledge.

Folstein, M. F., Folstein, S. E., & McHugh, P. R. (1975). 'Mini-Mental State': A practical method for grading the cognitive state of patients for the clinician. *Journal of Psychiatric Research, 12*, 189–198.

Gallagher-Thompson, D., Haley, W., Guy, D., Rupert, M., Trinidad Argüelles, L., Zeiss, L. M., et al. (2003). Tailoring psychological interventions for ethnically diverse caregivers. *Clinical Psychology: Science and Practice, 10*(4), 423–438.

Gallagher-Thompson, D., Gray, H., Tang, P., Pu, C. Y., Leung, L. Y. L., Wang, P.-C., et al. (2007). Impact of in-home intervention versus telephone support in reducing depression and stress of Chinese caregivers: Results of a pilot study. *The American Journal of Geriatric Psychiatry, 15*, 425–434.

Gallagher-Thompson, D., Wang, P.-C., Liu, W., Cheung, V., Peng, R., China, D., et al. (2010). Effectiveness of a psychoeducational skill training DVD program to reduce stress in Chinese American dementia caregivers: Results of a preliminary study. *Aging & Mental Health, 14*(3), 263–273.

Gerdner, L. A. (2008). Translating research findings into a Hmong American children's book to promote understanding of persons with Alzheimer's disease. *Hmong Studies Journal, 9*, 1–29.

Gerdner, L. A., Xiong, S. V., & Cha, D. (2006). Chronic confusion and memory impairment in Hmong elders: Honoring differing cultural beliefs in America. *Journal of Gerontological Nursing, 32*(3), 23–31.

Gerdner, L. A., Xiong, X. A. X., & Yang, D. (2006). Working with Hmong American Families. In G. Yeo & D. Gallagher-Thompson (Eds.), *Ethnicity and the dementias* (2nd ed., pp. 209–230). New York: Routledge/Taylor & Francis.

Gerdner, L. A., Sarah Langford with illustrations by Stuart Loughridge. (2008). *Grandfather's Story Cloth / Yawg Daim Paj Ntaub Dab Neeg*. Walnut Creek: Shen's Books.

Gerdner, L. A., Tripp-Reimer, T., & Yang, D. (2008). Perception and care of elder Hmong Americans with chronic confusion or tem toob. *Hallym International Journal of Aging, 10*(2), 111–138.

Graves, A. B., Larson, E. B., Edland, S. D., Bowen, J. D., McCormick, W. C., McCurry, S. M., et al. (1996). Prevalence of dementia and its subtypes in the Japanese American population of King County, Washington state. The Kame Project. *American Journal of Epidemiology, 144*(8), 760–771.

Green, R. C. (2005). *Diagnosis and management of Alzheimer's disease and other dementias* (2nd ed.). West Islip, NY: Professional Communications.

Han, H.-R., Choi, Y. J., Kim, M. T., Lee, J. E., & Kim, K. B. (2008). Experiences and challenges of informal caregiving for Korean immigrants. *Journal of Advanced Nursing, 63*(5), 517–526.

Hikoyeda, N. (2010). Assessment of Dementia and caregiving in Dementia with Japanese American elders. In *Ethnicity and the Dementias*, Stanford Geriatric Education Webinar Series.

Hikoyeda, N., Mukoyama, W. K., Liou, L. J., & Masterson, B. (2006). Working with Japanese American families. In G. Yeo & D. Gallagher-Thompson (Eds.), *Ethnicity and dementias* (2nd ed., pp. 231–244). New York: Taylor & Francis/Routledge.

Hinton, L., Franz, C. E., Yeo, G., & Levkoff, S. E. (2005). Conceptions of dementia in a multiethnic sample of family caregivers. *Journal of the American Geriatrics Society, 53*, 1405–1410.

Huang, Z.-B., Richard, R. N., Lidourezos, A., Breuer, B., Khaski, A., Milano, E., et al. (2003). Sociodemographic and health characteristics of older Chinese on admission to a nursing home: A cross-racial/ethnic study. *Journal of the American Geriatrics Society, 51*, 404–409.

Hughes, T. F., Borenstein, A. R., Schofield, E., Wu, Y., & Larson, E. B. (2009). Association between late-life body mass index and dementia: The Kame Project. *Neurology, 19*, 1741–1746.

Irie, F., Masaki, K. H., Petrovitch, H., Abbott, R. D., Ross, G. W., Taaffe, D. R., et al. (2008). Apolipoprotein E epsilon4 allele genotype and the effect of depressive symptoms on the risk of dementia in men: The Honolulu-Asia aging study. *Archives of General Psychiatry, 65*(8), 906–912.

Janevic, M. R., & Connell, C. M. (2001). Racial, ethnic, and cultural differences in the dementia caregiving experience: Recent findings. *The Gerontologist, 41*(3), 334–347.

Katzman, R., Zhang, M. Y., Ouang, Y.-Q., Wang, Z., Liu, W. T., Yu, E., et al. (1988). A Chinese version of the Mini-Mental State Examination; impact of illiteracy in a Shanghai dementia survey. *Journal of Clinical Epidemiology, 41*(10), 971–978.

Kempler, D., Teng, E. L., Taussig, M., & Dick, M. B. (2010). The common objects memory test (COMT): A simple test with cross-cultural applicability. *Journal of the International Neuropsychology Society, 16*, 537–545.

Kim, J., Jeong, I., Chun, J.-H., & Lee, S. (2003). The prevalence of dementia in a metropolitan city of South Korea. *International Journal of Geriatric Psychiatry, 18*, 617–622.

Kwon, O. (2003). *Buddhist and protestant Korean immigrants: Religious beliefs and socioeconomic aspects of life.* New York: LFB Scholarly Publishing LLC.

Kwon, Y.-C., & Park, J.-H. (1989). Standardization of minimental state examination – Korean version for the elderly (MMSE-K). *Journal of Korean Neuropsychiatric Association, 28*, 125–135 (in Korean).

Larson, E. B., & Imai, Y. (1996). An overview of dementia and ethnicity with special emphasis on the epidemiology of dementia. In G. Yeo & D. Gallagher-Thompson (Eds.), *Ethnicity and the dementias* (2nd ed., pp. 9–19). New York: Taylor & Francis/Routledge.

Lee, S. E., & Casado, B. L. (2011). Attitudes toward community services use in dementia care among Korean Americans. *Clinical Gerontologist, 34*, 4.

Lee, D. Y., Lee, J. H., Ju, Y.-S., Lee, K. U., Kim, K. W., Jhoo, J. H., et al. (2002). The prevalence of dementia in older people in an urban population of Korea: The Seoul study. *Journal of the American Geriatrics Society, 50*, 1233–1239.

Lee, J. H., Lee, K. U., Lee, D. Y., Kim, K. W., Jhoo, J. H., Kim, J. H., et al. (2002). Development of the Korean version of the consortium to establish a registry for Alzheimer's disease assessment packet (CERAD-K): Clinical and neuropsychological assessment batteries. *Journal of Gerontology B: Psychological and Social Sciences, 57*, P47–P53.

Lee, S., Diwan, S., & Yeo, G. (2010). Causal attributions of dementia among Korean American immigrants. *Journal of Gerontological Social Work, 53*(8), 743–759.

Lee, S. E., Lee, H. Y., & Diwan, S. (2010). What do Korean American immigrants know about Alzheimer's disease (AD)? The impact of acculturation and exposure to the disease on AD knowledge. *International Journal of Geriatric Psychiatry, 25*(1), 66–73.

Levkoff, S., Levy, B., & Weitzman, P. L. (1999). The role of religion and ethnicity in the help seeking of family caregivers of elders with Alzheimer's disease and related disorders. *Journal of Cross-Cultural Gerontology, 14*, 335–356.

Liu, D., Hinton, L., Tran, C., Hinton, D., & Barker, J. (2008). Reexamining the relationships among, dementia, stigma, and aging in immigrant Chinese and Vietnamese caregivers. *Journal of Cross-Cultural Gerontology, 23*, 283–299.

Mahoney, D. F., Cloutterbuck, J., Neary, S., & Zhan, L. (2005). African Americans, Chinese, and Latino family caregivers' impressions of the onset and diagnosis of dementia: Cross-cultural similarities and differences. *The Gerontologist, 45*, 783–792.

Marasigan, S. M. (2008, October). *The current status of dementia in Asia: Philippine situation.* Paper presented at combined conferences of 2nd Asian Society against Dementia Congress and 3rd Annual Meeting of Taiwan Dementia Society.

McBride, M. R. (2006). Working with Filipino American families. In G. Yeo & D. Gallagher-Thompson (Eds.), *Ethnicity and dementias* (2nd ed., pp. 189–207). New York: Routledge/Taylor Francis.

Moon, A. (2006). Working with Korean American families. In G. Yeo & D. Gallagher-Thompson (Eds.), *Ethnicity and the dementias* (2nd ed., pp. 245–261). Bristol, PA: Taylor & Francis/CRC Press.

Moua, W. (2005, August 11). Man is found after 21 days. *Hmong Today, 2*(16):1, 14.

Office of Minority Health and Health Disparities. (2009). Ten leading causes of death in Asian American and Pacific Islander Population, U.S., 2006. Retrieved March 18, 2011, from http://www.cdc.gov/omhd/Populations/definitionsREMP.htm.

Pfeifer, M. E., & Lee, T. P. (2005). Hmong religion. *Hmong Today, 2*(16), 24.

Porell, F. (2009). *Analysis of Medicare data from the U.S. Centers for Medicare and Medicaid Services.* Medicare Chronic Condition Warehouse.

Reeves, T. J., & Bennett, C. (2004). We the people: Asians in the United States. *Census 2000 special reports.* Retrieved April 30, 2011 http://www.census.gov/prod/2004pubs/censr-17.pdf.

Ross, G. W., Abbott, R. D., Petrovich, H., Masaki, K. H., Murdaugh, C., Trockman, C., et al. (1997). Frequency and characteristics of silent dementia among elderly Japanese-American Men: The Honolulu-Asia aging study. *Journal of the American Medical Association, 277*(10), 800–805.

Sanchez, F., & Gaw, A. (2007). Mental health care of Filipino Americans. *Psychiatric Services, 58*, 810–815.

Teng, E. L., Hassegawa, K., Homma, A., Imai, Y., Larson, E., Graves, A., et al. (1994). The cognitive abilities screening instrument (CASI): A practical test for cross-cultural epidemiological studies of dementia. *International Psychogeriatrics, 6*(1), 45–58.

Tran, J. N. U., Tran, C. G. U., & Hinton, L. (2006). Working with Vietnamese American families. In G. Yeo & D. Gallagher-Thompson (Eds.), *Ethnicity and the dementias* (2nd ed.). New York: Taylor & Francis.

Valle, R. (1998). *Caregiving across cultures: Working with dementing illness and ethnically diverse populations*. Washington D. C: Taylor & Francis.

Wang, P.-C., Tong, H.-Q., Liu, W., Long, S., Leung, L. Y. I., Yau, E., et al. (2006). In G. Yeo & D. Gallagher-Thompson (Eds.), *Ethnicity and the dementias* (2nd ed., pp. 55–69). Bristol, PA: Taylor & Francis/CRC Press.

White, L., Petrovich, H., Ross, G. W., Masaki, K. H., Abbot, R. D., Teng, E. L., et al. (1996). Prevalence of dementia in older Japanese-American in Hawaii: The Honolulu-Asia aging study. *Journal of the American Medical Association, 276*, 955–960.

Xu, G., Meyer, J. S., Huang, Y., Du, F., Chowdhury, M., & Quach, M. (2003). Adapting mini-mental state examination for dementia screening among illiterate or minimally educated elderly Chinese. *International Journal of Geriatric Psychiatry, 18*(7), 609–616.

Yeo, G. (2007). Healthy aging for California's immigrant and low income elders from diverse ethnic backgrounds: Policy issues and recommendations. Commissioned Paper by the California Endowment. In *Women, health, and aging: building a statewide movement*, p. 73. Los Angeles: The California Endowment. Retreived from http://www.calendow.org/uploadedFiles/women_health_aging.pdf.

Yeo, G. (2009). How will the U.S. health care system meet the challenge of the ethnogeriatric imperative? *Journal of the American Geriatrics Society, 57*(7), 1278–1285.

Yeo, G., & Gallagher-Thompson, D. (Eds.). (2006). *Ethnicity and the dementias* (2nd ed.). New York: Routledge/Taylor & Francis.

Yeo, G., Tran, J. N. U., Hikoyeda, N., & Hinton, L. (2001). Concepts of dementia among Vietnamese American caregivers. *Journal of Gerontological Social Work, 36*, 131–152.

Young, H. M., McCormick, W. M., & Vitaliano, P. P. (2002). Evolving values in community-based long term care services for Japanese Americans. *Advances in Nursing Science, 25*, 40–56.

Zhan, L. (2004). Caring for family members with Alzheimer's disease: Perspectives from Chinese American caregivers. *Journal of Gerontological Nursing, 30*(8), 19–29.

Zhang, M., Katzman, R., Salmon, D., Jin, H., Cai, G., Wang, Z., et al. (1990). The prevalence of dementia and Alzheimer's disease in Shanghai, China: Impact of age, gender, and education. *Annals of Neurology, 27*, 428–437.

Giang T. Nguyen

Asian Americans and Cancer

Introduction

Asian Americans, Native Hawaiians and Pacific
Islanders (known collectively as AA/NHPI) are
the only major racial group in America for which
cancer is the leading cause of death (Heron,
2007). Compared to other ethnicities in the U.S.,
there are disparities associated with Asian
Americans with regard to cancer incidence and
mortality, health information access and awareness, stage at cancer diagnosis, and treatment.

This phenomenon is not new. Between 1980
and 1993, AA/NHPI were noted to have experienced a greater increase in cancer deaths than any
other racial or ethnic group in the United States
(Miller et al., 1996). Despite the recognition of
this phenomenon in the 1990s, these cancer disparities persist in the twenty-first century.

The available data help illustrate the predica-
ment. AA/NHPI men and women experience
higher incidence rates of liver and stomach cancer
than other racial and ethnic groups (Miller, Chu,
Hankey, & Ries, 2008). The hepatocellular carcinoma (liver cancer) incidence rate for AA/NHPI
was four times higher than that for whites, with

rates being highest for people of Vietnamese and
Korean origin (Faruque et al., 2008).

Several AA/NHPI subgroups exhibit incongru-
encies with non-Hispanic Whites with regard to
timing of cancer diagnosis. Laotian women and
Laotian, Samoan, and Vietnamese men have lower
percentages of colorectal cancers diagnosed at
an early (localized) stage. Similarly, Laotian,
Samoan, and Tongan women have a smaller percentage of cases diagnosed at an earlier time.
Kampuchean (Cambodian), Laotian, and Samoan
women have smaller percentages of cervical cancers that are diagnosed early (Miller et al., 2008).

Asian Americans are the fastest growing of all
major racial/ethnic groups in the USA (U.S.
Census Bureau, 2011). It follows that as the Asian
American population continues to grow (and to
age), so too is the number of Asian American
cancer patients.

Cancer: Definitions, Screening, and Treatment

Cancer is a group of conditions characterized by
uncontrolled duplication and spread of abnormal
cells in the body. This can result in pain and disruption of normal body functioning which can be
fatal. Cancer can arise in different organs in the
body, attributed to inherent characteristics such
as a person's genetics, other internal factors such
as immune disorders and the body's hormones, or
external factors including infections, chemical

G.T. Nguyen (✉)
Department of Family Medicine and Community Health,
Center for Public Health Initiatives, University of
Pennsylvania, Philadelphia, PA, USA
e-mail: giang.nguyen@uphs.upenn.edu

G.J. Yoo et al. (eds.), *Handbook of Asian American Health*,
DOI 10.1007/978-1-4614-2227-3_15, © Springer Science+Business Media, LLC 2013

exposures, and radiation (American Cancer Society [ACS], 2010), among other possible influences. For most cancers, risk increases with age, and people age 50 and higher have the greatest risk of cancer. Symptoms of cancer can include fatigue, unintentional weight loss, and pain. Other symptoms may be more specific to the part of the body where the cancer originated or to which the cancer has spread. For example, skin cancer may present itself as a large dark mole, whereas liver cancer might cause jaundice (yellowed skin and eyes). Cancer that is only "localized" to only one part of the body usually causes fewer problems. By contrast, disease that has spread ("metastasized") to the bones can cause excruciating pain in the affected body parts.

Cancer screening refers to the detection of the disease before symptoms appear. Screening is not possible or even appropriate for every type of cancer. In some cases, early detection of cancer would result in no improvements in mortality or quality of life, yet at the same time could result in more invasive procedures, increased diagnostic testing, and added psychological distress. However, in situations where early detection could result in cure or longer survival times, screening could be a great benefit to a patient. Ideally, screening tests need to be fairly inexpensive and should be feasibly performed on a population level.

In the U.S., the most common causes of cancer death for men are lung, prostate and colorectal cancer, while for women, the most common are lung, breast, and colorectal cancer (ACS, 2010). A thorough discussion of every type of cancer is beyond the scope of this chapter, but it is important to know some basic information about some of the cancers that are most common or relevant to Asian American communities as well as the population at large.

Lung Cancer accounts for more than one in six cancer deaths worldwide. Tobacco smoking remains the leading cause of lung cancer. Symptoms may include chronic cough, chest pain, shortness of breath, coughing up blood, pneumonia, and swollen lymph nodes. Lung cancer may be identified first through a chest x-ray or other imaging test, but as with all cancers formal diagnosis requires a tissue sample (biopsy) in order to determine the nature of the abnormality (Hoffman, Mauer, & Vokes, 2000).

Breast Cancer is another very common cancer with over 200,000 cases diagnosed in the U.S. every year (ACS, 2010). Risk factors include gender, obesity, nulliparity (not having had children), estrogen exposure, early menarche (age of first menses), late menopause, alcohol consumption, and radiation exposure (Veronesi, Boyle, Goldhirsch, Orecchia, & Viale, 2005). Symptoms include breast pain, skin changes on the breast, nipple discharge, and lumps in the breast, in the armpit, or around the collarbone. Screening is accomplished using a mammogram (X-ray) which can begin at age 40 or 50, though controversy exists about whether mammograms ought to be performed before age 50 in women with average risk (Quanstrum & Hayward, 2010).

Prostate Cancer is the second most frequently diagnosed cancer in men who live in developed countries like the U.S. Symptoms can include difficulty with urination and blood in the urine. This disease affects only men, since women lack a prostate gland. Risk factors include older age, family history of prostate cancer, and ethnic origin (the risk is highest for African American men). Prostate cancer can be cured if treated early, and in many cases the disease progresses very slowly. Screening is typically done using the Prostate-Specific Antigen (PSA) blood test (Damber & Aus, 2008), but not all experts believe that screening for prostate cancer will actually result in greater longevity. As a result of the controversy, current recommendations are for healthcare providers to initiate a discussion about prostate cancer screening and to let the patients decide if they wish to proceed with screening.

Colorectal Cancer (cancer of the large intestine) is one of the most common cancers affecting both men and women, with about 140,000 new cases yearly in the U.S. (ACS, 2010). It can cause bloody stool, abdominal pain, other changes in bowel habits, and bowel obstruction.

Risk factors for colorectal cancer include family history, obesity, and red meat consumption. Decisions regarding screening are complicated by the number of options that exist. The most commonly recommended tests are colonoscopy every 10 years, flexible sigmoidoscopy every 5 years, or annual fecal occult blood testing, although double-contrast barium enema, computed tomographic (CT) colonography, fecal DNA testing, and ingestion of a Pillcam (wireless camera capsule) have also been used (Wilkins & Reynolds, 2008). Colonoscopy and flexible sigmoidoscopy both involve the insertion of a flexible tube into the colon; the tube houses a tiny camera that allows visualization of the inside of the colon. Flexible sigmoidoscopy ("flex sig") is limited to the lower portion of the colon (where the majority of colon cancers begin) and therefore does not offer as complete a view of the colon. Also, unlike colonoscopy, the flex sig does not allow collection of biopsy samples if an abnormality is identified.

Liver Cancer can be caused by cirrhosis (due to alcohol, for example) and by viral hepatitis (particularly Hepatitis B and C). Symptoms may include pain in the right upper portion of the abdomen, unexplained weight loss, abnormal liver enzyme levels in the blood, anemia (low red blood cell counts or low blood hemoglobin), jaundice, and fluid accumulation in the abdomen (El-Serag, Marrero, Rudolph, & Reddy, 2008). In general, screening for liver cancer is restricted to people who are at high risk (e.g., people already known to have liver cirrhosis or chronic hepatitis infection). This is particularly important because outcomes and options for liver cancer treatment are much more favorable in early stages of the disease (Tong et al., 2009).

Prevalence of hepatitis B virus (HBV) infection in the U.S. is 0.1%, but for foreign-born Americans, the prevalence is greater, from 1.0% to 2.6% of this subpopulation. Because HBV is endemic to all parts of Asia (at least a prevalence rate of 2% in all countries), it is a predominant cause of liver cancer for Asians residing in America, especially those who are immigrants. However, American-born Asians of immigrant parents are still at higher risk, since mothers can infect their children at time of birth. HBV is transmitted through exposure to infectious blood or other body fluids such as semen. The most common forms of transmission are through sex, from mother to child during childbirth, through sharing of hypodermic needles (e.g., recreational drug use or injuries in healthcare settings), and through close contact with infectious fluids such as sharing razors or toothbrushes (Weinbaum et al., 2008). The virus is tenacious, as it can survive for seven (7) days in the environment (e.g., on a table or doorknob), although it is important to note that day-to-day contact does not present a risk for HBV transmission from one person to another. The main risks are blood-to-blood contact and sexual activity. Risk of liver cancer is associated with chronic HBV infection, but not all people who are infected ultimately have chronic disease (some people are sick for a short period and then clear the virus from their bodies). Age of HBV infection is also a risk factor. Newborns infected with HBV have a 90% chance of chronic disease, yet this drops to 5% with adults that are infected (Lok & McMahon, 2009). Therefore, screening of pregnant women and treatment for newborns born to infected mothers is critical. For people who are not already infected with HBV, vaccination is important to prevent future infection and to reduce the spread of HBV through the community.

Stomach Cancer is the second leading cause of cancer-related death worldwide (Khushalani, 2008), although it is not so common in the general American population, only about 21,000 new cases reported per year (ACS, 2010). Although this text is focused on Asian Americans, it is important to understand the global epidemiology because so many Asian Americans are actually immigrants from countries where such diseases are more common. Incidence is especially high in Japan, China, Eastern Europe, and Latin America. Risk factors include Helicobacter pylori (*H. pylori*, a bacterial infection that also causes stomach ulcers), smoking, chronic gastritis, diets low in fruits/vegetables, and increased consumption of nitrates, salt, and smoked foods. Symptoms include an early sense of fullness when eating, abdominal pain, weight loss, gastrointestinal bleeding, and bowel obstruction. Screening can be done using ultrasound (a test that uses sound waves to generate images of internal organs) or upper endoscopy (a test similar to colonoscopy that is used to look at the upper parts of the gastrointestinal tract). Of note, screening programs for this disease exist in the Far East (e.g., Japan) but not in the U.S. (Khushalani, 2008).

Nasopharyngeal Cancer occurs in the lining of the nose and throat. It is a relatively rare cancer, but it is more common in southern China, northern Africa and Alaska. It can be caused by Epstein-Barr virus (EBV), the same virus that commonly causes mononucleosis in U.S. populations. Symptoms can include nosebleed, nasal obstruction, hearing problems, pain, involvement of cranial nerves, and neck tumors (Wei & Sham, 2005). Blood tests for EBV can be performed for screening in high-risk areas like southern China, but in general screening is not done.

Cervical Cancer occurs in the lower part of the uterus, or womb. Worldwide, it is the second most common cancer in women. Practically all cases of cervical cancer are caused by Human Papillomavirus (HPV), a common virus that exists in many genotypes, some of which are oncogenic (cancer-causing). Risk factors that increase the likelihood of cervical cancer include HIV infection, other immune suppression, a history of multiple sexual partners, smoking, low socioeconomic status, and history of sexually transmitted infection (Canavan & Doshi, 2000). With about 12,000 new cases per year, cervical cancer is relatively rare in the U.S. (ACS, 2010). This is largely due to effective screening methods that allow pre-cancerous lesions to be identified early and treated before they turn into cervical cancer. Screening is accomplished using the Papanicolaou (Pap) test, in which cells on the surface of the cervix are brushed off and examined under a microscope. If a patient has an abnormal Pap test, additional testing is necessary to determine whether cancer or precancer exists. Treatment may include surgery to remove the cancerous or precancerous tissue (Canavan & Doshi, 2000). For Asian American immigrants who come from countries where Pap screening is not routinely done, it can be a challenge to encourage the acceptance of this unfamiliar screening method. Cervical cancer also can potentially be prevented through vaccination against the most common oncogenic types of HPV (Franco & Harper, 2005).

Cancer treatment is complicated and specific to the anatomic site where the cancer originated, and explanations of site-specific treatments are beyond the scope of this chapter. Treatments may include surgery to remove the tumor, chemotherapy (medications meant to kill the cancer cells), radiation therapy directed to the tumor, and other measures such as hormone treatments. Some cancer therapies have substantial side effects, including nausea, vomiting, fever, neutropenia (depletion of the white blood cells that normally fight infection), anemia, hair loss, diarrhea, thrush (a fungal infection in the mouth), and fatigue. Patients may turn to complementary and alternative medicine (CAM) to treat their cancer or their symptoms. Many CAM therapies have not been proven effective through clinical trials, although some (such as massage and aromatherapy massage) have been shown effective in dealing with some symptoms (Smith & Toonen, 2007). Acupuncture, a therapeutic modality with an extensive history in Asia, can also be beneficial. Potential areas where acupuncture could play a role in cancer symptom management include pain, nausea and vomiting, hot flashes related to hormonal treatments, fatigue, anxiety, depression, insomnia, and xerostomia (dry mouth due to radiation or chemotherapy) (O'Regan & Filshie, 2010).

Unmet Needs of Cancer Patients. There remain many questions about the experiences of Asian American cancer survivors, including what needs are and are not currently being met by existing resources in family, community and healthcare settings. For example, consider older Asian

Americans of lower educational levels who are thyroid cancer survivors. These patients appear to experience a lower quality of life (Tan, Nan, Thumboo, Sundram, & Tan, 2007). In a study of Asian American breast cancer survivors conducted in English, Mandarin Chinese and Korean, acculturation did not appear to explain differences in health-related quality of life. After controlling for acculturation and other potential factors, Korean ethnicity persisted to be associated with lower scores for quality of life when compared to other Asian American subgroups (Kim, Ashing-Giwa, Singer, & Tejero, 2006). Prayer emerged as one potentially useful method for addressing the needs of Asian American cancer survivors. In one multiethnic study, AA/NHPI breast cancer survivors were found more likely to pray than Caucasian and Latina cancer survivors (Levine, Aviv, Yoo, Ewing, & Alfred, 2009).

Epidemiology of Cancer Among Asian Americans

Because of inconsistent data collection for Asian American subgroups, small numbers of Asians in some regions of the country, and poor recruitment of Asian Americans into research, data regarding Asian Americans are often unreported or difficult to interpret. However, a body of literature has grown over the past several decades, ever since Chen and Hawks wrote one of the first papers to debunk the myth that Asian

Americans are at low risk for cancer (Chen & Hawks, 1995). Indeed, Asian Americans and Pacific Islanders suffered a cancer incidence rate of 335 per 100,000 population (males) and 276 per 100,000 population (females), according to 2002–2006 national statistics (ACS, 2010). While this is lower than the rates for Caucasian men and women (550 and 420, respectively), it certainly is not an inconsequential number. Consider, a 2009 Census-estimated population of seven million Asian American males and 7.5 million Asian American females; this would equate to 44,150 *new* cases of cancer among Asian Americans in that 1 year alone.

Even more important, the aggregated figures (combining all Asian American and Pacific Islander subgroups into a single category) fail to describe the full impact of cancer on the Asian American population. When the data are disaggregated, a clearer picture emerges. Seven states (California, Hawaii, Illinois, New Jersey, New York, Texas, and Washington) require the inclusion of expanded Asian/Pacific Islander racial categories on their death certificates, allowing more careful analysis of cancer deaths. The most recent analysis of this type was conducted with data collected from 1998 to 2002 (Miller et al., 2008). The following table, based on the work by Miller and colleagues, shows the top five causes of cancer death for some Asian American subgroups, by sex. The table also shows cancer mortality (per 100,000), by subgroup and sex.

	Sex (mortality)	#1 rank	#2 rank	#3 rank	#4 rank	#5 rank
Asian Indian and Pakistani	Male (82.8)	Lung	Prostate	Pancreatic	Liver	Leukemia
	Female (67.4)	Breast	Lung	Colorectal	Ovarian	Pancreatic
Chinese	Male (167.8)	Lung	Liver	Colorectal	Stomach	Prostate
	Female (107.7)	Lung	Colorectal	Breast	Liver	Stomach
Filipino	Men (155.6)	Lung	Prostate	Colorectal	Liver	Non-Hodgkin's Lymphoma
	Women (96.1)	Breast	Lung	Colorectal	Pancreatic	Ovarian
Korean	Men (196.5)	Lung	Stomach	Liver	Colorectal	Pancreatic
	Women (108.2)	Lung	Stomach	Colorectal	Liver	Breast
Vietnamese	Men (159.9)	Lung	Liver	Stomach	Pancreatic	Colorectal
	Women (97.8)	Lung	Liver	Breast	Colorectal	Stomach
Japanese	Men (173.7)	Lung	Colorectal	Stomach	Prostate	Pancreatic
	Women (117.0)	Lung	Colorectal	Breast	Pancreatic	Stomach

The table points out the fact that, for some ethnic subgroups, liver and stomach cancer – somewhat rare for the general U.S. population – are major causes of cancer death. Though mortality data are not available for Kampuchean/Cambodian and Laotian Americans, the available cancer incidence data nonetheless suggests that liver and stomach cancer are important for these subgroups as well.

While it is useful to look at data concerning cancer deaths (*mortality*), it is also important to examine cancer *incidence* (new cases). This information would not be available from death certificates, so one would need to rely on state and regional cancer registries, which track new cancer diagnoses rather than deaths. Several cancer registries include detailed racial subgroup data: Atlanta, Detroit, Seattle/Puget Sound and the states of Connecticut, Hawaii, Iowa, Kentucky, Louisiana, New Jersey, New Mexico, and Utah (Miller et al., 2008). Looking at incidence rates, consider now the disproportionate impact of liver and stomach cancer on Asian Americans. While liver cancer incidence for non-Hispanic Whites (NHW) men in the U.S. is 6.7 per 100,000, the incidence is 8.7 for Asian Indian and Pakistani, 11.4 for Japanese, 17.2 for Filipino, 24.0 for Chinese, 35.9 for Korean, and a staggering 55.5 for Vietnamese American men. Similar disparities exist for women. Likewise, stomach cancer incidence is 4.5 per 100,000 NHW women, while it is 4.7 for Asian Indian/Pakistani, 5.6 for Filipino, 11.1 for Chinese, 13.8 for Vietnamese, 15.0 for Japanese, and 35.9 for Korean American women.

Consequently, American physicians, less accustomed to diagnosing these cancers among most of their patients of other ethnicities, need to be more vigilant about diagnosing (and perhaps screening for) these specific cancers in higher-risk Asian American patients. Medical students and other health professional trainees should be educated about how these nuances in the data could affect the differential diagnosis of the Asian patients they will evaluate.

Current Context

Cancer Awareness and Screening Among Asian Americans. A number of studies have suggested that there is low cancer awareness among Asian Americans. Several examples have been documented.

A study of 1,174 Asian Americans showed that the majority of Asians surveyed were aware of the connection between smoking and cancer (82%) (Ma, Tan, Feeley, & Thomas, 2002). However, it is disconcerting that this percentage was not even higher. Moreover, cancer awareness was lower among Southeast Asians. Lower education was also associated with lack of cancer awareness.

Colon cancer screening rates among Asian Americans are lower than for NHW. In a large study in California (36,660 NHW; 1,298 Chinese; 944 Filipino; 803 Korean; 857 Vietnamese; and 1,036 other Asians), colon cancer screening rates were 61.1% for NHW, as compared to 49.2% for Chinese, 46.3% for Filipino, 41.3% for Korean, 42.2% for Vietnamese, and 54.3% for other Asians (Kandula, Wen, Jacobs, & Lauderdale, 2006).

Mammography rates are low among Asian American women. In one study of 2,239 Asian American women, 67.7% reported having had a mammogram in the past two years. Rates were even lower for some Asian subgroups: 53.2% among Korean and 56.6% among Cambodian American women (Kagawa-Singer, Wellisch, & Durvasula, 2007).

The number of Asian American women getting screened for cervical cancer is less than ideal. In one study of NHW, Chinese, Vietnamese, Korean, Filipino, and Japanese women, Pap testing was reported at only 70% among Asian women as compared to 81% for NHW. Vietnamese had the lowest screening rates, with just over half (55%) being screened (Wang, Sheppard, Schwartz, Liang, & Mandelblatt, 2008). With low cervical cancer screening rates among Asians and high rates of cervical cancer among some of these same populations (e.g., Korean and Vietnamese), it is concerning that general knowledge is also low with regard to this disease. For example, a study of young Korean, Vietnamese and Filipino adults revealed that many had not heard of HPV, cervical cancer, and Pap testing (Gor, Chilton, Camingue, & Hajek, 2010).

As previously noted, Hepatitis B-related liver cancer disproportionately affects many AA/NHPI communities, yet for many immigrant communities knowledge about, screening for, and vaccination against Hepatitis B remains low. (Please refer to the separate chapter in this book that focuses specifically on Hepatitis B.).

Although vaccines do not exist to prevent most cancers, two important cancer-preventing vaccines are available. Specifically, immunizations are available for Human Papillomavirus and Hepatitis B virus, which can prevent infections leading to cervical cancer and liver cancer. Unfortunately, awareness of anti-cancer vaccines among Asian Americans is low, particularly among those with limited English proficiency (LEP). A study of 380 Asian American women, conducted in six languages, showed that LEP women were less likely than non-LEP women to be aware of vaccines for preventable cancers and more likely to think that there are vaccines to prevent other cancers, when no such vaccines exist (Nguyen, Leader, & Hung, 2009).

Efforts to Improve Cancer Awareness and Screening Among Asian Americans. Several strides have been made in the effort to increase cancer awareness and screening in Asian American communities. The Asian American Network for Cancer Awareness, Research, and Training (AANCART), for example, has brought together collaborators from Boston, New York, Houston, Seattle, San Francisco, Los Angeles, Hawaii, and Sacramento to address cancer disparities affecting Asian Americans (Chen et al., 2006). In the mid-Atlantic region, the Asian Tobacco Education, Cancer Awareness and Research (ATECAR) center has also utilized community partnership to address cancer needs of Asian communities (Ma, Toubbeh, Su, & Edwards, 2004). In the San Francisco/San Jose area, the *Health Is Gold* program has been very effective in mobilizing community members and increasing awareness through mass media campaigns, lay health workers, and academic-community coalition building (McPhee et al., 1996; Nguyen, Vo, McPhee, & Jenkins, 2001).

Asian Americans and Clinical Trial Participation. Asian Americans have limited engagement with clinical trials. Generally, only 3–20% of eligible participants participate in clinical trials across all races. Minority participation in these trials is even lower. For Asians, the primary reasons for lack of participation are linguistic (limited English proficiency), structural (work conflicts, family decision-making), and cultural (beliefs about asymptomatic states, fatalism, collectivism). Mistrust of research and the medical system, fear, and lack of knowledge about the origin of cancer can also play a role in decisions about cancer clinical trials (Giuliano et al., 2000; Nguyen, Somkin, Ma, Fung, & Nguyen, 2005).

A study on clinical trial participation with 132 oncologists found that language and cultural support through interpreters or patient navigators are key facilitators for trial participation (Nguyen, Somkin, Ma, Fung, & Nguyen, 2005). Meanwhile, physician-specific barriers to clinical trial participation by Asian American patients include lack of study knowledge and the effort required to establish eligibility and to explain risks and benefits (Nguyen, Somkin, & Ma, 2005).

A mixed-methods study involving newly diagnosed cancer patients and their caretakers showed that Asians were less likely to be aware of the term "clinical trial" and were more likely to equate a clinical trial with the term "experiment" or "a test procedure in a clinic" than non-Asians. Asians were also less likely to have participated in or to know someone in a clinical trial. Moreover, they were less willing than white respondents to consider participation in a clinical trial. Meanwhile, qualitative observations from this report showed that Asians who were interested in clinical trial participation were turned away because of ineligibility for the available trials (Paterniti et al., 2005).

Issues in Cancer Survivorship Among Asian Americans. There are different considerations in assessing cancer survivors of Asian descent. Survivorship appears to be poorer for foreign-born Asian Americans as compared to those born in the U.S. Data from the California Cancer Registry and the Surveillance, Epidemiology, and End Results (SEER) program were analyzed. Chinese, Japanese, Filipino, Korean, South Asian, and Vietnamese women diagnosed with breast cancer between 1988–2005 were then followed through 2007 (Gomez et al., 2010). Investigators found that U.S.-born women had similar mortality rates across all Asian ethnic groups with the exception of U.S.-born Vietnamese, who had a lower mortality risk. Meanwhile, foreign-born women (except for foreign-born Japanese) had higher mortality.

Since AA/NHPI communities often suffer from delayed cancer diagnosis due to low screening rates, such delay could result in levels of unmet psychosocial needs among AA/NHPI cancer survivors. Except for limited research on breast cancer survivors, there are not extensive studies of the psychological stress and needs for emotional support and practical assistance among AA/NHPI cancer patients. Compared to white females with breast cancer, AA/NHPI women with this disease were less likely to seek help for psychological distress (Kagawa-Singer, Wellisch, & Durvasula, 1997). For AA/NHPI women, their primary concern was fear of emotionally burdening their families with their illness (Ashing-Giwa, Padilla, Tejero, & Kim, 2004; Kagawa-Singer et al., 1997). Still, many stated they would have desired additional emotional support during the process of diagnosis and treatment (Giwa, Padilla, Tejero, & Kim, 2004).

Asian American patients have a high likelihood of using complementary and alternative medicine (CAM) in general (Nguyen & Bowman, 2007). Cancer patients with unmet needs often turn to CAM therapies as well (Mao et al., 2008). The degree to which these factors intermingle within the population of Asian American cancer survivors is uncertain. Although some Asian American cancer survivors do turn to CAM therapies, white patients actually appear to have the highest reported use of CAM therapies among cancer survivors (Shumay, Maskarinec, Gotay, Heiby, & Kakai, 2002). Of note, there are differences between Asian ethnicities. CAM use is highest among Filipinos, intermediate for Chinese and Native Hawaiians, and much lower for Japanese. Specific types of CAM also vary according to ethnicity, specifically herbal medicines for Chinese, Hawaiian healing for Native Hawaiians, and religious healing for Filipinos (Maskarinec, Shumay, Kakai, & Gotay, 2000). For women diagnosed with breast cancer, the role of prayer seems to be more prominent among Asian Americans and African Americans than among other ethnic groups (Levine et al., 2009).

Some Asian-specific cancer support groups do exist in the U.S., and many of them are affiliated with the Asian and Pacific Islander National Cancer Survivors Network (APINSCN), a national organization that works to link cancer survivors, advocates, and support groups.

Future Directions in Research and Care

It has been written that the "Asian American cancer burden is unique, unusual, and, to a certain extent, unnecessary" (Chen, 2005). Asian Americans are the only racial group for whom cancer is the leading cause of death. They also face a higher proportion of cancers of infectious origin than other groups (e.g., HBV, HPV, H. pylori, EBV) while at the same time facing new cancers associated with the adoption of more Western lifestyles. Cultural and linguistic barriers add another challenge for these populations and for the providers who care for them.

Data Advocacy. Researchers such as those involved in AANCART and ATECAR, as well as advocate groups such as the Asian and Pacific Islander American Health Forum (APIAHF) and the Asian and Pacific Islander National Cancer Survivors Network (APINCSN) have been pushing for more inclusive data collection and reporting from the federal government. Recognizing that most policy decisions rely upon data reported by government agencies, these advocates have stressed the need to oversample Asian American communities, apply best practices to maximize study recruitment in understudied populations, and report data in a disaggregated form. Moving into the future, this will continue to be an area of emphasis.

Cultural Competency and Language Access. As the Asian American population continues to grow and age, healthcare providers will need to pay increasingly more attention to the cultural and linguistic needs of this very diverse population. Lay health workers who come from these minority communities can play an important role in engaging community members in the process of health education and cancer screening (Nguyen et al., 2006). *Patient navigators* can also be important in assisting patients with limited health literacy as they attempt to find their way through the complex healthcare environment, especially after the diagnosis of cancer (Freeman, Muth, & Kerner, 1995). Finally, cancer centers and larger health systems will need to find more effective ways to implement the established guidelines for culturally and linguistically appropriate services so that equitable care is provided to all patients (Office of Minority Health, 2001).

Cancer Survivorship Research. Despite the need to understand more about the unmet needs of AA/NHPI cancer survivors, studies of the needs of Asian American cancer survivors have largely been qualitative and have focused on breast cancer alone (Ashing-Giwa, Padilla, Tejero 2004; Ashing-Giwa et al., 2004). Moreover, there are no broad-scale national studies focusing on the experiences of Asian American cancer survivors. This will be an area of continued interest for researchers.

Clinical Trials Recruitment. Differences do exist between racial and ethnic groups. One example is the variation due to genetic polymorphisms among the drug metabolizing cytochrome P450 enzymes (e.g., CYP2C9, CYP2C19, CYP2D6), resulting in variations in pharmacodynamics. Specifically, 18–23% of Asians exhibit poor drug metabolism by the CYP2C19 enzyme (as compared to 1–5% of Blacks and 2–5% of Whites), resulting in much higher blood concentrations of drugs that are metabolized in this pathway. Meanwhile, up to 21% of Asians might be ultrarapid metabolizers with regard to CYP2D6, as compared to about 5% of Blacks and Whites (Belle & Singh, 2008).

This example demonstrates that scientists need to include Asian American participants in cancer clinical trials in order to understand whether treatments will work effectively in ethnic patient populations. Cancer prevention trials also need to use effective recruitment methods to ensure participation of Asian American patients, especially for cancers that affect large numbers of Asians. Community-based participatory approaches may be helpful in engaging these understudied communities.

While great progress has been made over the past several decades in treating and screening for cancer within the Asian American population, there is clearly more that remains to be done. However, due to increasing awareness among community leaders and researchers alike, there is great hope that collaboration between the ethnic and scientific communities will bring improvements in our understanding of how best to fight cancer in this diverse population.

References

American Cancer Society. (2010). *Cancer facts and figures 2010*. Atlanta, GA: American Cancer Society.

Ashing-Giwa, K. T., Padilla, G., Tejero, J., & Kim, J. (2004). Breast cancer survivorship in a multiethnic sample: Challenges in recruitment and measurement. *Cancer, 101*, 450–465.

Ashing-Giwa, K. T., Padilla, G., Tejero, J., Kraemer, J., Wright, K., Coscarelli, A., et al. (2004). Understanding the breast cancer experience of women: A qualitative study of African American, Asian American, Latina and Caucasian cancer survivors. *Psycho-Oncology, 13*, 408–428.

Belle, D. J., & Singh, H. (2008). Genetic factors in drug metabolism. *American Family Physician, 77*, 1553–1560.

Canavan, T. P., & Doshi, N. R. (2000). Cervical cancer. *American Family Physician, 61*, 1369–1376.

Chen, M. S., Jr. (2005). Cancer health disparities among Asian Americans: What we do and what we need to do. *Cancer, 104*, 2895–2902.

Chen, M. S., Jr., & Hawks., B. L. (1995). A debunking of the myth of healthy Asian Americans and Pacific Islanders. *American Journal of Health Promotion, 9*, 261–268.

Chen, M. S., Jr., Shinagawa, S. M., Bal, D. G., Bastani, R., Chow, E. A., Ho, R. C., et al. (2006). Asian American network for cancer awareness, research, and training's legacy. The first 5 years. *Cancer, 107*, 2006–2014.

Damber, J.-E., & Aus, G. (2008). Prostate cancer. *The Lancet, 371*, 1710–1721.

El-Serag, H. B., Marrero, J. A., Rudolph, L., & Reddy, K. R. (2008). Diagnosis and treatment of hepatocellular carcinoma. *Gastroenterology, 134*, 1752–1763.

Faruque, A., Perz, J. F., Kwong, S., Jamison, P. M., Friedman, C., & Bell, B. P. (2008). National trends and disparities in the incidence of hepatocellular carcinoma, 1998-2003. *Preventing Chronic Disease, 5*, A74.

Franco, E. L., & Harper, D. M. (2005). Vaccination against human papillomavirus infection: A new paradigm in cervical cancer control. *Vaccine, 23*, 2388–2394.

Freeman, H. P., Muth, B. J., & Kerner, J. F. (1995). Expanding access to cancer screening and clinical follow-up among the medically underserved. *Cancer Practice, 3*, 19–30.

Giuliano, A. R., Mokuau, N., Hughes, C., Tortolero-Luna, G., Risendal, B., Ho, R. C. S., et al. (2000). Participation of minorities in cancer research: The influence of structural, cultural, and linguistic factors. *Annals of Epidemiology, 10*, S22–S34.

Gomez, S. L., Clarke, C. A., Shema, S. J., Chang, E. T., Keegan, T. H. M., & Glaser, S. L. (2010). Disparities in breast cancer survival among Asian women by ethnicity and immigrant status: a population-based study. *American Journal of Public Health, 100*, 861–869.

Gor, B. J., Chilton, J. A., Camingue, P. T., & Hajek, R. A. (2010). Young Asian Americans' knowledge and perceptions of cervical cancer and the human papillomavirus. *Journal of Immigrant and Minority Health, 13*(1), 81–86.

Heron, M. P. (2007). *Deaths: Leading causes for 2004.* (National Vital Statistics Reports 56). Hyattsville, MD: National Center for Health Statistics.

Hoffman, P. C., Mauer, A. M., & Vokes, E. E. (2000). Lung cancer. *The Lancet, 355*, 479–485.

Kagawa-Singer, M., Pourat, N., Breen, N., Coughlin, S., McLean, T. A., McNeel, T. S., & Ponce, N. A. (2007). Breast and cervical cancer screening rates of subgroups of Asian American women in California. *Medical Care Research and Review, 64*, 706–730.

Kagawa-Singer, M., Wellisch, D. K., & Durvasula, R. (1997). Impact of breast cancer on Asian American and Anglo American women. *Culture, Medicine and Psychiatry, 21*, 449–480.

Kandula, N. R., Wen, M., Jacobs, E. A., & Lauderdale, D. S. (2006). Low rates of colorectal, cervical, and breast cancer screening in Asian Americans compared with non-Hispanic Whites: Cultural influences or access to care? *Cancer, 107*, 184–192.

Khushalani, N. I. (2008). Cancer of the esophagus and stomach. *Mayo Clinic Proceedings, 83*, 712–722.

Kim, J., Ashing-Giwa, K., Singer, M., & Tejero, J. (2006). Breast cancer among Asian Americans: Is acculturation related to health-related quality of life? *Oncology Nursing Forum, 33*, E90–E99.

Levine, E. G., Aviv, C., Yoo, G., Ewing, C., & Alfred, A. (2009). The benefits of prayer on mood and well-being of breast cancer survivors. *Supportive Care in Cancer, 17*, 295–306.

Lok, A. S., & McMahon, B. J. (2009). Chronic hepatitis B: Update 2009. *Hepatology, 50*, 661–662.

Ma, G. X., Tan, Y., Feeley, R. M., & Thomas, P. (2002). Perceived risks of certain types of cancer and heart disease among Asian American smokers and nonsmokers. *Journal of Community Health, 27*, 233–246.

Ma, G. X., Toubbeh, J. I., Su, X., & Edwards, R. L. (2004). ATECAR: An Asian American community-based participatory research model on tobacco and cancer control. *Health Promotion Practice, 5*, 382–394.

Mao, J. J., Palmer, S. C., Straton, J. B., Cronholm, P. F., Keddem, S., Knott, K., et al. (2008). Cancer survivors with unmet needs were more likely to use complementary and alternative medicine. *Journal of Cancer Survivorship, 2*, 116–124.

Maskarinec, G., Shumay, D. M., Kakai, H., & Gotay, C. C. (2000). Ethnic differences in complementary and alternative medicine use among cancer patients. *Journal of Alternative and Complementary Medicine, 6*, 531–538.

McPhee, S. J., Bird, J. A., Ha, N.-T., Jenkins, C. N., Fordham, D., & Le, B. (1996). Pathways to early cancer detection for Vietnamese women: Suc Khoe La Vang! (Health Is Gold!). *Health Education Quarterly, 23*, S60–S75.

Miller, B. A., Chu, K. C., Hankey, B. F., & Ries, L. A. G. (2008). Cancer incidence and mortality patterns among specific Asian and Pacific Islander populations in the U.S. *Cancer Causes & Control, 19*, 257–258.

Miller, B. A., Kolonel, L. N., Bernstein, L., Young, J. L., Jr., Swanson, G. M., West, D., et al. (1996). *Racial/ethnic patterns of cancer in the United States 1988-1992.* Bethesda, MD: National Cancer Institute.

Nguyen, G. T., & Bowman, M. A. (2007). Culture, language, and health literacy: Communicating about health with Asians and Pacific Islanders. *Family Medicine, 39*, 208–210.

Nguyen, G. T., Leader, A. E., & Hung, W. L. (2009). Awareness of anticancer vaccines among Asian American women with limited English proficiency: An opportunity for improved public health communication. *Journal of Cancer Education, 24*, 280–283.

Nguyen, T. T., McPhee, S. J., Bui-Tong, N., Luong, T.-N., Ha-Iaconis, T., Nguyen, T., et al. (2006). Community-based participatory research increases cervical cancer screening among Vietnamese-Americans. *Journal of Health Care for the Poor and Underserved, 17*, 31–54.

Nguyen, T. T., Somkin, C. P., & Ma, Y. (2005). Participation of Asian-American women in cancer chemoprevention research. *Cancer, 104*, 3006–3014.

Nguyen, T. T., Somkin, C. P., Ma, Y., Fung, L.-C., & Nguyen, T. (2005). Participation of Asian-American women in cancer treatment research: A pilot study. *Journal of the National Cancer Institute. Monographs, 35*, 102–105.

Nguyen, T., Vo, P. H., McPhee, S. J., & Jenkins, C. N. (2001). Promoting early detection of breast cancer among Vietnamese-American women. Results of a controlled trial. *Cancer, 91*, 267–273.

O'Regan, D., & Filshie, J. (2010). Acupuncture and cancer. *Autonomic Neuroscience-Basic & Clinical, 157*, 96–100.

Office of Minority Health. (2001). *National standards for culturally and linguistically appropriate services in health care: Final report.* Washington, DC: U.S. Department of Health and Human Services.

Paterniti, D. A., Chen, M. S., Jr., Chiechi, C., Beckett, L. A., Horan, N., Turrell, C., et al. (2005). Asian Americans and cancer clinical trials: A mixed-methods approach to understanding awareness and experience. *Cancer, 104*, 3015–3024.

Quanstrum, K. H., & Hayward, R. A. (2010). Lessons from the mammography wars. *The New England Journal of Medicine, 363*, 1076–1079.

Shumay, D. M., Maskarinec, G., Gotay, C. C., Heiby, E. M., & Kakai, H. (2002). Determinants of the degree of complementary and alternative medicine use among patients with cancer. *Journal of Alternative and Complementary Medicine, 8*, 661–671.

Smith, G. F., & Toonen, T. R. (2007). Primary care of the patient with cancer. *American Family Physician, 75*, 1207–1214.

Tan, L. G., Nan, L., Thumboo, J., Sundram, F., & Tan, L. K. (2007). Health-related quality of life in thyroid cancer survivors. *Laryngoscope, 117*, 507–510.

Tong, M. J., Chavalitdhamrong, D., Lu, D. S., Raman, S. S., Gomes, A., Duffy, J. P., et al. (2009). Survival in Asian Americans after treatments for hepatocellular carcinoma: A seven-year experience at UCLA. *Journal of Clinical Gastroenterology, 44*(3), e63–e70.

U.S. Census Bureau. (2011). Overview of Race and Hispanic Origin: 2010. *2010 Census Briefs.*

Veronesi, U., Boyle, P., Goldhirsch, A., Orecchia, R., & Viale, G. (2005). Breast cancer. *The Lancet, 365*, 1727–1741.

Wang, J. H., Sheppard, V. B., Schwartz, M. D., Liang, W., & Mandelblatt, J. S. (2008). Disparities in cervical cancer screening between Asian American and non-Hispanic white women. *Cancer Epidemiology, Biomarkers & Prevention, 17*, 1968–1973.

Wei, W. I., & Sham, J. S. T. (2005). Nasopharyngeal carcinoma. *The Lancet, 365*, 2041–2054.

Weinbaum, C. M., Williams, I., Mast, E. E., Wang, S. A., Finelli, L., Wasley, A., et al. (2008). Recommendations for identification and public health management of persons with chronic hepatitis B virus infection. *MMWR. Morbidity and Mortality Weekly Report, 57*, 1–20.

Wilkins, T., & Reynolds, P. L. (2008). Colorectal cancer: A summary of the evidence for screening and prevention. *American Family Physician, 78*, 1385–1392.

Heterogeneity in Cardiovascular Health among Asian American Subgroups: Risk Factors, Outcomes, Treatment and Prevention, and Future Research Opportunities

Ariel T. Holland and Latha P. Palaniappan

Introduction

Cardiovascular disease (CVD), including heart and cerebrovascular diseases, represents the leading cause of death in Asian Americans as a group (Heron, 2010; National Center for Health Statistics, 2009b). Much of our knowledge of CVD in Asian Americans has been based on studies that have either grouped Asian Americans together, or examined one Asian American subgroup alone. The results from these previous studies are often inappropriately interpreted and extrapolated – in many cases the findings based on the aggregated Asian American group or one subgroup alone are presumed to be applicable for all other subgroups. Japanese have been the focus of most early CVD research in Asian Americans.

The Ni-Hon-San study has tracked CVD in Japanese men living in Japan (Nippon – Ni), Honolulu, Hawaii (Hon), and San Francisco, CA (San) since 1965 (Marmot et al., 1975). This landmark study demonstrated the importance of environmental factors in the development of CVD by showing varying prevalence rates of CVD for Japanese men depending on their location, with Japanese in Japan having the highest rates of stroke, and Japanese in San Francisco having the highest rates of heart disease. Further,

this study highlights the limitations of relying only on studies of native Asian populations for estimates of disease risk, as prevalence and progression of CVD is likely to differ for immigrant Asians compared to native Asian populations.

Not only is it important to study immigrant Asian Americans separately from native Asian populations, but Asian American subgroups should be studied separately due to differences in language, culture, and religion which can influence lifestyle practices, values and beliefs, and ultimately risk of CVD. In recent years more studies have acknowledged these differences and have examined CVD among Asian American subgroups. One of the first large scale epidemiologic cohorts in the U.S. to include an Asian American subgroup in addition to other racial/ethnic groups is the Multi-ethnic Study of Atherosclerosis (MESA), which recruited 797 Chinese Americans (11% of the total study sample). The MESA, which began in July 2000, aims to investigate the prevalence, correlates, and progression of pre-symptomatic CVD in a population-based sample of 6,500 men and women aged 45–84 years (Bild et al., 2002). Interest in studying Asian Indians in the U.S. has increased due to findings from recent studies in India documenting greater risk for coronary artery disease (CAD) compared to European populations (Yusuf et al., 2004). Higher risk of CAD has also been found for Filipinos compared to Non-Hispanic Whites (NHWs), spurring greater interest in this population as well. As a result of their more recent immigration history and smaller population

A.T. Holland (✉) • L.P. Palaniappan
Health Policy Research Department,
Palo Alto Medical Foundation Research Institute,
Palo Alto, CA, USA
e-mail: hollanda@pamfri.org; lathap@stanford.edu

G.J. Yoo et al. (eds.), *Handbook of Asian American Health*,
DOI 10.1007/978-1-4614-2227-3_16, © Springer Science+Business Media, LLC 2013

numbers, fewer studies have examined CVD in Koreans and Vietnamese. The majority of studies have focused on CVD risk factors and patient knowledge of CVD rather than heart disease and stroke rates (Ton et al., 2010; Choi, Rankin, Stewart, & Oka, 2008; Han et al., 2007; Coronado et al., 2008; Nguyen et al., 2009). These and other studies suggest marked heterogeneity in the prevalence of CVD and its risk factors among various Asian American subgroups. In this chapter, we will present our current understanding of CVD in Asian Americans with respect to disease definitions, prevalence and epidemiology, cultural and structural barriers to health care, lifestyle and prevention, and future directions for research.

What is Cardiovascular Disease?

Cardiovascular diseases are the conditions that affect the heart and blood vessels. The most common cardiovascular diseases are coronary artery disease (CAD) and stroke, and peripheral arterial disease (Hirsch et al., 2001; Lloyd-Jones et al., 2010; Pleis, Lucas, & Ward, 2009).

Coronary Artery Disease

Coronary artery disease (CAD) is a condition that occurs when the arteries that bring blood to the heart muscle become hardened and narrowed, preventing the muscle from getting adequate blood flow and oxygen. The main cause of CAD is atherosclerosis, which occurs when plaque, made up of fat, cholesterol, calcium, and fibrous elements from muscle cells, forms on the inside walls of the blood vessels, causing them to stiffen and narrow (Lusis, 2000). Atherosclerosis begins with the inflammatory immune response to the accumulation of fat particles and lipids in the blood stream (Corrado et al., 2010; Lusis, 2000). Lipoproteins, responsible for transporting lipids, such as low-density lipoprotein (LDL) and lipoprotein(a), accumulate in the inner-most layer of the blood vessel wall. In response to this aggregation of lipoproteins, immune cells called monocytes, a type of white blood cell, adhere to and cross the blood vessel wall. The monocytes form

foam cells as they pick up lipoproteins. Those lipoproteins that are not taken up by the monocytes, undergo modifications, including oxidation which contributes to the inflammatory immune response. As the foam cells die, the lipid contents combine with muscle fibers and other cellular material to form plaques. A thrombus, or blood clot, usually forms as the result of a plaque rupture. Thrombosis, the occlusion of the blood vessel due to thrombus, leads to heart attack (myocardial infarction) or stroke (Lusis, 2000). Two markers of inflammation, high sensitivity C-reactive protein (hsCRP) and fibrinogen, have been identified as possible predictors of atherosclerosis. Hs-CRP is known to play a role in the adhesion of immune cells to the blood vessel wall, activation of the coagulation system, and low density lipoprotein oxidation. Fibrinogen is involved in the formation and growth of atherosclerotic plaques (Corrado et al., 2010).

The symptoms of CAD vary, often depending on the severity of the atherosclerosis. A patient in the early stages of CAD may be asymptomatic, or may report symptoms of chest pain (angina). A heart attack, an acute form of CAD, results when plaque in the arteries breaks apart causing a blood clot to form which prevents blood from reaching the heart muscle. This lack of oxygen can cause myocardial ischemia which can lead to death of myocardial cells and permanent damage to the heart (myocardial infarction). Acute coronary syndrome refers to any condition brought on by sudden, reduced blood flow to the heart, and includes ischemia and myocardial infarction. Common symptoms of an acute coronary syndrome include shortness of breath, chest pain, pain in one or both arms, discomfort, nausea, vomiting, and faintness.

Stroke

While CAD is a condition that affects the blood vessels' ability to deliver blood to the heart, stroke is a condition that interferes with the blood vessels' ability to deliver blood to the brain. Stroke occurs either due to a blocked blood vessel, which prevents blood from reaching the brain (ischemic stroke), or a burst blood vessel, which causes bleeding in or around the brain (hemorrhagic stroke). Both ischemic and hemorrhagic stroke impede the supply of oxygen and nutrients to the brain, leading to brain cell death. Transient ischemic attack is caused by a temporary blood clot that causes the same symptoms of stroke, but only last a short time. Typical symptoms of stroke include sudden onset of the following: weakness or numbness (especially on one side of the body), confusion, trouble speaking or understanding speech, difficulty seeing in one or both eyes, and/or loss of balance.

Peripheral Arterial Disease

Peripheral arterial disease refers to disease of the blood arteries outside of the heart and brain. The peripheral blood arteries carry blood to the arms, legs, stomach and kidneys. When they become narrow or clogged, they interfere with blood flow to these parts of the body. Similar to CAD, the most common cause of peripheral arterial disease is atherosclerosis. Symptoms of peripheral arterial disease may be harder to recognize than those for CAD and stroke. Some patients may not present any symptoms, and disease may be detected by routine measures of ankle and brachial (upper arm) blood pressures (ABI). Symptoms vary and may include pain or cramping in the arms and legs, limping, sores on the legs and arms, and/or a change in color of the arms and legs.

Understanding CVD in Asian Americans: Advantages and Limitations of Data Sources

Many guidelines for treatment and prevention of CVD for all sex and racial/ethnic groups are based on findings from studies of Non-Hispanic White men, such as the Framingham Heart Study, which was initiated in the 1950s. Since then, research studies have established sex and racial/ethnic differences in the prevalence of CVD and its risk factors (Dawber, Meadors, & Moore, 1951; Hemann, Bimson, & Taylor, 2007). We now know that CVD risk factors and rates are different in men and women (Eastwood & Doering, 2005; Ren & Kelley, 2009) and in different racial/

ethnic groups (Cossrow & Falkner, 2004; Davis, Vinci, Okwuosa, Chase, & Huang, 2007; Kuzawa & Sweet, 2009), with some groups at higher (Cossrow & Falkner, 2004; Davis et al., 2007; Eastwood & Doering, 2005; Kuzawa & Sweet, 2009; Ren & Kelley, 2009) and others at lower risk (Cossrow & Falkner, 2004; Davis et al., 2007; Eastwood & Doering, 2005; Ren & Kelley, 2009). While some work has been done to elucidate these differences among women (Eastwood & Doering, 2005; Ren & Kelley, 2009), African Americans (Davis et al., 2007; Kuzawa & Sweet, 2009), and Hispanics (Cossrow & Falkner, 2004; Davis et al., 2007) in the U.S., there have been fewer studies in Asian Americans (Davis et al., 2007; Narayan et al., 2010; Palaniappan, Araneta, Assimes, et al., 2010). It is necessary to collect cardiovascular disease data for individual Asian American subgroups, as disease prevalence and risk factors may differ. Results from one Asian American subpopulations may not necessarily be extrapolated to another subpopulations. In addition, the diverse cultural, genetic, and environmental factors that influence the cardiovascular health of Asian American subgroups provide a unique opportunity to contribute to the understanding of cardiovascular disease.

There are different sources of epidemiologic data (national surveys, disease registries, and cohort studies, among others) that can inform us about risk factor and disease rates in Asian Americans, and each data source has its own set of advantages and limitations, as shown in Table 16.1.

National surveys, such as the U.S. Decennial Census and the American Community survey can provide demographic information about the whole population, and currently collect detailed race/ethnicity information by Asian American subgroups (Asian Indian, Chinese, Filipino, Japanese, Korean, Vietnamese, and Other Asian) (U.S. Census Bureau, 2008, 2010). These surveys also provide accurate information on the size of the Asian American subgroup populations, percent foreign born, education level, and household income. Using these surveys, we can obtain excellent "denominator" information – how many people are at risk, and their demographic

Table 16.1 Sources of epidemiologic data

Data source	Population coverage	Advantages	Disadvantages	Asian race/ethnicity collection
National surveys				
U.S. Decennial Census (U.S. Census Bureau, 2001; U.S. Census Bureau, 2010)	• In 2000, collected information on ~281.4 million people across the United States	• Collects demographic information from all U.S. citizens • Education, labor, income, housing, and population questions were asked of a sample (~1/6 persons) reflective of national population	• Self-reported data is subject to recall limitations, misinterpretation of questions, etc. • Data is only collected every ten years and therefore may not be representative of the changing population	• Collects Asian subgroup information
American Community Survey, U.S. Census (U.S. Census Bureau, 2008)	• Random sample of ~3 million addresses	• Reflective of national population • Collects annual demographic, income, benefits, health insurance, education, veteran status, disabilities, occupation, residential status, and essential expenses information	• Self-reported data is subject to recall bias, misinterpretation of questions, etc. • Based on a sample and may not reflect the actual characteristics of the entire population (e.g., often excludes institutionalized persons and active military personnel)	• Collects Asian subgroup information
National health interview survey (NHIS) (Pleis et al., 2009)	• ~75,000–100,000 persons are sampled each year • Oversamples African Americans, Hispanics and Asians	• Reflective of national population • Interview participants with a set of basic health and demographic health status, health care services, and health behavior questions • Useful for determining prevalence rates of disease and disease risk factors • Useful for monitoring national population health	• Self-reported data is subject to recall limitations, misinterpretation of questions, etc. • Based on a sample and may not reflect the actual characteristics of the entire population (e.g., often excludes institutionalized persons and active military personnel)	• Collects Asian subgroup information, but limited by one group only, or small sample size
National health and nutrition examination survey (NHANES) (National Center for Health Statistics, 2007)	• ~5,000 persons are sampled each year • Over-samples persons 60 and older, African Americans, and Hispanics	• Reflective of the national population • Provides demographic, socioeconomic, dietary, and health-related information • Provides detailed medical, dental, and laboratory tests (i.e., cholesterol, blood pressure) • Useful for determining prevalence rates of disease and disease risk factors	• Self-reported data is subject to recall limitations, misinterpretation of questions, etc. • Lab data subject to measurement variation • Based on a sample and may not reflect the actual characteristics of the entire population (e.g., often excludes institutionalized persons and active military personnel)	• Collects only aggregated Asian race/ethnicity information

Death and disease registries

Death records (National Center for Health Statistics, 2001)	• U.S. states collect data on deaths for a given year	• For each death, demographic information and cause of death are collected • As of 2003, all states collect race/ethnicity by Asian American subgroup • Prior to 2003, seven states collected race/ethnicity by Asian American subgroup: California, Hawaii, Illinois, New Jersey, New York, Texas, and Washington	• As of 2003, all states collect race/ethnicity by Asian American subgroup • Prior to 2003, not all states collected race/ethnicity by Asian American subgroup
National registry of myocardial infarction (Fonarow, French, & Frederick, 2009)	• Pharmaceutical industry sponsored • ~200,000 acute myocardial infarction (AMI) patients per year • ~2.1 million patients with AMI since 2006	• Hospitals report detailed demographic data, risk factors for coronary artery disease, presenting clinical characteristics, initial diagnosis, medications within 24 hours, medications at discharge, CVD procedures, and hospitals characteristics (facilities and services) • Useful in assessing care provided by participating hospitals • Useful in examining characteristics of patients with MI	• Hospital selection was not random, and therefore the findings are not generalizable • Data is not always uniformly available for all patients	• Collects only aggregated Asian race/ethnicity information
Paul coverdell national acute stroke registry (PCNASR) (George et al., 2009)	• Centers for disease control funded four U.S. states to recruit hospitals during 2005–2007 (Georgia, Illinois, Massachusetts, and North Carolina) • ~57,000 patients with stroke	• Hospitals report data on hospital characteristics (facilities and services), cases of stroke, and patient characteristics • Data are useful in assessing care provided by participating hospitals • Data are useful in examining characteristics of patients with stroke	• Hospital selection was not random, and therefore the findings are not generalizable or representative of the national population • The number of Hispanic cases is limited; therefore, statistical comparison of data on Hispanics should be interpreted with caution • Stroke definition is based on clinical diagnosis and ICD-9-CM codes	• Collects only aggregated Asian race/ethnicity information

(continued)

Table 16.1 (continued)

Data source	Population coverage	Advantages	Disadvantages	Asian race/ethnicity collection
Cohort studies				
Multi-ethnic study of atherosclerosis (MESA) (Bild et al., 2002)	• Cohort study that recruited sample of ~6,500 (38% White, 28% African-American, 23% Hispanic, and 11% Chinese)	• Data are useful in determining risk factors and prevalence of disease • Detailed diet, physical activity, laboratory and medical examination data is collected (including CT and MRI scans, carotid ultrasound, among others) • Characterization of subclinical disease will inform more precise and valid phenotypic characterization of CVD	• Patients must be followed over time to determine outcomes • Only Chinese Americans were recruited, no other Asian subgroup data are available	• Limited to one Asian subgroup only
Ni-Hon-San Study (Marmot et al., 1975)	• Cohort study of ~10,800 Japanese Americans and ~2,100 Japanese from Japan	• Detailed medical and laboratory data was collected • Used to determine prevalence of CVD (CAD and stroke), CVD risk factors, and CVD mortality in Japanese living in the U.S. and Japan	• Patients must be followed over time to determine outcomes • There were no other racial/ethnic groups sampled for comparison, making it difficult to compare findings with other studies	• Limited to one Asian subgroup only

characteristics. Unfortunately, these surveys do not ask any questions about health, and therefore do not provide "numerator" information – how many people have disease and what kind of disease. We can calculate disease rate estimates in a certain population by dividing the numerator by the denominator.

The National Health Interview Survey (NHIS) attempts to provide numerator information by calling over 100,000 people per year, and asking questions about their health (i.e. "Have you ever been told by a doctor or other health professional that you had coronary heart disease?") (National Center for Health Statistics, 2009a). While this survey provides some information on a relatively small proportion (<0.003%) of the whole U.S. population, there are important limitations to this survey. Health data reported by people (self-report) is often inaccurate, due to recall bias (i.e. someone forgets the doctor told them they had high cholesterol) and possible misclassification of disease (i.e. someone reports they had a stroke when they actually had a transient ischemic attack). The little information we have on Asian Americans and CVD comes from the NHIS telephone survey self-report data from approximately 800 Asian Americans each year, representing <0.00005% of the Asian American population (Oza-Frank, Ali, Vaccarino, & Narayan, 2009).

The National Health and Nutrition Examination Survey is a more in-depth survey, a nationally representative sample of fewer people (5,000 per year), and provides detailed medical, dental, and laboratory tests. An approximately equal number of NHWs, African Americans, and Hispanics are included in this survey (National Center for Health Statistics, 2010). Unfortunately, there are extremely few Asian Americans in this survey, and there is no subgroup information. Fewer than 500 participants are sampled from Asian, Native Hawaiian or Pacific Islander, Native American or Alaskan Native, and other racial/ethnic groups (National Center for Health Statistics, 2006, 2010). These data are not released for public analysis by individual Asian subgroups to protect the privacy of the participants, since participants may be identifiable due to the small sample sizes in each sex/race/ethnic group.

Thus, nationally representative, in-depth health data is not currently available for Asian American subgroups.

Disease registries are another way of providing numerator information (i.e. number of people with a disease or number of deaths due to a disease). None of the death or disease registries in the U.S. uniformly collect Asian subgroup information. Prior to 2003, there were only a few states that disaggregated death record data on Asian Americans (National Center for Health Statistics, 2001). It is from these states that have provided Asian subgroup information that we are able to discern notable differences in death rates among Asian American subgroups (Palaniappan, Wang, & Fortmann, 2004; Wild, Laws, Fortmann, Varady, & Byrne, 1995). There are two national registries for CVD – the National Registry of Myocardial Infarction (NRMI) (Canto et al., 1998; Fonarow et al., 2009) and the Paul Coverdell National Acute Stroke Registry (PCNASR) (George et al., 2009), Both of these only report data for aggregated Asian Americans.

Cohort studies, like the Framingham Heart Study (Dawber et al., 1951), are an excellent way to study CVD risk factors, incidence, and progression. Many people need to be followed over long periods of time to generate accurate information. The few cohort studies that include Asian subgroups include only one, such as Japanese (Marmot et al., 1975) or Chinese (Bild et al., 2002). The prevailing wisdom, that Asians in general are at lower risk of CVD, comes from these cohort studies of East Asian subgroups. Newer cohort studies, including other Asian subgroups, are needed to more accurately assess the range of CVD risks and rates across all Asian subgroups.

There are many sources of data on CVD in Asian Americans. Each data source has its strengths and limitations. While the U.S. Census Bureau has collected data on Asian subgroups separately since the mid 19th century, the only nationally representative data on CVD for Asian American subgroups are self-reported data from the NHIS (Barnes, Adams, & Powell-Griner, 2008; Pleis et al., 2009). National registries of CVD, such as the National Registry of Myocardial

Infarction (NRMI) (Canto et al., 1998; Fonarow et al., 2009) and the Paul Coverdell National Acute Stroke Registry (PCNASR) (George et al., 2009), which only report data for aggregated Asian Americans. Due to small sample sizes, Asian Americans are often aggregated to allow for statistically significant comparisons. However, these aggregated comparisons may be misleading, given the heterogeneity across the different subgroups. As a result, CVD research in Asian Americans is often opportunistically conducted in geographic areas with high Asian population concentration. We should keep in mind these limitations when interpreting the current data on CVD in Asian Americans, and future studies should strive to improve our knowledge by addressing these limitations.

Prevalence and Epidemiology

The number of Asian Americans in the U.S. has grown rapidly, especially in the latter half of the twentieth century. As different Asian American subgroups have increased in numbers more research has been dedicated to studying these populations separately. Recent research suggests that there is substantial variability in cardiovascular risk and incidence of CAD, stroke, peripheral arterial disease across subgroups.

Coronary Artery Disease
The national self-reported prevalence rate of CAD for all Asian Americans (2.9%) is lower than the rate for NHWs (6.5%) (Pleis et al., 2009). However, Asian Americans as an aggregated group have been shown to have a higher percentage of premature deaths due to heart disease compared to Whites (Centers for Disease Control and Prevention, 2004). While most data on CAD is presented for Asian Americans as a group, there appears to be substantial variability for CAD risk by Asian American subgroup. Precise estimates of CAD prevalence for Asian American subgroups are not available. However, self-reported telephone survey data from NHIS on the prevalence of heart disease for Asian Americans ranged from 4.4% for Koreans to 9.2% for Asian

Indians, for the years 2004–2006 (Barnes et al., 2008). Higher rates of hospitalization for CAD have been shown in Asian Indian men and Filipino women, and lower rates in Chinese (Klatsky & Tekawa, 2005). A similar study using outpatient clinical data, found that Asian Indian men and Filipino women had higher prevalence of CAD, while Chinese had lower prevalence of CAD (Holland et al., 2011).

Few studies have examined leading causes of mortality among Asian American subgroups, since few states collect Asian subgroup information on death records (Palaniappan et al., 2004; Wild et al., 1995). In 2003, the Secretary of the Department of Health and Human Services approved the separation of Asian race category from the Pacific Islander race category and added the following Asian subcategories on U.S. death and birth certificates and reports: Asian Indian, Chinese, Filipino, Japanese, Korean, Vietnamese, Other Asian (specify) (National Center for Health Statistics, 2001). Prior to 2003, only seven states required reporting of specific Asian racial/ethnic subgroups (California, Hawaii, Illinois, New Jersey, New York, Texas, and Washington) (National Center for Health Statistics). Most studies of mortality in Asian American subgroups have been conducted using California mortality records, due to the high concentration of Asian Americans in the geographic region, and availability of Asian subgroup information on this state's death records. A higher proportion of deaths due to CAD were found for Asian Indians and lower proportion for Japanese and Chinese in California, compared to NHWs (Palaniappan et al., 2004; Wild et al., 1995). Using California mortality records, Palaniappan and colleagues found that CAD is the leading cause of death in Asian Indians, further highlighting the burden of CAD in this population (Palaniappan, Mukherjea, Holland, & Ivey, 2010).

The Ni-Hon-San study was the first population based study to examine CAD mortality in one Asian American subgroup, documenting lower CAD mortality rates in Japanese living in the U.S., compared to Whites, but higher rates compared to those living in Japan (Benfante, 1992). This landmark study demonstrated the important role of environmental and cultural factors in disease risk for populations of the same racial/ethnic background.

There appears to be marked heterogeneity among Asian American subgroups with respect to CAD morbidity and mortality. Asian Indians and Filipinos appear to be at higher risk for CAD, and Chinese and Japanese at lower risk compared to other groups.

Stroke

It is widely accepted that strokes are more prevalent among cohorts of persons of Asian descent, when compared to persons of European descent. However, the epidemiology of stroke among Asians living in the U.S. is less well known. According to NHIS data, national self-reported prevalence rates of stroke are lower among Asian Americans (1.8%) compared to NHWs (2.7%) (Pleis et al., 2009). Stroke prevalence estimates for Asian American subgroups, however, are much less reliable due to small sample sizes, and reliance on self-report telephone survey data. The only Asian American subgroup with a large enough sample size to produce reliable stroke prevalence rates in NHIS was Chinese (2.4%), who reported identical rates to NHWs (2.4%) (Barnes et al., 2008).

Epidemiologic research indicates that Asian Americans may experience higher prevalence rates for different subtypes of stroke, such as hemorrhagic, compared to NHWs. Studies have found more hemorrhagic strokes for Asian Americans as a group (Ayala et al., 2002; Gonzalez-Fernandez, Kuhlemeier, & Palmer, 2008; Klatsky et al., 2005) compared to NHWs. Chinese Americans are reported to have strokes at a younger age, with a greater proportion of hemorrhagic strokes, compared to NHWs (Fang, Foo, Jeng, Yip, & Alderman, 2004). No research has examined prevalence rates of ischemic stroke among Asian American subgroups. In addition, complications due to stroke, such as problems with swallowing, may be more common in Asian Americans (as an aggregated group), (Gonzalez-Fernandez et al., 2008) compared to NHWs (Nguyen-Huynh & Johnston, 2005; Fang, Foo, Fung, Wylie-Rosett, & Alderman, 2006).

Little research has been dedicated to examining stroke mortality in Asian American subgroups. The Ni-Hon-San study first reported intermediate stroke mortality rates for Japanese in Hawaii, compared to lower rates for Japanese living in San Francisco and higher rates for native Japanese in 1977 (Benfante, 1992). This study demonstrated that Japanese living in the U.S. had different rates of disease, despite similar ancestry. More recently, Wild et al. (1995), using California census and 1985–1990 death data, found that while Chinese and Japanese had fewer total deaths, they had higher proportions of deaths due to stroke, compared to NHWs.

While stroke mortality may decrease with duration in the U.S. for some subgroups, it is still a leading cause of death in Asian Americans, particularly Chinese and Japanese. These findings indicate that combining Asian American subgroups into one race/ethnicity category may be inappropriate (Gonzalez-Fernandez et al., 2008; Klatsky et al., 2005). Some Asian American subgroups may be at greater risk for stroke, particularly for certain subtypes of stroke. However, further studies are needed to determine differences in stroke incidence and risk factors among the various Asian American subgroups.

Peripheral Arterial Disease

Peripheral arterial disease poses a significant health threat, afflicting over eight million Americans, and increasing risk of stroke and heart attack (Hirsch et al., 2001). National prevalence rates are not reported by NHIS, with most of our understanding coming from epidemiologic studies. In the MESA study, the prevalence of peripheral arterial disease for Chinese (2.0%) was identified to be nearly half that of NHWs (3.6%) and a fourth that of African-Americans (7.2%) (Allison et al., 2006). Studies that have aggregated Asians have shown lower incidence of peripheral arterial disease compared to NHWs (Criqui et al., 2005). It is unknown whether this aggregation (due to limitations in data collection methods) may mask higher risks in some subgroups. Despite findings that risk for peripheral arterial disease appears to be lower, more research should be dedicated to examining peripheral arterial disease prevalence and incidence in Asian American subgroups.

In summary, few studies of CVD have examined Asian American subgroups separately. The studies that have examined specific subgroups have shown higher rates of CAD in Asian Indians, and stroke among Chinese and Japanese, and lower rates of CAD in Chinese and Japanese, and lower rates of peripheral arterial disease among Chinese.

Cultural, Language, and Structural Barriers to Cardiovascular Health Care

There is great cultural diversity among Asian Americans, which is important in the context of cardiovascular health as culture defines perceptions of health, self-care behaviors, and lifestyle risk factors (Kagawa-Singer & Kassim-Lakha, 2003). Culture is a multi-dimensional construct, encompassing language, social structure, environment, economy, technology, religion/world view, and belief and values, which is passed on from one generation to the next (Kagawa-Singer & Kassim-Lakha). Acculturation is defined as the changes that occur when culturally dissimilar people, groups, and social influences come together (Schwartz, Unger, Zamboanga, & Szapocznik, 2010). While earlier definitions of acculturation were conceptualized as a spectrum from the retention of an individual's heritage culture to the acquisition of the new culture, more recently a two-dimensional definition of acculturation has been proposed, in which receiving-culture acquisition and heritage-culture retention intersect to form four categories: *assimilation* (adopts the receiving culture and discards the heritage culture), *separation* (rejects the receiving culture and retains the heritage culture), *integration* (adopts the receiving culture and retains the heritage culture), and *marginalization* (rejects both the heritage and receiving cultures) (Schwartz et al., 2010).

In the context of health care, language is often the most easily identifiable cultural difference between patient and health care provider. In the U.S., 62% of Vietnamese, 50% of Chinese, 24% of Filipinos, and 23% of Asian Indians are not fluent in English (Office of Minority Health, 2010). Language is cited as a common barrier to health care by Chinese patients (Bryant et al., 2010; Ton et al., 2010), Vietnamese (Bryant et al., 2010; Ton et al., 2010; Nguyen et al., 2009) and Korean (Bryant et al., 2010; Ton et al., 2010). Studies have shown that limited English proficient (LEP) patients receive fewer preventive health screenings and demonstrate lower rates of medication adherence (Flores, 2006). Bilingual physicians and professional interpreters, as opposed to family or friends, have been shown to improve care delivery to LEP patients (Diamond, Wilson-Stronks, & Jacobs, 2010). While translation and interpretation services can improve communication between patient and physician, they may not resolve cultural differences. Asian Americans report frustration with translated education materials that often only provide Western examples for lifestyle changes such as diet or physical activity (Bryant et al., 2010). Few studies have examined cultural and language barriers to cardiovascular care in Asian Americans specifically. However, recent studies indicate that cultural and language barriers may impede knowledge of CVD symptoms among Asian Americans. New immigrant Asian populations were found to have incomplete knowledge about CVD, compared with those who had lived in the U.S. longer (Bryant et al., 2010; Nguyen et al., 2009). Limited knowledge of CVD symptoms and risk factors may prevent patients from seeking proper medical care and ultimately lead to poor health outcomes.

In addition to cultural and language barriers, Asian Americans are more likely to face structural barriers to care, such as lack of health insurance or a regular care provider. Employer-sponsored health insurance coverage ranges from as low as 49% among Koreans to a high of 77% among Asian Indians (The Kaiser Family Foundation, 2008). According to the NHIS, Korean adults (25%) were most likely to be without a regular provider for health care, compared to NHWs (12.9%) (Barnes et al., 2008), with rates for the other Asian subgroups ranging from 12% for both Japanese and Filipino adults to 16% for both Chinese and Vietnamese adults. Not having a regular care provider, regardless of insurance status, has been found to be associated with untreated hypertension or hypercholesterolemia, major risk factors for CVD (Spatz, Ross, Desai, Canavan, & Krumholz, 2010). Among Asian adults who have access to a regular care provider, Vietnamese adults (23%) were more likely to consider a clinic or health center – versus a doctor's office /HMO, a hospital ER/outpatient department, or some other – as their usual place for health care, compared to NHWs (15.2%) (Barnes et al., 2008).

The practices of hospitals (and doctors) may mediate the relationship between race/ethnicity and receipt of CVD treatment. One study found that Asian Americans were less likely to receive coronary artery bypass graft surgery or coronary angiography when controlled for age, gender, insurance type, and income. When differences in cardiac procedures performed and volume of procedures performed at hospitals were controlled for, the differences in rates of cardiac procedures disappeared (Carlisle, Leake, & Shapiro, 1995). These findings indicate that Asian patients may be more likely to receive care at hospitals that are unable to or are too overwhelmed to give proper cardiovascular care.

(a) Culturally competent care has been implemented in many healthcare settings to improve health care for racial/ethnic minorities, including Asian Americans. A report addressing health care disparities in Asian American and Pacific Islander populations stated:

(b) "Culturally competent providers consistently and systematically: understand and respect their patients' values, beliefs, and expectations; understand the disease-specific epidemiology and treatment efficacy of different population groups; (and) adapt the way they deliver care to each patient's needs and expectations" (Office of Minority Health and Bureau of Primary Health Care, 2005).

Research to assess and address cultural, language, and structural barriers is needed to advance CVD care among Asian Americans.

Prevention and Lifestyle

Several lifestyle behaviors (e.g., diet, physical activity, smoking, drinking) have been associated with increased CVD risk and these risk factors are the first targets of CVD prevention efforts by clinicians and healthcare professionals. In considering CVD prevention for Asian Americans, it is important to consider that lifestyle behaviors are tied closely to cultural beliefs and values. Acculturation (assimilation) has generally been associated with adverse changes in CVD risk factors in Chinese and Japanese Americans (Taylor et al., 2007; Marmot & Syme, 1976). The aforementioned Ni-Hon-San study, one of the most comprehensive studies of immigration, acculturation, and CVD risk in Asian Americans, showed that CAD and stroke mortality rates in Hawaii were intermediate between the high rates of stroke in Japan and high rates of CAD in California. They found that levels of CVD risk factors, such as blood pressure and cholesterol, correlated to the rates of disease (Benfante, 1992). However, Western acculturation is not always associated with increases in CVD rates. Stroke prevalence has been reported to decrease with acculturation among Japanese men (Rodriguez et al., 2002) as well as Chinese immigrants (Fang et al., 2006), compared to their native counterparts. Acculturation may mediate the relationship between risk factors and disparate CVD outcomes, altering practices in diet, physical activity, smoking, and drinking.

Diet

The characteristic East Asian (Chinese, Korean, and Japanese) diet appears to be protective of CVD. The East Asian diet is generally lower in animal protein, total and saturated fat, and greater in quantities of rice, vegetables, seafood, tea, and red yeast rice. Fatty fish, such as mackerel and salmon, which are high in omega-3 fatty acids, may reduce CVD risk. A study in King County, Washington showed seafood consumption was higher among Asian Americans, as a group, compared to the general U.S. population (Sechena et al., 2003). Fish consumption decreases among subsequent generations of Asian Americans (Sechena et al., 2003). Tea consumption has been shown to reduce CVD risk as well. Both black and green teas have also been implicated in CVD prevention, resulting in favorable cholesterol and blood pressure levels, as well as anti-inflammatory effects. Further, it was found that those who consumed seven or more cups of tea daily had lower incidence of stroke and CAD (Higdon & Frei, 2003).

In contrast to the typical East Asian diet, the Asian Indian diet is generally characterized by high consumption of refined carbohydrates and saturated fat through clarified butter, hydrogenated oils, and coconut products. A study of Asian Indians in the United Kingdom (UK) found lower intake of omega-3 fatty acids and fiber, and higher intake of carbohydrates, saturated fat, and trans-fatty acids compared to UK Caucasians (Misra & Khurana, 2009). High intake of carbohydrates and uneven meal distribution (no breakfast and large evening meals) has been associated with CAD risk (Yagalla, Hoerr, Song, Enas, & Garg, 1996). In the Canadian Study of Health Assessment and Risk in Ethnic groups (SHARE) study, higher intake of saturated and trans fats were associated with subclinical atherosclerosis (measured by carotid ultrasound) among participants of Chinese or Asian Indian ancestry (Merchant et al., 2008).

Adoption of Western culture may result in unhealthy dietary practices, which has been shown both in Asia (Popkin, Horton, Kim, Mahal, & Shuigao, 2001), as well as in the U.S., where Chinese immigrants report a healthier diet compared to Chinese Americans who reside in the U.S. for more than 10 years (Taylor et al., 2007). Acculturation may alter dietary practices resulting in weight gain, with one study documenting higher BMI with greater acculturation for Korean men, although this did not hold true for Korean women (Song et al., 2004).

Physical Activity

Physical inactivity has been reported more often in Asian Americans as compared with U.S. NHWs, Hispanics, and African Americans

(Kandula & Lauderdale, 2005). Insufficient physical activity has important health implications, with higher prevalence of obesity, insulin resistance, and hypertension found in Asian Americans who report no or limited physical activity (Hwu et al., 2004). Studies of Japanese American men have shown that lower levels of activity are associated with a higher incidence of diabetes, and CVD morbidity (Burchfiel et al., 1995). Differences in socioeconomic status, perceived barriers and benefits of activity, and access to spaces to participate in activity (Kandula & Lauderdale, 2005), have been found to mediate the role of acculturation and physical activity behaviors. Intervention studies have been done in Chinese American population to increase physical activity, and these suggest that CVD risk factors can be favorably modified in Chinese Americans, despite generally lower initial BMI (Taylor-Piliae et al., 2006).

Smoking and Drinking Behaviors

Smoking and alcohol consumption are significant risk factors for CVD morbidity and mortality (Ueshima et al., 2008; Yusuf et al., 2004). Asian Americans are much less likely to be current smokers than NHWs, African Americans, and Native Americans (Ye, Rust, Baltrus, & Daniels, 2009). However, smoking prevalence compared to other Asian American subgroups has been shown to be highest in Korean and Vietnamese males (Tang, Shimizu, & Chen, 2005), and Filipinos (Ye et al., 2009). Alcohol abstinence is generally higher for Asian Americans. Vietnamese adults (68%) have the highest percentage of lifetime abstinence from alcohol use, with rates for other Asian subgroups ranging from 32% for Japanese to 57% for Asian Indian (Barnes et al., 2008). Acculturation may influence smoking practices differently according to gender. Among Korean Americans, men smoked less and women smoked more the longer they lived in the U.S. (Song et al., 2004).

These studies highlight the variable effect of acculturation on CVD risk factors in across Asian subgroups, and suggest gender differences may also exist. Future studies should strive to assess and address lifestyle risk factors for CVD in Asian subgroups, with targeted intervention strategies.

Future Directions in Research

Until recently, few research studies have been devoted to examining CVD in Asian Americans. According to a study conducted in 2003, only 0.2% of federal funding was given to health research in Asian Americans and Pacific Islanders between 1986 and 2000 (Ghosh, 2003). Despite efforts by national organizations, such as the American Heart Association to devote more resources to examining CVD in Asian Americans, (Palaniappan, Araneta, Assimes, et al., 2010) there is still a lack of data and research regarding this topic. To address this gap, President Obama signed an Executive Order, in 2009, calling for strategies to improve the health of and seeking data on health disparities in Asian American subgroups (U.S. White House Office of the Press Secretary 2009).

The study of Asian Americans offers important opportunities and challenges for CVD research. Much of the existing work highlights the variability among Asian subgroups, and reinforces the need to study individual Asian subgroups separately. With over 1.1 billion people living in India, and over 1.3 billion in China (Central Intelligence Agency, 2010), there are remarkable opportunities for cardiovascular disease research in Asian Americans to have a global impact. Specific improvements can be made to better assess the health of Asian Americans, including but are not limited to improvement of data collection and the development of new research studies.

Improvement of Data Collection

The existing data have many limitations which affect the study of CVD in Asian Americans. National surveys should oversample Asian Americans and ensure representation across the six largest subgroups of country of origin. Sampling should recognize the wide range of socioeconomic status among Asian American subgroups and focus on underserved populations, such as Korean and Vietnamese, and on very high-risk groups such as Asian Indians and Filipinos. Studies that do include Asian Americans should be expanded to include at least the six largest Asian American subgroups. Researchers should make sure that findings for one Asian subgroup should not be generalized to another. Race/ethnicity collection changes also need to be made within the healthcare system. Asian American subgroups should be identified on death certificates, hospital discharge information, and population-based studies. The National Registry of Myocardial Infarction should identify specific Asian American subgroups on data collection forms. In addition, a Stroke Registry should be established that identifies the various Asian American subgroups in order to determine differences in stroke incidence and risk factors (Klatsky et al., 2005; Nguyen-Huynh & Johnston, 2005).

Research Opportunities

There is a dearth of data on CVD in Asian Americans, particularly for Asian American subgroups. Research studies should be developed that examine the following areas: treatment patterns and outcomes, risk prediction models that account for the different prevalence and relative importance of CVD risk factors in Asian American subgroups, cultural and structural barriers to CVD care, and culturally specific lifestyle and medical interventions to address CVD risk factors in Asian American subgroups.

As the Asian American population continues to grow, it is imperative to accurately assess and address CVD health disparities in Asian American subgroups. The limited data currently available suggest substantial variability in CVD risk and incidence across Asian American subgroups. Opportunities to study health disparities in this diverse population will improve CVD prevention and treatment of Asians in the United States.

References

Allison, M. A., Criqui, M. H., McClelland, R. L., Scott, J. M., McDermott, M. M., Liu, K., et al. (2006). The effect of novel cardiovascular risk factors on the ethnic-specific odds for peripheral arterial disease in the Multi-Ethnic Study of Atherosclerosis (MESA). *Journal of the American College of Cardiology, 48,* 1190–1197.

Ayala, C., Croft, J. B., Greenlund, K. J., Keenan, N. L., Donehoo, R. S., Malarcher, A. M., et al. (2002). Sex differences in US mortality rates for stroke and stroke subtypes by race/ethnicity and age, 1995-1998. *Stroke, 33,* 1197–1201.

Barnes, P. M., Adams, P. F., & Powell-Griner, E. (2008). Health characteristics of the Asian adult population: United States, 2004-2006. *Advance Data No., 394*, 1–22.

Benfante, R. (1992). Studies of cardiovascular disease and cause-specific mortality trends in Japanese-American men living in Hawaii and risk factor comparisons with other Japanese populations in the Pacific region: A review. *Human Biology, 64*, 791–805.

Bild, D. E., Bluemke, D. A., Burke, G. L., Detrano, R., Roux, A. V. D., Folsom, A. R., et al. (2002). Multi-ethnic study of atherosclerosis: Objectives and design. *American Journal of Epidemiology, 156*, 871–881.

Bryant, L. L., Chin, N. P., Cottrell, L. A., Duckles, J. M., Fernandez, I. D., Garces, D. M., et al. (2010). Perceptions of cardiovascular health in underserved communities. *Preventing Chronic Disease, 7*, A30.

Burchfiel, C. M., Sharp, D. S., Curb, J. D., Rodriguez, B. L., Hwang, L.-J., Marcus, E. B., et al. (1995). Physical activity and incidence of diabetes: The Honolulu heart program. *American Journal of Epidemiology, 141*, 360–368.

Canto, J. G., Taylor, H. A., Jr., Rogers, W. J., Sanderson, B., Hilbe, J., & Barron, H. V. (1998). Presenting characteristics, treatment patterns, and clinical outcomes of non-black minorities in the National Registry of Myocardial Infarction 2. *American Journal of Cardiology, 82*, 1013–1018.

Carlisle, D. M., Leake, B. D., & Shapiro, M. F. (1995). Racial and ethnic differences in the use of invasive cardiac procedures among cardiac patients in Los Angeles County, 1986 through 1988. *American Journal of Public Health, 85*, 352–356.

Centers for Disease Control and Prevention. (2004). Disparities in premature deaths from heart disease-50 States and the District of Columbia, 2001. *MMWR Morbidity and Mortality Weekly Report, 53*, 121–125.

Central Intelligence Agency. (2010). The world fact book. Retrieved December 14, 2010, from https://www.cia.gov/library/publications/the-world-factbook/index.html.

Choi, S., Rankin, S., Stewart, A., & Oka, R. (2008). Perceptions of coronary heart disease risk in Korean immigrants with type 2 diabetes. *Diabetes Educator, 34*, 484–492.

Coronado, G. D., Woodall, E. D., Do, H., Li, L., Yasui, Y., & Taylor, V. M. (2008). Heart disease prevention practices among immigrant Vietnamese women. *Journal of Women's Health, 17*, 1293–1300.

Corrado, E., Rizzo, M., Coppola, G., Fattouch, K., Novo, G., Marturana, I., et al. (2010). An update on the role of markers of inflammation in atherosclerosis. *Journal of Atherosclerosis and Thrombosis, 17*, 1–11.

Cossrow, N., & Falkner, B. (2004). Race/ethnic issues in obesity and obesity-related comorbidities. *The Journal of Clinical Endocrinology & Metabolism, 89*, 2590–2594.

Criqui, M. H., Vargas, V., Denenberg, J. O., Ho, E., Allison, M., Langer, R. D., et al. (2005). Ethnicity and peripheral arterial disease: The San Diego population study. *Circulation, 112*, 2703–2707.

Davis, A. M., Vinci, L. M., Okwuosa, T. M., Chase, A. R., & Huang, E. S. (2007). Cardiovascular health disparities: A systematic review of health care interventions. *Medical Care Research and Review, 64*, 29S–100S.

Dawber, T. R., Meadors, G. F., & Moore, F. E., Jr. (1951). Epidemiological approaches to heart disease: The Framingham study. *American Journal of Public Health Nations Health, 41*, 279–281.

Diamond, L. C., Wilson-Stronks, A., & Jacobs, E. A. (2010). Do hospitals measure up to the national culturally and linguistically appropriate services standards? *Medical Care, 48*, 1080–1087.

Eastwood, J.-A., & Doering, L. V. (2005). Gender differences in coronary artery disease. *Journal of Cardiovascular Nursing, 20*, 340–351.

Fang, J., Foo, S. H., Fung, C., Wylie-Rosett, J., & Alderman, M. H. (2006). Stroke risk among Chinese immigrants in New York city. *Journal of Immigrant Minority Health, 8*, 387–393.

Fang, J., Foo, S. H., Jeng, J.-S., Yip, P.-K., & Alderman, M. H. (2004). Clinical characteristics of stroke among Chinese in New York City. *Ethnicity & Disease, 14*, 378–383.

Flores, G. (2006). Language barriers to health care in the United States. *The New England Journal of Medicine, 355*, 229–231.

Fonarow, G. C., French, W. J., & Frederick, P. D. (2009). Trends in the use of lipid-lowering medications at discharge in patients with acute myocardial infarction: 1998 to 2006. *American Heart Journal, 157*, 185–194.

George, M. G., Tong, X., McGruder, H., Yoon, P., Rosamond, W., Winquist, A., et al. (2009). Paul Coverdell national acute stroke registry surveillance – four states, 2005–2007. *Morbidity and Mortality Weekly Report: Surveillance Summaries, 58*, 1–23.

Ghosh, C. (2003). Healthy people 2010 and Asian Americans/Pacific Islanders: Defining a baseline of information. *American Journal of Public Health, 93*, 2093–2098.

Gonzalez-Fernandez, M., Kuhlemeier, K. V., & Palmer, J. B. (2008). Racial disparities in the development of dysphagia after stroke: Analysis of the California (MIRCal) and New York (SPARCS) inpatient databases. *Archives of Physical Medicine and Rehabilitation, 89*, 1358–1365.

Han, H.-R., Kim, K. B., Kang, J., Jeong, S., Kim, E.-Y., & Kim, M. T. (2007). Knowledge, beliefs, and behaviors about hypertension control among middle-aged Korean Americans with hypertension. *Journal of Community Health, 32*, 324–342.

Hemann, B. A., Bimson, W. F., & Taylor, A. J. (2007). The Framingham risk score: An appraisal of its benefits and limitations. *The American Heart Hospital Journal, 5*, 91–96.

Heron, M. (2010). Deaths: Leading causes for 2006. *National Vital Statistics Reports, 58*, 1–95.

Higdon, J. V., & Frei, B. (2003). Tea catechins and polyphenols: Health effects, metabolism, and antioxidant functions. *Critical Reviews in Food Science and Nutrition, 43*, 89–143.

Hirsch, A. T., Criqui, M. H., Treat-Jacobson, D., Regensteiner, J. G., Creager, M. A., Olin, J. W., et al. (2001). Peripheral arterial disease detection, awareness, and treatment in primary care. *Journal of the American Medical Association, 286*, 1317–1324.

Holland, Ariel T., Wong, Eric C., Lauderdale, Diane S., & Palaniappan, Latha P. (2011). Spectrum of cardiovascular diseases in Asians-American racial/ethnic subgroups. *Annals of Epidemiology, 21*, 608–614.

Hwu, C. M., Hsiao, C.-F., Kuo, S.-W., Wu, K.-D., Ting, C.-T., Quertermous, T., et al. (2004). Physical inactivity is an important lifestyle determinant of insulin resistance in hypertensive patients. *Blood Pressure, 13*, 355–361.

Kagawa-Singer, M., & Kassim-Lakha, S. (2003). A strategy to reduce cross-cultural miscommunication and increase the likelihood of improving health outcomes. *Academic Medicine, 78*, 577–587.

Kandula, N. R., & Lauderdale, D. S. (2005). Leisure time, non-leisure time, and occupational physical activity in Asian Americans. *Annals of Epidemiology, 15*, 257–265.

Klatsky, A. L., Friedman, G. D., Sidney, S., Kipp, H., Kubo, A., & Armstrong, M. A. (2005). Risk of hemorrhagic stroke in Asian American ethnic groups. *Neuroepidemiology, 25*, 26–31.

Klatsky, A. L., & Tekawa, I. (2005). Health problems and hospitalizations among Asian-American ethnic groups. *Ethnicity Disease, 15*, 753–760.

Kuzawa, C. W., & Sweet, E. (2009). Epigenetics and the embodiment of race: Developmental origins of US racial disparities in cardiovascular health. *American Journal of Human Biology, 21*, 2–15.

Lloyd-Jones, D., Adams, R. J., Brown, T. M., Carnethon, M., Dai, S., De Simone, G., et al. (2010). Heart disease and stroke statistics–2010 update: A report from the American Heart Association. *Circulation, 121*, e46–e215.

Lusis, A. J. (2000). Atherosclerosis. *Nature, 407*, 233–241.

Marmot, M. G., & Syme, S. L. (1976). Acculturation and coronary heart disease in Japanese-Americans. *American Journal of Epidemiology, 104*, 225–247.

Marmot, M. G., Syme, S. L., Kagan, A., Kato, H., Cohen, J. B., & Belsky, J. (1975). Epidemiologic studies of coronary heart disease and stroke in Japanese men living in Japan, Hawaii and California: Prevalence of coronary and hypertensive heart disease and associated risk factors. *American Journal of Epidemiology, 102*, 514–525.

Merchant, A. T., Kelemen, L. E., de Koning, L., Lonn, E., Vuksan, V., Jacobs, R., et al. (2008). Interrelation of saturated fat, trans fat, alcohol intake, and subclinical atherosclerosis. *American Journal of Clinical Nutrition, 87*, 168–174.

Misra, A., & Khurana, L. (2009). The metabolic syndrome in south Asians: Epidemiology, determinants, and prevention. *Metabolic Syndrome Related Disorders, 7*, 497–514.

Narayan, K. M. V., Aviles-Santa, L., Oza-Frank, R., Pandey, M., Curb, J. D., McNeely, M., et al. (2010). Report of a National Heart, Lung, and Blood Institute Workshop: Heterogeneity in cardiometabolic risk in Asian Americans in the U.S. opportunities for research. *Journal of the American College of Cardiology, 55*, 966–973.

National Center for Health Statistics, Centers for Disease Control and Prevention. (2001). Report to evaluate the U.S. standard certificates.

National Center for Health Statistics, Centers for Disease Control and Prevention. (2006). National Health and Nutrition Examination Survey: Screener module #1.

National Center for Health Statistics, Centers for Disease Control and Prevention. (2007). *National Health and Nutrition Examination Survey, 2007-2008: Let's improve our health.* Hyattsville, MD: National Center for Health Statistics, Centers for Disease Control and Prevention.

National Center for Health Statistics, Centers for Disease Control and Prevention. (2009a). 2008 NHIS questionnaire – sample adult adult identification.

National Center for Health Statistics, Centers for Disease Control and Prevention. (2009b). *Health, United States, 2008 with special feature on the health of young adults* (Vol. DHHS publication No. 2009-1232). Hyattsville, MD: National Center for Health Statistics.

National Center for Health Statistics, Centers for Disease Control and Prevention. (2010). National Health and Nutrition Examination Survey: Note on 2007-2008 sampling methodology. Retrieved February 15, 2010, from http://www.cdc.gov/nchs/nhanes/nhanes2007-2008/sampling_0708.htm.

Nguyen, T. T., Liao, Y., Gildengorin, G., Tsoh, J., Bui-Tong, N., & McPhee, S. J. (2009). Cardiovascular risk factors and knowledge of symptoms among Vietnamese Americans. *Journal of General Internal Medicine, 24*, 238–243.

Nguyen-Huynh, M. N., & Johnston, S. C. (2005). Regional variation in hospitalization for stroke among Asians/Pacific Islanders in the United States: A nationwide retrospective cohort study. *BMC Neurology, 5*, 21.

Office of Minority Health and Bureau of Primary Health Care, Health Resources and Services Administration. (2005). Reducing health disparities in Asian American & Pacific Islander populations: What is cultural competence. Retrieved February 8, 2011, from http://erc.msh.org/aapi/cc4.html.

Office of Minority Health, U.S. Department of Health and Human Services. (2010). Asian American/Pacific Islander profile. Retrieved February 8, 2011, from http://minorityhealth.hhs.gov/templates/browse.aspx?lvl=3&lvlid=29.

Oza-Frank, R., Ali, M. K., Vaccarino, V., & Narayan, K. M. V. (2009). Asian Americans: Diabetes prevalence across U.S. and World Health Organization weight classifications. *Diabetes Care, 32*, 1644–1646.

Palaniappan, L. P., Araneta, M. R., Assimes, T. L., Barrett-Connor, E., Carnethon, M. R., Criqui, M. H., et al.

(2010). Call to action: Cardiovascular disease in Asian Americans: A science advisory from the American Heart Association. *Circulation, 122,* 1242–1252.

Palaniappan, L. P., Mukherjea, A., Holland, A., & Ivey, S. L. (2010). Leading causes of mortality of Asian Indians in California. *Ethnicity & Disease, 20,* 53–57.

Palaniappan, L., Wang, Y., & Fortmann, S. P. (2004). Coronary heart disease mortality for six ethnic groups in California, 1990-2000. *Annals of Epidemiology, 14,* 499–506.

Pleis, J. R., Lucas, J. W., & Ward, B. W. (2009). Summary health statistics for U.S. adults: National Health Interview Survey, 2008. *Vital Health Statistics, 10,* 1–157.

Popkin, B. M., Horton, S., Kim, S., Mahal, A., & Shuigao, J. (2001). Trends in diet, nutritional status, and diet-related noncommunicable diseases in China and India: The economic costs of the nutrition transition. *Nutrition Reviews, 59,* 379–390.

Ren, J., & Kelley, R. O. (2009). Cardiac health in women with metabolic syndrome: Clinical aspects and pathophysiology. *Obesity, 17,* 1114–1123.

Rodriguez, B. L., D'Agostino, R., Abbott, R. D., Kagan, A., Burchfiel, C. M., Yano, K., et al. (2002). Risk of hospitalized stroke in men enrolled in the Honolulu Heart Program and the Framingham study: A comparison of incidence and risk factor effects. *Stroke, 33,* 230–236.

Schwartz, S. J., Unger, J. B., Zamboanga, B. L., & Szapocznik, J. (2010). Rethinking the concept of acculturation: Implications for theory and research. *American Psychologist, 65,* 237–251.

Sechena, R., Liao, S., Lorenzana, R., Nakano, C., Polissar, N., & Fenske, R. (2003). Asian American and Pacific Islander seafood consumption – a community-based study in King county, Washington. *Journal of Exposure Analysis and Environmental Epidemiology, 13,* 256–266.

Song, Y. J., Hofstetter, C. R., Hovell, M. F., Paik, H. Y., Park, H. R., Lee, J., et al. (2004). Acculturation and health risk behaviors among Californians of Korean descent. *Preventive Medicine, 39,* 147–156.

Spatz, E. S., Ross, J. S., Desai, M. M., Canavan, M. E., & Krumholz, H. M. (2010). Beyond insurance coverage: Usual source of care in the treatment of hypertension and hypercholesterolemia. Data from the 2003-2006 National Health and Nutrition Examination Survey. *American Heart Journal, 160,* 115–121.

Tang, H., Shimizu, R., & Chen, M. S., Jr. (2005). English language proficiency and smoking prevalence among California's Asian Americans. *Cancer, 104,* 2982–2988.

Taylor, V. M., Yasui, Y., Tu, S.-P., Neuhouser, M. L., Li, L., Woodall, E., et al. (2007). Heart disease prevention among Chinese immigrants. *Journal of Community Health, 32,* 299–310.

Taylor-Piliae, R. E., Haskell, W. L., & Froelicher, E. S. (2006). Hemodynamic responses to a community-based Tai Chi exercise intervention in ethnic Chinese adults with cardiovascular disease risk factors. *European Journal of Cardiovascular Nursing, 5,* 165–174.

The Kaiser Family Foundation. (2008). Health coverage and access to care among Asian Americans, Native Hawaiians, and Pacific Islanders. *Race, Ethnicity, & Health Care Fact Sheet.* Menlo Park, CA: Kaiser Family Foundation.

Ton, T. G., Steinman, L., Yip, M.-P., Ly, K. A., Sin, M.-K., Fitzpatrick, A. L., et al. (2010). Knowledge of cardiovascular health among Chinese, Korean and Vietnamese immigrants to the US. *Journal of Immigrant Minority Health, 13*(1), 127–139.

U.S. White House Office of the Press Secretary. (2009, October 14). Executive Order: Increasing Participation of Asian Americans. Retrieved from http://www.whitehouse.gov/the-press-office/executive-order-asian-american-and-pacific-islander-community.

U.S. Census Bureau. (2001). Introduction to Census 2000 Data Products.

U.S. Census Bureau. (2008). B02006. Asian alone by selected groups. American Community Survey, 2006-2008.

U.S. Census Bureau. (2010). What is the census? Retrieved December 12, 2010, from http://2010.census.gov/2010census/about/.

Ueshima, H., Sekikawa, A., Miura, K., Turin, T. C., Takashima, N., Kita, Y., et al. (2008). Cardiovascular disease and risk factors in Asia: A selected review. *Circulation, 118,* 2702–2709.

Wild, S. H., Laws, A., Fortmann, S. P., Varady, A. N., & Byrne, C. D. (1995). Mortality from coronary heart disease and stroke for six ethnic groups in California, 1985 to 1990. *Annals of Epidemiology, 5,* 432–439.

Yagalla, M. V., Hoerr, S. L., Song, W. O., Enas, E., & Garg, A. (1996). Relationship of diet, abdominal obesity, and physical activity to plasma lipoprotein levels in Asian Indian physicians residing in the United States. *Journal of the American Dietetic Association, 96,* 257–261.

Ye, J., Rust, G., Baltrus, P., & Daniels, E. (2009). Cardiovascular risk factors among Asian Americans: Results from a National Health Survey. *Annals of Epidemiology, 19,* 718–723.

Yusuf, S., Hawken, S., Ounpuu, S., Dans, T., Avezum, A., Lanas, F., et al. (2004). Effect of potentially modifiable risk factors associated with myocardial infarction in 52 countries (the INTERHEART study): Case-control study. *Lancet, 364,* 937–952.

Diabetes: A Growing Concern in the Asian American Community

17

Ranjita Misra

Introduction

Diabetes is a chronic disorder characterized by high blood glucose and either insufficient or ineffective insulin, depending on the type of diabetes. The prevalence and incidence of diabetes and pre-diabetes [as defined by impaired fasting glucose (IFG) or impaired glucose tolerance (IGT)] are rapidly increasing both in developed and developing countries (Chiasson, Brindisi, & Rabasa-Lhoret, 2005). Diabetes is a serious disease that is associated with long-term complications that may affect a person's quality of life (Chandie Shaw et al., 2002). Overall, diabetes incidence and prevalence rates have been increasing for all racial groups in the US (Manson et al., 1991). Compared to whites and the general US population, Asian Americans in the US have had a consistently higher rates of new cases of diabetes (termed as incidence rate that arise during a specific period of time) over the last decade, with 9.5 new cases of diabetes per 1,000 Asian Americans in 2006 compared to 7.6 new cases per 1,000 in the general population (OMH, 2006; Tong et al., 2007). Likewise, prevalence rates for diabetes (defined as the total number of cases with diabetes) have also increased for Asians

over the past decade, and have overtaken those of whites and the general US population (see chart 17.1: Prevalence of diabetes by race). While diabetes was less prevalent among Asian Americans compared to the general population in 1999 (at 34/1,000 vs. 41/1,000 respectively), the 2006 prevalence figures show there is a reverse in trend, and that diabetes has become more prevalent among Asian Americans (61/1,000) than in the general population (57/1,000). By 2006, both the incidence and prevalence of diabetes in the Asian American community have escalated beyond the rates of the general US population.

Types of Diabetes

Type 1 diabetes also known as insulin dependent diabetes or juvenile onset diabetes typically strikes around the ages of 8–12 years but can occur at any age (Ramachandran, Snehalatha, Tuomilehto-Wolf, et al., 1999). The disease has a strong genetic link. The pancreas cannot synthesize insulin thereby altering the body's metabolism. Insulin is required to assist the cells in taking up the needed fuels from the blood.

By contrast, type 2 diabetes is characterized by high blood glucose and insulin resistance (Fujimoto et al., 2000). This disease usually begins after the second decade of life. However the widespread changes in lifestyle and dietary practices have resulted in the appearance of this disease at a much younger age. The person may actually have insulin levels that are higher than

R. Misra (✉)
Department of Health and Kinesiology,
College of Education and Human Development,
Center for the Study of Health Disparities (CSHD),
College Station, TX, USA
e-mail: Ranjita.misra@osumc.edu

G.J. Yoo et al. (eds.), *Handbook of Asian American Health*,
DOI 10.1007/978-1-4614-2227-3_17, © Springer Science+Business Media, LLC 2013

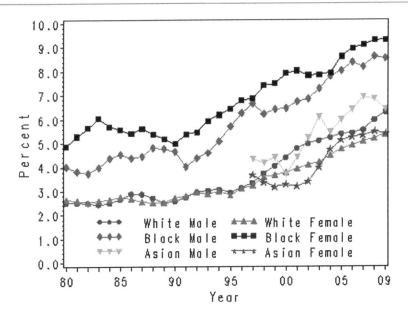

Chart 17.1 Prevalence of diabetes by race (age adjusted per 1,000 standard population) (*Source*: Centers for Disease Control, Healthy People 2010 Database (http://wonder.cdc.gov/))

average, but the receptor cells are either fewer in number or are malfunctioning. Consequently, the blood glucose levels increase thereby stimulating the pancreas to produce insulin. This exhausts the cells and reduces their ability to function. Generalized weight gain particularly in the abdominal region aggravates the condition because the higher body fat necessitates higher insulin production.

The main etiological (causal) risk factors for type 2 diabetes are older age, obesity, family history, physical inactivity and dietary factors such as a high proportion of energy consumed as saturated fat and low intake of fruit and vegetables (Chiasson et al., 2005). The rapid rise and epidemiological transition in Asian countries like India and China, especially in urban areas, is associated with westernized lifestyle. Changes in the traditional lifestyles, dietary patterns and technological advancement has resulted in a pronounced physical inactivity and the affluence of society has lead to consumption of diets rich in fat, sugar and calories. There is also an association between low birth weight and the risk of diabetes in later life has also led to the development of an alternative to

the thrifty genotype hypothesis. It is hypothesized that the risk of type 2 diabetes is programmed by fetal nutrition and the pattern of early growth (McNeely & Boyko, 2004). The causal nature of these associations is strengthened by studies that show the incidence of diabetes is reduced by interventions aimed at reducing weight, increasing activity and improving diet (Bajaj & Banerji, 2004). Symptoms of diabetes include frequent urination, excessive thirst, extreme hunger, unusual weight loss, increased fatigue, irritability, and blurred vision.

Criteria for diagnosis includes:

– Symptoms of diabetes together with casual (any time of day) plasma glucose concentrations of >200 mg/dl.
– Fasting plasma glucose (At least 8 h following no caloric intake) >26/dl.
– Two hour plasma glucose >200 mg/dl during an oral glucose tolerance test.

Criteria for *impaired glucose levels* includes:

– Fasting plasma glucose levels of > 100–126 mg/dl or post-prandial glucose levels (2 h after meals) of > than 140 mg/dl during an oral glucose tolerance test can be considered to be in the Impaired blood glucose range.

While the overall risk for diabetes is now higher among Asian Americans than in the general population, important subgroup differences exist within the larger Asian American community. Asian Americans are comprised of approximately 50 subgroups (OMH, 2006). Some of the Asian subgroups, e.g., Filipino, multiple-race Asians, and South Asians have been reported to have significantly higher rates of diabetes (generally over 10%) and diabetes-related mortality than Caucasians and other ethnic groups in the United Kingdom, Canada, Singapore, and South Africa.

Despite limited data, adjusted prevalence of diabetes is higher among Asian Americans that in the general U.S. population. Similarly, gestational diabetes is observed in women who exhibit high blood glucose levels during pregnancy without previously diagnosed diabetes. This condition was more often observed in a survey of South and Central Asian populations residing in New York, including women from Afghanistan, Bangladesh, Bhutan, Ceylon, India, Kashmir, Kazakhstan, Maldives, Nepal, Pakistan, Sri Lanka, Tajikistan, Turkmenistan, Uzbekistan, or others of Hindu or Sikh ancestry (Thorpe et al., 2005). However, self-report data for diabetes is lower for these individuals compared to other individuals, suggesting a higher rate of undiagnosed diabetes in this group (Bhopal et al., 1999).

The risk factors – or variables or conditions that increases one's risk for developing a disease – for type 2 diabetes (previously known as adult onset diabetes) includes age, obesity, body fat distribution, physical inactivity, family history of diabetes, previous gestation diabetes, being a member of a minority group, elevated fasting glucose levels, impaired glucose tolerance, and insulin resistance. These risk factors have not been systematically assessed in migrant Asian Americans, nor have changes in these factors as they acculturate to western society received attention. Current national surveys are incapable of assessing risk factors and disease prevalence in specific Asian sub-populations because multiple ethnic groups are aggregated into the general category of "Asian and Pacific Islander," and because sample sizes of individual Asian sub-groups are small.

Insulin Resistance and Diabetes

Insulin resistance occurs when the pancreas produces insulin, but the individual's body cannot use the insulin properly. A genetic antecedent for the disease is likely as insulin resistance tends to run in families. Excess fat interferes with the ability of muscles to use insulin, so that weight gain also contributes to insulin resistance. Lack of exercise further reduces muscles' ability to use insulin. Many people with insulin resistance and high blood glucose have excess weight around the waist, high LDL (bad) blood cholesterol levels, low HDL (good) cholesterol levels, high levels of triglycerides (another fat in the blood), and high blood pressure (Esperat, Inouye, Gonzalez, Owen, & Feng, 2004). All of these conditions also put the heart at risk. This combination of problems is referred to as the metabolic syndrome, or the insulin resistance syndrome (formerly called Syndrome X). Metabolic syndrome is defined as a clustering of risk factors with the presence of three or more of the following: abdominal obesity, low levels of HDL, high levels of serum triglyceride, high blood pressure, and high blood glucose levels.

Metabolic Syndrome

Metabolic syndrome is a condition closely related to insulin resistance (Tillin et al., 2005). Abdominal obesity and insulin resistance aggravate the disease along with hypertension and abnormal lipid levels (Razak et al., 2005).

Diagnostic criteria put out by the International Diabetes Federation include a waist circumference of >90 cm for men and 80 cm for women; a triglyceride level of >150 mg/dl; a HDL-cholesterol level of <40 mg/dl for men and <50 mg/dl for women; a blood pressure of >130/85 mmHg and a fasting plasma glucose of >100 mg/dl or previously diagnosed type 2 Diabetes (Ford, 2005).

Complications of Diabetes

The accumulation of glucose in the blood leads to acute and chronic complications. Therefore early, aggressive treatment to control blood glucose significantly reduces the risk of long term diabetes related complications. Diabetes related complications include diseases involving:

- large blood vessels such as atherosclerosis.
- small blood vessels resulting in loss of kidney function as seen in kidney diseases, retinal degeneration and blindness.
- nerves resulting in loss of sensation, increased infections stemming from unnoticed injuries, and gastrointestinal problems.

Higher Risk at Lower Body Mass Index

Many studies suggest that "healthy" adult Asian Americans have abnormal body composition characterized by an excessive percentage of total body fat and abdominal fat, which may contribute to certain risk factors. Other abnormalities include higher fat in the abdomen area and around the buttocks. Further, Asian Americans have lower waist circumferences but comparable ratios of waist-to-hip circumference compared to Caucasians (Deurenberg, Yap, & van Staveren, 1998). Such abnormalities may contribute to the development of insulin resistance and high levels of blood cholesterol and/or triglyceride levels (sometimes referred to as dyslipidemia). Hence in 2000, the World Health Organization Western Pacific Region (WHO-WPR) and the International Association for the Study of Obesity and International Obesity Task Force jointly recommended a revised cutoff of body mass index (BMI; a ratio of weight to height) ≥ 23 and ≥ 25 kg/m^2 for redefining overweight and obesity, respectively, in Asian populations (World Health Organization Western Pacific Region, 2000). First-generation Asian Americans tend to have lower body mass when compared to other ethnic groups. As a result, many Asian Americans are not routinely screened for diabetes during a doctor's visit even though some subgroups have higher prevalence of type 2 diabetes than the general population. However,

second-generation Asian Americans actually have abnormal body compositions mass and a greater risk of developing type 2 diabetes at a younger age. For example, Japanese Americans are twice as likely to develop type 2 diabetes as compared to non-Hispanic whites even though they are less obese (Fujimoto et al., 2000).

The average body mass index in Asian Americans is lower than in white Caucasians, Mexican Americans and African Americans. BMI increases as individuals become affluent and westernized. Among several Asian subgroups, being born in the US is associated with having a higher BMI. Further, a high prevalence of abdominal obesity is a risk factor and is characteristic of South Asians. Importantly, increased abdominal adiposity has been reported in those with BMI <25 kg/m^2. Although the average waist circumference in some Asian subgroups appears to be lower than in Caucasians, abdominal adiposity is significantly greater among the former group. The impact of a "westernized" lifestyle, physical inactivity, information on chronic diseases as well as access to health care upon the body fat patterning of US Asian Americans has not been investigated.

Behavioral, Environmental, and Cultural Factors Related to Diabetes Among Asian Americans

Important cultural factors impacting diabetes risk include ethnic customs and cultural and health beliefs that influence dietary intake and physical activity (Hsu & Yoon, 2007). Environmental factors that impact the incidence and complications of diabetes include socioeconomic status (assessed by income and educational level of individuals) and health care access and utilization. Socioeconomic status plays a decisive role in an individual's access to open spaces, sports equipment, and exercise facilities. Lack of opportunities for physical activity is only one indicator supporting the observation that low-income populations, across all age groups, experience higher rates of disease and deaths associated with diabetes and CVD (Pradeepa et al., 2003). An individual's degree of acculturation influences dietary intake and utilization of health care. Immigrants who have lived in the US for longer periods of time and with higher degrees of acculturation (defined as adoption of behavior and assimilation into the host culture) may have different lifestyles than those who report fewer years of residence or lesser degrees of acculturation (Patel et al., 2005). Second generation and acculturated Asian Americans have higher body mass mostly due to their western lifestyle (Lv & Cason, 2004).

As Asian Americans adapt to the American culture, dietary changes (i.e. the "Americanization" of traditional Asian diets) occur with increased fat, saturated fat and protein and fewer grains and vegetables that impact on the risk of developing chronic diseases such as type 2 diabetes and cardiovascular disease among other conditions (Misra, Wasir, & Vikram, 2005a). These dietary changes have been noted among Korean Americans and Japanese Americans with immigration to the United States (Yang, Chung, Kim, Bianchi, & Song, 2007). Use of the Diabetes Food Pyramid can help individuals with diabetes.

It is noteworthy that inherent in the Asian diet is white rice. Unfortunately, rice is high on the glycemic index, a measurement of the effect of carbohydrates on blood glucose levels. The consumption of rice can cause a rapid spike, then a drop in blood glucose (Yang et al, 2007). In contrast, high fiber foods tend to be lower on the glycemic index and have a more gradual effect on blood glucose (Jonnalagadda, Diwan, & Cohen, 2005; Snehalatha, Sivasankari, Satyavani, Vijay, & Ramachandran, 2000). A diet that includes more vegetables would provide a good source of fiber.

Food habits are changing among Asian Americans in the US, particularly among adolescents, due to the attractive and aggressive advertisement campaigns of the fast food industry, low cost, and peer pressure to "fit in." The changes include consuming fast foods such as hamburgers and pizza while increasing dietary fat, calories and salt (Raj, Ganganna, & Bowering, 1999). Each of these practices results in a less than adequate intake of foods of appropriate nutritional value. Furthermore, teenagers also show a preference for sedentary activities such as watching TV and playing video games (Misra, Patel, Davies, & Russo, 2000). Activity

profiles of individuals also vary based on socioeconomic status, location of residence, and years of residence in the US. Families who are less acculturated might be more likely to live in low-income neighborhoods where safe areas for physical activity are not available, fast-food restaurants are more prevalent, and healthy foods are less easily available. While some have become more aware of the benefits of physical activity and exercise, physical inactivity is still more common among Asian American immigrants than other ethnic groups (Ramachandran, Snehalatha, Shobana, Vidyavathi, & Vijay, 1999). Increased years in the US tend to increase the risk for obesity-related behaviors among Asian Americans (Yang et al., 2007).

Among lifestyle factors, physical activity, alcohol and tobacco use are important determinants of an adverse metabolic profile. Smoking is highly prevalent in some subgroups, especially the Vietnamese, Filipino, and Japanese Americans at an earlier age. Activity levels of most immigrant Asians are less as compared to their white peers. Sedentary lifestyle is a critical factor for the development of insulin resistance and excess cardiovascular risk in South Asians, but one that has been sparsely investigated. Obesity is also linked to diet and physical activity. The genetic predisposition of some Asian subgroups (e.g., South Asians) coupled with physical inactivity, abdominal obesity, and lifestyle changes can lead to early onset of chronic diseases (Merchant, et al., 2005; Misra, Wasir, & Vikram, 2005b).

Dietary Recommendations for Type 1 Diabetes

Nutrition is an important part of the treatment regimen. Focus is on meal intake patterns and consistency in carbohydrate intake to minimize glucose fluctuations.

Nutritional therapy should focus on:
- Maintaining optimal nutrition for growth and development in the child
- Educating clients about portion sizes
- Modifying recipes
- Controlling blood glucose
- Preventing and treating related complications

Dietary Recommendations for Type 2 Diabetes

The American Diabetes Association recommends that the distribution of calories between fats and carbohydrates should be individualized according to the individual's assessment and treatment plan.

- Calories should be prescribed to maintain a reasonable body weight ideal for the person's age, sex and lifecycle needs.
- Protein intake is recommended at 10–20% of caloric intake with a focus on plant based sources such as lentils and beans, cereal lentil combinations and the use of smaller portions of lean meats, poultry and fish.
- Total fat, saturated fat and cholesterol intakes must be tailored to meet individual requirements based on blood lipid profiles. Focus on healthy fats rather than saturated fats and emphasize avoidance of trans-fats.
- Diet should focus on the consumption of complex carbohydrates such as whole grains, fruits and vegetables. Consistent and evenly spaced carbohydrate intake throughout the day should be emphasized. In this respect carbohydrate counting and exchange lists provided in this book will help.
- Current guidelines advise moderation of salt intake that is <1,500 mg. of sodium/day and no more than 2,300 mg. of sodium/day.

Diabetic patients can seek help from a trained nutrition professional i.e., a registered dietitian (RD) (visit www.eatright.org and click on the link to "Find a Nutrition Professional" to find a RD). A dietitian can help you focus on dietary modification and therapeutic lifestyle changes (e.g., increasing physical activity, smoking cessation, alcohol consumption in moderation, stress reduction).

Future Research

There are several myths about Asian Americans and diabetes addressed in this chapter. With current national studies incapable of assessing prevalence and risk factors for Asian subgroups, national (epidemiological) studies on Asian Americans can help achieve the Healthy People 2010 goal of eliminating health disparities as well as quantify the incidence/prevalence rates and understand the risk factors and disease mechanisms in this group. With their high growth rate and disproportionately high risk of diabetes in some Asian subgroups, baseline data can help to develop culturally competent interventions with a view to reducing the burden of diabetes and improve their quality of life.

There are many programs (clinic and community-based) to help individuals prevent the early onset and/or help in better self-management. The Diabetes Prevention Program and the UK Prospective Diabetes Study have shown that lifestyle intervention is the most cost-effective strategy to prevent or manage type 2 diabetes. Prevention of the disease should be emphasized through a healthy diet, physical activity, and improved knowledge of risk factors; wellness screening can help identify asymptomatic individuals who are likely to have diabetes. The National Diabetes Education Program (NDEP) provides patient education materials and diabetes education resources in several Asian languages (Cambodian, Chamorro, Chinese, Gujarati, Hindi, Hmong, Korean, Japanese, Laotian, Samoan, Tagalog, Thai, Tongan and Vietnamese) that can be downloaded for free at http://www.ndep.nih.gov/diabetes/prev/prevention.htm. Proper management of the disease and reaching the ABC goals (A1c less than 7.0; Blood pressure less than 130/80, and cholesterol (LDL) less than 100) can help to avoid long-term complications associated with the disease. NDEP provides information on steps to control diabetes for life. Self-management is key in order to stay healthy and requires that an individual use a diabetes meal plan, eat healthy food (more fiber and less fat, sugar, and salt), maintain a healthy weight, learn to cope with stress, do not smoke, take medications, check blood glucose and blood pressure regularly, and report changes to eyesight and sores in the feet and mouth to a health care professional. Barriers and challenges to manage and control among those who have diabetes includes poor health care access, low income and education, acceptable social norms (such as smoking among Vietnamese males), language barriers, mental health conditions related to physical and mental trauma, and dealing with other chronic diseases simultaneously (Lee & Cheng, 2006). Cultural differences in understanding western medical beliefs and practices and lack of interpreter services are obstacles that need to be overcome to provide quality medical care for this ethnic group.

References

Bajaj, M., & Banerji, M. A. (2004). Type 2 diabetes in South Asians: A pathophysiologic focus on the Asian-Indian epidemic. *Current Diabetes Reports, 4,* 213–218.

Bhopal, R., Unwin, N., White, M., Yallop, J., Walker, L., Alberti, K. G., et al. (1999). Heterogeneity of coronary heart disease risk factors in Indian, Pakistani, Bangladeshi, and European origin populations: Cross sectional study. *BMJ, 319,* 215–220.

Chandie Shaw, P. K., Vandenbroucke, J. P., Tjandra, Y. I., Rosendaal, F. R., Rosman, J. B., Geerlings, W., et al. (2002). Increased end-stage diabetic nephropathy in Indo-Asian immigrants living in the Netherlands. *Diabetologia, 45,* 337–341.

Chiasson, J. L., Brindisi, M. C., & Rabasa-Lhoret, R. (2005). The prevention of type 2 diabetes: What is the evidence? *Minerva Endocrinologica, 30,* 179–191.

Deurenberg, P., Yap, M., & van Staveren, W. A. (1998). Body mass index and percent body fat: A meta analysis among different ethnic groups. *International Journal of Obesity and Related Metabolic Disorders, 22,* 1164–1171.

Dhawan, J., Bray, C. L., Warburton, R., Ghambhir, D. S., & Morris, J. (1994). Insulin resistance, high prevalence of diabetes, and cardiovascular risk in immigrant Asians. Genetic or environmental effect? *British Heart Journal, 72,* 413–421.

Esperat, M. C., Inouye, J., Gonzalez, E. W., Owen, D. C., & Feng, D. (2004). Health disparities among Asian Americans and Pacific Islanders. *Annual Review of Nursing Research, 22,* 135–159.

Ford, E. S. (2005). Prevalence of the metabolic syndrome defined by the International Diabetes Federation among adults in the U.S. *Diabetes Care, 28,* 2745–2749.

Fujimoto, W. Y., Bergstrom, R. W., Boyko, E. J., Chen, K., Kahn, S. E., Leonetti, D. L., et al. (2000). Type 2 diabetes and the metabolic syndrome in Japanese Americans. *Diabetes Research and Clinical Practice, 50*(Suppl. 2), S73–S76.

Hsu, W., & Yoon, H. (2007). Bridging Cultural Competency for Improved Diabetes Care: Asian Americans and Diabetes. *Journal of Family Practice, September,* S7–S13.

Jonnalagadda, S. S., Diwan, S., & Cohen, D. L. (2005). U.S. Food Guide Pyramid food group intake by Asian Indian immigrants in the U.S. *The Journal of Nutrition, Health & Aging, 9,* 226–231.

Lee, S. K., & Cheng, Y. Y. (2006). Reaching Asian Americans: Sampling strategies and incentives. *Journal of Immigrant and Minority Health, 8,* 245–250.

Lv, N., & Cason, K. L. (2004). Dietary pattern change and acculturation of Chinese Americans in Pennsylvania. *Journal of the American Dietetic Association, 104,* 771–778.

Manson, J. E., Colditz, G. A., Stampfer, M. J., Willett, W. C., Krolewski, A. S., Rosner, B., et al. (1991). A prospective study of maturity-onset diabetes mellitus and risk of coronary heart disease and stroke in women. *Archives of Internal Medicine, 151,* 1141–1147.

McNeely, M. J., & Boyko, E. J. (2004). Type 2 diabetes prevalence in Asian Americans: Results of a national health survey. *Diabetes Care, 27,* 66–69.

Merchant, A. T., Anand, S. S., Vuksan, V., Jacobs, R., Davis, B., Teo, K., et al. (2005). Protein intake is inversely associated with abdominal obesity in a multi-ethnic population. *Journal of Nutrition, 135,* 1196–1201.

Misra, R., Patel, T. G., Davies, D., & Russo, T. (2000). Health promotion behaviors of Gujurati Asian Indian immigrants in the United States. *Journal of Immigrant Health, 2,* 223–230.

Misra, A., Wasir, J. S., & Vikram, N. K. (2005a). Carbohydrate diets, postprandial hyperlipidaemia, abdominal obesity and Asian Indians: A recipe for atherogenic disaster. *Indian Journal of Medical Research, 121,* 5–8.

Misra, A., Wasir, J. S., & Vikram, N. K. (2005b). Waist circumference criteria for the diagnosis of abdominal obesity are not applicable uniformly to all populations and ethnic groups. *Nutrition, 21,* 969–976.

Office of Minority Health. (2006). Asian American profile. Retrieval from http://minorityhealth.hhs.gov/templates/browse.aspx?lvl=3&lvlid=29.

Patel, J. V., Vyas, A., Cruickshank, J. K., Prabhakaran, D., Hughes, E., Reddy, K. S., et al. (2005). Impact of migration on coronary heart disease risk factors: Comparison of Gujaratis in Britain and their contemporaries in villages of origin in India. *Atherosclerosis, 185*(2), 297–306.

Pradeepa, R., Deepa, R., Rani, S. S., Premalatha, G., Saroja, R., & Mohan, V. (2003). Socioeconomic status and dyslipidaemia in a South Indian population: The Chennai Urban Population Study (CUPS 11). *The National Medical Journal of India, 16,* 73–78.

Raj, S., Ganganna, P., & Bowering, J. (1999). Dietary habits of Asian Indians in relation to length of residence in the United States. *Journal of the American Dietetic Association, 99,* 1106–1108.

Ramachandran, A., Snehalatha, C., Shobana, R., Vidyavathi, P., & Vijay, V. (1999). Influence of life style factors in development of diabetes in Indians–scope for primary prevention. *The Journal of the Association of Physicians of India, 47,* 764–766.

Ramachandran, A., Snehalatha, C., Tuomilehto-Wolf, E., Vidgren, G., Ogunkolade, B. W., Vijay, V., et al. (1999). Type 1 diabetes in the offspring does not increase the risk of parental type 2 diabetes in South Indians. *Diabetes/Metabolism Research and Reviews, 15*, 328–331.

Razak, F., Anand, S., Vuksan, V., Davis, B., Jacobs, R., Teo, K. K., et al. (2005). Ethnic differences in the relationships between obesity and glucose-metabolic abnormalities: A cross-sectional population-based study. *International Journal of Obesity and Related Metabolic Disorders, 29*, 656–667.

Snehalatha, C., Sivasankari, S., Satyavani, K., Vijay, V., & Ramachandran, A. (2000). Postprandial hypertriglyceridaemia in treated type 2 diabetic subjects –the role of dietary components. *Diabetes Research and Clinical Practice, 48*, 57–60.

Thorpe, L. E., Berger, D., Ellis, J. A., Bettegowda, V. R., Brown, G., Matte, T., et al. (2005). Trends and racial/ethnic disparities in gestational diabetes among pregnant women in New York City, 1990-2001. *American Journal of Public Health, 95*, 1536–1539.

Tillin, T., Forouhi, N., Johnston, D. G., McKeigue, P. M., Chaturvedi, N., & Godsland, I. F. (2005). Metabolic syndrome and coronary heart disease in South Asians, African-Caribbeans and white Europeans: A UK population-based cross-sectional study. *Diabetologia, 48*, 649–656.

Tong, J., Boyko, E. J., Utzschneider, K. M., McNeely, M. J., Hayashi, T., Carr, D. B., et al. (2007). Intra-abdominal fat accumulation predicts the development of the metabolic syndrome in non-diabetic Japanese-Americans. *Diabetologia, 50*, 1156–1160.

World Health Organization Western Pacific Region. (2000). *The Asia-Pacific perspective: Redefining obesity and its treatment*. Melbourne: Health Communications.

Yang, E. J., Chung, H. K., Kim, W. Y., Bianchi, L., & Song, W. O. (2007). Chronic diseases and dietary changes in relation to Korean Americans' length of residence in the United States. *Journal of the American Dietetic Association, 107*, 942–950.

Obesity and Asian Americans: Prevalence, Risk Factors, and Future Research Directions

18

May C. Wang

Introduction

About a year ago, a classmate from my high school days came to California for a visit, bringing with him his wife and children. 'Peter' was an athlete in high school but I had not seen him in 30 years. Before he came, he sent me a picture of himself to warn me that he had "gained a lot of weight." I was glad he prepared me. Even with the unlikely image of him in my mind, I was still unprepared for our first meeting. Peter must have gained at least 250 pounds. As he slowly climbed the three steps that led to our house, I wondered how he had gained so much weight. With a small Asian frame of no taller than 5 feet 6 inches, he was having difficulty breathing and walking. Over the next few days, as we took him and his family around town, I realized that I knew little about the daily challenges faced by those who are obese, despite being an obesity researcher.

Obesity is a serious health condition that unfortunately, is not often taken seriously enough. It is often misunderstood to be an individual problem due simply to "eating too much" or "being lazy." Obesity is not just an individual problem but a societal one. The current obesity epidemic is prompted by many factors that are often not within the control of individuals – economics, politics, and a changing socio-cultural environment – which influences the amount of time we spend on activities that affect what we eat and how much we exercise. Many people with busy work lives or parents trying to balance work and family life find little time or energy to prepare a healthy meal. The food supply has changed drastically over the past few decades, partially in response to the increasing demand for more convenience foods. Fast and processed foods, which are usually high in fat, salt, and sugar, are readily accessible to all Americans. Food that is naturally fresh tastes good, while food that is processed needs flavor enhancers (added salt, fat, sugar) to enhance palatibilty.

In this chapter, we will discuss how obesity is defined and measured and if current obesity definitions apply to Asian Americans, how prevalent obesity is among Asian Americans, what factors increase risk for obesity especially in the Asian American population, why obesity is such a major public health concern today, and some ideas for future research.

Definition and Measurement of Obesity

Obesity has been defined as "abnormal or excessive (body) fat accumulation that may impair health" (Garrow, 1988; World Health Organization, 2000). Current studies state that it is not just total body fat that may impair health but that the distribution of body fat may also be harmful

M.C. Wang (✉)
Department of Community Health Sciences,
UCLA School of Public Health, Los Angeles,
CA, USA
e-mail: maywang@ucla.edu

G.J. Yoo et al. (eds.), *Handbook of Asian American Health*,
DOI 10.1007/978-1-4614-2227-3_18, © Springer Science+Business Media, LLC 2013

(Canoy, 2010; Després, Arsenault, Côté, Cartier, & Lemieux, 2008). The term "abdominal obesity" refers to excessive accumulation of visceral fat which is found within the peritoneal cavity of the abdomen.

There are several ways to measure body fat directly but these are either invasive or expensive. For example, hydrostatic underwater weighing is a relatively well-accepted method for measuring body fat but requires the person to be under water for a short period of time, Dual-energy X-ray absorptiometry and computerized tomography measure total body fat as well as the distribution of body fat but are relatively expensive (Heymsfield, Lohman, Wang, & Going, 2005).

For clinical purposes and population surveys, a more practical measure of obesity is Body Mass Index (BMI). BMI is calculated from weight and height using the following formula: weight (kg)/height (m)^2. For example, an adult who is 5 ft (= 1.524 m) tall and weighs 130 lbs (= 59.1 kg) has a

$$BMI = 59.1 / (1.524 \times 1.524) = 25.45 kg / m^2.$$

The Centers for Disease Control and Prevention (CDC, 2012), uses BMI to define two categories of 'excessive' body fat for adults (1) overweight, which is defined as having a BMI between 25 and 29.9 kg/m^2, and (2) obese, which is defined as having a BMI of 30 kg/m^2 or higher (http://www.cdc.gov/obesity/defining.html). It is important to keep in mind that these are simply operational definitions that help to screen for individuals who may be at higher risk for obesity-related chronic diseases. Because BMI is calculated from weight, which measures not only fat mass but also lean mass, BMI may incorrectly classify a heavy muscular athlete as being overweight or obese.

For children aged 2 years and older, CDC also uses BMI to define overweight and obesity. However, because children are growing and there are gender differences in growth patterns, the definitions of overweight and obesity are based on sex- and age-specific BMI cut-points derived from growth charts. Overweight is defined as having a

BMI that is ≥85th percentile but <95th percentile, while obesity is defined as having a BMI ≥95th percentile. There are two sets of widely used growth charts, specifically the Centers for Disease Control and Prevention (CDC, 2010) growth charts (http://www.cdc.gov/growthcharts/cdc_charts.htm) and the World Health Organization (WHO, n.d) growth charts (http://www.who.int/childgrowth/en/). Currently, the American Academy of Pediatrics recommends the use of CDC's growth charts for children aged two years and older. For children younger than two years, the WHO growth charts are recommended but weight-for-height rather than BMI is the preferred measure of growth (Grummer-Strawn, Reinold, & Krebs, 2010).

Some Issues with Applying CDC's Definitions to Asian Americans

While it would be impractical to have ethnically specific BMI cut-points to define overweight and obesity, it should be noted that the appropriateness of CDC's cut-points for Asian adults has been questioned. In particular, at any given BMI level, Asians may have a higher percentage of body fat and risk for cardiovascular disease than Whites (Odegaard et al., 2009; Palaniappan, Wong, Shin, Fortmann, & Lauderdale, 2010; Razak et al., 2005, 2007; Wang et al., 1994). This increased risk for cardiovascular disease may also be partially due to ethnic differences in the *distribution of body fat* (Kohli, Sniderman, Tchernof, & Lear, 2010; Lear et al., 2007). Because studies have shown that the lowest all-cause mortality in Asian populations is associated with a BMI of 23.0–24.9 kg/m^2 (Gu et al., 2006; Jee et al., 2006; Tsugane, Sasaki, & Tsubono, 2002) lower BMI cut-points for defining overweight and obesity for Asians have been recommended: <15.5 kg/m^2 (underweight), 15.5–22.9 kg/m^2 (normal weight), 23.0–24.9 kg/m^2 (overweight) and 25 kg/m^2 (obesity). These cut-points have not been adopted (WHO, 2000).

Since most of the research studies supporting lower cut-points for Asians were those living in

Asia or of mostly Asian immigrants born and raised in Asia, it is not clear if the recommended lower BMI cut-points apply to Asian Americans born and raised in the United States. In a study involving a small convenience sample of young adult Asian women living in California, Wang & Crespi (2011) observed that the association between BMI and percent body fat differed between women who had lived 12 or more years in the United States and women who had lived fewer years in the United States. Controlling for BMI, women who had lived 12 years or more in the United States had higher percent body fat than Caucasians for BMIs less than 20.5 kg/m^2, but lower percent body fat than Caucasians for higher BMIs. These findings suggest that early childhood environment may influence the relation between percent body fat and BMI. Future research will help clarify how childhood environment influences body fat accumulation and distribution later in life.

Obesity Prevalence Among Asian Americans

Obesity has been declared a global epidemic by the World Health Organization (2000). Obesity rates are highest in western industrialized countries, averaging over 30% among adults, 18% among 12–19 year olds, and 10% among 2–5 year olds in the United States (Flegal, Carroll, Ogden, & Curtin, 2010; Ogden & Carroll, 2010). Obesity rates in Asian Americans are lower than in other racial/ethnic groups. However, there is evidence to suggest that these rates are climbing rapidly (Harrison et al., 2005). The latest Los Angeles County Health Survey reported that adult obesity rates among Asian Americans and Pacific Islanders more than doubled, increasing from 4% in 1997 to 9% in 2007 (Los Angeles County Department of Public Health, 2010). It should also be noted that there is considerable variation in obesity rates among the various Asian ethnic subgroups, and that this variation differs between children and adults, as discussed below.

Children: A recent study of about 670,000 children attending 5th, 7th and 9th grades in public schools in Los Angeles County between 2006 and 2007 found wide variation in obesity rates among the various Asian ethnic subgroups, with Pacific Islanders having the highest rate of 36%, Filipinos and Laotians following with rates of 18% and 17% respectively, and Chinese and Japanese trailing with rates of 10% and 8% respectively (Shabbir, Kwan, Wang, Shih, & Simon, 2010). While there were not enough Hmong in the sample, it should be noted that child obesity has been observed to be a problem among this subpopulation (Hyslop, Deinard, Dahlberg-Luby, & Himes, 1996). Another study of low-income 3 to 4-year-olds participating in the Special Supplemental Nutrition Program for Women, Infants and Children in Los Angeles County, 2003–2009, reported an obesity prevalence rate of 12% among Asians, and 14% among Whites in 2009. While the rate for Whites increased from 2003 to 2009, that for Asians showed a slight decrease by about 1% point (The Public Health Foundation Enterprises [PHFE] Women Infants and Children [WIC], 2010). On a national level, using data from the National Survey of Children's Health 2003, Singh, Kogan, & Yu, (2009) reported obesity and overweight prevalence rates of 15% and 32% respectively for 10–17 year old first generation Asian immigrant children.

Adults: Using data from the California Health Interview Survey, Wang, Quan, Kanaya, and Fernandez (2010) estimated the combined prevalence of overweight and obesity among Asian Americans to be 50% among men and 34% among women. In an analysis of data from the National Health Interview Survey, Ye, Rust, Baltrus, and Daniels (2009) reported unadjusted obesity prevalence rates varying from 4% among Chinese to 13% among Filipinos. In Chicago, Shah et al. (2010) found obesity rates varying from 2% to 4% in Chinese and Vietnamese to 12% in Cambodians among nearly 800 lower income adults living in Chicago. A summary of

Table 18.1 Summary of studies reporting obesity prevalence rates in Asian Americans

Author, year	Location	Subjects	Obesity definition	Obesity prevalence (OB = obese; OW = overweight)
Shabbir et al. (2010)	Los Angeles County, CA	670,352 children (49% girls) 5th, 7th and 9th grade students (9–17 yo) attending public schools in Los Angeles County in 2006 and 2007 [data from CDE's Physical Fitness Test (PFT)]	OW ≥85th <95th percentile of sex-and age-specific BMI growth reference values (CDC) OB >95th percentile	OB (Asians only): 12.1% OB (Pacific Islanders): 35.6% OB (Filipinos): 17.5% – highest OB (Laotian): 16.8% – highest OB (Cambodians): 15.4% – highest OB (Chinese): 9.5% – lowest OB (Japanese): 8.4% – lowest OW (Asians only): 15.5% OW (Pacific Islanders): 20.3% OW (Korean): 17.3% – highest OW (Japanese): 12.8% – lowest
Shah et al. (2010)	Chicago	380 randomly selected Chinese adults, 250 Cambodian and 150 Vietnamese adults recruited through respondent-driven sampling	BMI ≥30 kg/m² based on self-reports of height and weight	OB (Chinese): 3.5% OB (Cambodian): 11.4% OB (Vietnamese): 1.9%
Wang et al. (2010)	California	5,704 Asian American adults (traditional, bicultural, and acculturated groups[a], which included Chinese, Vietnamese, and Korean ethnicities) over the age of 18 year, from combined 2005 and 2007 CHIS data	OW or OB: BMI ≥25 kg/m²	OW or OB (Traditional, male): 33.74% OW or OB (Bicultural, male): 32.95% OW or OB (Acculturated, male): 50.02% OW or OB (Traditional, female): 18.54% OW or OB (Bicultural, female): 12.52% OW or OB (Acculturated, female): 33.95%

(continued)

Table 18.1 (continued)

Author, year	Location	Subjects	Obesity definition	Obesity prevalence (OB=obese; OW=overweight)
Ye et al. (2009)	National Health Interview Survey (2003–2005)	534 Asian Indian, 550 Chinese, 633 Filipino, and 1,117 other Asian	BMI ≥30 kg/m^2 based on self-reports of height and weight	OB (Asian Indian) 6.1% OB (Chinese) 4.2% OB (Filipino) 13.2% OB (Other Asian) 6.9%
Anderson and Whitaker (2009)	Nationally representative sample of US children born in 2001	8,550 children age 4 – from the Early Childhood Longitudinal Study, Birth Cohort – 2005 data	OB >95th percentile of sex-and age-specific BMI growth reference values (CDC) Extreme OB >97th percentile	OB Asian boys (>95th): 15.8% OB Asian girls (>95th): 10.0% OB Asian both sexes (>95th): 12.8% OB Asian boys (>97th): 11.3% OB Asian girls (>97th): 5.2% OB Asian both sexes (>97th): 8.1%
Au, Kwong, Chou, Tso, and Wong (2009)	New York City, NY	4,695 Chinese American children (55.5% of subjects US born, 47.8% girls) aged 6–19 years old from a community health center stationed at Manhattan and Queens, NY serving low income medically underserved Chinese immigrants in New York City	OW ≥85th <95th percentile of sex-and age-specific BMI growth reference values (CDC) OB ≥95th percentile	OB (all-both sexes, US and Foreign born): 10.2% OB (both sexes, US born, ages 6–19): 13.3% OB (both sexes, Foreign born): 6.3% OB (Boys, 6–19, US born): 17.9% OB (Boys, 6–19, Foreign Born): 9.9% OB (Girls, 6–19, US born): 8.4% OB (Girls, 6–19, Foreign born): 2.3% OW (all- both sexes, US and Foreign born): 24.6% OW (both sexes, US born, ages 6–19): 29.8% OW (both sexes, Foreign born): 18.1% OW (Boys, 6–19, US born): 37.4% OW (Boys, 6–19, Foreign Born): 25.4% OW (Girls, 6–19, US born): 21.5% OW (Girls, 6–19, Foreign born): 10.1%

(continued)

Table 18.1 (continued)

Author, year	Location	Subjects	Obesity definition	Obesity prevalence (OB = obese; OW = overweight)
Nelson, Gortmaker, Subramanian, Cheung, and Wechsler (2007)	119 US colleges	24,613 full time college students (of all ethnicities) attending a 4 year college. Data from Harvard School of Public Health's College Alcohol Study (CAS), which used data from surveys in 1993 (849 Asian students), and 1999 (978 Asian students)	OW: BMI $\geq$25 kg/m^2 OB: BMI $\geq$30 kg/m^2 Class II OB: BMI $\geq$ 35 kg/m^2	OW (Asian, 1993): 13.6% OW (Asian, 1999): 16.4% OB (Asian, 1993): 2.0% OB (Asian, 1999): 2.3% OB II (Asian, 1993): 0.2% OB II (Asian, 1999): 0.6%

[a]Traditional: foreign-born, speaking English "not well" or "not well at all"; Bicultural: foreign-born, speaking English "well" or "very well"; Acculturated: U.S.-born, speaking English "well" or "very well"

studies reporting obesity prevalence rates in Asian Americans is provided in Table 18.1.

Risk Factors for Obesity

Obesity is directly caused by an imbalance between energy intake and energy expenditure (Redinger, 2009). Hence, behavioral factors associated with increased obesity risk are diet and physical activity, which determine energy intake and expenditure respectively. In the general American population, specific dietary and physical activity factors that have been associated with obesity development include frequent soda and fast food consumption as well as a sedentary lifestyle (Jeffery & French, 1998; Ludwig, Peterson, & Gortmaker, 2001; Jeffery & Utter, 2003). In addition, obesity prevalence is inversely associated with socioeconomic status (SES) (McLaren, 2007; Ogden, Lamb, Carroll, & Flegal, 2010a; 2010b). The question is whether such risk factors also apply to Asian Americans. Are soda and fast food consumption and sedentary behavior important contributors to obesity development among Asian Americans or are other dietary and physical activity factors more relevant?

To answer this question, we begin by comparing obesity rates between Asian Americans born in the U.S. and Asians born outside the U.S. We find that Asians born in the U.S. have higher obesity rates than Asians born outside the U.S., suggesting that length of stay in the U.S. influences diet and physical activity in ways that lead to energy imbalance (Au, Kwong, Chou, Tso, & Wong, 2009; Singh, Kogan, & Yu, 2009). The following sections will discuss how dietary behavior and physical activity change among Asian American immigrants as they adapt to the U.S.

Dietary Behavior

Similar to Latinos and other emigrating groups to the United States, many Asian immigrants increase their risk of diet-related chronic diseases as a result of eating more convenience foods high in fat, sugar, and / or salt (Norman, Castro, Albright, & King, 2004; Yang, Chung, Kim, Bianchi, & Song, 2007). In studies of Japanese, Korean, Thai, Hmong and Chinese Americans, immigrants tend to consume greater amounts of "American" foods such as fast food, sweets, and soda (Franzen & Smith, 2009; Kim & Chan, 2004; Kudo, Falciglia, & Couch, 2000; Lv & Brown, 2010; Sukalakamala & Brittin, 2006; Yang et al., 2007), the longer they live in the U.S. As immigrants acculturate, they may also show increased dietary variety but lower dietary moderation (Liu, Berhane, & Tseng, 2010). The adoption of westernized (American) foods is most prevalent during breakfast and lunch, while dinners still often feature traditional Asian foods (Lv & Brown, 2010).

These observations are consistent with what is known about the extent to which new foods replace traditional foods among those who relocate or emigrate to a new socio-cultural environment. Foods that are eaten daily as part of a main meal such as rice in the Asian diet are less susceptible to change, whereas foods that are not eaten as part of the main meal (e.g. fast food, sweets, beverages) are more likely modified. (Jerome, Kandel, & Pelto, 1980; Satia, 2010). The extent to which new foods replace traditional foods may also depend on the availability of culturally familiar foods. Immigrants who move to locales where few residents are of the same ethnic background may be forced to replace traditional foods more quickly than immigrants who move to places where there is an existing community of the same ethnic background. In addition, convenient access to cheap fast food in many parts of the U.S., aggressive marketing of processed foods as being "preferable," and unfamiliarity to discriminate between healthy and unhealthy choices for American cuisine may also influence unhealthy choices.

Dietary behavioral changes of Asian immigrants may also differ among subgroups. Ethnic background, country of origin, and socio-demographic factors such as income, education, and occupation may influence the dietary acculturation experience of Asian immigrants. The dietary acculturation experience of the Hmong, who suffer from high rates of poverty and whose food assistance usage has been noted to increase with length of residence in the United States (Franzen & Smith, 2009). Consequently, the diet changes with Hmong immigrants can be expected to be different compared to Chinese immigrants with higher levels of education (Lv & Brown, 2010).

Segmented assimilation theory which posits that the assimilation process may differ for different groups of immigrants, leading to upward assimilation, downward assimilation, or upward mobility and biculturalism (Portes & Zhou, 1993), could

help explain why the dietary acculturation process may differ between socio-demographically different subgroups. Biculturalism as measured by Asian language retention has been shown to be protective against obesity among Asian American adults (Wang, 2010). Unfortunately, there are few studies of the mechanisms by which socio-demographic factors influence dietary acculturation. In the general American population, socioeconomic factors such as income and education are known to be powerful determinants of health behaviors (Winkleby Marilyn, Jatulis, Frank, & Fortmann, 1992). Income determines a family's resources, and hence its ability to purchase healthy foods, which are often more expensive than less healthy alternatives (Drenowski, 2010). Education as well as occupation may influence social networks and hence an individual's exposure to social norms affecting food behaviors including meal patterns and health-related information. Education and/or occupation also influence where a person lives and works. Given that recent studies show that access to healthy or unhealthy foods in the U.S. varies between neighborhoods (Lovasi, Hutson, Guerra, & Neckerman, 2009; Morland, Wing, Diez-Roux, & Poole, 2002), where a person lives and works may be an important determinant of the types of food that are readily accessible (Inagami, Cohen, Finch, & Asch, 2006).

Physical Activity Behavior

It is not clear how physical activity changes among Asian American immigrants as they acculturate the findings of studies on physical activity acculturation among Asian American immigrants are inconsistent. Among of Korean American men and women, Lee, Sobal, and Frongillo (2000) observed that higher acculturation was associated with higher levels of light physical activity (e.g., walking, gardening, bowling, dancing), but not with levels of vigorous physical activity (e.g., aerobics, running, swimming, bicycling). In contrast, using data from the California Health Interview Survey, Afable-Munsuz, Ponce, Rodríguez, and Perez-Stable (2010) reported that the percentage of Chinese adults meeting recommended leisure-time physical activity increased from 20% among the first generation to 32% among 3rd generation adults. Filipino adults meeting recommended non-leisure time physical activity decreased significantly from 30% in the first generation to 20% in the second generation and then increased to 43% in the third generation. Clearly, more research is needed to understand how physical activity changes among immigrants of various socio-demographic groups, and what factors influence these changes.

Socio-Cultural Beliefs

Beliefs about and attitudes toward obesity could influence dietary and physical activity behaviors (Liou & Bauer, 2007). There may be a preference for "chubby" babies and young children, making it challenging for health educators to convince mothers not to overfeed their young children. Furthermore, Asian immigrants may believe that obesity is a non-Asian problem and hence, interventions are not necessary.

Chronic Stressors

Diet and physical activity are considered the primary behavioral determinants of obesity development. However, there is emerging research that suggests a role for chronic stressors such as major life events, and exposure to stressful social and physical environments including racial discrimination and unsafe neighborhoods (Block, He, Zaslavsky, Ding, & Ayanian, 2009; Björntorp & Rosmond, 2000; Chambers et al., 2004; Chandola, Brunner, & Marmot, 2006; Gee, 2008; Hill, Ross, & Angel, 2005; Mattei, Demissie, Falcon, Ordovas, & Tucker, 2010). Chronic stressors are not merely individually experienced phenomena, as stressors can vary systematically by social group and neighborhood. Youth from low-income families are more likely to encounter negative life events, and extraneous and daily hassles than youth from higher-income families (McNamara, 2000; Timko, Moos, & Michelson, 1993). Furthermore,

these stressors differ by community, with racially and socioeconomically segregated neighborhoods more likely to encounter violence, and are often exposed to toxic chemicals and poor air quality (Gee & Payne-Sturges, 2004). In an analysis of data from the 2002 to 2003 National Latino and Asian American Study involving nearly 2000 adults, Gee, Ro, Gavin, and Takeuchi (2008) found that racial discrimination was associated with increased BMI and obesity after controlling for weight discrimination, social desirability bias, and other factors. The strength of this association increased with duration of residence in the U.S.

Chronic stressors may influence obesity in several ways. First, stressors may directly contribute to obesity by increasing the body's ability to retain fat, especially around the abdominal region (Björntorp & Rosmond, 2000). Second, stressors can affect dietary behavior. Evidence from both animal and human research finds that stressors may encourage the eating of "comfort foods" (Dallman, Pecoraro, & la Fleur, 2005; Lemmens, Rutters, Born, & Westerterp-Plantenga, 2011). Third, stressors have been associated with lower physical activity levels (Taylor & Dorn, 2006). These pathways are, however, not unidimensional. Chronic stressors may lead to weight gain in some individuals and weight loss in others (Kivimäki et al., 2006).

Why Obesity is a Major Public Health Concern

Medical costs resulting from obesity in the United States are estimated at a staggering $147 billion in 2008 dollars (Finkelstein, Trogdon, Cohen, & Dietz, 2009). Obesity is associated with increased risk of many chronic conditions including heart disease, hypertension and stroke, some types of cancer such as breast cancer and colorectal cancer, non-insulin-dependent diabetes mellitus, gallbladder disease, osteoarthritis and gout, and pulmonary diseases (NIH and NHLBI Obesity Education Initiative, 1998; Conway & Rene, 2004). Obesity is also associated with poorer mental health in some populations

(Kivimaki et al., 2009; Scott, McGee, Wells, & Browne, 2008).

Obesity *in childhood* is also a major public health concern. Overweight and obesity in childhood track into adulthood, with overweight children being at least twice as likely to become overweight adults as normal weight children (Singh, Mulder, Twisk, van Mechelen, & Chinapaw, 2008). Obese children are also more likely to suffer from diabetes and other metabolic conditions (Abrams & Katz, 2011), and to be bullied with psychosocial consequences (Lumeng et al., 2010).

Future Directions

While obesity rates are generally lower in Asian Americans compared to Hispanic and non-Hispanic Whites and Blacks, there is considerable variation in obesity rates among the various Asian ethnic subgroups. Rates appear to be higher among Filipinos, Laotians, Cambodians and Hmong, and among those who are born in the U.S. It should also be noted that the especially high rates of obesity among Pacific Islanders are often hidden by the frequent practice of aggregating data for Pacific Islanders with Asians.

SES, which is inversely associated with obesity risk in the general American population especially among women, may influence obesity risk, however, the relation of SES to obesity risk in Asian American populations may vary with migrant status and country of origin. It is likely that among newer Asian immigrants from developing countries, higher SES may be associated with higher risk of obesity, a relation that has been observed in Asian societies such as China and India (Cui, Huxley, Wu, & Dibley, 2010; Goyal et al., 2010). Among Asian Americans who are more acculturated, biculturalism appears to be protective against obesity (Wang, 2010).

More studies are needed to investigate obesity and obesity-related conditions in the various Asian American socio-demographic groups so that appropriate interventions can be tailored to meet the needs of Asian Americans. Current obesity rates for Asian Americans (not including Pacific Islanders) are relatively lower than for other major ethnic/racial groups in the United States. However, increasing exposure to an environment that markets unhealthy processed and fast foods and promotes sedentary behaviors, makes Asian American immigrants vulnerable to the unhealthy effects of acculturation. There are few published reports of evidence-based interventions to promote healthy eating and physical activity behaviors, and address chronic stressors, tailored specifically for the various Asian American subgroups. Such interventions will address not only obesity but also the many chronic diseases that are associated with unhealthy lifestyles and chronic stressors. Socio-ecological and acculturation models (Bronfenbrenner, 1979; Portes & Zhou, 1993; Satia, 2010), which recognize the contributions of cultural, psychological, social, economic, political, and physical factors to the health and well-being of individuals and populations, are relevant for developing etiologic studies and tailored interventions for Asian Americans.

References

Abrams, P., & Katz, L. E. L. (2011). Metabolic effects of obesity causing disease in childhood. *Current Opinion in Endocrinology, Diabetes, and Obesity, 18*(1), 23–27.

Afable-Munsuz, A., Ponce, N. A., Rodríguez, M., & Perez-Stable, E. J. (2010). Immigrant generation and physical activity among Mexican, Chinese & Filipino adults in the U.S. *Social Science & Medicine, 70*(12), 1997–2005.

Anderson, S. E., & Whitaker, R. C. (2009). Prevalence of obesity among U.S. preschool children in different racial and ethnic groups. *Archives of Pediatrics & Adolescent Medicine, 163*(4), 344–348.

Au, L., Kwong, K., Chou, J. C., Tso, A., & Wong, M. (2009). Prevalence of overweight and obesity in Chinese American children in New York City. *Journal of Immigrant and Minority Health, 11*(5), 337–341. Epub 2009 Jan 21.

Björntorp, P., & Rosmond, R. (2000). Obesity and cortisol. *Nutrition, 16*(10), 924–936.

Block, J. P., He, Y., Zaslavsky, A. M., Ding, L., & Ayanian, J. Z. (2009). Psychosocial stress and change in weight among U.S. adults. *American Journal of Epidemiology, 170*(2), 181–192.

Bronfenbrenner, U. (1979). *The ecology of human development: Experiments by nature and design.* Cambridge, MA: Harvard University Press.

Canoy, D. (2010). Coronary heart disease and body fat distribution. *Current Atherosclerosis Reports, 12*(2), 125–133.

Centers for Disease Control and Prevention [CDC]. (2012). *Obesity and overweight for professionals: Adult defining*. Retrieved (n.d.) from http://www.cdc.gov/obesity/adult/defining.html

Centers for Disease Control and Prevention [CDC]. (2011). *Web-based injury statistics query and reporting system (WISQARS)*. Retrieved (n.d.).

Centers for Disease Control and Prevention [CDC]. (2010). *Growth charts*. Retrieved (n.d.) from http://www.cdc.gov/growthcharts/cdc_charts.htm

Chambers, E. C., Tull, E. S., Fraser, H. S., Mutunhu, N. R., Sobers, N., & Niles, E. (2004). The relationship of internalized racism to body fat distribution and insulin resistance among African adolescent youth. *Journal of the National Medical Association, 96*(12), 1594–1598.

Chandola, T., Brunner, E., & Marmot, M. (2006). Chronic stress at work and the metabolic syndrome: A prospective study. *British Medical Journal, 332*(7540), 521–525.

Conway, B., & Rene, A. (2004). Obesity as a disease: No lightweight matter. *Obesity Reviews, 5*(3), 145–151.

Cui, Z., Huxley, R., Wu, Y., & Dibley, M. J. (2010). Temporal trends in overweight and obesity of children and adolescents from nine Provinces in China from 1991-2006. *International Journal of Pediatric Obesity, 5*(5), 365–374.

Dallman, M. F., Pecoraro, N. C., & la Fleur, S. E. (2005). Chronic stress and comfort foods: Self-medication and abdominal obesity. *Brain, Behavior, and Immunity, 19*(4), 275–280.

Després, J.-P., Arsenault, B. J., Côté, M., Cartier, A., & Lemieux, I. (2008). Abdominal obesity: The cholesterol of the 21st century? *The Canadian Journal of Cardiology, 24*(Suppl. D), 7D–12D [Review].

Drenowski, A. (2010). The cost of U.S. foods as related to their nutritive value. *The American Journal of Clinical Nutrition, 92*(5), 1181–1188.

Finkelstein, E. A., Trogdon, J. G., Cohen, J. W., & Dietz, W. (2009). Annual medical spending attributable to obesity: Payer- and service-specific estimates. *Health Affairs, 28*(5), w822–w831.

Flegal, K. M., Carroll, M. D., Ogden, C. L., & Curtin, L. R. (2010). Prevalence and trends in obesity among U.S. adults, 1999-2008. *Journal of the American Medical Association, 303*(3), 235–241.

Franzen, L., & Smith, C. (2009). Acculturation and environmental change impacts dietary habits among adult Hmong. *Appetite, 52*(1), 73–83.

Garrow, J. S. (1988). *Obesity and related diseases*. New York: Churchill Livingstone.

Gee, G. C., & Payne-Sturges, D. C. (2004). Environmental health disparities: A framework integrating psychosocial and environmental concepts. *Environmental Health Perspectives, 112*(17), 1645–1653.

Gee, G. C., Ro, A., Gavin, A., & Takeuchi, D. T. (2008). Disentangling the effects of racial and weight discrimination on body mass index and obesity among Asian Americans. *American Journal of Public Health, 98*(3), 493–500.

Goyal, R. K., Shah, V. N., Saboo, B. D., Phatak, S. R., Shah, N. N., Gohel, M. C., Raval, P. B., et al. (2010). Prevalence of overweight and obesity in Indian adolescent school going children: Its relationship with socioeconomic status and associated lifestyle factors. *Journal of Association of Physicians of India, 58*, 151–158.

Grummer-Strawn, L. M., Reinold, C., & Krebs, N. F. (2010). Use of World Health Organization and CDC growth charts forchildren aged 0-59 months in the United States. *Morbidity and Mortality Weekly Report. Recommendations and Reports, 59*(RR-9), 1–15.

Gu, D., He, J., Duan, X., Reynolds, K., Wu, Z., Chen, J., Guangyong, H., et al. (2006). Body weight and mortality among men and women in China. *Journal of the American Medical Association, 295*(7), 776–783.

Harrison, G. G., Kagawa-Singer, M., Foerster, S. B., Lee, H., Kim, L. P., Nguyen, T.-U., Fernandez-Ami, A., et al. (2005). Seizing the moment: California's opportunity to prevent nutrition-related health disparities in low-income Asian American population. *Cancer, 15*(Suppl. 12), 2962–2968.

Heymsfield, S., Lohman, T., Wang, Z., & Going, S. (2005). *Human body composition* (2nd ed.). Champaign, IL: Human Kinetics.

Hill, T. D., Ross, C. E., & Angel, R. J. (2005). Neighborhood disorder, psychophysiological distress, and health. *Journal of Health and Social Behavior, 46*(2), 170–186.

Hyslop, A. E., Deinard, A. S., Dahlberg-Luby, E., & Himes, J. H. (1996). Growth patterns of first-generation Southeast Asian Americans from birth to 5 years of age. *The Journal of the American Board of Family Practice, 9*(5), 328–335.

Inagami, S., Cohen, D. A., Finch, B. K., & Asch, S. M. (2006). You are where you shop: Grocery store locations, weight, and neighborhoods. *American Journal of Preventive Medicine, 31*(1), 10–17.

Jee, S. H., Sull, J. W., Park, J., Lee, S.-Y., Ohrr, H., Guallar, E., & Samet, J. M. (2006). Body-mass index and mortality in Korean men and women. *The New England Journal of Medicine, 355*(8), 779–787.

Jeffery, R. W., & French, S. A. (1998). Epidemic obesity in the United States: Are fast foods and television viewing contributing? *American Journal of Public Health, 88*(2), 277–280.

Jeffery, R. W., & Utter, J. (2003). The changing environment and population obesity in the United States. *Obesity Research, 11*(Suppl.), 12S–22S.

Jerome, N. W., Kandel, R. F., & Pelto, G. H. (1980). *Nutrition anthropology. Contemporary approaches to diet and culture*. Pleasantville, NY: Redgrave.

Kim, J., & Chan, M. M. (2004). Acculturation and dietary habits of Korean Americans. *British Journal of Nutrition, 91*(3), 469–478.

Kivimäki, M., Batty, G. D., Singh-Manoux, A., Nabi, H., Tabak, A. G., Akbaraly, T. N., Vahtera, J., et al. (2009). Association between common mental disorder and obesity over the adult life course. *The British Journal of Psychiatry, 195*(2), 149–155.

Kivimäki, M., Head, J., Ferrie, J. E., Shipley, M. J., Brunner, E. J., Vahtera, J., et al. (2006). Work stress, weight gain and weight loss: Evidence for bidirectional effects of job strain on body mass index in the Whitehall II study. *International Journal of Obesity, 30*, 982–987.

Kohli, S., Sniderman, A. D., Tchernof, A., & Lear, S. A. (2010). Ethnic-specific differences in abdominal subcutaneous adipose tissue compartments. *Obesity, 18,* 2177–2183.

Kudo, Y., Falciglia, G. A., & Couch, S. C. (2000). Evolution of meal patterns and food choices of Japanese-American females born in the United States. *European Journal of Clinical Nutrition, 54*(8), 665–670.

Lear, S. A., Humphries, K. H., Kohli, S., Chockalingam, A., Frohlich, J. J., & Birmingham, C. L. (2007). Visceral adipose tissue accumulation differs according to ethnic background: Results of the Multicultural Community Health Assessment Trial (M-CHAT). *American Journal of Clinical Nutrition, 86*(2), 353–359.

Lee, S. K., Sobal, J., & Frongillo, E. A., Jr. (2000). Acculturation and health in Korean Americans. *Social Science & Medicine, 51*(2), 159–173.

Lemmens, S. G., Rutters, F., Born, J. M., & Westerterp-Plantenga, M. S. (2011). Stress augments food 'wanting' and energy intake in visceral overweight subjects in the absence of hunger. *Physiology and Behavior, 103*(2), 157–163.

Liou, D., & Bauer, K. D. (2007). Exploratory investigation of obesity risk and prevention in Chinese Americans. *Journal of Nutrition Education and Behavior, 39*(3), 134–141.

Liu, A., Berhane, Z., & Tseng, M. (2010). Improved dietary variety and adequacy but lower dietary moderation with acculturation in Chinese women in the United States. *Journal of the American Dietetic Association, 110*(3), 457–462.

Los Angeles County Department of Public Health. (2010). Trends in diabetes: A reversible public health crisis. Retrieved April 28, 2011, from http://www.publichealth.lacounty.gov/ha/reports/habriefs/2007/diabetes/Diabetes_Secure/Diabetes_2010_6pg_Sfinal.pdf.

Lovasi, G. S., Hutson, M. A., Guerra, M., & Neckerman, K. M. (2009). Built environments and obesity in disadvantaged populations. *Epidemiologic Reviews, 31*(1), 7–20.

Ludwig, D. S., Peterson, K. E., & Gortmaker, S. L. (2001). Relation between consumption of sugar-sweetened drinks and childhood obesity: A prospective, observational analysis. *The Lancet, 357*(9255), 505–508.

Lumeng, J. C., Forrest, P., Appugliese, D. P., Kaciroti, N., Corwyn, R. F., & Bradley, R. H. (2010). Weight status as a predictor of being bullied in third through sixth grades. *Pediatrics, 125,* e1301–e1307.

Lv, N., & Brown, J. L. (2010). Chinese American family food systems: Impact of Western influences. *Journal of Nutrition Education and Behavior, 42*(2), 106–114.

Mattei, J., Demissie, S., Falcon, L. M., Ordovas, J. M., & Tucker, K. (2010). Allostatic load is associated with chronic conditions in the Boston Puerto Rican Health Study. *Social Science & Medicine, 70*(12), 1988–1996.

McLaren, L. (2007). Socioeconomic status and obesity. *Epidemiologic Reviews, 29*(1), 29–48.

McNamara, S. (2000). *Stress in young people: What's new and what can we do?* London: Continuum.

Morland, K., Wing, S., Diez-Roux, A., & Poole, C. (2002). Neighborhood characteristics associated with the location of food stores and food service places. *American Journal of Preventive Medicine, 22*(1), 23–29.

Nelson, T. F., Gortmaker, S. L., Subramanian, S. V., Cheung, L., & Wechsler, H. (2007). Disparities in overweight and obesity among US college students. *American Journal of Health Behavior, 31*(4), 363–373.

NIH, & NHLBI Obesity Education Initiative. (1998). Clinical guidelines on the identification, evaluation, and treatment of overweight and obesity in adults. Retrieved http://www.nhlbi.nih.gov/guidelines/obesity/ob_gdlns.pdf.

Norman, S., Castro, C., Albright, C., & King, A. (2004). Comparing acculturation models in evaluating dietary habits among low-income Hispanic women. *Ethnicity & Disease, 14*(3), 399–404.

Odegaard, A. O., Koh, W.-P., Vazquez, G., Arakawa, K., Lee, H.-P., Yu, M. C., & Pereira, M. A. (2009). BMI and diabetes risk in Singaporean Chinese. *Diabetes Care, 32*(6), 1104–1106.

Ogden, C., & Carroll, M. (2010). Prevalence of obesity among children and adolescents: United States, trends 1963–1965 through 2007–2008. *NCHS Health E-Stat.*

Ogden, C. L., Lamb, M. M., Carroll, M. D., & Flegal, K. M. (2010a). Obesity and socioeconomic status in children and adolescents: United States, 2005-2008. *National Center for Health Statistics Data Brief, 51,* 1–8.

Ogden, C. L., Lamb, M. M., Carroll, M. D., & Flegal, K. M. (2010b). Obesity and socioeconomic status in adults: United States, 2005-2008. *National Center for Health Statistics Data Brief, 50,* 1–8.

Palaniappan, L. P., Wong, E. C., Shin, J. J., Fortmann, S. P., & Lauderdale, D. S. (2010). Asian Americans have greater prevalence of metabolic syndrome despite lower body mass index. *International Journal of Obesity (London), 35*(3), 393–400.

PHFE WIC. (2010, August). *WIC data 2003-2009: A report on low-income families with young children in Los Angeles County.*

Portes, A., & Zhou, M. (1993). The new second generation: Segmented assimilation and its variants. *Annals of American Academy of Political and Social Sciences, 530,* 74–96.

Razak, F., Anand, S. S., Shannon, H., Vuksan, V., Davids, B., Jacobs, R., McQueen, M., et al. (2007). Defining Obesity Cut Points in a Multiethnic Population. *Circulation, 115*(16), 2111–2118.

Razak, F., Anand, S. S., Vuksan, V., Davids, B., Jacobs, R., Teo, K. K., et al. (2005). Ethnic differences in the relationships between obesity and glucose-metabolic abnormalities: A cross-sectional population-based study. *International Journal of Obesity and Related Metabolic Disorders, 29*(6), 656–667.

Redinger, R. N. (2009). Fat storage and the biology of energy expenditure. *Translational Research, 154*(2), 52–60. Epub 2009 Jun 11.

Satia, J. A. (2010). Dietary acculturation and the nutrition transition: An overview. *Applied Physiology, Nutrition, and Metabolism, 35*(2), 219–223.

Scott, K. M., McGee, M. A., Wells, J. E., & Browne, M. A. O. (2008). Obesity and mental disorders in the adult general population. *Journal of Psychosomatic Research, 64*(1), 97–105.

Shabbir, S., Kwan, D., Wang, M. C., Shih, M., & Simon, P. A. (2010). Asians and Pacific Islanders and the growing childhood obesity epidemic. *Ethnicity & Disease, 20*(2), 129–135.

Shah, A. M., Guo, L., Magee, M., Cheung, W., Simon, M., LaBreche, A., & Liu, H. (2010). Comparing selected measures of health outcomes and health-seeking behaviors in Chinese, Cambodian, and Vietnamese communities of Chicago: Results from local health surveys. *Journal of Urban Health, 87*(5), 813–826.

Singh, G. K., Kogan, M. D., & Yu, S. M. (2009). Disparities in obesity and overweight prevalence among US immigrant children and adolescents by generational status. *Journal of Community Health, 34*(4), 271–281.

Singh, A. S., Mulder, C., Twisk, J. W., van Mechelen, W., & Chinapaw, M. J. M. (2008). Tracking of childhood overweight into adulthood: A systematic review of the literature. *Obesity Reviews, 9*(5), 474–488.

Sukalakamala, S., & Brittin, H. C. (2006). Food practices, changes, preferences, and acculturation of Thais in the United States. *Journal of the American Dietetic Association, 106*(1), 103–108.

Taylor, A. H., & Dorn, L. (2006). Stress, fatigue, health, and risk of road traffic accidents among professional drivers: The contribution of physical inactivity. *Annual Review of Public Health, 27,* 371–391.

Timko, C., Moos, R. H., & Michelson, D. J. (1993). The contexts of adolescents' chronic life stressors. *American Journal of Community Psychology, 21*(4), 397–420.

Tsugane, S., Sasaki, S., & Tsubono, Y. (2002). Under- and overweight impact on mortality among middle-aged Japanese men and women: A 10-y follow-up of JPHC study cohort I. *International Journal of Obesity and Related Metabolic Disorders, 26*(4), 529–537.

Wang, M. C., & Crespi, C. M. (2011). The influence of childhood and adolescent environmental exposure to a west-ernized environment on the relationship between BMI and adiposity in young Asian American women. *The American Journal of Clinical Nutrition* Mar 9. [Epub ahead of print] PubMed PMID: 21389179.

Wang, S., Quan, J., Kanaya, A. M., & Fernandez, A. (2010). Asian Americans and obesity in California: A protective effect of biculturalism. *Journal of Immigrant and Minority Health, 13*(2), 276–283.

Wang, J., Thornton, J. C., Russell, M., Burastero, S., Heymsfield, S., & Pierson, R. N., Jr. (1994). Asians have lower body mass index (BMI) but higher fat% than whites: Comparisons of anthropometric measurements. *The American Journal of Clinical Nutrition, 60*(1), 23–28.

WHO/IASO/IOTF. (2000). WHO: The Asia-Pacific perspective: Redefining obesity and its treatment. Geneva: World Health Organization, Western Pacific Regional Office.

Winkleby Marilyn, A., Jatulis, D. E., Frank, E., & Fortmann, S. P. (1992). Socioeconomic status and health: How education, income, and occupation contribute to risk factors for cardiovascular disease. *American Journal of Public Health, 82*(6), 816–820.

World Health Organization. (2000). Obesity: Preventing and managing the global epidemic. Report of a WHO Consultation. *WHO Technical Report Series 894.*

World Health Organization. (n.d.). *The WHO Child Growth Standards.* Retrieved (n.d.) from http://www.who.int/childgrowth/en/

Yang, E. J., Chung, H. K., Kim, W. Y., Bianchi, L., & Song, W. O. (2007). Chronic diseases and dietary changes in relation to Korean Americans' length of residence in the United States. *Journal of the American Dietetic Association, 107*(6), 942–950.

Ye, J., Rust, G., Baltrus, P., & Daniels, E. (2009). Cardiovascular risk factors among Asian Americans: Results from a National Health Survey. *Annals of Epidemiology, 19*(10), 718–723.

Hepatitis B and Asian Americans

19

Tung T. Nguyen, Vicky Taylor, Annette E. Maxwell,
Moon S. Chen Jr., Roshan Bastani,
and Susan Stewart

Introduction

Suppose you learned that for every ten of your friends, one has been sentenced to death, and that death is related to their Asian ancestry? Unfortunately, other than having been born in Asia or having a parent from an Asian country there might be no other warning sign. In fact, in the great majority of cases, there are no apparent symptoms. Consider Mark Lim, a young physician in the prime of his life, who one day suddenly doubled over with pain, was diagnosed with liver cancer at the age of 30, and died from it. On the surface, Dr. Lim was a healthy young man, and neither he nor his doctors knew he had "chronic hepatitis B." The causative agent, the hepatitis B virus, had been in his liver for years and eventually resulted in liver cancer. This same infection is also implicated in liver inflammation and liver failure. Yet there is a simple blood test that can diagnose hepatitis B and medications that prevent complications from hepatitis B in those who have it. There is even a vaccine that can prevent the infection in those who do not have hepatitis B so that they will not later develop liver failure and liver cancer. In fact, the vaccine to prevent hepatitis B is the first vaccine ever developed that can prevent cancer.

In spite of these medical advances, many Asian Americans do not know enough nor have done enough to lower their chances of being harmed by hepatitis B. In a recent study of college students who self-identified themselves as Asian American or Pacific Islander (AAPI), the rate of persistent hepatitis B infection was three times higher among U.S.-born AAPI students and 11 times higher among foreign-born AAPI students compared to the general population. Additionally, about one-third of all students were unaware of their hepatitis B vaccination status (Quang et al., 2010).

T.T. Nguyen (✉)
Vietnamese Community Health Promotion Project,
School of Medicine, University of California, Asian
American Network for Cancer Awareness, Research,
and Training (AANCART), San Francisco, CA, USA
e-mail: tung.nguyen@ucsf.edu

V. Taylor
Department of Health Services, Cancer Prevention
Program at Fred Hutchinson Cancer Research Center,
University of Washington, Seattle, WA, USA

A.E. Maxwell
School of Public Health, University of California,
Los Angeles, CA, USA

M.S. Chen Jr.
University of California, Davis Cancer Center,
Davis, CA, USA

R. Bastani
Department of Health Services, University of California,
Los Angeles (UCLA) School of Public Health,
Los Angeles, CA, USA

S. Stewart
School of Medicine, UCSF Helen Diller Family
Comprehensive Cancer Center Biostatistics Core,
University of California, San Francisco, CA, USA

G.J. Yoo et al. (eds.), *Handbook of Asian American Health*,
DOI 10.1007/978-1-4614-2227-3_19, © Springer Science+Business Media, LLC 2013

This chapter defines what hepatitis B is, why it is perhaps the most important health challenge and health disparity affecting Asian Americans, what factors promote hepatitis B viral infections, what can be done to reduce the transmission and impact of this infection including vaccination and screening for the hepatitis B virus. This chapter also describes the research on what demographic, socio-cultural and behavioral factors are associated with hepatitis B infections and prevention among Asian Americans and a framework to understand these issues. Current activities to address hepatitis B being implemented by various governmental, academic, and community organizations are also described. Finally, further research and policy needs to understand and reduce the impact of hepatitis B among Asian Americans are discussed.

Hepatitis B: Pathophysiology and Clinical Considerations

The generally accepted definition of hepatitis is inflammation of the liver. An insult such as alcohol or a virus can cause acute hepatitis. The severity of acute hepatitis can range from no significant findings (asymptomatic) to significant liver damage leading to coma or death. Symptoms can include vomiting, jaundice, and abdominal swelling. Following acute hepatitis, some affected persons may have no further problems. Others who are continually exposed to alcohol or to a persistent virus may eventually develop chronic hepatitis (Khalili, Liao, & Nguten, 2009). Chronic hepatitis can later result in fibrosis (scarring), cirrhosis (liver failure), and/or hepatocellular carcinoma (a type of liver cancer).

There are five major hepatitis viruses (A, B, C, D, and E) (Khalili et al., 2009). Each virus is associated with different transmission pathways and varying symptoms. Hepatitis A virus (HAV) and hepatitis E virus (HEV) are ribonucleic acid (RNA) viruses that only cause acute hepatitis. They are transmitted through the fecal-oral route infection usually results from ingesting food or liquids prepared by an infected person. After

recovery, the patient gains immunity against further infection. Hepatitis C virus (HCV) is an RNA virus that is primarily transmitted through blood. HCV can cause acute hepatitis and chronic hepatitis. Hepatitis D virus (HDV) is a defective RNA virus that requires the presence of hepatitis B virus (HBV) to cause infection and thus is usually found in only those who are infected with HBV. There is currently an effective vaccine against HAV but not against HDV, HCV, or HEV.

Much of the attention centers on the Hepatitis B virus (HBV), a DNA virus with eight major genotypes (Colvin & Mitchell, 2010) that can cause acute and chronic hepatitis. In addition, the virus can exist as a carrier state, in which the virus persists in the liver but causes no inflammation. Highly infectious, HBV is transmitted through contact with blood, semen, and other bodily fluids. Transmission of the virus can occur in several ways, including birthing of a child as he/she passes through the birth canal of an infected mother (vertical transmission), sexual contact with an infected person, or sharing of contaminated needles, syringes, medical instruments, razors, and toothbrushes (Colvin & Mitchell, 2010).

The likelihood of developing chronic hepatitis B or being a carrier depends on the age at infection. Over 90% of infected infants and 25–50% of children age 1–5 years will be chronically infected or become carriers. By comparison, only 6–10% of older children and adults will develop chronic disease (Colvin & Mitchell, 2010). Those who have been infected with hepatitis B but had complete recovery (no chronic hepatitis B or carrier state) may have evidence of previous exposure and/or immunity to HBV in their blood. Most people infected chronically with HBV are asymptomatic for long periods; however, 15–25% of those chronically infected will eventually die from cirrhosis, liver failure, or hepatocellular carcinoma (Colvin & Mitchell, 2010). Even those who are carriers are at high risk for liver cancer.

There is an effective method to prevent hepatitis B infection. Specifically, the hepatitis B vaccine is safe and highly effective in preventing

HBV infection and its sequelae, including liver cancer (Chang et al., 1997; Lee & Ko, 1997; Maynard, Kane, & Hadler, 1989). In the U.S., vaccination is recommended for all children age 0–18 years. For adults, vaccination is recommended for those at high-risk for exposure including health care workers, dialysis patients, those with multiple sexual partners, injection drug users, men who have sex with men, and household or sexual contacts of those infected with hepatitis B. Also, any adult who request hepatitis B vaccination regardless of their risk status should be vaccinated (Mast et al., 2006). The vaccine is most effective when given based on an appropriate schedule, typically three shots over 6 months. There is also a blood test that can show that there is immunity to HBV infection as a result of the vaccine. However, the vaccine does not prevent complications in those who already have persistent hepatitis B infection. Consequently, it is important that those who are from high-risk populations, such as Asian Americans, should be screened for hepatitis B at least once even if they have had vaccinations, since they may have had the infection prior to getting the vaccination.

Screening is an effective method of limiting the spread of hepatitis B. Screening for hepatitis B is recommended for individuals in the aforementioned high-risk categories, as well as all foreign-born Americans from hyperendemic areas, such as Asia and the South Pacific Islands (Lok & McMahon, 2009). Screening is important because approximately 65 percent of those who are infected with hepatitis B do not know that they are infected (Colvin & Mitchell, 2010). The standard test for hepatitis B infection involves the detection of the hepatitis B surface antigen (HBsAg), which if positive indicates acute or chronic infection (Khalili et al., 2009). An additional test for HBV, the HBV DNA viral load, may also be used by some physicians for screening and monitoring. Other key tests for HBV include the hepatitis B surface antibody (HBsAb) test, which documents immunity to further HBV infection and the hepatitis B core antibody (HBcAb) test, which shows prior infection. All of these tests can be done on a small

sample of blood taken from the vein through a simple blood draw.

A variety of treatments are available for individuals who have chronic hepatitis B. Medications such as interferon alpha, lamivudine, adefovir, entecavir, tenofovir, and telbivudine decrease liver inflammation and may prevent cirrhosis among those chronically infected (Lok & McMahon, 2009). Lamivudine prevents liver cancer in Asian patients with advanced hepatitis B (Liaw et al., 2004). With the exception of interferon alpha, which is given by injection, the medications to treat chronic hepatitis B are given orally. Decisions about when to treat chronic hepatitis B, how long to continue treatment, and which medications to utilize are complex and evolving; patients with chronic hepatitis B should discuss various options with the treating physician. Those who are carriers do not need treatment but should receive close medical monitoring. People with persistent hepatitis B should engage in behaviors that minimize liver damage. This includes refraining from consuming alcohol, obtaining medical advice about what medications or herbs that will not adversely affect the liver, and getting vaccinated for hepatitis A if needed. Hepatitis B patients should encourage all of their immediate family and household members as well as their sexual contacts to get tested. Any individual who is a household member or sexual contact of those with persistent hepatitis B infection should get vaccinated after getting tested.

Screening for liver cancer may benefit patients with chronic HBV infection (Lok & McMahon, 2009; Zhang, Yang, & Tang, 2004). The American Association for the Study of Liver Diseases recommend that liver cancer screening be done using liver ultrasound tests every 6–12 months on those with persistent hepatitis B who are considered high-risk for liver cancer. High-risk categories for liver cancer include Asian men over 40 years and Asian women over 50 years of age, persons with cirrhosis, persons with a family history of liver cancer, Africans over 20 years of age, and anyone over 40 years of age with persistent evidence of liver inflammation in the blood or high viral loads (Lok & McMahon, 2009).

Hepatitis B and Liver Cancer Among Asian Americans

Approximately 350 million people have persistent hepatitis B infection worldwide. Areas with intermediate or high rates of hepatitis B include all countries in Asia, Africa, and the South Pacific and parts of the Arctic, the Middle East, Central and South America, Mediterranean and Eastern Europe, and the Caribbean (Lok & McMahon, 2009). There are approximately 1.25 million people with persistent hepatitis B living in the U.S., with the majority of chronic infection occurring among Asian and Pacific Islanders (API) (Lok & McMahon, 2009; Mast et al., 2006). Thus, hepatitis B is an important health disparity for APIs.

Having been born in an HBV-endemic country is strongly associated with chronic HBV infection in the API population and should be viewed as a risk factor (Lin, Chang, & So, 2007). Accordingly, up to two-thirds of Asian immigrants have been exposed to HBV (Tong & Hwang, 1994). The rate of having a positive HBsAg test in the general U.S. population is less than 1% (Centers for Disease Control and Prevention [CDC], 1991a, 1991b). By contrast, among Asian Americans, the rate of having a positive HBsAg test ranges from 6.1% to 14.8% (Hu, 2008). Certain Asian American subgroups report markedly high rates of infection, including estimates of 7–14% among Vietnamese Americans, (CDC, 1991a, 1991b; Goodman & Sikes, 1984; Klontz, 1987), 9–14% among Chinese Americans (Tong & Hwang, 1994), and up to 28% among Laotians and Hmong Americans age 15–19 (Gjerdingen & Lor, 1997).

Asian Americans also differ in how they become infected and at what age. While most infections in the general U.S. population occur in adults through use of injection drugs or sexual contact, most Asian Americans are exposed at birth from an infected mother or through childhood contacts. Infection at younger ages mean that, compared to the general U.S. population, Asian Americans are more likely to have persistent HBV infection and have complications such as cirrhosis or liver cancer at a very young age, approximately 20 years earlier than what is commonly observed in the general U.S. population (Hsieh et al., 1992; Hwang et al., 1996; Nguyen & Keeffe, 2003).

The relationship between HBV and liver cancer is highly disconcerting for Asian Americans. As a group, HBV accounted for 80% of the liver cancer cases among Asian Americans compared to 19% for non-Latino Whites (Hwang et al., 1996). Because of hepatitis B, liver cancer is the most significant cancer disparity for the Asian Americans population, who experience much higher rates of liver cancer than non-Hispanic whites (Chen, 2005). From 1998 to 2002, the age-adjusted incidence rate, or new cases, of liver cancer per 100,000 people each year among non-Hispanic white males was 6.7 (Miller, Chu, Hankey, & Ries, 2008). By contrast, the rates for Japanese, Filipino, Chinese, and Korean American males were 11.4, 17.2, 24.0, and 35.9 respectively. Similarly, while the age-adjusted incidence rate among non-Latino White females were 2.6 per 100,000, the rates for Japanese, Filipino, Chinese, and Korean American women were 7.9, 5.1, 8.2, and 14.4, respectively. The disparity is greatest among Southeast Asians. The incidence rate of liver cancer among Cambodian, Laotian, and Vietnamese men are 49.1, 79.4, and 55.5 and 14.1, 23.1, and 16.8, respectively for women (Miller et al., 2008). While survival rates for those with liver cancer are dismal (less than 10% still alive after 5 years), among Californians of Asian ancestry, the median survival for Laotian/Hmong is significantly short, only about 1 month from diagnosis (Kwong, Stewart, Aoki, & Chen, 2010).

Behavioral Research on Hepatitis B and Asian Americans

Early behavioral research efforts addressing hepatitis B in Asian American communities focused on "catch-up" vaccinations for children and adolescents not vaccinated as infants (Chen et al., 2001; Euler, 2001; Jenkins, McPhee, Wong, Nguyen, & Euler, 2000; Liu, Hynes, Lim, & Chung, 2001; McPhee et al., 2003; Nguyen et al., 2007). Over the last decade, researchers have begun focusing on hepatitis B testing and vaccination among adults from highly endemic geographic areas of Asia such as China, Korea, and Vietnam. Finally, several recent research initiatives have focused on hepatitis B-related knowledge and clinical practices among health care providers serving Asian American patients (Khalili et al., 2010; Upadhyaya et al., 2010).

McPhee et al. (2003) designed and tested two hepatitis B "catch-up" vaccination campaigns for Vietnamese children and adolescents in the 3–18 age group. The different campaigns included a media-led information and education campaign in Houston, a community mobilization strategy in Dallas, while Washington, DC served as a control site for the study (Jenkins et al., 2000; McPhee et al., 2003). A pre-intervention telephone survey found that older children, children who had lived in the U.S. for a longer time, and children whose provider was Vietnamese were less likely to have been vaccinated. Both the tested interventions significantly increased Vietnamese American parents' knowledge about hepatitis B vaccination and improved the numbers of children receiving hepatitis B vaccinations. It was further noted that these strategies proved cost-effective interventions for this community (McPhee et al., 2003; Zhou et al., 2003).

Researchers have used qualitative methods to explore knowledge of hepatitis B infection, hepatitis B testing, and barriers (and facilitators) of vaccination among Asian American adults (Burke et al., 2004; Chang, Nguyen, & So, 2008; Chen et al., 2006; Choe et al., 2005). An ethnographic study of Vietnamese Americans residing in the Seattle area revealed unanticipated information about socio-cultural influences on hepatitis B-related health beliefs and practices. As examples, this study indicated that traditional Vietnamese and Chinese medicine theories influence beliefs about liver illness and health. Further, beliefs about hepatitis B transmission are embedded in personal experiences and socio-historical circumstances (Burke et al., 2004). Focus group research found that Chinese Americans residing in San Francisco are often discouraged from hepatitis B testing and vaccination by costs, lack of health insurance, fear of side effects, worries about reliability or efficacy, poor patient-doctor communication, and lack of symptoms and apparent good health (Chen et al., 2006).

Quantitative studies using surveys have provided details about levels of hepatitis B testing and vaccination among Asian American adults (Bastani, Glenn, Maxwell, & Jo, 2007; Coronado et al., 2007; Grytdal et al., 2009; Hwang, Huang, & Yi, 2008; Juon, Choi, Park, Kwak, & Lee, 2009; Levy, Nguyen, & Nguyen, 2010; Ma et al., 2007a; Ma et al., 2007b, 2008; Nguyen et al., 2010; Taylor et al., 2009; Taylor, Seng, Acorda, Sawn, & Li, 2009; Thompson et al., 2002; Wu, Lin, So, & Chang, 2007). For example, an analysis of the 2006 Racial and Ethnic Approaches to Community Health survey data described hepatitis B testing and vaccination levels among Cambodian American and Vietnamese Americans in four communities. Three-fifths (60%) of the survey respondents reported being tested for hepatitis B and over one-third (35%) reported being vaccinated against hepatitis B. Ethnic Cambodians were less likely than Vietnamese to have been tested for hepatitis B. Level of education was also a factor, as respondents with at least a high school education were more likely to have been tested. Respondents born in the United States, younger individuals, and respondents with at least some college education were more likely to have been vaccinated against hepatitis B (Grytdal et al., 2009).

Several community programs have reported findings from hepatitis B and liver cancer control demonstration programs for Asian Americans (Bailey et al., 2010; Chang, Sue, Zola, & So, 2009; Chao et al., 2009; Hsu et al., 2007):

• The Jade Ribbon Campaign is a culturally targeted, community-based outreach program targeting Asian American adults in California and elsewhere. In 2001, 476 Chinese attended a hepatitis B screening clinic and educational seminar in San Francisco. After one year, two-thirds (67%) of participants with chronic hepatitis B infection had consulted a physician for liver cancer screening, and 78% of all participants had encouraged family members to be tested for hepatitis B (Chao et al., 2009).
• The Hepatitis B Initiative-DC conducted a faith-based hepatitis B program that included education, hepatitis B testing, and hepatitis B vaccination at Korean and Chinese churches in

the Baltimore-Washington DC metropolitan area. During 2003–2006, a total of 1,775 individuals were successfully tested for hepatitis B infection through this initiative, and 79% of the participants who were eligible for vaccination completed the three-dose vaccination series (Hsu et al., 2007).

- Most recently, Bailey et al. (2010) reported preliminary results from the San Francisco Hep B Free Campaign, a local effort to eliminate hepatitis B by building a broad, community-wide coalition reaching out to the AAPI community, health care providers, policy-makers, businesses, and the general public in San Francisco, California. Mass-media and grassroots messaging raised citywide awareness of hepatitis B and promoted use of the existing health care system for hepatitis B screening and follow-up. From 2007 to 2009, over 150 organizations contributed approximately $1,000,000 in resources. Activities included 40 educational events for healthcare providers with 50 percent of primary care physicians pledging to screen AAPIs for hepatitis B and numerous community events that reached over 200,000 community members. Over 3,300 AAPI community members have been tested at stand-alone screening sites (Bailey et al., 2010).

To date, few controlled studies have evaluated hepatitis B intervention programs for Asian American adults. However, one recent randomized controlled trial found that a lay health worker approach for individuals of Chinese ancestry that included home visits and the use of culturally appropriate educational materials, was effective in improving hepatitis-B related knowledge, but had only a very limited impact on hepatitis B testing levels (Taylor et al., 2009).

Khalili and associates (2010) recently surveyed health care providers serving large Asian populations in the San Francisco area about their hepatitis B and liver cancer screening practices. Only 76% of the respondents had screened over half of their Asian patients for hepatitis B, 43% had vaccinated over half of their eligible patients against hepatitis B, and 79% had screened over half of their patients who were chronically infected with hepatitis B for liver cancer. Hepatitis B screening was positively associated with famil-

iarity with clinical guidelines, while liver cancer screening was positively associated with having a higher proportion of Asian patients and higher levels of knowledge about liver cancer (Khalili et al., 2010).

Social, Cultural, and Behavioral Factors Related to Hepatitis B Testing

The high rates of chronic hepatitis B infection among Asians should result in a substantial number of cases detected by hepatitis B testing. The results of the testing efforts should lead to better and more informed decision-making with respect to treatment for hepatitis B and screening for liver cancer, as well as counseling to help arrest the spread of the disease. In addition, case identification would allow vaccination of household members to prevent further transmission. Those who are found to be seronegative can still be counseled on the risks and benefits of hepatitis B vaccination. Vaccination of all infants and children under the age of 18 years is recommended. However, vaccination of Asian immigrant adults without testing for the disease is not considered an adequate public health strategy, since vaccination without testing will deny health providers the opportunity to offer treatment to those in need as well as inform and educate patients about transmission. Additionally, vaccinations would be wasted on those individuals already exposed to the virus yet have resolved the infection and are now immune. Consequently, hepatitis B research among Asian Americans has focused on hepatitis B testing within the population.

To date, most studies have tried to understand why so few Asian Americans are being tested for hepatitis B. A few studies have tested various interventions to encourage hepatitis B testing. Individuals and their families, the health care system and the broader geographic, social and political environment interact in complex ways to influence behavior related to hepatitis B testing, vaccination and treatment in Asian Americans. A sound conceptual framework can provide a roadmap for systematically addressing the multiple and complex determinants of the health behavior in which change is desired. The Health

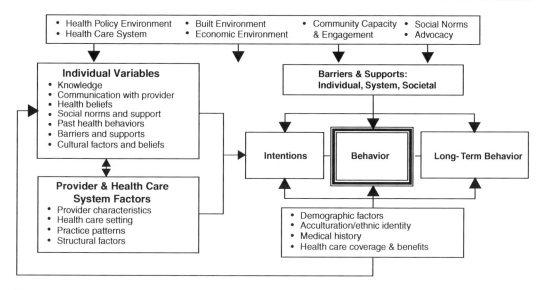

Fig. 19.1   Health Behavior Framework

Behavior Framework is one of the conceptual models that have been used to systematically examine these factors (Bastani et al., 2010; Maxwell et al., 2010).

The Health Behavior Framework (HBF) is based on the premise that multi-faceted behaviors can only be influenced and changed by using a multi-dimensional model based on different theoretical orientations (Fig. 19.1). The HBF represents a synthesis of some of the major theoretical formulations in the area of health behavior, such as *Social Cognitive Theory* (Bandura, 1989, 2004), the *Health Belief Model* (Becker & Maiman, 1974) the *Theory of Planned Behavior* (Ajzen, 2002; Ajzen & Madden, 1986; Fishbein & Ajzen, 1975; Madden, Ellen, & Ajzen, 1992), the *Transtheoretical Model of Change* (Prochaska, 1992; Prochaska & DiClemente, 1983), and *Social Influence Theory* (Greer, 1988; Lomas & Haynes, 1988; Mittman, Tonesk, & Jacobson, 1992). In addition, the model considers the context within which the desired behavior and behavior change are enacted, including characteristics of the provider and the health care setting (Wagner, 1998; Zapka & Lemon, 2004), as well as larger community and societal influences (Babey, Hastert, Yu, & Brown, 2008; Ponce, Huh, & Bastani, 2005).

The HBF assumes that Individual Variables and Provider and Health Care System Factors influence behavioral intentions, which in turn influence health behavior. It should be emphasized that intentions do not automatically translate into behavior. Rather, this connection depends on the absence of barriers and/or presence of supports, which may function at the level of the individual (e.g., cultural beliefs), the health system (e.g., practice patterns), or society (e.g., impoverished neighborhood). Supports and barriers may also bypass intentions and exert direct influence on health behaviors. The model also considers a broader context within which the desired behavior and behavior change are enacted. These are the broader socio-ecological conditions under which people lead their lives and include the health policy environment, community capacity and engagement, social norms, social deprivation, discrimination, and physical environmental influences.

Individual variables, such as *knowledge/ awareness of hepatitis B and its transmission routes* have been assessed in previous studies. Such knowledge about hepatitis B testing has been evaluated with different Asian American subpopulations, including Chinese (Thompson et al., 2003), Vietnamese (Levy, Nguyen, &

Nguyen, 2010; Taylor et al., 2004, 2005), Cambodians (Taylor et al., 2009) and Korean Americans (Bastani, Glenn, Maxwell, & Jo, 2007). *Communication with a provider* or a recommendation by a provider to get tested are associated with greater hepatitis B testing in these and other studies (Bastani et al., 2007; Coronado et al., 2007; Hislop et al., 2007; Ma et al., 2007a; Nguyen et al., 2010; Taylor et al., 2004, 2005; Tu et al., 2009). *Health beliefs* can facilitate hepatitis B testing in the expected direction; that is, those who believed that people from their ethnic background were more likely to be infected with hepatitis B than Whites (*perceived susceptibility*) would consider testing. Further, individuals who believe hepatitis B can cause liver cancer (*perceived severity*) were more likely to be tested than respondents who did not hold belief. Other beliefs that have been reported to motivate individuals to get tested and/or vaccinated for hepatitis B include achieving peace of mind, prevention of transmission to others and protection of one's future health (Chang, Nguyen, & So, 2008).

There are also several barriers to hepatitis B testing that have been described, including the cost of screening and difficulty of taking the time off work to get tested (Chang et al., 2008; Choe et al., 2006; Ma et al., 2007a). Several other barriers that may be particularly salient for Asian American immigrants include lack of interpreter services/language barriers (Choe et al., 2006; Ma et al., 2007a) and the belief that blood tests can deplete the body of energy (Taylor et al., 2004). Testing, vaccination and treatment can be discouraged by the Buddhist belief that suffering is an integral part of life, or Taoism that teaches that perfection is achieved when events are allowed to take their natural course (Tran, 2009).

In some Asian groups, people with hepatitis B are avoided and shunned by others. The stigma of hepatitis B infection can interfere with getting tested or, among those chronically infected with hepatitis B virus, getting necessary treatment (Bastani et al., 2007; Tran, 2009). However, there is little data asserting that such beliefs are actually related to lower rates of hepatitis B testing, vaccination or treatment. It may well be that

many Asian Americans who hold these beliefs will nevertheless undergo testing and treatment if they have access to care, understand the issues at stake, and if they have a strong recommendation from a trusted provider.

Provider and health care system factors can also influence hepatitis B testing. Surprisingly, many primary care providers are not aware of the CDC recommendations for hepatitis B testing, cannot correctly identify the screening test for hepatitis B, and do not generally recommend hepatitis B testing to their patients (Bailey et al., 2010). Other researchers stated that the majority of patients with chronic hepatitis B infection that they studied received insufficient evaluation and treatment. The authors suggest that this is because many physicians may be unaware of treatment and evaluation guidelines (Jung et al., 2010). San Francisco Hep B Free, a grassroots community coalition, is working to address these shortcomings by creating awareness about the importance of testing and vaccination among health care providers, by promoting routine hepatitis B testing and vaccination in the medical community and by ensuring access to treatment for chronically infected individuals (Bailey et al., 2010).

Most of the individual and provider and health care system factors described above are *mutable,* potential and practical targets for interventions. Individual-level interventions can promote good health behaviors by increasing knowledge or reducing barriers. Provider-level interventions can influence practice norms by providing physician education or addressing structural barriers such as opening evening or weekend clinics and having interpreters available. Although factors at the macro-level such as the health policies and community characteristics are theoretically mutable, they are unlikely targets for community-based efforts (Bastani et al., 2010).

Other factors of the Health Behavior Framework are considered *immutable*, such as demographic factors and health care coverage. However, immutable factors at all levels are still important, requiring assessment when possible. Demographics can be used to target or tailor intervention content (e.g., crafting messages specific for certain ethnic or age groups) at the individual-level. Higher levels of education and being married are positively associated with testing for the disease (Grytdal et al., 2009; Taylor, Jackson, Kuniyuki, & Yasui, 2002; Taylor et al., 2000; Thompson et al., 2003). Age may serve to provide contradictory data between groups. While some studies have found higher level of hepatitis B testing among older Vietnamese and Cambodian adults (Taylor et al., 2002, 2004, 2005) others found that younger age was associated with hepatitis B testing in Chinese adults (Thompson et al., 2002; Tu et al., 2009), though differences in age distribution, length of residence in the United States, and level of income may explain the findings. The availability of insurance – or lack thereof – is another example of an immutable factor that can also moderate the effect of the intervention (Jung et al., 2010).

Using a common theoretical framework such as the Health Behavior Framework allows for comparison of predictors of testing, vaccination and treatment across population groups. If the major predictors are similar across populations, the field can begin to move in the direction of developing common interventions for multiple populations as opposed to the inefficient approach of having to develop specialized interventions for specific sub-populations in the community (Bastani et al., 2010).

Community Efforts to Address Hepatitis B in Asian American Communities

Over the last decade, there has been increasing awareness within the Asian American communities about hepatitis B and a wide range of efforts to address this health disparity. Table 19.1 lists ongoing efforts to address hepatitis B in different regions of the U.S. (Additional organizations can be found at http://www.hepprograms.org/apia/). More resources with up-to-date information about organizations that are active working on hepatitis B with Asian Americans can be accessed through the National Hepatitis B Task Force and the Hepatitis B Foundation. The Hepatitis B Foundation (HBF) is a national non-profit organization dedicated to finding a cure and improving the quality of life for those affected by hepatitis B worldwide. The foundation is committed to funding focused research, promoting disease awareness, supporting immunization and treatment initiatives and serving as the

Table 19.1 List of community organizations working on hepatitis B and Asian Americans

Name	Website
National Hepatitis B Task force	hepbtaskforce.wordpress.com
Hepatitis B Foundation	www.hepb.org
California Hepatitis Alliance	www.calhep.org
Hepatitis B Coalition of Washington State and International Community Health Services	www.hepbwa.org hwww.ichs.com/index.php?page=HepB
B Free CEED	hepatitis.med.nyu.edu
Asian Liver Center at Stanford University	liver.stanford.edu
Hepatitis B Initiative of Washington DC, Inc.	www.hepbinitiative.org/dcmetro/index.html
San Francisco Hep B Free	www.sfhepbfree.org
Hepatitis Outreach Network	hwww.mssm.edu/research/programs/hepatitis-outreach-network/about-us
Hep B Free Philadelphia	www.hepbfreephiladelphia.org
Asian Community Alliance, Inc of Cincinnati (ACA)	www.acacinci.org
Asian Pacific Health Foundation	www.aphfoundation.net
Laotian American National Alliance, Inc. (LANA)	www.lana-usa.org
Hep B Moms	www.HepBMoms.org

primary source of information for patients and their families, the medical and scientific community and the general public.

In 1997, the National Task Force on Hepatitis B: Focus on Asian and Pacific Islander Americans was established. The Task Force gathered scientists, health professionals, non–profit organizations, and concerned citizens in a concerted effort to eliminate hepatitis B in the United States by 2015. The mission of the Task Force, which currently has nearly 200 members, is to eradicate hepatitis B by empowering and mobilizing communities, enabling national networking and policy development, advocating for education, and improving access to comprehensive care and affordable treatment for all AAPIs.

Statewide efforts include the California Hepatitis Alliance (CalHEP), which include more than 90 organizations dedicated to reducing the scope and consequences of the hepatitis B and C epidemics in California through advocacy for sound policies, promotion of evidence-based education, and increasing access to services. The Hepatitis B Coalition of Washington State (HBCW) is dedicated to reducing hepatitis B disease and its complications through innovation, education, and community partnership. HBCW and International Community Health Services (ICHS), a non-profit community health center in King County, WA are collaborating on the Hepatitis B Community Engagement Project, which seeks to raise and expand awareness and action among high-risk populations for chronic hepatitis B. In New York, B Free CEED is a partnership of New York University School of Medicine and local and national coalition members. B Free CEED is committed to eliminating hepatitis B disparities in AAPI communities by developing, evaluating, and disseminating evidence-based practices.

Some local efforts, such as the Jade Ribbon Campaign in Northern California led by the Asian Liver Center at Stanford, San Francisco Hep B Free, and Hepatitis B Initiative of Washington, DC have published their activities and findings in research journals and were discussed in the preceding sections (Bailey et al., 2010; Chang et al., 2009; Chao et al., 2009; Hsu et al., 2007; Hsu,

Zhang, Yan, Shang, & Le, 2010). The Asian Liver Center at Stanford University is the first non-profit organization in the United States that addresses the high incidence of hepatitis B and liver cancer in Asians and Asian Americans. Founded in 1996, the center uses a three-pronged approach towards fighting hepatitis B through outreach and education, advocacy, and research. The Hepatitis B Initiative of Washington DC, Inc. (HBI-DC) is a non-profit organization founded in 2002 with a mission to mobilize communities to prevent HBV infection and its consequences among at-risk groups in the Washington DC metropolitan area. HBI-DC serves the community by providing community education, screening tests, immunization, treatment referrals, by building partnerships, and by gathering relevant data. San Francisco Hep B Free is a city-wide campaign to turn San Francisco into the first hepatitis B free city in the nation. The campaign provides free and low-cost hepatitis B testing and vaccinations to AAPI adults. SF Hep B Free campaign's goals are to create public and healthcare provider awareness about the importance of testing and vaccinating AAPIs for hepatitis B, to promote routine hepatitis B testing and vaccination within the primary care medical community, and to ensure access to treatment for chronically infected individuals.

The Hepatitis Outreach Network (HONE) is a collaboration between faculty of The Mount Sinai Medical Center and community physicians who care for minority patients at high risk for chronic hepatitis in New York. HONE aims to raise awareness about chronic hepatitis B and C, offers free HBV and HCV screening, and links people to appropriate vaccinations and treatments. Hep B Free Philadelphia is a public awareness and education campaign to increase testing and vaccination to fight hepatitis B and liver cancer in Philadelphia. Hep B Free Philadelphia uses a community-organizing approach to established multi-disciplinary partnerships across the city. In Cincinnati, Ohio, hepatitis B control efforts are led by Asian Community Alliance, Inc of Cincinnati (ACA). ACA provides education to Asian Americans as well as health providers, collaborates with others to provide free screening as well as vaccinations and follow-up treatment. In

San Diego, CA, the Asian Pacific Health Center and the Asian Pacific Health Foundation has been working on hepatitis B issues since 2003 by providing outreach and screening to nearly 3,000 people. Other efforts to address hepatitis include the Asian Center – Southeast Michigan in Michigan, Laotian American National Alliance, Inc. (LANA) which has been developing educational materials for Laotians and conducting outreach in California, and HepBMoms, a non-profit organization dedicated to the prevention of perinatal transmission of hepatitis B.

Future Directions for Efforts to Eliminate Hepatitis B in Asian American Communities

One priority area for research is to identify more effective treatments to control and/or eradicate hepatitis B in those who are infected. Current strategies to eliminate hepatitis B in Asian American communities need to focus on screening to identify those who are infected, ensuring that they receive appropriate health care, and vaccinating those who are at-risk but not yet infected. The Institute of Medicine (IOM) published a national strategy for the prevention and control of viral hepatitis in 2010 (Colvin & Mitchell, 2010). The IOM review committee found that the main barriers to current efforts to prevent and control viral hepatitis were lack of knowledge and awareness about chronic viral hepatitis on the part of health-care, social-service providers, at-risk populations, and policy-makers and inadequate public resources allocated to prevention, control, and surveillance programs (Colvin & Mitchell, 2010). The IOM made a series of recommendations for governmental organizations and service providers, including:

- Expand community-based programs that provide hepatitis B screening, testing, and vaccination services that target foreign-born populations.
- Develop educational programs for health-care and social-service providers.
- Conduct effective outreach and education programs to target at-risk populations.

- Ensure that infants are vaccinated appropriately against hepatitis B.
- Mandate that the hepatitis B vaccine series be completed or in progress as a requirement for school attendance.
- Increase resources to vaccinate against hepatitis B among at-risk adults including expanding insurance coverage.
- Incorporate guidelines for appropriate screening and treatment of those infected as a core component of health care.

Although hepatitis B is a scourge among Asian Americans, we already know in large part how to diagnose it, how to treat it, and how to prevent it. There is a burgeoning literature on what is keeping Asian Americans from receiving appropriate screening, treatment, and vaccination. In addition, there are many active local efforts to address hepatitis B control, particularly through collaborative partnerships to promote and deliver hepatitis B screening. However, there remains a paucity of rigorous research showing which interventions work and how they may work among various Asian American populations, and how to address health care provider and health care systems barriers preventing appropriate screening, treatment, and vacci-nation.

We still need to know what works best to increase the rates of screening and vaccination in various Asian American communities. An ongoing program project funded by the National Cancer Institute is using rigorous scientific methods to evaluate the effect of three behavioral interventions to increase levels of hepatitis B testing among Asian populations in California: a media-based intervention for Vietnamese, a lay health educator intervention for Hmong, and a group educational intervention for Korean church attendees (Bastani et al., 2010; Chen, Nguyen, & Bastani, 2007; Maxwell et al., 2010; Nguyen et al., 2010). Findings from this and other ongoing research as well as active community efforts to address hepatitis B will ensure that the goal of eliminating hepatitis B from Asian American communities will be achieved.

Acknowledgments This work was supported in part by grants from the National Cancer Institute (U54 CA153499) and co-funding by the National Cancer Institute and the National Institute on Minority Health and Health Disparities (P01 CA109091-A1). The views expressed do not necessarily represent the views of the National Institutes of Health.

References

Ajzen, I. (2002). Perceived behavioral control, self-efficacy, locus of control, and the theory of planned behavior. *Journal of Applied Social Psychology, 32*, 665–683.

Ajzen, I., & Madden, T. (1986). Prediction of goal-directed behavior: Attitudes, intentions and perceived behavioral control. *Journal of Experimental Social Psychology, 22*, 453–474.

Babey, S. H., Hastert, T. A., Yu, H., & Brown, R. (2008). Physical activity among adolescents. When do parks matter? *American Journal of Preventive Medicine, 34*(4), 345–348.

Bailey, M. B., Shiau, R., Zola, J., Fernyak, S. E., Fang, T., So, S. K. S., et al. (2010). San Francisco Hep B free: A grassroots community coalition to prevent hepatitis B and liver cancer. *Journal of Community Health* [epub ahead of print]

Bandura, A. (1989). Human agency in social cognitive theory. *American Psychologist, 44*(9), 1175–1184.

Bandura, A. (2004). Health promotion by social cognitive means. *Health Education & Behavior, 31*(2), 143–164.

Bastani, R., Glenn, B. A., Maxwell, A. E., & Jo, A. M. (2007). Hepatitis B testing for liver cancer control among Korean Americans. *Ethnicity & Disease, 17*(2), 365–373.

Bastani, R., Glenn, B. A., Taylor, V. M., Chen, M. S., Jr., Nguyen, T. T., Stewart, S. L., et al. (2010). Integrating theory into community interventions to reduce liver cancer disparities: The Health Behavior Framework. *Preventive Medicine, 50*(1–2), 63–67.

Becker, M., & Maiman, L. A. (1974). The health belief model: Origins and correlates in psychological theory. *Health Education Monographs, 2*, 336–353.

Burke, N. J., Jackson, C. J., Thai, H. C., Stackhouse, F., Nguyen, T., Chen, A., et al. (2004). 'Honoring tradition, accepting new ways': Development of a hepatitis B control intervention for Vietnamese immigrants. *Ethnicity and Health, 9*(2), 153–169.

Centers for Disease Control and Prevention. (1991a). Hepatitis B virus: A comprehensive strategy for eliminating transmission in the United States through universal childhood vaccination: Recommendations of the immunization practices advisory committee (ACIP). *MMWR Recommendations and Reports, 40*(RR-13), 1–19.

Centers for Disease Control and Prevention. (1991b). Screening for hepatitis B virus infection among refugees arriving in the United States, 1979-1991. *MMWR. Morbidity and Mortality Weekly Report, 40*(45), 784–786.

Chang, M.-H., Chen, C.-J., Lai, M.-S., Hsu, H.-M., Wu, T.-C., Kong, M.-S., et al. (1997). Universal hepatitis B vaccination in Taiwan and the incidence of hepatocellular carcinoma in children. Taiwan Childhood Hepatoma Study Group [see comments]. *The New England Journal of Medicine, 336*(26), 1855–1859.

Chang, E. T., Nguyen, B. H., & So, S. K. (2008). Attitudes toward hepatitis B and liver cancer prevention among Chinese Americans in the San Francisco Bay Area, California. *Asian Pacific Journal of Cancer Prevention, 9*(4), 605–613.

Chang, E. T., Sue, E., Zola, J., & So, S. K. (2009). 3 For life: A model pilot program to prevent hepatitis B virus infection and liver cancer in Asian and Pacific Islander Americans. *American Journal of Health Promotion, 23*(3), 176–181.

Chao, S. D., Chang, E. T., Le, P. V., Propong, W., Kiernan, M., & So, S. K. S. (2009). The jade ribbon campaign: A model program for community outreach and education to prevent liver cancer in Asian Americans. *Journal of Immigrant and Minor Health, 11*(4), 281–290.

Chen, M. S., Jr. (2005). Cancer health disparities among Asian Americans: What we do and what we need to do. *Cancer, 104*(Suppl. 12), 2895–2902.

Chen, M. S. Jr., Nguyen, T., & Bastani, R., Y. (2007). Liver cancer control interventions for Asian Americans: A first community-based program project to reduce cancer health disparities. AACR Proceedings, 2007, 120–121. http://owl.english.purdue.edu/owl/resource/583/03/

Chen, Q. S., Jr., Ngo-Metzger, Q., Tran, L. Q., Sugrue-McElearney, E., Levy, E. R., Williams, G., et al. (2001). Hepatitis B vaccination among Vietnamese-American children in a Boston community clinic. *Asian American and Pacific Islander Journal of Health, 9*(2), 179–187.

Chen, H., Tu, S.-P., Yip, M.-P., Choe, J. H., Teh, C. Z., Hislop, T. G., et al. (2006). Lay beliefs about hepatitis among North American Chinese: Implications for hepatitis prevention. *Journal of Community Health, 31*(2), 94–112.

Choe, J. H., Chan, N., Do, H., Woodall, E., Lim, E., & Taylor, V. M. (2005). Hepatitis B and liver cancer beliefs among Korean immigrants in Western Washington. *Cancer, 104*(Suppl. 12), 2955–2958.

Choe, J. H., Taylor, V. M., Yasui, Y., Burke, N., Nguyen, T., Acorda, E., et al. (2006). Health care access and sociodemographic factors associated with hepatitis B testing in Vietnamese American men. *Journal of Immigrant and Minority Health, 8*(3), 193–201.

Colvin, H. M., & Mitchell, A. E. (Eds.). (2010). Hepatitis and liver cancer: A national strategy for prevention and control of hepatitis B and C. Washington, DC: National Academies Press.

Coronado, G. D., Taylor, V. M., Tu, S.-P., Yasui, Y., Acorda, E., & Woodall, E. (2007). Correlates of hepatitis B testing among Chinese Americans. *Journal of Community Health, 32*(6), 379–390.

Euler, G. L. (2001). The epidemiology of hepatitis B vaccination catch-up among AAPI children in the United States. *Asian American and Pacific Islander Journal of Health, 9*(2), 154–161.

Fishbein, M., & Ajzen, I. (1975). Belief, attitude, intention, and behavior :An introduction to theory and research. Reading, MA: Addison-Wesley.

Gjerdingen, D. K., & Lor, V. (1997). Hepatitis B status of Hmong patients. *The Journal of the American Board of Family Practice, 10*(5), 322–328.

Goodman, R. A., & Sikes, R. K. (1984). Hepatitis B markers in Southeast Asian refugees [letter]. *Journal of the American Medical Association, 251*(16), 2086.

Greer, A. L. (1988). The state of the art versus the state of the science. The diffusion of new medical technologies into practice. *International Journal of Technology Assessment in Health Care, 4*(1), 5–26.

Grytdal, S. P., Liao, Y., Chen, R., Garvin, C. C., Grigg-Saito, D., Kagawa-Singer, M., et al. (2009). Hepatitis B testing and vaccination among Vietnamese- and Cambodian-Americans. *Journal of Community Health, 34*(3), 173–180.

Hislop, T. G., Teh, C. Z., Low, A., Tu, S.-P., Yasui, Y., Coronado, G. D., et al. (2007). Predisposing, reinforcing and enabling factors associated with hepatitis B testing in Chinese Canadians in British Columbia. *Asian Pacific Journal of Cancer Prevention, 8*(1), 39–44.

Hsieh, C.-C., Tzonou, A., Zavitsanos, X., Kaklamani, E., Lan, S.-J., & Trichopoulos, D. (1992). Age at first establishment of chronic hepatitis B virus infection and hepatocellular carcinoma risk. A birth order study. *American Journal of Epidemiology, 136*(9), 1115–1121.

Hsu, C., Liu, L. C.-H., Juon, H.-S., Chiu, Y.-W., Bawa, J., Tillman, U., et al. (2007). Reducing liver cancer disparities: A community-based hepatitis-B prevention program for Asian-American communities. *Journal of the National Medical Association, 99*(8), 900–907.

Hsu, C. E., Zhang, G., Yan, F. A., Shang, N., & Le, T. (2010). What made a successful hepatitis B program for reducing liver cancer disparities: An examination of baseline characteristics and educational intervention, infection status, and missing responses of at-risk Asian Americans. *Journal of Community Health, 35*(3), 325–335.

Hu, K. Q. (2008). Hepatitis B virus (HBV) infection in Asian and Pacific Islander Americans (APIAs): How can we do better for this special population? *American Journal of Gastroenterology, 103*(7), 1824–1833.

Hwang, J. P., Huang, C.-H., & Yi, J. K. (2008). Knowledge about hepatitis B and predictors of hepatitis B vaccination among Vietnamese American college students. *Journal of American College Health, 56*(4), 377–382.

Hwang, S.-J., Tong, M. J., Lai, P. P., Ko, E. S., Ko, R. L., Chien, D., et al. (1996). Evaluation of hepatitis B and C viral markers: Clinical significance in Asian and Caucasian patients with hepatocellular carcinoma in the United States of America. *Journal of Gastroenterology and Hepatology, 11*(10), 949–954.

Jenkins, C. N., McPhee, S. J., Wong, C., Nguyen, T., & Euler, G. L. (2000). Hepatitis B immunization coverage among Vietnamese-American children 3 to 18 years old. *Pediatrics, 106*(6), E78.

Jung, C. W., Tan, J., Tan, N., Kuo, M. N., Ashok, A., Eells, S. J., et al. (2010). Evidence for the insufficient evaluation and undertreatment of chronic hepatitis B infection in a predominantly low-income and immigrant population. *Journal of Gastroenterology and Hepatology, 25*(2), 369–375.

Juon, H.-S., Choi, K. S., Park, E.-C., Kwak, M.-S., & Lee, S. (2009). Hepatitis B vaccinations among Koreans: Results from 2005 Korea National Cancer Screening Survey. *BMC Infectious Diseases, 9*, 185.

Khalili, M., Guy, J., Yu, A., Li, A., Diamond-Smith, N., Stewart, S., et al. (2010). Hepatitis B and hepatocellular carcinoma screening among Asian Americans: Survey of safety net healthcare providers. Digestive Diseases and Sciences.

Khalili, M., Liao, C. E., & Nguten, T. (2009). Liver disease. In G. D. Hammer & S. J. McPhee (Eds.), Pathophysiology of disease: An introduction to clinical medicine. New York: Lange Medical Books/McGraw-Hill.

Klontz, K. C. (1987). A program to provide hepatitis B immunoprophylaxis to infants born to HBsAg-positive Asian and Pacific Island women. *The Western Journal of Medicine, 146*(2), 195–199.

Kwong, S. L., Stewart, S. L., Aoki, C. A., & Chen, M. S. (2010). Disparities in hepatocellular carcinoma survival among Californians of Asian ancestry, 1988 to 2007. *Cancer Epidemiology, Biomarkers & Prevention, 19*(11), 2747–2757.

Lee, C.-L., & Ko, Y.-C. (1997). Hepatitis B vaccination and hepatocellular carcinoma in Taiwan. *Pediatrics, 99*(3), 351–353.

Levy, J. D., Nguyen, G. T., & Nguyen, E. T. (2010). Factors influencing the receipt of hepatitis B vaccination and screenings in Vietnamese Americans. *Journal of Health Care for the Poor and Underserved, 21*(3), 851–861.

Liaw, Y.-F., Sung, J. J. Y., Chow, W. C., Farrell, G., Lee, C.-Z., Yuen, H., et al. (2004). Lamivudine for patients with chronic hepatitis B and advanced liver disease. *The New England Journal of Medicine, 351*(15), 1521–1531.

Lin, S. Y., Chang, E. T., & So, S. K. (2007). Why we should routinely screen Asian American adults for hepatitis B: A cross-sectional study of Asians in California. *Hepatology, 46*(4), 1034–1040.

Liu, H., Hynes, K., Lim, J. M., & Chung, H. I. (2001). Hepatitis B catch-up project: Analysis of 1999 data from the Chicago public schools. *Asian American and Pacific Islander Journal of Health, 9*(2), 205–210.

Lok, A. S., & McMahon, B. J. (2009). Chronic hepatitis B: Update 2009. *Hepatology, 50*(3), 661–662.

Lomas, J., & Haynes, R. B. (1988). A taxonomy and critical review of tested strategies for the application of clinical practice recommendations: From "official" to "individual" clinical policy. *American Journal of Preventive Medicine, 4*(Suppl. 4), 77–94 discussion 95-77.

Ma, G. X., Fang, C. Y., Shive, S. E., Toubbeh, J., Tan, Y., & Siu, P. (2007a). Risk perceptions and barriers to Hepatitis B screening and vaccination among Vietnamese immigrants. *Journal of Immigrant and Minority Health, 9*(3), 213–220.

Ma, G. X., Shive, S. E., Fang, C. Y., Feng, Z., Parameswaran, L., Pham, A., et al. (2007b). Knowledge, attitudes, and behaviors of hepatitis B screening and vaccination and liver cancer risks among Vietnamese Americans. *Journal of Health Care for the Poor and Underserved, 18*(1), 62–73.

Ma, G. X., Shive, S. E., Toubbeh, J. I., Tan, Y., & Wu, D. (2008). Knowledge, attitudes, and behaviors of Chinese hepatitis B screening and vaccination. *American Journal of Health Behavior, 32*(2), 178–187.

Madden, T. J., Ellen, P. S., & Ajzen, I. (1992). A comparison of the Theory of Planned Behavior and the Theory of Reasoned Action. *Personality and Social Psychology Bulletin, 18*, 3–9.

Mast, E. E., Weinbaum, C. M., Fiore, A. E., Alter, M. J., Bell, B. P., Finelli, L., et al. (2006). A comprehensive immunization strategy to eliminate transmission of hepatitis B virus infection in the United States: Recommendations of the Advisory Committee on Immunization Practices (ACIP) Part II: Immunization of adults. *MMWR Recommendations and Reports, 55*(RR-16), 1–33; quiz CE31-34.

Maxwell, A. E., Bastani, R., Chen, M. S., Jr., Nguyen, T. T., Stewart, S. L., & Taylor, V. M. (2010). Constructing a theoretically based set of measures for liver cancer control research studies. *Preventive Medicine, 50*(1–2), 68–73.

Maynard, J. E., Kane, M. A., & Hadler, S. C. (1989). Global control of hepatitis B through vaccination: role of hepatitis B vaccine in the Expanded Programme on Immunization. *Reviews of Infectious Diseases, 11*(Suppl. 3), S574–S578.

McPhee, S. J., Nguyen, T., Euler, G. L., Mock, J., Wong, C., Lam, T., et al. (2003). Successful promotion of hepatitis B vaccinations among Vietnamese-American children ages 3 to 18: Results of a controlled trial. *Pediatrics, 111*(6 Pt 1), 1278–1288.

Miller, B. A., Chu, K. C., Hankey, B. F., & Ries, L. A. G. (2008). Cancer incidence and mortality patterns among specific Asian and Pacific Islander populations in the U.S. *Cancer Causes & Control, 19*(3), 227–256.

Mittman, B. S., Tonesk, X., & Jacobson, P. (1992). Implementing clinical practice guidelines: Social influence strategies and practitioner behavior change. QRB. *Quality Review Bulletin, 18*(12), 413–422.

Nguyen, M. H., & Keeffe, E. B. (2003). Chronic hepatitis B and hepatitis C in Asian Americans. *Reviews in Gastroenterological Disorders, 3*(3), 125–134.

Nguyen, T. T., McPhee, S. J., Stewart, S., Gildengorin, G., Zhang, L., Wong, C., et al. (2010). Factors associated with hepatitis B testing among Vietnamese Americans. *Journal of General Internal Medicine, 25*(7), 694–700.

Nguyen, T. T., Taylor, V., Chen, M. S., Bastani, R., Maxwell, A. E., & Mcphee, S. J. (2007). Hepatitis B awareness, knowledge, and screening among Asian Americans. *Journal of Cancer Education, 22*(4), 266–272.

Ponce, N. A., Huh, S., & Bastani, R. (2005). Do HMO market level factors lead to racial/ethnic disparities in colorectal cancer screening? A comparison between high-risk Asian and Pacific Islander Americans and high-risk whites. *Medical Care, 43*(11), 1101–1108.

Prochaska, J. O. (1992). A transtheoretical model of behavior change: Learning from mistakes with majority populations. In D. M. Becher, D. R. Hill, S. Jackson, et al. (Eds.), Health behavior research in minority populations: Access, design and implementation (pp. 105–111). Washington, DC: National Institutes of Health.

Prochaska, J. O., & DiClemente, C. (1983). Stages and processes of self-change of smoking: Toward an integrative model of change. *Journal of Consulting and Clinical Psychology, 51*(3), 390–395.

Quang, Y. N., Vu, J., Yuk, J., Li, C.-S., Chen, M., & Bowlus, C. L. (2010). Prevalence of hepatitis B surface antigen in US-born and foreign-born Asian/Pacific Islander college students. *Journal of American College Health, 59*(1), 37–41.

Taylor, V. M., Hislop, T. G., Tu, S.-P., Teh, C., Acorda, E., Yip, M.-P., et al. (2009). Evaluation of a Hepatitis B lay health worker intervention for Chinese Americans and Canadians. *Journal of Community Health, 34*(3), 1625–1672.

Taylor, V. M., Jackson, J. C., Kuniyuki, A., & Yasui, Y. (2002). Hepatitis B knowledge and practices among Cambodian American women in Seattle, Washington. *Journal of Community Health, 27*(3), 151–163.

Taylor, V. M., Jackson, J. C., Pineda, M., Pham, P., Fischer, M., & Yasui, Y. (2000). Hepatitis B knowledge among Vietnamese immigrants: Implications for prevention of hepatocellular carcinoma. *Journal of Cancer Education, 15*(1), 51–55.

Taylor, V. M., Seng, P., Acorda, E., Sawn, L., & Li, L. (2009). Hepatitis B knowledge and practices among Cambodian immigrants. *Journal of Cancer Education, 24*(2), 100–104.

Taylor, V. M., Yasui, Y., Burke, N., Choe, J. H., Acorda, E., & Jackson, J. C. (2005). Hepatitis B knowledge and testing among Vietnamese-American women. *Ethnicity & Disease, 15*(4), 761–767.

Taylor, V. M., Yasui, Y., Burke, N., Nguyen, T., Chen, A., Acorda, E., et al. (2004). Hepatitis B testing among Vietnamese American men. *Cancer Detection and Prevention, 28*(3), 170–177.

Thompson, M. J., Taylor, V. M., Jackson, J. C., Yasui, Y., Kuniyuki, A., Tu, S.-P., et al. (2002). Hepatitis B knowledge and practices among Chinese American women in Seattle, Washington. *Journal of Cancer Education, 17*(4), 222–226.

Thompson, M. J., Taylor, V. M., Yasui, Y., Hislop, T. G., Jackson, J. C., Kuniyuki, A., et al. (2003). Hepatitis B knowledge and practices among Chinese Canadian women in Vancouver, British Columbia. *Canadian Journal of Public Health, 94*(4), 281–286.

Tong, M. J., & Hwang, S. J. (1994). Hepatitis B virus infection in Asian Americans. *Gastroenterology Clinics of North America, 23*(3), 523–536.

Tran, T. T. (2009). Understanding cultural barriers in hepatitis B virus infection. *Cleveland Clinic Journal of Medicine, 76*(Suppl. 3), S10–S13.

Tu, S.-P., Li, L., Tsai, J. H.-C., Yip, M.-P., Terasaki, G., Teh, C. Z., et al. (2009). A cross-border comparison of hepatitis B testing among Chinese residing in Canada and the United States. *Asian Pacific Journal of Cancer Prevention, 10*(3), 483–490.

Upadhyaya, N., Chang, R., Davis, C., Conti, M. C., Salinas-Garcia, D., & Tang, H. (2010). Chronic hepatitis B: Perceptions in Asian American communities and diagnosis and management practices among primary care physicians. *Postgraduate Medicine, 122*(5), 165–175.

Wagner, E. H. (1998). Chronic disease management: What will it take to improve care for chronic illness? *Effective Clinical Practice, 1*(1), 2–4.

Wu, C. A., Lin, S. Y., So, S. K., & Chang, E. T. (2007). Hepatitis B and liver cancer knowledge and preventive practices among Asian Americans in the San Francisco Bay Area, California. *Asian Pacific Journal of Cancer Prevention, 8*(1), 127–134.

Zapka, J. G., & Lemon, S. C. (2004). Interventions for patients, providers, and health care organizations. *Cancer, 101*(Suppl. 5), 1165–1187.

Zhang, B.-H., Yang, B.-H., & Tang, Z.-Y. (2004). Randomized controlled trial of screening for hepatocellular carcinoma. *Journal of Cancer Research and Clinical Oncology, 130*(7), 417–422.

Zhou, F., Euler, G. L., McPhee, S. J., Nguyen, T., Lam, T., Wong, C., et al. (2003). Economic analysis of promotion of hepatitis B vaccinations among Vietnamese-American children and adolescents in Houston and Dallas. *Pediatrics, 111*(6 Pt 1), 1289–1296.

Severe Mental Illnesses in Asian Americans: Schizophrenia and Bipolar Disorder

20

Russell F. Lim and Francis G. Lu

Mr. W. is a 23 year old Chinese American man who was in his normal state of good health until he moved to Boston one year ago. He went to live in Boston to establish Massachusetts state residency for the purpose of qualifying for in-state tuition at a state college in Boston. He was a straight-A student, had a part-time job, and was close to his family.

Before leaving San Francisco for Boston, Mr. W. could be described as a loner. He rented an apartment, where he lived alone for the first time in his life. He began to hear voices telling him that he should stay in his apartment. Within six months, he was a virtual recluse in his apartment. He became preoccupied about imaginary threats to his life and how he should protect himself. He put together a notebook with sheet protectors and black backgrounds, covering each page with both recurring motifs of Xeroxed Greek statues, and meandering text that wrapped around the outside of each page and around the statues. After getting a taxi, he was unable to articulate where he wanted to go, fearful of his life outside of his house.

He was then eventually hospitalized in a psychiatric inpatient unit where he was diagnosed with schizophrenia. Anti-psychotic medications were administered to reduce the frequency and

volume of the voices and his fears of others trying to hurt him. He returned home to his parents in California, and was taking an antipsychotic medication when he was seen at a community mental health center for follow-up. His voices were less intrusive than before, but he still remains unable to work or go back to school.

Introduction

A wide variety of psychological disturbances are associated with the term *mental illness*. The Surgeon General of the United States (1999) defined mental illness as "the term that refers collectively to all diagnosable mental disorders. Mental disorders are health conditions that are characterized by alterations in thinking, mood, or behavior (or some combination thereof) associated with distress and/or impaired functioning" (p. 5). Furthermore, the Surgeon General stated: "Persons suffering from any of the severe mental disorders present with a variety of symptoms that may include inappropriate anxiety, disturbances of thought and perception, disregulation of mood, and cognitive dysfunction. Many of these symptoms may be relatively specific to a particular "diagnosis or cultural influence" (p. 40). In short, they are illnesses that cause significant loss of functioning. These disorders can include psychotic disorders, schizophrenia and schizoaffective disorder, and bipolar disorders.

These disorders have been studied for many years in many different cultural contexts, including

R.F. Lim (✉) • F.G. Lu, MD
School of Medicine, Department of Psychiatry & Behavioral Sciences, University of California, Sacramento, CA, USA
e-mail: rflim@ucdavis.edu; francis.lu@ucdmc.ucdavis.edu

G.J. Yoo et al. (eds.), *Handbook of Asian American Health*, DOI 10.1007/978-1-4614-2227-3_20, © Springer Science+Business Media, LLC 2013

Asian societies. An early example includes the writings of Emil Kraeplin, who is credited with defining schizophrenia as a unique malady, having studied the disease in Java in 1904 to learn about schizophrenia in a non-western country. There are also differences in the criteria used to identify psychopathological. In some Asian (as well as some African and Latin) cultures, auditory and visual hallucinations may be considered "culturally normative" rather than psychopathological (Jenkins, 1998). In some other cultures, experiences that would be considered as symptoms of a psychotic disorder are instead viewed as something that is spiritual, positive, and acceptable, and are encouraged in rituals performed by shamans. Consequently, it is generally agreed that the content of psychosis is determined by cultural beliefs (Stompe et al., 2006).

The Prevalence of Schizophrenia Among Asian Americans

The most recent edition of the Diagnostic and Statistical Manual, Fourth Edition, Text Revision (DSM-IV-TR) (American Psychiatric Association [APA], 2000) currently defines schizophrenia as the presence of two of the following symptoms for a one month period, or only delusions if they are bizarre: delusions, hallucinations, disorganized speech (e.g., frequent derailment or incoherence), or grossly disorganized or catatonic behavior and negative symptoms, (i.e., affective flattening, alogia, poverty of speech, avolition, or lack of motivation). Also required is some social or occupational dysfunction, as shown by a disturbance in one or more major areas of functioning such as work, interpersonal relations, or self-care that are markedly below the level achieved prior to the onset of the illness, or when the onset is in childhood or adolescence, a failure to achieve the expected level of interpersonal, academic, or occupational achievement.

The duration of the symptoms must last six months without a marked affective/mood component. There are several subtypes of schizophrenia of note: *paranoid*, in which the individual believes that he or she is in danger; *catatonic*, in which

the patient is withdrawn to the point of not moving; *disorganized*, characterized by speech and thinking patterns lacking typical organization; *undifferentiated*, which does not meet the criteria for the first three types; and *residual*, in which the active symptoms are significantly less pronounced than at the peak of symptoms.

Understanding the prevalence of schizophrenia among Asian Americans and immigrants is difficult, as there are no large-scale studies in the United States specifying this community. The Epidemiologic Catchment Area (ECA) study in 1984 remains the benchmark study of psychiatric diagnoses in the U.S., but researchers did not actively sample or recruit enough individuals to state how prevalent schizophrenia was among Asian Americans.

Generally, schizophrenia was measured at 0.6% in the rural areas, and 1.1% in the urban areas. It is worth considering whether schizophrenia among Asians Americans can be extrapolated using international studies in Taiwan, Korea, and China to assess the prevalence of schizophrenia in these Asian countries. The Taiwan Psychiatric Epidemiological Project, surveying 11,004 patients, reported the incidence of schizophrenia being 0.3% in urban areas, and 0.23% in rural areas. In Korea, among 5,100 subjects, the incidence was 0.34% in rural areas, and 0.65% in urban areas. The data was gathered by using a translated and back-translated Diagnostic Interview Schedule (DIS). In China, a total of five psychiatric epidemiological studies were conducted between 1981 and 1996 with different Chinese ethnic groups, including Han Chinese, Baima Tibetans and Uygurs. The occurrence of schizophrenia in these combined populations was reported between 0.19% and 0.47%. In Japan the rate of the illness is estimated between 0.19% and 1.79% (Gee & Ishii, 1997). Admittedly, the application of this data to Asian Americans is limited at best.

Goldner, Hsu, Waraich, and Somers (2002) reported geographical variations in prevalence. In reviewing the ECA data, Taiwan was compared to other countries. The rate of schizophrenia in New Zealand, in the Netherlands, and in rural villages in Taiwan was assessed at 0.9 per 100 in the U.S.

ECA study. Other comparisons include the life-time prevalence rates for schizophrenia, ranging from 0.12 per 100 in Hong Kong to 1.6 per 100 in Puerto Rico, a difference of over 13-fold. It is notable that low lifetime prevalence rates were reported in all reviewed studies conducted in Hong Kong, Taiwan, and Korea.

A brief report showed that in a population of 219 inpatients diagnosed with schizophrenia, 71 of the patients (56%) were classified as Chinese American, with 95% of this group originally from China (Chang, Newman, D'Antonio, McKelvey & Serper, 2011). These patients had significantly fewer symptoms of psychosis compared to Latino and African Americans and slightly fewer symptoms that seen in European Americans.

Kaplan, Sadock, and Grebb (1994) stated about 0.025–0.05% of the total U.S. population is treated for schizophrenia within any one year period. While most of those diagnosed treated require inpatient care, only about half of all individuals with schizophrenia actually obtain treatment, in spite of the severity of the disorder.

The World Health Organization (WHO) found that lack of insight, delusions, flat affect, auditory hallucinations, and experiences of control were common in schizophrenic patients throughout the world. The typical patient with schizophrenia is a loner, who lives on the fringes of his or her group. Around the age of 20, the individual's functioning level drops, and they may have to drop out of college. They are increasingly unable to care for themselves, become more withdrawn and emotionless, and eventually start talking to themselves, dressing oddly, and writing which can perseverate on themes that may be considered peculiar.

There are distinct characteristics associated with Asian Americans with severe mental issues, particularly as it relates to patient care. Asian Americans diagnosed with schizophrenia experience their illness differently than others. Asian American patients are less likely to be found on street corners and under bridges, and more likely to be taken care of by their families. Interestingly, the prognosis for patients in developing countries is better than for those patients from developed countries. It is thought that the emphasis in industrialized countries on individualism, competition and self-reliance makes it difficult for patients with schizophrenia to function within its structure. The rural environment, with its emphasis on the village structure, long-term relationships, stability, supportiveness, and interdependence would better support recovery from schizophrenia. In general, extended families, such as seen in most non-Western societies, are thought to contribute to better outcomes, whereas may be correlated with worse outcomes (Tseng & Strelzer, 1997).

As previously noted, there are very limited studies on Asian Americans and schizophrenia. Still, there has been conducted abroad that can help shed some light on the issues that Asians Americans face with schizophrenia. Bhugra, Corridan, Rudge, Leff, and Mallett (1999) found that in the United Kingdom there were differences in symptom manifestations between Asians and Caucasians and in the mode of onset. The London study found that Asians were more likely to commit suicide than Caucasians and that auditory hallucinations were more often reported in Asians than in Caucasians. Asians were more likely to show neglect of activities, to lose appetite, and to be irritable. In contrast, Caucasians were twice as likely to have somatic complaints and perform violent acts compared to Asians. The study also found that Caucasians were more likely to suggest that others are responsible for the onset of the mental illness of the individual compared to Asians who were more likely to take responsibility for the onset and treatment of the disorder, suggesting higher pre-morbid functioning (Bhugra, Corridan, Rudge, Leff, & Mallett, 1999). These findings may reflect the Western cultural expectations for Asians to be more stoic and controlled than other cultural groups.

Other studies conducted abroad also speculate that Asians might experience schizophrenia differently than those in the West. Tateyama, Asai, Hashimoto, Bartels, and Kasperm (1998) compared patients with schizophrenia in Germany and Japan, and found that patients with schizophrenia in Japan felt that they were "being slandered by surrounding people." A 26 year old Japanese patient complained, "My fellows speak ill of me" and "they do spiteful things to me." Another Japanese patient, 36 years old, stated, "my father and neighbors conspire together and are doing something secretly behind my back." Because the Japanese culture is group-oriented (also observed in other Asian cultures), patients may be concerned about what others think of them.

Many patients experience anxiety that they may disgrace themselves in public, which is a culture bound syndrome known as *Taijin Kyofusho* (APA, 2000). The behavior of schizophrenic patients in Western Europe differ, expressing their anxiety towards others and stating concerns about specific and direct harm by others, such as "I am being poisoned by others," and thinking of their "house catching fire or exploding," whereas more amorphous delusions of reference such as "being slandered by others" are frequent among Japanese patients. Since guilt and sin are western constructs from Christianity, western Europeans were more likely to have delusions of guilt, as seen in over a third of German and Austrian patients, among patients reporting religious delusions. By comparison, guilt was an issue for only 10% of Japanese patients.

Treatment has historically been medication-based with typical anti-psychotics, such as haloperidol and fluphenazine, sometimes in a depot formulation that can be administered monthly with an injection. Atypical anti-psychotics, such as risperidone, olanzipiene, quetiapiene, ziprasadone, arapiperazole, and clozapine can also be used in conjunction with other medications. Newer drugs, including paloperidone, asenapine, iloperidone, and lurasidone, are less susceptible to the side effects of irreversible tardive dyskinesia (involuntary movements of the mouth, lips, and tongue), associated with long-term use of these anti-psychotic medications (Eon & Durham, 2009; Medilexicon, 2011a, 2011b). Risperidone, olanzipiene, and paliperidone are available in a depot injection, which can improve adherence in patients with frequent hospitalizations due to forgetting to take their medicine.

Some patients may require electroconvulsive therapy (ECT) to recover from catatonic symptoms (APA, 2004). The treatment plan includes non-medication therapies, such as psychoeducation to reduce stigma, psychosocial rehabilitation, family therapy, cognitive behavioral therapy, individual therapy, art therapy, and social skills training.

Bipolar Disorder in Asian Americans

Bipolar disorder is a condition characterized by periods of mood elevation or irritability. The disorder is characterized by distinct mood episodes, one of which has to be a manic or hypomanic episode, marked by euphoric or irritable mood, rapid speech, racing thoughts, insomnia, euphoria, and an increase in goal directed activity. Complicating the diagnosis of bipolar disorder is the presence of depressive episodes that are identical to those seen in major depressive disorders, embodied by depressed mood, anhedonia, or lack of pleasure, fatigue, insomnia, and a sense of a foreshortened future. Patients with Bipolar I disorder have sustained episodes of mania when the mood elevation or irritability persists at least 1 week or leads to hospitalization. In addition, many bipolar I patients experience depressive episodes. Patients with bipolar II disorder have one or more major depressive episodes, with at least one hypomanic episode when the mood elevation or irritability continues for at least three days.

By and large, the disorder has not been well documented within the Asian American population. A re-analysis of the ECA data with respect to Asian Americans showed that they are less likely to have bipolar disorder than Caucasians (Zhang & Snowden, 1999). Lifetime prevalence of bipolar spectrum disorder in the U.S. is 4.4%, compared to Japan's 0.7%, and China's 1.5%. We can again attempt to use the international data to hypothesize that the lifetime prevalence of bipolar spectrum disorder is less than found in the general population (Merikangas et al., 2011).

Different findings were offered by Hwang (2010), who examined the prevalence of bipolar disorder in Asian Americans in a university clinic. Asian American patients were 20% more likely to be diagnosed with bipolar disorder than whites, were more likely to exhibit psychosis, while less likely to have received psychotherapy. The findings substantiate previous observations about the underutilization of services by Asian Americans, as well as their tendency to wait until the illness is very severe before seeking services. Kilbourne, Bauer, and Pincus, (2005) suggested that Asian Americans with bipolar disorder are more likely to have a substance use disorder as well.

The mainstays of treatment are biological treatments involving mood stabilizers, such as lithium, and anti-seizure medications such as divalproex or carbamazepine. More recent options include anticonvulsants such as oxcarbazepine, lamotrigine, and atypical antipsychotics such as quetiapine, olanzipiene, and risperidone (Mayo Clinic, 2011). In addition, non-medication types of therapies, such as those for schizophrenia, are also important as part of the comprehensive biopsychosocial treatment plan.

Severe Mental Illness: Barriers and Challenges

Asian Americans face several barriers and challenges to accessing mental health services including cultural beliefs about the causation of mental illness. Fundamental Asian American explanatory models for illnesses that may affect mental health treatment include imbalance of *yin* and *yang*, and the corresponding conditions of "hot" and "cold." Illness may be attributed to an upset in this balance of forces (Salimbene, 2000). In Eastern societies, the explanatory models of psychiatric symptoms as supernatural or social (Landrine & Klonoff, 1994) differs from that in Western societies, which emphasizes the biomedical model and a separation of mental and physical conditions.

Assessing Asian American patients can be facilitated by the clinician's use of the DSMIV-TR Outline for Cultural Formulation (OCF) (APA, 2000), which includes a section on cultural health beliefs. The formulation has five parts. Part A asks the clinician to understand the cultural identity of the individual, which includes such dimensions as the patient's ethnicity, country of origin, years in the U.S., languages spoken, religious and cultural beliefs and practices, sexual orientation, gender identity, socioeconomic status, geographic location, and disabilities. Part B of the OCF is the

cultural explanations of the individual's illness. Examples include: 1) a spiritual explanation, where an individual was being punished for his sins or possessed by an evil spirit, 2) a magical explanation, such as an evil eye, 3) an imbalance of hot and cold caused by not enough of one kind of food or the other, 4) a weakness of will, or 5) an imbalance in *Qi*, or vital energy. Kleinman and others suggested a list of eight questions (Kleinman, Eisenberg, & Good, 1978) that help to assess the patient's explanatory model of their illness, as well as their ideas about its treatment and prognosis. The questions include:

1. What do you call your illness? What name does it have?
2. What do you think has caused the illness?
3. Why and when did it start?
4. What do you think the illness does? How does it work?
5. How severe is it? Will it have a short or long course?
6. What kind of treatment do you think the patient should receive? What are the most important results you hope she receives from this treatment?
7. What are the chief problems the illness has caused?
8. What do you fear most about the illness?

Inquiring about the use of complementary or alternative medicine practices is appropriate for Asian American patients. Part C of the OCF are the cultural factors related to psychosocial environment and levels of functioning and helps the clinician to determine both stressors, such as financial difficulty, peer pressure, unemployment, homelessness, or parental disapproval, and supports in the patient's life such as their religion, family or ethnic community. Part D includes the cultural elements of the relationship between the individual and the clinician, and pertains to the interactional effect of the cultural identity of both the individual and the clinician on areas such as their religion, family or ethnic community. Part D includes the cultural elements of the relationship between the individual and the clinician, and pertains to the interactional effect of the cultural identity of both the individual and the clinician on areas such as communication (both verbal and nonverbal) rapport, and the therapeutic relationship. Finally, Part E is the overall cultural formulation, and it asks the clinician to summarize the information assessed in the previous four sections for developing both the differential diagnosis and the treatment plan that incorporates the patient's explanatory models. The treatment plan should also address the patient's role in the family and community system. The use of OCF should help the clinician to make a more accurate diagnosis as well as to negotiate a treatment plan that will be acceptable to the patient. For further details, the reader is referred to the *Clinical Manual of Cultural Psychiatry* (Lim, 2006), Chapters 1, 3, 6, and Appendix A, which pertain to the general evaluation and treatment of ethnically diverse patients, as well as some specific material about selected Asian cultural groups.

The mismatch between the Eastern and Western models of illness can cause a disconnection between physicians and patients, and the two models need to be skillfully bridged by the clinician to ensure the patient's cooperation with treatment. Gee and Ishii (1997) described various Asian cultures' attitudes towards schizophrenia. Filipinos may see schizophrenia as being caused by a weak will that can be inherited by other family members. Denial of the illness and secrecy to protect the family reputation and other members from the stress of shame is a common response. Japanese may see mental illness as deviating from conformity to society, and view such illness as a family dishonor. Traditionally oriented Filipinos and Southeast Asians may consider spirit possession as the main etiology of schizophrenia, so an indigenous healer, such as a shaman, will be consulted before a physician.

Chinese families may view a severe mental illness from a multidimensional perspective, making diagnosis and treatment acutely complex. Moral, religious, physiological, psychological, social, and genetic factors are all possible etiologies. Morally, the patient's behavior can be regarded as volitional deviation from conformity to family and society. Schizophrenia or the symptomatology of a psychosis can disrupt social functioning and dishonor a family's reputation. Of particular concern are family members who

spend time caring for the patient to the detriment of performing their normal duties within society. Mental illness can be seen as punishment from the gods or ancestors for past wrongs in current or former lives. Auditory hallucinations may be regarded as the manifestation of ghosts and spirits and/or communication from ancestors. Schizophrenia and other mental illnesses can represent a physiological imbalance between *yin* and *yang*. Psychologically, Chinese families believe that stress can cause mental issues. As Chinese families often believe that mental illnesses are inherited, potential partners will not marry into the family of the afflicted.

One strategy that a clinician can consider is creating a "bridge" between the patient's perceptions and medically-based explanatory model by using parts of the patient's belief structure. A physician can advise a patient "you may feel that you are having a spirit taking over your body. We might explain this by saying that thoughts that you hear appear to you to be outside of your body. We believe that medications will help you to see where the 'spirits' are really coming from."

Stigma and Other Barriers to Mental Illness in Asian Americans

Though there has been much progress made in the realm of mental health, perceived disgrace and dishonor can still deter patients and their families from seeking needed treatment and therapy. It can be even more of an ignominy within the Asian American community, where people with schizophrenia and other severe psychoses can be viewed as bringing shame upon their families, thus presenting even greater barriers to seeking treatment. Culture shapes the way in which families construe schizophrenia and other mental illness. A treatment plan that does not consider the unique family system of the patient can create additional barriers to treatment. An understanding of a client's cultural heritage can improve the quality of the relationship between the mental health professional and client.

Strategies in dealing with these stigmas include psychoeducation and emphasizing the importance of patient confidentiality during treatment. Patients and families need to understand that severe mental illnesses are chronic brain disorders and are treated in ways that are similar to any other physical or medical illness, easing patients and their families from having to find someone or something to blame or fault for the illness. Knowing the chronic nature and prognosis of these disorders can help patients and their families to accept rather than deny their situation. Patients and families can also learn the importance of maintaining medication even when psychotic symptoms and behaviors have waned. Clinicians can help patients navigate through the cultural stigma and discriminatory behaviors often associated with mental illness.

The Asian American community is known for the family inclination to provide direct care for a patient. Like many non-Western cultures, the preference of families is to care for the individual within the home over institutionalizing the patient. Males generally experience earlier onset of illness, they are more likely still living in the family home, and can benefit from this approach. The collectivist nature of Asian culture values the extended family, so that working with other relatives besides immediate family members is also useful. Galanti (2004) recommends that family members be included to allow them to fulfill their familial duty by spending as much time with the patient as possible, and not labeling such behavior as necessarily dependency inducing. Mental health professionals should be mindful that decision-making varies with kinship structure so that an elder, and not the patient, may be the designated decision-maker.

Bae and Brekke (2002) stated that Asian families are more likely to accompany the patient with schizophrenia on clinic visits and to actively participate in treatment decisions. In reviewing previous studies, the authors noted that geographical location, acculturation levels, and diagnostic criteria may account for variations and sometimes conflicting findings in the literature. Socio-centric individuals with collectivistic cultural orientation tend to emphasize family integrity, harmonious relationships, and sociability. Bae and Brekke noted the importance of incorporating cultural characteristics into the

intervention process. Interventions that are designed to involve families in a collaborative effort may be more appropriate for Asian American patients because of the interdependent nature of their family dynamics.

Bae and Kung (2000) describe a family intervention for traditionally oriented Asian American families. The intervention consists of a five-stage model involving preparation, engagement, psycho-educational (i.e., survivor skills) workshop, family sessions, and termination. The effectiveness of this program would be enhanced by the use of bicultural and bilingual staff to deliver culturally appropriate services. Key elements of this model include community outreach, home visits, and an educational approach focusing on practical ways of dealing with stress and anxiety.

Communication and problem solving approaches have been found to be highly applicable to Asian American families. Shin and Lukens (2002) described a model used in a community clinic in New York with Korean American patients. Patients were given ten 90-min psycho-educational group sessions while a control group received ten 45-min supportive sessions. The psycho-educational groups were given in Korean, involving lectures, question and answer sessions, and discussion. The content included modules on the definitions of illness, medications and side effects, relapse prevention, crisis and illness management, stigma, communication and stress management, self-help, and community resources. Information was also provided about traditional disease concepts, such as shamanism, ailments, distress, diseases, fortune and misfortune, psyche and soma, and life and death. Patients attending the psycho-educational groups showed a decrease in both psychiatric symptoms and reported stigma as well as an increase in coping skills compared to the control group.

Getting patients to stay on their anti-psychotic medications is often challenging, and it can be particularly difficult with Asian American patients experiencing severe mental illness. Gilmer et al., (2009) compared adherence with medication in Asians and Latinos with limited English proficiency versus those with normal language proficiency. The authors reported Asians with limited English proficiency were less likely than English-proficient Asians to be adherent to medication protocols (40% vs. 45%) and more likely to be non-adherent (29% vs. 22%). More than three-quarters of Latinos and Asians with limited English proficiency resided independently (78% of each). These proportions are higher than those of English-proficient Latinos or Asians (65% and 69%, respectively). In contrast, Asians with limited proficiency were less likely than English-proficient Asians to be adherent, although they were also less likely to be hospitalized and had lower costs.

Although antipsychotic medications are the mainstay of treatment for the positive symptoms of schizophrenia, some patients will either refuse medication or respond poorly to these drugs. In such instances, a cognitive approach may be effective (Beck-Sander, Birchwood, & Chadwick, 1979) and can be an alternative for Asian American and other patients who choose not to take medications. Some patients use distraction techniques (for example, listening to music, talking with someone, or thinking about something else). In recent years, an increasing body of literature has suggested that cognitive-behavioral therapy, in conjunction with treatment with antipsychotic medications, benefits patients with chronic delusions and hallucinations, even those with early psychosis (Haddock, Morrison, Hopkins, Lewis, & Tarrier, 1998). Each patient's individual coping methods should be explored and enhanced. In addition, traditionally oriented Asian American patients often will use herbs or other non-Western medical treatments, such as acupuncture or medical preparations, from their home country. Such alternatives should be acknowledged, and checked for the possibility of interactions with medications or other therapies.

Research on Disparities: Future Directions

In the *Supplement to the Report on Mental Health: Culture, Race, and Ethnicity* published by the Office of the Surgeon General (USDHHS, 2001), six ways to improve mental health services are recommended to help to reduce disparities in mental health care for Asian Americans:

- Continue to expand the science base
- Improve access to treatment
- Reduce barriers to mental health care
- Improve quality of mental health service
- Support capacity development
- Promote mental health.

A continued challenge has been the under-representation of all racial and ethnic minorities in research studies as well as the need for community-based research. In addition to the under representation of patients in the research studies, other challenges include: (1) lack of analyses on the impact of ethnic, linguistic, or cultural factors; (2) limited resources devoted to the research of culturally specific practices; (3) lack of development of theory related to the relationships between culture, mental health disorders, and treatment; (4) the absence of culturally relevant treatment outcomes; (5) the limited involvement of ethnically and culturally diverse researchers. To deal with these challenges, Isaacs, Huang, Hernandez, & Echo-Hawk (2005) advocate for the inclusion of Practice Based Evidence (PBE) as "a range of treatment approaches and supports that are derived from, and supportive of, the positive cultural attributes of the local society and traditions. PBE services are accepted as effective by the local community, through community consensus, and address the therapeutic and healing needs of individuals and families from a culturally-specific framework…" (p. 16).

Research on Asian American mental health disparities also needs better developed infrastructure support. In September 2007, the Asian American Center for Disparities Research (2007) opened at University of California, Davis, headed by Nolan Zane, Ph.D. The Center obtained funding from the National Institute of Mental Health (NIMH) for 5 years at 3.9 million dollars. It is the only NIMH-funded, Asian-specific center on Asian American mental health disparities. Partnering with the National Asian American and Pacific Islander Mental Health Association (NAAPIMHA) and other community-based organizations, its objectives include conduct programmatic, problem-oriented research toward the empirical testing of effective clinical treatments for Asian American populations; conduct research that has theoretical and policy significance for Asian Americans in particular and the mental health field in general; promote and conduct research that addresses key methodological issues involved in the study of diversity and disparities; serve as the focal point and stimulus for researchers conducting Asian American disparities research on a national level by maintaining and enhancing a network of researchers, service providers, and policy makers to facilitate theory and methodology development; bridge science into mental health practice, in particular, concerning cultural influences that affect critical problems of treatment and service delivery such as medical non-adherence and premature dropout.

More study needs to be done on the diverse Asian American population to characterize how schizophrenia and bipolar disorder present differently within different subpopulations, and how to develop culturally appropriate diagnostic criteria and treatment, such as possible ethnic matching of therapist and patient. Clinical research is necessary to show that Asian American patients may require different approaches to treatment. There should be attention directed toward assessing biological differences, which may affect the rates of the metabolism of psychotropic medications. Differences in worldview, such as the group orientation that is the polar opposite to Western individualism and its effects on patient and family cooperation with treatment protocols should also be reviewed. Such studies also will facilitate a better understanding of how factors such as acculturation, help-seeking behaviors, stigma, ethnic identity, racism, and spirituality provide protection from, or increase risk for, mental illness in racial and ethnic minority populations. In terms of the promotion of mental health and the prevention of mental and behavioral disorders, important opportunities exist for researchers to study cultural differences in stress, coping, and resilience as part of the complex of factors that influence mental health. Such work will lay the groundwork for developing new prevention and treatment strategies that build upon community

strengths to foster mental health and restructure negative health outcomes.

Sue and McKinney (1975), in their landmark article, made many of the recommendations discussed in this chapter. With the increasing larger Asian American population 35 years later, there is an even greater imperative to improve mental health services for Asian Americans by increasing access to services with better language and insurance access and through the use of ethnic specific techniques and treatments.

Conclusions

Asian Americans are a heterogeneous group with over 43 distinct subethnic groups, each with their own language, cultural beliefs, and medical traditions. Severe mental illness in Asian Americans can present differently than in the mainstream population, and thus requires different approaches to diagnosis and treatment, as well as service delivery. The DSM-IV-TR OCF can be helpful with diagnosis and treatment planning with Asian American mental health patients. Clinicians working with Asian Americans with schizophrenia and bipolar disorder need to work with their families during assessment and treatment planning, and effectively address the issue of the stigma of mental health in Asian Americans with the patient and family members. There are some published treatment protocols for the treatment of schizophrenia, and none for bipolar disorder in Asian American families. More research needs to be done to characterize schizophrenia and bipolar disorder in Asian Americans, its prevalence, phenomenology, and document effective treatment strategies for those populations because they have not been well represented in recent or past studies. Appropriately trained interpreters should be made available, with the community needing to be engaged in the importance of mental health. Such engagement can assist in reducing barriers to mental health treatment, such as stigma, lack of insurance, or linguistic difficulties. There are many organizations that can offer technical assistance in developing such programs, such as NAAPIMHA (National Asian American Pacific

Islander Mental Health Association), NAMI (National Alliance for the Mentally Ill) and its Multicultural Action Center, NAWHO (National Asian Women's Health Organization), AAPCHO (Association of Asian Pacific Community Health Organizations), NAPAFASA (National Association of Pacific Asian Families Against Substance Abuse), NCAPA (National Council of Asian Pacific Americans), APIAHF (Asian and Pacific Islander Health Forum), and AHC-AMHPI (Asian Health Coalition-Asian Mental Health Partnership Initiative). The Asian American community must come together to support the development of mental health treatment services, as well as empowering its members to become advocacy leaders and mental health providers to provide culturally appropriate, effective mental health services that are available to all Asian Americans.

References

American Psychiatric Association (APA). (2000). *Diagnostic and statistical manual of mental disorders DSM-IV-TR Fourth Edition* (4th ed.). Washington, DC: American Psychiatric Press Incorporated.

American Psychiatric Association (APA). (2004). *Practice guidelines for the treatment of schizophrenia* (2nd ed.). Washington, DC: American Psychiatric Press, Incorporated. Retrieved April 25, 2011, from http://www.psychiatryonline.com/content.aspx?aID=46733.

Asian American Center for Disparities Research (AACDR) at University of California, Davis. (2007). Retrieved June 5, 2011, from http://psychology.ucdavis.edu/aacdr.

Bae, S. W., & Brekke, J. S. (2002). Characteristics of Korean-Americans with schizophrenia: A cross-ethnic comparison with African-Americans, Latinos, and Euro-Americans. *Schizophrenia Bulletin, 28*(4), 703–717.

Bae, S. W., & Kung, W. W. M. (2000). Family intervention for Asian Americans with a schizophrenic patient in the family. *The American Journal of Orthopsychiatry, 70*(4), 532–541.

Beck-Sander, A., Birchwood, M., & Chadwick, P. (1979). Acting on command hallucinations: A cognitive approach. *British Journal of Clinical Psychology, 36*, 139–148.

Bhugra, D., Corridan, B., Rudge, S., Leff, J., & Mallett, R. (1999). Early manifestations, personality traits and pathways into care for Asian and white first-onset case of schizophrenia. *Social Psychiatry, 34*, 595–599.

Chang, N., Newman, J., D'Antonio, E., McKelvey, J., & Serper, M. (2011). Ethnicity and symptom expression

in patients with acute schizophrenia. *Psychiatry Research, 185*(3), 453–455.

Eon, S., & Durham, J. (2009). Schizophrenia: A review of pharmacologic and nonpharmacologic treatments. *US Pharmacist, 34*(11), 1–5.

Galanti, G. A. (2004). *Caring for patients from different cultures* (3rd ed.). Philadelphia: University of Pennsylvania Press.

Gee, K., & Ishii, M. (1997). Assessment and treatment of schizophrenia among Asian Americans. In E. Lee (Ed.), *Working with Asian Americans: A guide for clinicians* (pp. 227–252). New York: Guilford Press.

Gilmer, T. P., Ojeda, V. D., Concepcion-Barrio, C., Dahlia, F., Piedad, G., Nicole, M. L., & Kelly, C. L.(2009). Adherence to antipsychotics among Latinos and Asians with schizophrenia and limited English proficiency. Psychological Services, 60(2), 175–182.

Goldner, E. M., Hsu, L., Waraich, P., & Somers, J. M. (2002). Prevalence and incidence studies of schizophrenic disorders: A systematic review of the literature. *Canadian Journal of Psychiatry, 47*(9), 833–843.

Haddock, G., Morrison, A., Hopkins, R., Lewis, S., & Tarrier, N. (1998). Individual cognitive-behavioural interventions in early psychosis. *The British Journal of Psychiatry, 172*(Suppl. 33), 101–106.

Hwang, S. H. J., Childers, M. E., Wang, P. W., Nam, J. Y., Keller, K. L., Hill, S. J., et al. (2010). Higher prevalence of bipolar I disorder among Asian and Latino compared to Caucasian patients receiving treatment. *Asia-Pacific Psychiatry, 2*(2010), 156–165.

Isaacs, M. R., Huang, L. N., Hernandez, M., & Echo-Hawk, H. (2005). *The road to evidence: The intersection of evidence-based practices and cultural competence in children's mental health.* Washington, DC: The National Alliance of Multi-Ethnic Behavioral Health Associations.

Jenkins, J. H. (1998). Diagnostic criteria for schizophrenia and related psychotic disorders: Integration and suppression of cultural evidence in DSM-IV. *Transcultural Psychiatry, 35*, 357–376.

Kaplan, H. I., Sadock, B. J., & Grebb, J. A. (1994). *Kaplan and Sadock's synopsis of psychiatry: Behavioral sciences, clinical psychiatry* (7th ed.). Baltimore: Williams & Wilkins.

Kilborne, A. M., Bauer, M. S., & Pincus, H. (2005). Clinical, psychosocial, and treatment differences in minority patients with bipolar disorder. *Bipolar Disorders, 7*, 89–97.

Kleinman, A., Eisenberg, L., & Good, B. (1978). Culture, illness, and care: Clinical lessons from anthropologic and cross-cultural research. *Annals of Internal Medicine, 88*(2), 251–258.

Landrine, H., & Klonoff, E. A. (1994). Cultural diversity in causal attribution for illness; the role of the supernatural. *Journal of Behavioral Medicine, 17*, 181–193.

Lee, T. M. Y., Chong, S. A., Huat, Y., & Sathyadevan, G. (2004). Command hallucinations among Asian patients with schizophrenia. *Canadian Journal of Psychiatry, 49*(12), 838–842.

Lim, R. F. (2006). *Clinical manual of cultural psychiatry.* Arlington, VA: APPI.

Mayo Clinic. (2011). *Bipolar disorder: Treatment and drugs.* Retrieved May 1, 2011, from http://www.mayoclinic.com/health/bipolar-disorder/DS00356/DSECTION=treatments-and-drugs.

Medilexicon. (2011a). *Latuda (lurasidone).* Retrieved May 1, 2011, from http://www.medilexicon.com/drugs/latuda.php.

Medilexicon. (2011b). *Saphris (Asenapine).* Retrieved May 1, 2011, from http://www.medilexicon.com/drugs/saphris.php.

Merikangas, K. R., Jin, R., He, J. P., Dahlia, F., Piedad, G., Nicole, M. L., & Kelly, C. L. (2011). Prevalence and correlates of bipolar spectrum disorder in the world mental health survey initiative. *Archives of General Psychiatry, 68*(3), 241–251.

Salimbene, S. (2000). *What language does your patient hurt in? A practical guide to culturally competent patient care* (2nd ed.). Amherst, MA: Diversity Resources.

Shin, S. K., & Lukens, E. P. (2002). Effects of psychoeducation for Korean Americans with chronic mental illness. *Psychiatric Services, 53*(9), 1125–1131.

Stompe, T., Karakula, H., Rudalevičiene, P., Okribelashvili, N., Chaudhry, H. R., Idemudia, E. E., & Gscheider, S. (2006). The pathoplastic effect of culture on psychotic symptoms in schizophrenia. *World Cultural Psychiatry Research Review, 1*(3/4), 157–163. July/October.

Sue, S., & McKinney, H. (1975). Asian Americans in the community mental health care system. *The American Journal of Orthopsychiatry, 45*(1), 111–118.

Tateyama, M., Asai, M., Hashimoto, M., Bartels, M., & Kasperm, S. (1998). Transcultural study of schizophrenic delusions: Tokyo versus Vienna and Tübingen (Germany). *Psychopathology, 31*, 59–68.

Tseng, W. S., & Strelzer, J. (1997). *Culture and psychopathology.* New York: Brunner/Mazel.

U.S. Department of Health and Human Services (USDHHS). (1999). *Mental health: A report of the surgeon general.* Rockville, MD: U.S. Department of Health and Human Services. Retrieved March 19, 2011, from http://www.surgeongeneral.gov/library/mentalhealth/home.html.

USDHHS. (2001). *Mental health: Culture, race and ethnicity: A supplement to mental health: A report to the Surgeon General.* Rockville, MD: U.S. Department of Health and Human Services. Retrieved March 15, 2011, from http://www.surgeongeneral.gov/library/mentalhealth/cre/

Zhang, A. Y., & Snowden, L. R. (1999). Ethnic characteristics of mental disorders in five U.S. Communities. *Cultural Diversity and Ethnic Minority Psychology, 5*(2), 134–146.

Asian American Violence: Scope, Context, and Implications

21

Deborah A. Goebert, Thao N. Le,
and Jeanelle J. Sugimoto-Matsuda

Within hours of releasing the identity of the gunman that terrorized Virginia Polytechnic Institute in 2007, messages of hate against Asian Americans and immigrants began appearing on blogs and Internet forums, and acts of violence against Asian Americans increased. Rather than focusing on the wrongful actions of one individual, media attention centered on the ethnicity of the gunman. For example, several major newspapers used "Korean" or "Asian" in headlines. This placed emphasis on all Asians, thereby enabling the spread of a message of hate. As a result, the media and a portion of the public quickly latched onto the killer's race, making the incident a race issue. Some suggested that all Asians, especially Asian immigrants, be given psychological testing prior to college admission. Others described the killer's childhood and parental expectations, indicating the killer's sister epitomized the immigrant success story, while the gunman represented its failure (Daugherty, 2007). This event is fraught with stereotypes, prejudice and racism.

D.A. Goebert (✉) • J.J. Sugimoto-Matsuda
Asian/Pacific Islander Youth Violence Prevention Center,
Department of Psychiatry, John A. Burns School
of Medicine, University of Hawaii, Honolulu, HI, USA
e-mail: GoebertD@dop.hawaii.edu

T.N. Le
College of Tropical Agriculture and Human Resources,
Family and Consumer Sciences, University of Hawaii
at Manoa, Honolulu, HI, USA
e-mail: tle@cahs.colostate.edu

Stereotypes, Racism, and the Myth of the "Model Minority"

The concepts of "stereotype," "prejudice," and "racism" are often confused. A stereotype is a popular belief or simplified conception of a group based on some prior assumptions. A prejudice is a prejudgment made about someone or something before having adequate knowledge. Used herein, the word prejudice refers to preconceived judgments toward a people or a person because of race. Racism is the belief that there are inherent differences in people's traits and capacities which are entirely due to their race. Specifically, institutional racism can be defined as an oppressive system(s) of racial relations, justified by ideology, in which one racial group benefits from dominating another through harmful and degrading beliefs and actions (Krieger, Rowley, Herman, Avery, & Phillips, 1993). Institutional racism is used to justify the practice of differential social and legal treatment.

For decades the overriding stereotype of Asian Americans, and especially Asian American students, has been that of the model minority. Model minority refers to a minority group whose members achieve greater success than the population average. Violence is not part of the image; neither is help-seeking. Members of a model minority group such as Asian Americans are expected to be outstanding and driven scholars, diligent, respectful, and have strong family ties. Relative to other minority groups, Asian

Americans generally have a higher mean level of education, lower rates of poverty and unemployment, and are underrepresented in official crime statistics (Bridges & Steen, 1998; Reeves & Bennett, 2004; Sampson & Lauritsen, 1997). However, the model minority stereotype accentuates the idea that Asian Americans will succeed under any circumstance because of their cultural attributes such as strong work ethics, close family ties, and perseverance against adversities (Gym, 2011). The model minority stereotype implies that Asian Americans do not need targeted services, resources, and political or cultural attention.

Health Status of Asian Americans

Consequently, the model minority stereotype has been detrimental to the Asian American community. It masks the needs of Asian American communities for access to services and assistance programs, and glosses over their difficulties in communication, psychological stress, and discrimination (Sun & Starosta, 2006; Wong & Haglin, 2006; Yang, 2004). Indeed, Asian Americans face many of the same barriers to health and wellbeing as other minority groups. For instance, two out of five Asian Americans do not speak English well or at all (Reeves & Bennett, 2004). However, this number varies significantly by ethnic group (Africa & Carrasco, 2011). Among Asian American groups, 62% of Vietnamese, 50% of Chinese, 24% of Filipinos and 23% Asian Indians are not fluent in English (U.S. Census Bureau, 2003). A growing literature suggests language barriers can lead to poor quality of health care delivery, and as a result, lower health status (DuBard & Gizlice, 2008; Pippins, Alegría, & Haas, 2007; Woloshin, Bickell, Schwartz, Gany, & Welch, 1995; Woloshin, Schwartz, Katz, & Welch, 1997). While poverty rates as a whole for Asian Americans are similar to the US population, rates for certain Asian groups are significantly higher (Reeves & Bennett, 2004). Living in poverty or being uninsured has been associated with limited access to health care (Hughes, 2002).

Studies on ethnic differences in help seeking behaviors suggest that Asian ethnic groups generally present later for evaluation of medical symptoms (Ayalon & Arean, 2004; Low & Anstey, 2009). Cultural beliefs about health and illness may not match Western medicine concepts, influencing whether some Asian Americans seek help for symptoms, particularly those that are not physical. In addition, perceptions of disease may be influenced not only by culture, but also education and acculturation. For instance, Asian Americans and Pacific Islanders are significantly less likely than Caucasians to mention their mental health concerns to a friend or relative (12% vs. 25%); a physician (2% vs. 13%); or a mental health professional (4% vs. 26%) (Zhang, Snowden, & Sue, 1998). Furthermore, only one in sixteen Asian Americans with mental illness seeks help compared to one in four Caucasians (Chen & Mak, 2008). Asian Americans may avoid seeking help because of the cultural stigma placed on mental illness, or for fear of bringing shame to the family (U.S. Department of Health and Human Services [DHHS], 2001). Akutsu and Chu (2006) found that when they do seek counseling, Asian Americans show higher levels of psychological distress, possibly due to the fact that they spend the least time in treatment relative to other groups. This may be due to either underestimating the importance of their condition, or perceiving that no options exist to treat their symptoms (Chu, Hsieh, & Tokars, 2011).

This model minority myth in relation to Asian Americans has led to the notion that they are not the typical minority, but in fact represent a highly privileged group that has evoked fear and competition among American educators. As such, this stereotype also creates and widens divisions between Asian Americans and other people of color. Endorsement of the stereotype of Asian American competence has been associated with both positive and negative attitudes and emotions toward them (Ho & Jackson, 2001; Maddux, Galinsky, Cuddy, & Polifroni, 2008); for example, as highly successful and respected, but also not sociable thus building resentment and envious prejudice (Lin, Kwan, Cheung, & Fiske, 2005). In addition, Ho & Jackson, (2001) found that individuals who believed Asian Americans had traits consistent with the model minority stereotype (such as intelligent, ambitious, and obedient), indicated they admired and respected Asian Americans but also reported feeling hostile and jealous. As a result, Asian Americans have been the target of bullying and racism from other races due to the model minority stereotype (Ancheta, 2006).

Hate Crimes

Asian minorities and immigrants to the United States experience racial discrimination and prejudice. As stated by U.S. Conference of Catholic Bishops (2002, p. 12): "Throughout history, Asians in the United States, native-born and immigrant, have been characterized as permanent aliens, a race of foreigners given externally imposed labels and racial identities and only referred to in passing or even omitted altogether in classic immigration history." It is important to understand the historical context of racism, particularly since it is an emotionally charged issue, in order to move beyond imposed limitations, advance change and create new expectations. It can only be undone through increased understanding of what it is, where it comes from, how it functions, and why it persists.

Hate Crimes Against Asians: The Past

Racism against Asians in the United States dates back to the 1800s, and includes restrictive laws ranging from those that affected all non-white populations, to those that targeted specific Asian groups. Most notably, Executive Order 9066 of 1942 forced Japanese immigrants, including two-thirds of who were American citizens mainly from the west coast, into internment camps under the guise of military necessity. Also, unlike other immigrants to the United States, Asian immigrants were denied the right to become naturalized citizens until the 1950s. For example, the Chinese Exclusion Law of 1882 barred additional Chinese laborers from entering the United States and prevented Chinese aliens from obtaining American citizenship. Furthermore, laws in many

states forbade marriages between non-whites (including Asians) and whites. Where it was permitted, social pressures were immense.

Racist acts again Asian Americans have persisted to current times. In 1982, Vincent Chin was beaten to death at his bachelor party in Detroit, Michigan by two unemployed auto workers. These men blamed the Japanese auto industry for taking their jobs away and killed Chin, a Chinese American, because of his racial appearance. His assailants did not serve time for their crime, and instead received 3 years of probation. Such judicial leniency led to outrage from the Asian American community. Despite changes in legal provisions, discriminatory actions by individuals and groups persist. Hate crimes against Asian Americans continue to plague the community 25 years after Chinese-American draftsman Chin was beaten to death because of his race. His case was a turning point for Asian American activism for fighting hate crimes and finding justice within their communities. Chin's case has been cited by some Asian Americans to support the continued existence of such hate crimes. In parallel, however, the national immigration debate is driving up the number of hate groups in the country that are perpetrated against immigrants (Southern Poverty Law Center, 2011).

In 1990, the Hate Crime Statistics Act was enacted in response to growing concerns surrounding this issue. According to this Act, data collection as part of the Uniform Crime Reporting (UCR) program was mandated for hate crimes defined as, "Crimes that manifest evidence of prejudice based on race, religion, sexual orientation, or ethnicity, including where appropriate the crimes of murder and non-negligent manslaughter; forcible rape; aggravated assault, simple assault, intimidation; arson; and destruction, damage or vandalism of property (Federal Bureau of Investigation [FBI], 1999, p. 1)." Disabilities, both physical and mental, were added to the list in 1994 via the Violent Crime Control and Law Enforcement Act (FBI). The Matthew Shepard and James Byrd, Jr. Hate Crimes Prevention Act (formerly the Local Law Enforcement Hate Crimes Prevention Act of 2009) brought more progressive legislation, and was signed into law on

October 28, 2009. The Act criminalized willfully causing bodily injury, and authorized the federal government to investigate and prosecute bias-motivated crimes (FBI, 2011). The Act also gave the federal government jurisdiction to prosecute hate crimes in states where the current law is inadequate, or when local authorities are unwilling or do not have the resources to do so themselves.

Hate Crimes Against Asians: The Present

April 16, 2007 will forever be infamous as the day at Virginia Polytechnic Institute when Seung-Hui Cho murdered 32 people and injured 23 others before turning the gun on himself. A week before the 2-year anniversary of the shooting, Jiverly Wong, an immigrant from Vietnam, killed 13 people at an immigration center in New York before committing suicide. It was reported that in their last messages, both Cho and Wong mentioned that they had been treated badly by dominant society. Cho was repeatedly taunted for being Asian, and Wong mentioned policy brutality.

In 2009, 3.9% of all reported hate crimes (188 out of 7,624) were committed against Asian Americans and Pacific Islanders, a ratio that over the past decade has declined slightly relative to other groups, but is nearly double the rate reported in 2007 (Leadership Conference on Civil Rights Education Fund, 2009). Furthermore, an independent audit in 2002 found that hate crimes against Asian Americans display a disturbingly high level of violence. The most commonly reported hate crime offense against Asian Americans were assault and/or battery (29%), followed by vandalism (27%), harassment (21%), and threats (16%) (National Asian American Pacific Legal Consortium [NAAPLC], 2002). While the nature of the majority of the crimes remains unknown due to underreporting by state UCR agencies and fear of reporting by victims, the overall percentage of assault and battery crimes against Asian Americans increased from 12% in 2001 to 15% in 2002 (NAAPLC, 2002). Furthermore, the NAAPLC study discussed that in general, hate crimes occurring immediately after September 11th demonstrated a high degree

of physical violence, with perpetrators wielding baseball bats, metal poles, and guns as weapons while attacking their victims. For Asian Americans, this violent trend continued beyond 2001 including two murders in Brooklyn, New York and a hate rape in Kansas.

Many hate crimes perpetrated against Asian Americans involve youth, frequently instigated by classmates and occurring in the school setting (NAAPLC, 2002). Occurring at both the high school and college levels, the attacks are generally perpetrated by a group of students who target individual Asian American students. In an article titled, "Asian Youth Persistently Harassed by U.S. Peers," the Associated Press (2005) chronicled hate crimes committed against Asian American youth:

• In 2004, 16 year-old Vietnamese American student Bang Mai from Boston was killed in a massive brawl between white and Vietnamese American youths. The basketball court brawl was the result of weeks of tension between the two groups. Mai was fatally stabbed as he attempted to walk away from the brawl. The student who stabbed him was convicted of manslaughter.
• In 2005, Hmong American students from Fresno, California were taunted and had food thrown at them during lunch. On February 25, 2005, the taunts escalated into fights involving at least 30 students and resulting in numerous injuries, suspensions, and expulsions. Eight students were convicted of misdemeanor assault.
• In 2005, 18 year-old Chen Tsu from New York was accosted by four high school classmates who demanded his money. After Tsu showed his classmates his pockets were empty, they assaulted him, taking turns beating his face. At his school, Chinese immigrant students had been harassed and bullied so routinely that school officials agreed to a Department of Justice consent decree to curb alleged severe and pervasive harassment directed at Asian American students.

Hate Crimes, Health, and Wellbeing

The Associated Press (2005) found that Asian American students from across the nation were saying they are often beaten, threatened, and called ethnic slurs by other young people. School safety data suggest that the problem may be worsening. Asian American teens, stereotyped as high-achieving students who rarely fight back, have for years suffered the most from ethnic tension as formerly segregated communities expand and neighborhoods become more ethnically diverse. In areas with an influx of Asian Americans, culture clashing may lead to youth harassment. The 2002–2003 National Latino and Asian American Study found that 74% of Asian Americans reported experiencing some form of routine unfair treatment in their lifetime, and 62% reported being disliked, treated unfairly, or seeing friends being treated unfairly because they were Asian (Chae et al., 2008). Among youth, more Asian American adolescents report experiencing discrimination from their peers than adolescents from other ethnic groups (Fisher, Wallace, & Fenton, 2000; Greene, Way, & Pahl, 2006; Rosenbloom & Way, 2004).

Recent research suggests that racism is one of the mechanisms explaining and expanding racial disparities in health. Although many Asian Americans face racial and anti-immigrant discrimination, the effects of such experiences have not been well understood. Gee, Ro, Shariff-Marco, and Chae (2009) identified 62 empirical articles assessing the relationship between discrimination and health among Asian Americans. Most studies found that discrimination was associated with mental health issues. For example, Gee (2008) found that individual-level discrimination has more of an influence on health status than does institutional discrimination among Chinese Americans. Self-reported racial discrimination was shown to predict poor health status overall, poor mental health, and higher levels of psychological symptomatology. Conversely, segregation predicted better health status. In this context, segregation into ethnic enclaves may represent the clustering of resources and services such as indigenous medical practices and political advocacy, and help to ameliorate "culture shock" and other stressors including discrimination.

Youth Violence

Disaggregation of Data

At a brief glance, Youth Risk Behavior Survey (YRBS) data from 1991 through 1997 suggest that significantly fewer Asian American/Pacific Islander students (31.3%) participated in a fight in the year preceding the survey, relative to non-Hispanic Black (46.4%) and Hispanic (43.1%) students. The prevalence estimates were also significantly less than non-Hispanic Whites for boys (37.4% vs. 46.8%), but not for girls (27.6% vs. 23.6%). However when looking more carefully, social science researchers suggest that the model minority stereotype is an unfounded myth, and that a bimodal pattern of behaviors exists (Choi & Lahey, 2006; Zhou & Bankston, 1994). This bimodal distribution is not readily apparent when viewing statistics for all Asian Americans in aggregate, who are also commonly lumped together with Pacific Islanders, hence the "model minority" branding; but it can be imputed from a closer examination of data.

One of the first prevalence studies that disaggregated sub-ethnicities within Asian Americans and Pacific Islanders, using survey data collected in Hawai'i, showed Filipino American youths experienced significantly higher rates than Japanese American on overall indicators of high-risk behavior related to violence (Mayeda, Hishinuma, Nishimura, Garcia-Santiago, & Mark, 2006). Choi and Lahey (2006) used a nationally representative dataset, the multi-year National Longitudinal Study of Adolescent Health, and found that while Asian American youth report better school performance and less engagement in aggressive offenses than their Black and Latino counterparts, they report higher non-aggressive (e.g., graffiti) and aggressive offenses than do White youth. Compared to Black youth, they also report more non-aggressive offenses and substance use. Under a more accurate bimodal distribution, some Asian American students do very well in school, do not engage in substance use, and avoid behaviors such as risky sex; while others perform very poorly in schools and engage in maladaptive behaviors such as delinquency, gang associations, and violence. These studies emphasize the need to acknowledge group differences, and that Asian American communities are not immune to problems of youth gangs and violence.

The few studies that disaggregate the official records of Asian Americans into the various sub-ethnic groups reveal a disproportionate representation for the Southeast Asian Americans groups (i.e., Cambodian, Lao/Mien, Hmong, Vietnamese). In California's Alameda and San Francisco counties, Southeast Asian Americans group had higher rates of delinquency than East Asians, Latinos, and Whites (Le & Arifuku, 2005; Le, Arifuku, Louie, & Krisberg, 2001; Le, Arifuku, Louie, Krisberg, & Tang, 2001). Vietnamese American adolescents experienced one of the highest rates of increase in probation (67% from 1990 to 1995) which further illustrates the differences in delinquency prevalence between Asian American sub-ethnic groups (Le & Arifuku, 2005). Other studies support these findings. For example, sociologist Baba (2001) found that Vietnamese American youth were the fourth-largest group on probation in California, followed by Blacks, Latinos, and Whites. Hung (2002) reported that in Contra Costa County, despite representing only 2% of the overall population, highland Laotians comprise 10% of all juveniles on probation. The finding that these Asian sub-ethnic groups do experience high rates of delinquency stands in sharp contrast to the "model minority" stereotype attributed to Asian Americans earlier, which as an aggregated group had the lowest delinquency rate.

Youth Violence Among Asian Americans: A More Complete Picture

Research methods that rely on self-report have been useful to counter the model minority myth. Self-reported studies are those which, using surveys, questionnaires, and interviews, allow respondents to describe their own behaviors. Unlike grades, police reports, criminal justice data, and other official statistics, these generally anonymous and smaller/more localized studies can provide a more granular view into the world of the respondent. In particular, most self-report studies presenting statistics for Asian American youth delinquency rely more on regional, clinical, or convenience samples and thus can specify more sub-ethnic groups than more traditional, large or nationally representative samples. Although self-report data can be somewhat less reliable due to representational biases (i.e., the respondent wishing to minimize their perceived delinquent actions, or, in some cases, exaggerate them), they are still generally considered reliable when reporting youths' own behaviors (Johnston, O'Malley, & Bachman, 2001).

A number of studies using self-reported data have demonstrated that Asian American youth of Southeast Asian ancestry report more engagement in delinquent activities and violence than their East Asian counterparts (Bui & Thongniramol, 2005; Huang & Ida, 2004; Jang, 2002; Le & Arifuku, 2005; Le, Monfared, & Stockdale, 2005). In Hawai'i, Filipino American youth reported higher rates of delinquent behavior than Japanese American youth (Mayeda et al., 2006). Using a national sample, Choi, He, and Harachi (2008) found that Filipino American, other Asian/Pacific Islander, and multi-ethnic Asian youth reported higher engagement in risk factors such as delinquency, substance use, and sex as compared to Chinese American, Korean American, and Vietnamese American youth. Choi suggested that examining the different conditions in which these groups develop, as well as the context of their immigration patterns, can help lead to the identification and quantification of how each group responds to these different risk factors.

Studies have also shown variability with respect to victimization among the different Asian and Pacific Islander sub-groups. It is well known that victimization and bullying is a far too common experience among adolescents; in fact, three out of four youth experience bullying by their peers (Bosworth, Espelage, & Simon, 1999; Nansel et al., 2001). Given that interpersonal violence is occurring at high rates among youth, adolescence is clearly a period of elevated risk behavior for all youth. Numerous studies have demonstrated the relationship between violence exposure and adverse psychological outcomes such as major depressive episodes, posttraumatic stress disorder (PTSD), and substance abuse and dependence (Kilpatrick et al., 2000, 2003). Despite strong associations between violence and adverse outcomes, however, many exposed youth have exhibited resilience as evidenced by their abilities to maintain high levels of adaptive behavior and psychological functioning (Cichetti & Lynch, 1993). Thus, violence exposure in youth does not always lead to adverse outcomes, suggesting moderating factors may be involved (Holmbeck, 1997).

Several sources have reported Asian Americans to have lower rates of victimization. A national survey of adolescents in the U.S. reported lower prevalence for Asian youth regarding sexual assault, physical assault, and witnessing violence, compared to African American, Native American, and Hispanic adolescents (Kilpatrick, Saunders, & Smith, 1995). The National Crime Victimization Survey, in which violent victimization includes homicide, assault, robbery and rape, showed the average rate of victimization for Asian youth to be 5%, compared with 11% for other ethnicities (Rennison, 2001). The Office of Juvenile Justice and Delinquency Prevention (OJJDP) estimates the average annual victimization rates for violent crimes among Asians was 55.0 per 1,000, and simple assaults was 33.5 per 1,000, compared to 108.7 and 78.2 for White youth, respectively (Menard, 2002). Likewise, official statistics collected by the Oakland Police Department show the rate of victimization for Asian youth to be lower than the rates for Black and White youth (Le, 2005).

On the other hand, Chu and Sorenson (1996) suggested that homicide rates for Hispanics and Asians are not only higher than other ethnicities, but are increasing when other groups are experiencing decreases. Le and Wallen (2009), using self-report data from a community sample, found that the percentage of youth victimization is much higher for Southeast Asian American youth. Kilpatrick et al. (1995) found that one in four Cambodian American and one in five Lao/Mien American youth reported experiencing violent physical victimization. These rates approximate other high risk groups in the U.S. such as Native American, African American, and Hispanic youth. In particular, Asian immigrants

have a significantly higher risk of homicide than their native born counterparts (Sorenson & Shen, 1996). Asian Americans already represent a very heterogeneous group with more than three dozen different sub-groups and cultures. New arrivals coming to the U.S. (e.g., Mongolians, Sri Lankans, Tibetans) will continue to change the sub-ethnic characteristic of the existing population, further complicating matters. While at an aggregate level Asian American youth may have overall lower rates of delinquency compared to Blacks or Latinos, there is clearly disproportionate representation across the component sub-groups, with Southeast Asians tending to have higher rates and East Asian youth the lowest rates.

Risk and Protective Factors

The goals of delinquency studies are not simply to measure current rates, but also to help determine factors and root causes. Identifying those factors can help us to better target our limited resources to focus on programs that are most effective in alleviating these conditions. One of the main risk factors for youth violence among Asian Americans is acculturation. Acculturation has been recognized as a critical factor in Asian American wellbeing (Liu, Pope-Davis, Nevitt, & Toporek, 1999; Mehta, 1998; Wong-Stokem, 1998), and refers to the manner in which individuals negotiate two or more cultures where one culture is considered dominant while the other culture is perceived to have less cultural value (Berry, 1998; LaFromboise, Coleman, & Gerton, 1993). The culture of origin is referred to as the national culture, while the culture of contact is referred to as the "host culture" (Ward & Kennedy, 1994). The process of acculturation is influenced by how individuals maintain or let go of their national culture in the presence of competing cultural values (Berry, Kim, Minde, & Mok, 1987). While numerous studies have investigated Asian American acculturation (Atkinson, Lowe, & Matthews, 1995; Gim Chung, 2001; Iwamasa, 1996; Liem, Lim, & Liem, 2000; Liu et al., 1999; Ryder, Alden, & Paulhus, 2000; Yeh, 2003), only a few studies have examined the relationship between violence and acculturation.

Le (2002) examined 34 studies of delinquency among Asian American and Pacific Islander youth, and Smokowski, David-Ferdon, and Stroupe (2009) examined an additional 13 studies on acculturation and interpersonal or self-directed violence among Asian American and Pacific Islander youth. Most of the studies on Asian American youth indicate that high adolescent acculturation (e.g., generation, time in the U.S., English language use, U.S. cultural involvement or individualism scales) is a risk factor for adolescent problem behavior, aggression, and violence. Of these studies, 69% of the investigations indicated a relationship between acculturation and youth violence. The relationship between high acculturation and youth violence was robust across studies that included Asian American youth, even when acculturation and youth violence were measured in different ways. For example, using a national sample of more than 15,000 students in the sixth through tenth grades, Yu, Zhihuan, Schwalberg, Overpeck, and Kogan (2003) showed that relative to English-only speaking peers, Asian American youth who spoke another language at home were significantly more likely to be bullied. Low acculturated youth may have increased vulnerability within a new cultural system that he or she does not fully understand. In this context, many youths may see physically fighting as the only way that they can maintain their dignity, especially when language difficulties limit communication (Bacallao & Smokowski, 2007).

Attributes and outcomes related to immigration and acculturation status have also been linked to youth violence. Discrimination, individualism and intergenerational/intercultural conflict has been shown to enhance the impact of certain stressors (e.g., emotional hardship, physical abuse, emotional abuse) to predict violent behavior. After examining data from 217 Korean American students in Los Angeles, Shrake and Rhee (2004) reported that perceived discrimination showed a strong positive effect on both internalizing and externalizing problem behaviors. Ngo and Le (2007) reported that increased levels of acculturation, intergenerational/intercultural conflict, and individualism placed youth at increased risk for serious violence (e.g., aggravated assault, robbery, rape, and gang fights). Similarly, in a sample of 329 Southeast Asian Americans youth from Oakland, Le and Stockdale (2005) found that individualism was positively related to self-reported delinquency, with partial mediation through peer delinquency. In another study using the same sample, acculturative dissonance was found as significantly predictive of serious violence, with full mediation through peer delinquency (Le & Stockdale, 2008).

When looking specifically at generation, it has been found that controlling for immigrant generational status can either eliminate or magnify some of the differences between the groups, suggesting the need to consider immigrant status as a factor in delinquency prevalence. Perhaps surprisingly or not surprisingly, second generation youth who are born in the U.S. generally have higher rates of delinquency than do first generation who immigrated themselves. Among Filipino American youth for example, second generation adolescents had significantly higher delinquency than first generation youth (Willgerodt & Thompson, 2006); however, there were no differences relative to third generation peers. As such, in addition to all other factors which need to be considered for every group, immigrant status is a potential confounding factor when studying youth violence in the Asian American population. These issues, combined with the lack of disaggregated official statistics (aside from a handful of Californian counties) and the relatively few studies that use a national representative samples, make it challenging to gain an accurate pulse on the prevalence of delinquency for the varied Asian Americans sub-groups.

Preventing Youth Violence Among Asian Americans

In order to develop culturally appropriate and effective prevention and intervention youth violence programs for Asian American youth, an understanding of the relevant risk and protective factors specific to Asian Americans is needed. Prevention and intervention programs also need to be grounded in empirical research and theory. The research thus far highlights the importance of family, culture, and the acculturation process for Asian Americans. Cultural assets, such as culture-of-origin involvement, ethnic identity, and collectivism, may counterbalance the risk factors associated with lack of acculturation. Two out of three studies that tested ethnic identity or collectivism found these cultural assets to be related to lower youth violence in Asian American youth. The only caveat was that Go and Le (2005) also reported that (1) ethnic identity was a positive predictor of delinquency for male, but not female, Cambodian American youth; and (2) a sense of ethnic belonging was unrelated to delinquency for Cambodian American youth. Regardless, these initial findings are encouraging because they reflect a growing body of literature showing the positive effect ethnic identity, enculturation, and culture-of-origin involvement on minority adolescents' self-esteem and overall positive development (Phinney, Cantu, & Kurtz, 1995; Phinney, Chavira, & Tate, 1997; Phinney & Flores, 2002).

Intimate Partner Violence

According to the Centers for Disease Control and Prevention (CDC), the lifetime prevalence rate of intimate partner violence for women in the US is approximately 25% (CDC, 2008). National data indicate that women are nearly three times more likely to be victims than men. The National Institute of Justice's National Violence Against Women (NVAW) Survey has put forth the following statistics to describe the extent of the issue: (1) As a whole, violence against women is primarily intimate partner violence, in than 64% of women who reported being assaulted were victimized by a current or former partner, boyfriend, husband, or date; (2) Among women who were raped, 54% were younger than the age of 18; (3) Women who reported they were raped before the age of 18 were twice as likely to report being raped as an adult; and (4) Only 30–35% of women who are assaulted receive medical treatment after the

event (Tjaden & Thoennes, 2000). Other studies indicate that intimate partner violence among Asian American women is even greater. For example, a statewide study in Massachusetts showed that 18% of residents killed by and intimate partner were Asian American women (Foo, 2002). However, they comprised only 2% of the State's population, indicating a nine-fold increase in risk.

Intimate Partner Violence Among Asian Americans

The overall rates of intimate partner violence among Asian American women reported in the literature is low, due at least in part to under-reporting (Rennison, 2001; Tjaden & Thoennes, 2000). While national surveys have suggested that the prevalence of intimate partner violence among Asian American women is low, community-based studies have not consistently supported such findings. In fact, research has shown that Asian American women are more likely than other ethnic groups to face intimate partner violence in their lifetime (e.g., Kim, Lau, & Chang, 2006). These studies indicate that intimate partner violence is a significant concern among Asian Americans. Forty one to sixty percent of Asian American women report experiencing physical and/or sexual violence by an intimate partner during their lifetime (Asian and Pacific Islander Institute on Domestic Violence, 2005; Raj & Silverman, 2002; Yoshihama, 1999). This is higher than the prevalence for other ethnic groups: Euro-Americans (21.3%), African Americans (26.3%), Hispanic of any race (21.2%), mixed race (27.0%), and American Indians and Alaskan Natives (30.7%) (Tjaden & Thoennes, 2000). It is also higher than the 12.8% rate reported for Asians and Pacific Islanders in the same national survey, which again may be attributed to under-reporting arising from language and socio-cultural barriers.

One in four adolescents report verbal, physical, emotional, or sexual abuse from a dating partner each year (Foshee et al., 1996). Studies focusing on interpersonal or dating violence among minority adolescents are limited, but some investigators have suggested that adolescents from minority groups experience high rates of victimization. Using longitudinal data, Halpern, Oslak, Young, Martin, and Kupper (2001) examined physical and psychological dating violence, finding that Hispanic, Asian/Pacific Islander, White, and Black youth had a relatively equal likelihood of experiencing psychological abuse. However, Asian/Pacific Islander male adolescents were two times more likely to experience dating abuse, compared to Whites. Baker and Helm (2011), using an ethnically diverse adolescent population in Hawai'i, found that the most frequently reported type of violence was monitoring and controlling behaviors, particularly cybercontrol, followed by emotional violence.

Risk and Protective Factors

One of the fastest growing areas of research in intimate partner violence among Asian Americans concerns immigrant status (Ahmad, Riaz, Barata, & Stewart, 2004; Dasgupta, 2000; Tran, 1997; Tjaden & Thoennes, 2000). These studies show even higher rates for this population, and also increased severity of abuse and decreased knowledge of how to report or seek services for intimate partner violence (e.g., Raj & Silverman, 2003). The migration experience, which encompasses the circumstances around departure, period of transit, and settlement in the destination country, can increase an individual's risk for intimate partner violence (Wong et al., 2011). For example, Tran (1997) found that more than half of women refugees from Vietnam had been victims of intimate partner violence. A study by Song-Kim (1992) with abused Korean immigrant women found that while spousal abuse often began prior to immigration, frequency and severity tended to worsen in the initial years after arrival in the U.S.

Many hypotheses have been posited in the literature to explain this disparity. Raj and Silverman's (2003) study put forth several explanations. Social isolation, in particular, was associated with an increased likelihood of experiencing severe intimate partner violence. In other words,

women reporting no family in the U.S. were three times more likely to have been physically injured by their current partner, compared to those with family in the U.S. Similarly, another study which examined the effects of intimate partner violence on Asian women showed a strong direct effect of violence on psychological outcomes, which occurred without mediators to filter the impact such as social support and coping skills that existed for Caucasian women (Lee et al., 2007). This may imply that Asian women are more vulnerable to adverse psychological outcomes after experiencing abuse. Recent immigration, which would indicate increased retention of social norms from the woman's culture-of-origin, has also been suggested as contributing to higher levels of intimate partner violence. For example, a survey conducted by Yoshioka, DiNoia, and Ullah (2001) found that Vietnamese respondents were the most likely to agree with the statement, "A husband should have the right to discipline his wife." Tran's (1997) study supported this finding, in that Vietnamese wives generally felt it was acceptable for husbands to physically discipline them if there was a failure to meet the husband's expectations.

Similar to intimate partner violence, dating violence studies with minority youth frequently discuss immigration and acculturation as a contributor to increased or decreased risk. Silverman, Decker, and Raj's (2007) analysis of Youth Risk Behavior Survey data documented that being an immigrant was found to be protective against dating violence (OR 0.77, CI 0.60–0.98). Chung-Do and Goebert (2009) examined the influence of three acculturation components (parental role, gender role attitudes, and ethnic identity) on Filipino and Samoan youths' experiences of dating violence in Hawai'i. Their study demonstrated that parental role (punishment) and gender roles (appearance, female empowerment) were associated with verbal abuse victimization. Furthermore, gender role (appearance) and ethnic identity (out-group orientation) were associated with controlling victimization. On the other hand, having a strong commitment to one's ethnic identity served as a protective factor for Filipina youth.

Several studies have investigated the relationship between intimate partner violence and psychopathology (e.g., Callahan, Tolman, & Saunders, 2003; Coker et al., 2000; Hurwitz, Gupta, Liu, Silverman, & Raj, 2006; Molidor & Tolman, 1998; Silverman et al., 2001), and found a moderate empirical link. For example, Hurwitz et al., (2006) showed that South Asian women who experience intimate partner violence were significantly more likely to report poor physical health (95% CI=1.3–12.0), depression (95% CI=1.8–9.3), anxiety (95% CI=1.3–6.4), and suicidal ideation (95% CI=1.9–25.1), compared to those with no history of intimate partner violence. These findings were supported by qualitative data that indicated women who experienced intimate partner violence that resulted in injury, also reported chronic health concerns and disturbances in sleep patterns, appetite, energy, and overall wellbeing. Dating violence in adolescence has been linked with suicidality, distress, depression, and posttraumatic stress disorder (PTSD) symptoms, and this is link is also observed for Asian Americans (Chung-Do & Goebert, 2009; Decker, Raj, & Silverman, 2007; Silverman et al., 2007; Wolitzky et al., 2008).

Treating and Preventing Intimate Partner Violence Among Asian Americans

Certainly intimate partner violence is a salient issue in Asian American communities. However, barriers to help-seeking among Asian American victims must first be elucidated, acknowledged, and overcome. Several barriers have already been alluded to, such as difficulty in patient-provider communication due to language barrier, and overall communication style. However, many other barriers exist under the umbrella cultural norms and expectations. These may include one's commitment to children and family unity, perceived shame and "loss-of-face" related to the abuse, and a cultural stigma of divorce and fear of subsequent social isolation that may be accentuated by discrimination and/or fears of deportation (Bauer, Rodriguez, Quiroga, & Flores-Ortiz, 2000). Weil and Lee (2004) elaborated on these factors, commenting that a woman's decision to leave any

relationship, despite enduring physical and/or emotional abuse, may elicit an unsympathetic response from the victim's community. This phenomenon stems from traditional cultural values, and adds to the shame and stigma that together can minimize the gravity of intimate partner violence. Chang, Shen, and Takeuchi (2009) noted that while not condoned in Asian communities, certain cultural norms may even find intimate partner violence acceptable in certain situations or contexts. Furthermore, Asian American women generally find it difficult to discuss stressors in their lives, especially issues such as mental health, sexuality, or personal and bodily integrity (National Asian Women's Health Organization, 1997, 2002). Medical and social service providers, as well as policymakers, may improve the quality of care for Asian American women by understanding and addressing these barriers, and integrating potential solutions into more culturally competent practice.

Patterns of help-seeking behaviors among women experiencing intimate partner violence indicate that they don't use services, use informal care networks, or seek services but not use then (Rodríguez, Valentine, Son, & Muhammad, 2009). These are heightened among minority women (Chow, Jaffee, & Snowden, 2003). Despite underutilization of mental health care services, the vast majority of women that experience intimate partner violence, including Asian American women, express interest in psychosocial care and treatment (Chow et al., 2003; Wong et al., 2007). There are few programs developed for Asian American women in crisis, such as shelters and hotlines, however, these have limited resources to operate (Ingram et al., 2007). Cultural competency becomes even more crucial when dealing with intimate partner violence, enhancing accurate assessment and effective intervention (Campbell & Lewandowski, 1997). Cultural competence is about engagement with respect and reinforcing the strengths of the patient, family, community or population, its differences, and the process of this engagement (Betancourt, Green, Carrillo, & Ananeh-Firempong, 2003). It refers to an acceptance and respect for difference, a continuing self-assessment regarding culture, a regard for and attention to the dynamics of difference, engagement in ongoing development of cultural knowledge, and resources and flexibility within service models to work towards better meeting the needs of minority populations (Substance Abuse and Mental Health Services Administration [SAMSHA], 2000).

Recognizing the need for interpersonal violence prevention and intervention programs that address specific ethnic minority populations, the Centers for Disease Control and Prevention (CDC) funded demonstration projects that would develop, implement, and evaluate culturally competent prevention strategies (Whitaker & Reese, 2007). One of these projects focused on Asian Americans. The "Breaking-the-Silence" Asian-American Women's Discussion Group is a curriculum-based intervention specifically for college-aged women and applied in California (Ingram et al., 2007). It consists of four modules: (1) cultural influences that confront Asian American women and involvement of these in sexual violence and intimate partner violence related experience; (2) information on sexual violence statistics, combating common assumption, and integrating specific barriers faced by Asian American women; (3) definition of intimate partner violence, its effects on women's health, barriers to reporting intimate partner violence, and barriers faced by Asian American women victims of intimate partner violence; and (4) effective strategies for sexual violence and intimate partner violence prevention, developing safety plans, and campus and community resources for sexual violence and intimate partner violence victims.

Suicide

Self-directed violence refers to a person intentionally inflicting violence on himself or herself, with the goal of causing harm that may or may not shorten or end his or her life (Smokowski et al., 2009). This includes suicidal ideation, making a suicide plan, attempting suicide, and actually committing suicide. Suicide is the eighth most common cause of death among Asian and Pacific Islander Americans, compared to the 11th most common cause of death in the overall US

population (U.S. Department of Health and Human Services, 2007). Compared with other ethnic groups, rates among Asian Americans are higher than African Americans, but lower than Native American and European Americans. Comparative studies over the last half century have shown that Japanese Americans have higher suicide rates than Chinese Americans and Filipino Americans, potentially due to differences in rates of historical acceptance (e.g., Iga, Yamamoto, Noguchi, & Koshinaga, 1978). However, while here has been an increase in the number of studies examining Asian Americans and suicide in the United States, a dearth of information remains on Asian American subgroups. The vast majority of the Asian American population is foreign born (U.S. Census Bureau, 2003), yet research on Asian American subgroups has primarily focused on groups that have lived in the US a significant amount of time. Comparative studies have focused mainly on Chinese, Japanese, and Filipino Americans (e.g., Fugita, 1990; Leong, Leach, Yeh, & Chou, 2007; Lester, 1994).

Generally, suicide risk among Asian Americans increases with age. However, suicide trends among Asian Americans shows some differences by age. Among primary care patients, older Asian American adults have been found to have the highest rates of death and suicide ideation (56.8%) as compared with African American, Caucasian, and Hispanic older adults (Bartels et al., 2002). The suicide rates among Asian and Pacific Islander American women aged 65 and above also exceed rates from the major US racial and ethnic groups, at 7.1 per 100,000 (CDC, 2011). Among Asian and Pacific Islander American women aged 15–24 years, the suicide rate was 4.25 per 100,000, exceeding the national suicide rate as well as the rates for all major racial/ethnic groups except Native Americans (CDC, 2011). Several studies with Asian American college students reported higher levels of suicidal ideation compared with White American college students (Brener, Hassan, & Barrios, 1999; Chang, 1998; Kisch, Leino, & Silverman, 2005; Muehlenkamp, Gutierrez, Osman, & Barrios, 2005). Among adolescents, Grunbaum, Lowry, Kann, and Pateman (2000) found that Asian American and Pacific Islander youth were less likely to engage in health risk behaviors such a drinking or substance use, but were as likely to attempt suicide. Lau, Jernewall, Zane, and Myers (2002) found that suicidal youths were more likely than non-suicidal youths to have been born outside of the US.

Risk and Protective Factors

Family relationships have been shown to be an important factor when considering suicide among Asian Americans. Among Asian Americans aged 65 and above for example, the two most commonly known correlates of suicide were the death of a family member, and feeling rejected or perceiving oneself to be a burden on family members (Blinn, 1997). Elders may not be treated with the level of respect of their native cultures and may feel burdensome (Range et al., 1999). Many Asian American men who are in the U.S. without their families are isolated not just from family but also culture. Family conflict, in general, is strongly related to an increased likelihood of suicidal behavior for Asian Americans. Individuals may engage in suicidal behaviors after they experience the shame associated with "loss-of-face" when they fail to meet expectations of their families or others (Zane & Mak, 2003). When an individual's behavior upsets group harmony, "loss-of-face" or social shame, is experienced. This phenomenon is more prominent in East Asians (i.e., Chinese and Japanese) and East Asian Americans, although it may also exist in other Asian groups (e.g., South Asians) to a lesser degree, and it persists despite acculturation. Loss-of-face can serve as a precipitant for suicidal behavior if the shame is perceived as intolerable, or if the group views suicide as an honorable way of dealing with difficulties. Alternatively if the group views suicide as dishonorable, the person may be less likely to attempt suicide, despite failure to meet desired expectations.

Increasingly, discrimination has been documented as an Asian American experience in a number of different social settings (Turner, Ross, Bednarz, Herbig, & Lee, 2003). Furthermore, evidence suggests that perceived discrimination is associated with mental health problems among Asian Americans (Gee, Spencer, Chen, Yip, &

Takeuchi, 2007). Ethnic minorities, including Asian American groups, may internalize experiences of racism and discrimination experienced from the dominant culture, resulting in low self-esteem as well as feelings of depression, rejection and isolation (Atkinson, Morten, & Sue, 1993; Livengood & Stodolska, 2004; Ying, Lee, & Tsai, 2000). Both depression and social isolation are connected with risk factors for suicidality. Hwang and Goto (2008) found that perceived discrimination was associated with negative mental health outcomes and suicidal ideation among Asian American college students. Perceived discrimination has also been shown to be associated with suicide attempts (Cheng et al., 2010).

Culture in general may affect help-seeking behaviors relating to mental health services, and the actual utilization of services for prevention or treatment of suicidal behaviors (Goldston et al., 2008). For example, recently immigrated Asian families may lack familiarity with the health care system, or may believe that problems such as suicidal behaviors should be managed within the family or faith community rather than by specialty mental health services. Findings from the Chinese American Psychiatric Epidemiologic Study revealed extremely low rates of service use, with only 4% of Chinese Americans with mental health problems consulting with their physician, whereas 8% consulted with a minister or priest (Young, 1998). Even when Asian Americans seek mental health treatment, they may not disclose suicidal ideation as readily as other non-ethnic-minority Americans (Morrison & Downey, 2000). This may be due, in part, to their tendency to focus on their somatic rather than psychological stressors (Lin & Cheung, 1999; Tseng et al., 1990).

Influence of Acculturation

Only a few studies have directly examined the relationship between suicide indicators and acculturation (e.g., Cho, 2003; Goldston et al., 2008; Kennedy, Parhar, Samra, & Gorzalka, 2005; Lau et al., 2002; Yang & Clum, 1994; Yeh, 2003). These studies indicate that Asian Americans are at increased risk if they identify more with their culture of origin, and are unable to identify or adjust to the new host culture. Additionally, acculturation has been shown to be strongly associated with depression (Chen, Guarnaccia, & Chung, 2003; Jonnalagadda & Diwan, 2005). Most of this research has focused on adults. For example, Asian American college students who reported that they seriously considered committing suicide in the past year listed family, academic, and financial problems as the top three most common events preceding the developing of their suicide ideation (Wong et al., 2011).

Studies with Asian American youth reveal that acculturative stressors may culminate in suicidal behaviors through a variety of mechanisms. Hyman, Vu, and Beiser (2000) documented the multiple acculturative stresses experienced by children of Southeast Asian refugees, including feelings of estrangement, frustrations with learning English, unequal language fluency between parents and youths, and high parental expectations. Particularly among Asian American adolescents, family conflict poses a greater suicide risk among less acculturated adolescents as compared with highly acculturated adolescents (Lau et al., 2002). Lau et al. (2002) studied factors related to suicidal behaviors among Asian American adolescents receiving outpatient treatment. When high parent–child conflict existed, Asian American youths who identified with being Asian were at greater risk for suicidal behavior than were their more Western-identified counterparts. They speculated that less acculturated youths may experience greater distress when faced with family conflict and threats to group harmony, and may have less non-familial support than more acculturated youth. Furthermore, Costigan and Dokis (2006) found that Chinese American adolescents tended to have more severe depression when their level of enculturation (i.e., identification with their own culture) was incongruent with that of their parents.

Treating and Preventing Suicidality Among Asian Americans

Research on suicidality among Asian Americans is needed to prevent suicide and guide practitioners in treating suicidal Asian American patients

(Cheng et al., 2010; Leong et al., 2007). The prevention literature for Asian Americans is sparse and those that exist have generally not been evaluated (Goldston et al., 2008). Takahashi (1989) recommended taking cultural practices into consideration. For example, Asian Americans are less likely to verbalize suicide thoughts or intent as readily as other groups (Goldston et al., 2008). One in three Asian Americans who attempted suicide had no evidence of depressive or anxiety disorders (Fortuna, Perez, Canino, Sribney, & Alegria, 2007). Asian Americans self-reported higher levels of depression than Euro Americans (Sue & Chu, 2003). Importantly, among those with a diagnosis of depressive disorder, Asian Americans still reported higher levels of somatization. In fact, Asian Americans rarely distinguish depressive affect from somatization, although the distinction is generally made by Euro Americans (Cheng et al., 2010). Thus, Asian Americans may be more likely to express psychological distress through somatic complaints. Unfortunately, Asian Americans who express psychological distress in terms of somatic complaints may not be identified as requiring treatment. Therefore, practitioners must look beyond depressive symptom scales to identify suicide risk among Asian Americans.

Future Directions

Research on interpersonal and self-directed violence among Asian Americans remains in its infancy (Goldston et al., 2008; Kim et al., 2006; Leong, Leach, & Gupta, 2008; Smokowski et al., 2009). Future studies are clearly warranted. More nationally representative information is needed on the epidemiology of interpersonal and self-directed violence among Asian Americans as a whole, as well as baseline prevalences among Asian sub-ethnic groups (particularly in light of differing cultural norms). There is also a need for more diverse research methodologies, such as (1) longitudinal studies; (2) utilization of advanced, contemporary data analysis strategies (e.g., structural equation modeling, hierarchical linear modeling); (3) mixed methods research that obtains data from multiple informants (e.g., youth, parents, community); (4) application of sophisticated, multidimensional measures of acculturation, identity, and culture; and (5) consideration multiple areas of violence (e.g., discrimination and hate crimes, peer violence, dating violence, family violence, suicide). Such research among Asian Americans can begin to empirically assess specific explanatory models of interpersonal and self-inflicted violence, especially with regard to identification of causal mechanisms and related risk contexts.

Culture, Acculturation, and Acculturative Stress

One consistent theme in violence prevention and health promotion among Asian Americans is that culture, acculturation, and acculturative stress play pivotal roles (Kim et al., 2006; Smokowski et al., 2009). However, it is still unclear as to whether acculturation acts as a risk or protective factor, and if so, to how strong its effects are. As emerging research has revealed somewhat contradictory findings, compared to previous studies which associated higher acculturation levels with higher levels of violence, this represents an area where further empirical investigation is required. Just in the studies reviewed in this chapter, acculturation was found to be both a risk and protective factor. Ethnic group identity and culture-of-origin involvement appeared to be cultural assets against violence, but more studies are needed to determine if this relationship holds for different Asian American sub-groups (Smokowski et al., 2009). In future studies, increased attention to the specific sub-groups and between-group analyses are needed to assess for potential differences in the association between acculturation and the outcomes of interest. Furthermore, additional research is needed to better understand sensitive, and potentially stigmatizing, issues such as suicidality in the context of different cultural backgrounds and acculturation. This would include considerations such as culture-specific triggers or processes leading to suicidal behavior, as well as culture-specific risk and protective factors in general (Goldston et al., 2008).

Prevention and Intervention

Given the limited research available, clinicians have struggled to find literature to guide identification and treatment of the unique factors associated with Asian American violence and suicide. There are generally few culturally sensitive prevention and treatment interventions, and even fewer that are tailored for Asian American groups. "Tailoring" refers to the creation of interventions that utilize information about a given individual to determine what specific content he/she will receive, the contexts surrounding that information, by whom it will be presented, and the manner in which it will be delivered (Hawkins et al., 2008). Overall, tailoring aims to enhance the relevance of the intervention and improve recipient response. Use of this approach has grown exponentially since the 1990s, especially in chronic disease and, to a lesser extent, with mental health. Cultural approaches have shown success in decreasing violence, and thus warrant further study.

Given that people from different cultures have different habits, values, and ways of relating to one another, tailoring appears to be a promising approach for Asian Americans. More refined studies are needed to determine whether violence and suicide prevention and intervention programs should attend to different predictive associations and risk and protective factors for various subgroups within the Asian American population (Smokowski et al., 2009). Therefore, more research is needed to compare the effectiveness of different models of care among Asian Americans. It is possible, however, that we are not accessing the key components of culture that are needed to improve outcomes through tailoring. For example, an understudied area is the degree to which interventions focused on reducing risk factors such as hopelessness in the community, and enhancing culturally relevant protective factors or supports such as ties to elders or cultural traditions. These are specific strategies that can reduce violence and suicidality among Asian Americans (Goldston et al., 2008).

A common thread that has appeared throughout this chapter, and one that would be key in

any prevention or intervention effort, is the overall importance of tradition and culture and how
these constructs intersect with health. Many traditional Asian Americans believe that illness
comes from an imbalance of harmony, whether
the imbalance is in their bodies or interpersonal
relationships (Chung-Do, Chung-Do, Huh, &
Kang, 2011; Purnell & Kim, 2003). Another
important consideration is the utilization and
effectiveness of informal or traditional sources
of help within Asian American communities
(Goldston et al., 2008). Some Asian Americans
may be more comfortable speaking with lay
helpers or traditional healers, in lieu of discussing difficulties with strangers in unfamiliar settings. Efforts developed by and implemented
within communities have a greater likelihood of
sustainability due to heightened individual and
community investment in the programs, and
because participants are able to experience first-
hand the positive changes that occur as a result
of interventions. Such community-based efforts
have not often been the subject of research scru-
tiny and evaluation, but have much promise in
reducing violence, suicidal behaviors and related
problems, particularly in Asian American neighborhoods. To ensure that well-intended prevention and intervention efforts have desired effects,
innovative approaches to evaluation are needed
that are designed around programs that have
been tailored to the specific needs and contexts
of Asian American populations.

References

Africa, J., & Carrasco, M. (2011). *Asian-American and Pacific Islander mental health*. Arlington, VA: National Alliance on Mental Illness.
Ahmad, F., Riaz, S., Barata, P., & Stewart, D. E. (2004). Patriarchal beliefs and perceptions of abuse among South Asian immigrant women. *Violence Against Women, 10*, 262–282.
Akutsu, P. D., & Chu, J. P. (2006). Clinical problems that initiate professional help-seeking behaviors from Asian Americans. *Professional Psychology: Research and Practice, 37*(4), 407–415.
Ancheta, A. N. (2006). *Race, rights, and the Asian American experience*. New Brunswick, NJ: Rutgers University Press.

Asian & Pacific Islander Institute on Domestic Violence. (2005). *Fact sheet: Domestic violence in Asian communities*, http://www.apiahf.org/apidvinstitute/PDF/Fact_Sheet.pdf
Associated Press. (2005, November 13). Asian youth persistently harassed by U.S. peers. *USA Today*
Atkinson, D. R., Lowe, S., & Matthews, L. (1995). Asian-American acculturation, gender, and willingness to seek counseling. *Journal of Multicultural Counseling and Development, 23*, 130–138.
Atkinson, D. R., Morten, G., & Sue, D. W. (1993). *Counseling American minorities: A cross-cultural perspective*. Madison, WI: W.C. Brown & Benchmark.
Ayalon, L., & Arean, P. A. (2004). Knowledge of Alzheimer's disease in four ethnic groups of older adults. *International Journal of Geriatric Psychiatry, 19*(1), 51–57.
Baba, Y. (2001). Vietnamese gangs, cliques and delinquents. *Journal of Gang Research, 8*(2), 1–20.
Bacallao, M. L., & Smokowski, P. R. (2007). The costs of getting ahead: Mexican family systems after immigration. *Family Relations, 56*, 52–66.
Baker, C. K., & Helm, S. (2011). Prevalence of intimate partner violence victimization and perpetration among youth in Hawai'i. *Hawai'i Medical Journal, 70*, 92–96.
Bartels, S. J., Coakley, E., Oxman, T. E., Constantino, G., Oslin, D., Chen, H., et al. (2002). Suicidal and death ideation in older primary care patients with depression, anxiety, and at-risk alcohol use. *The American Journal of Geriatric Psychiatry, 10*(4), 417–427.
Bauer, H. M., Rodriguez, M. A., Quiroga, S. S., & Flores-Ortiz, Y. G. (2000). Barriers to health care for abused Latina and Asian immigrant women. *Journal of Health Care for the Poor and Underserved, 11*(1), 33–44.
Berry, J. W. (1998). Acculturation stress. In P. Balls Organista, K. M. Chun, & G. Marin (Eds.), *Readings in ethnic psychology* (pp. 117–122). New York: Routledge.
Berry, J. W., Kim, U., Minde, T., & Mok, D. (1987). Comparative studies of acculturative stress. *International Migration Review, 21*, 491–511.
Betancourt, J. R., Green, A. R., Carrillo, J. E., & Ananeh-Firempong, O. (2003). Defining cultural competence: A practical framework for addressing racial/ethnic disparities in health. *Public Health Reports, 118*, 292–302.
Blinn, R. E., Jr. (1997). Asian-American and Chinese-American suicide in San Francisco. *Dissertation Abstracts International: Section B: The Sciences and Engineering, 57*(7-B), 4694.
Bosworth, K., Espelage, D. L., & Simon, T. R. (1999). Factors associated with bullying behavior in middle school students. *Journal of Early Adolescence, 19*, 341–362.
Brener, N. D., Hassan, S. S., & Barrios, L. C. (1999). Suicidal ideation among college students in the United States. *Journal of Consulting and Clinical Psychology, 67*, 1004–1008.
Bridges, G. S., & Steen, S. (1998). Racial disparities in official assessments of juvenile offenders: Attributional stereotypes as mediating mechanisms. *American Sociological Review, 63*, 554–570.

Bui, H. N., & Thongniramol, O. (2005). Immigration and self-reported delinquency: The interplay of immigration generations, gender, race, and ethnicity. *Journal of Crime and Justice, 28*, 71–99.

Callahan, M. R., Tolman, R. M., & Saunders, D. G. (2003). Adolescent dating violence victimization and psychological well-being. *Journal of Adolescent Research, 18*, 664–681.

Campbell, J. C., & Lewandowski, L. A. (1997). Mental and physical health effects of intimate partner violence on women and children. *Psychiatric Clinics of North America, 20*(2), 353–374.

Cauce, A. M., Domenech-Rodriguez, M., Paradise, M., Cochran, B. N., Shea, J. M., Srebnik, D., et al. (2002). Cultural contextual influences in minority mental health help seeking: A focus on ethnic minority youth. *Journal of Consulting and Clinical Psychology, 70*, 44–55.

Centers for Disease Control and Prevention [CDC]. (2008). Adverse health conditions and health risk behaviors associated with intimate partner violence: United States, 2005. *Morbidity and Mortality Weekly Report, 57*(5), 113–117, February 8.

Centers for Disease Control and Prevention [CDC]. (2011). *Web-based injury statistics query and reporting system (WISQARS)*. Retrieved January 25, 2011, from www.cdc.gov/ncipc/wisqars/default.htm

Chae, D. H., Takeuchi, D. T., Barbeau, E. M., Bennett, G. G., Lindsey, J., & Krieger, N. (2008). Unfair treatment, racial/ethnic discrimination, ethnic identification, and smoking among Asian Americans in the National Latino and Asian American Study. *American Journal of Public Health, 98*(3), 485–492.

Chang, E. C. (1998). Cultural differences, perfectionism, and suicidal risk in a college population: Does social problem solving still matter? *Cognitive Therapy and Research, 22*, 237–254.

Chang, D. F., Shen, B. J., & Takeuchi, D. T. (2009). Prevalence and demographic correlates of intimate partner violence in Asian Americans. *International Journal of Law and Psychiatry, 32*, 167–175.

Chen, H., Guarnaccia, P. J., & Chung, H. (2003). Self-attention as a mediator of cultural influences on depression. *The International Journal of Social Psychiatry, 49*, 192–203.

Chen, S. X., & Mak, W. W. S. (2008). Seeking professional help: Etiology beliefs about mental illness across cultures. *Journal of Counseling Psychology, 55*(4), 442–450.

Cheng, J. K. Y., Fancher, T. L., Ratanasen, M., Conner, K. R., Duberstein, P. R., Sue, S., et al. (2010). Lifetime suicidal ideation and suicide attempts in Asian Americans. *Asian American Journal of Psychology, 1*, 18–30.

Cho, Y.-B. (2003). Suicidal ideation, acculturative stress and perceived social support among Korean adolescents. *Dissertation Abstracts International: Section B: The Sciences and Engineering, 63*, 3907.

Choi, Y., He, M., & Harachi, T. W. (2008). Intergenerational cultural dissonance, family conflict, parent-child bonding, and youth antisocial behaviors among Vietnamese and Cambodian immigrant families. *Journal of Youth and Adolescence, 37*, 85–96.

Choi, Y., & Lahey, B. B. (2006). Testing the model minority stereotype: Youth behaviors across racial and ethnic groups. *The Social Service Review, 80*(3), 419–452.

Chow, J. C.-C., Jaffee, K., & Snowden, L. (2003). Racial/ethnic disparities in the use of mental health services in poverty areas. *American Journal of Public Health, 93*(5), 792–797.

Chu, J. P., Hsieh, K.-Y., & Tokars, D. A. (2011). Help-seeking tendencies in Asian Americans with suicidal ideation and attempts. *Asian American Journal of Psychology, 2*(1), 25–38.

Chu, L. D., & Sorenson, S. B. (1996). Trends in California homicide, 1970 to 1993. *The Western Journal of Medicine, 165*, 119–125.

Chung-Do, J. J., Chung-Do, J. J., Huh, J., & Kang, M. (2011). The Koreans. In J. F. McDermott, J. F. McDermott, & N. N. Andrade (Eds.), *People and cultures of Hawai'i: The evolution of culture and ethnicity* (pp. 176–200). Honolulu, HI: University of Hawai'i Press.

Chung-Do, J. J., & Goebert, D. A. (2009). Acculturation and dating violence victimization among Filipino and Samoan youths. *Journal of School Violence, 8*, 338–354.

Cichetti, D., & Lynch, M. (1993). Toward an ecological/transactional model of community violence and child maltreatment: Consequences for children's development. *Psychiatry, 56*, 96–118.

Coker, A. L., McKeown, R. E., Sanderson, M., Davis, K. E., Valois, R. F., & Huebner, E. S. (2000). Severe dating violence and quality of life among South Carolina high school students. *American Journal of Preventive Medicine, 19*, 220–227.

Costigan, C., & Dokis, D. P. (2006). Relations between parent-child acculturation differences and adjustment within immigrant Chinese families. *Child Development, 77*, 1252–1267.

Dasgupta, S. D. (2000). Charting the course: An overview of domestic violence in the South Asian community in the United States. *Journal of Social Distress and the Homeless, 9*, 173–185.

Daugherty, A. (2007). Dealing with anti-Asian sentiments after Virginia Tech tragedy. Retrieved http://virginiatech.healthandperformancesolutions.net/

Decker, M. R., Raj, A., & Silverman, J. G. (2007). Sexual violence against adolescent girls: Influences of immigration and acculturation. *Violence Against Women, 13*, 498–513.

DuBard, C. A., & Gizlice, Z. (2008). Language spoken and differences in health status, access to care, and receipt of preventive services among US Hispanics. *American Journal of Public Health, 98*(11), 2021–2028.

Federal Bureau of Investigation [FBI]. (1999). *Hate crime data collection: Uniform Crime Reporting*. Washington, DC: Criminal Justice Information Services Division, Federal Bureau of Investigation, U.S. Department of Justice.

Federal Bureau of Investigation [FBI]. (2011). *Matthew Shepard/James Byrd, Jr., Hate Crimes Prevention*

Act of 2009. Washington, DC: Federal Bureau of Investigation, U.S. Department of Justice.

Fisher, C. B., Wallace, S. A., & Fenton, R. E. (2000). Discrimination distress during adolescence. *Journal of Youth and Adolescence, 29*(6), 679–695.

Foo, L. J. (2002). *Asian American women: Issues, concerns and responsive human and civil rights advocacy.* New York: The Ford Foundation.

Fortuna, L. R., Perez, D. J., Canino, G., Sribney, W., & Alegria, M. (2007). Prevalence and correlates of lifetime suicidal ideation and suicide attempts among Latino subgroups in the United States. *The Journal of Clinical Psychiatry, 68*, 572–581.

Foshee, V. A., Linder, G. F., Bauman, K. E., Langwick, S. A., Arriaga, X. B., Heath, J. L., et al. (1996). The safe dates project: Theoretical basis, evaluation design, and selected baseline findings. *American Journal of Preventive Medicine, 12*(Suppl. 2), 39–47.

Fugita, S. S. (1990). Asian/Pacific-American mental health: Some needed research in epidemiology and service utilization. In F. C. Serafica, A. I. Schwebel, R. K. Russell, P. D. Isaac, & L. B. Myers (Eds.), *Mental health of ethnic minorities* (pp. 66–83). New York: Praeger.

Fugita, S. S., Schwebel, A. I., & Russell, R. K. (1990). Asian/Pacific-American mental health: Some needed research in epidemiology and service utilization. In F. C. Serafica, F. C. Serafica, P. D. Isaac, & L. B. Myers (Eds.), *Mental health of ethnic minorities* (pp. 66–83). New York: Praeger.

Gee, G. C. (2008). A multilevel analysis of the relationship between institutional and individual racial discrimination and health status. *American Journal of Public Health, 98*(Suppl. 9), S48–S56.

Gee, G. C., Ro, A., Shariff-Marco, S., & Chae, D. (2009). Racial discrimination and health among Asian Americans: Evidence, assessment, and directions for future research. *Epidemiological Review, 31*, 130–151.

Gee, G. C., Spencer, M., Chen, J., Yip, T., & Takeuchi, D. T. (2007). The association between self-reported racial discrimination and 12-month *DSM–IV* mental disorders among Asian Americans nationwide. *Social Science & Medicine, 64*, 1984–1996.

Gim Chung, R. H. (2001). Gender, ethnicity, and acculturation in intergenerational conflict of Asian American college students. *Cultural Diversity and Ethnic Minority Psychology, 7*, 376–386.

Go, C. G., & Le, T. N. (2005). Gender differences in Cambodian delinquency: The role of ethnic identity, parental discipline, and peer delinquency. *Crime and Delinquency, 51*, 220–237.

Goldston, D. B., Molock, S. D., Whitbeck, L. B., Murakami, J. L., Zayas, L. H., & Hall, G. C. N. (2008). Cultural considerations in adolescent suicide prevention and psychosocial treatment. *American Psychologist, 63*, 14–31.

Greene, M. L., Way, N., & Pahl, K. (2006). Trajectories of perceived adult and peer discrimination among Black, Latino, and Asian American adolescents: Patterns and psychological correlates. *Developmental Psychology, 42*(2), 218–236.

Grunbaum, J. A., Lowry, R., Kann, L., & Pateman, B. (2000). Prevalence of health risk behaviors among Asian American/Pacific Islander high school students. *Journal of Adolescent Health, 27*, 322–330.

Gym, H. (2011). Tiger Moms: The model minority stereotype and the impact on Asian youth in schools." In response to Amy Chua op-ed for the *Wall Street Journal* titled "Why Chinese Mothers are Superior." Retrieved February 16, 2011, from http://www.youngphillypolitics.com/tiger_moms_model_minority_stereotype_and_impact_asian_youth_schools

Halpern, C. T., Oslak, S. G., Young, M. L., Martin, S. L., & Kupper, L. L. (2001). Partner violence among adolescents in opposite-sex romantic relationships: Findings from the national longitudinal study of adolescent health. *American Journal of Public Health, 91*, 1679–1685.

Hawkins, J. D., Brown, E. C., Oesterle, S., Arthur, M. W., Abbott, R. D., & Catalano, R. F. (2008). Early effects of communities that care on targeted risks and initiation of delinquent behavior and substance use. *Journal of Adolescent Health, 43*, 15–22.

Ho, C., & Jackson, J. W. (2001). Attitudes towards Asian Americans: Theory and measurement. *Journal of Applied Social Psychology, 31*, 1553–1581.

Holmbeck, G. N. (1997). Toward terminological, conceptual, and statistical clarity in the study of mediators and moderators: Examples from the child-clinical and pediatric psychology literatures. *Journal of Consulting and Clinical Psychology, 65*(4), 599–610.

Huang, L. N., & Ida, D. J. (2004). *Promoting positive development and preventing youth violence and high-risk behaviors in Asian American/Pacific Islander communities: A social ecology perspective.* Denver, CO: National Asian American Pacific Islander Mental Health Association.

Hughes, D. L. (2002). Quality of health care for Asian Americans: Findings from the 2001 Commonwealth Fund Health Care Quality Survey. Retrieved www.commonwealthfund.org

Hung, M. (2002). Lost generation: Portrait of an Asian gang. Retrieved http://www.modelminority.com/joomla/index.php?option=com_content&view=article&id=379:lost-generation-portrait-of-an-asian-gang-&catid=47:society&Itemid=56

Hurwitz, E. J. H., Gupta, J., Liu, R., Silverman, J. G., & Raj, A. (2006). Intimate partner violence associated with poor health outcomes in U.S. South Asian women. *Journal of Immigrant and Minority Health, 8*(3), 251–261.

Hwang, W.-C., & Goto, S. (2008). The impact of perceived racial discrimination on the mental health of Asian American and Latino college students. *Cultural Diversity & Ethnic Minority Psychology, 14*, 326–335.

Hyman, I., Vu, N., & Beiser, M. (2000). Post-migration stresses among Southeast Asian refugee youth in

Canada: A research note. *Journal of Comparative Family Studies, 31*, 281–293.

Iga, M., Yamamoto, J., Noguchi, T., & Koshinaga, J. (1978). Suicide in Japan. *Social Science & Medicine, 12*, 507–516.

Ingram, E., Hoover, M., Kobayashi, A., Hayashi, M. C., Ingram, E., Hoover, M., et al. (2007). Culturally competent approach to violence prevention: The Asian American Women's Discussion Group. In D. J. Whitaker, L. E. Reese, & L. E. Reese (Eds.), *Preventing intimate partner violence and sexual violence in racial/ethnic minority communities: CDC's demonstration projects.* Atlanta, GA: Centers for Disease Control and Prevention, National Center for Injury Prevention and Control.

Iwamasa, G. Y. (1996). Acculturation of Asian American university students. *Assessment, 3*, 99–102.

Jang, S. J. (2002). Race, ethnicity, and deviance: A study of Asian and non-Asian adolescents in America. *Sociological Forum, 17*, 647–680.

Johnston, L. D., O'Malley, P. M., & Bachman, J. G. (2001). *Monitoring the future: National results on adolescent drug use – Overview of key findings, 2000.* (National Institute of Health Publication 01-4923). Bethesda, MD: National Institute on Drug Abuse.

Jonnalagadda, S. S., & Diwan, S. (2005). Health behaviors, chronic disease prevalence and self-rated health of older Asian Indian immigrants in the U.S. *Journal of Immigrant Health, 7*, 75–83.

Kennedy, M. A., Parhar, K. K., Samra, J., & Gorzalka, B. (2005). Suicide ideation in different generations of immigrants. *Canadian Journal of Psychiatry, 50*, 353–356.

Kilpatrick, D. G., Acierno, R., Saunders, B., Resnick, H., Best, C. L., & Schnurr, P. P. (2000). Risk factors for adolescent substance abuse and dependence: Data from a national sample. *Journal of Consulting and Clinical Psychology, 68*, 19–30.

Kilpatrick, D. G., Ruggiero, K. J., Acierno, R., Saunders, B. E., Resnick, H. S., & Best, C. L. (2003). Violence and risk of PTSD, major depression, substance abuse/dependence, and comorbidity: Results from the National Survey of Adolescents. *Journal of Consulting and Clinical Psychology, 71*, 692–700.

Kilpatrick, D. G., Saunders, B. E., & Smith, D. W. (1995). Youth victimization: Prevalence and implications: Who's at risk? *Population Trends and Public Policy, 21*, 1–20.

Kim, I. J., Lau, A. S., & Chang, D. F. (2006). Family violence. In F. T. Leon, A. G. Inman, A. Ebreo, L. Yang, L. M. Kinoshita, & M. Fu (Eds.), *Handbook of Asian American psychology* (2nd ed., pp. 363–378). Thousand Oaks, CA: Sage.

Kisch, J., Leino, E., & Silverman, M. M. (2005). Aspects of suicidal behavior, depression, and treatment in college students: Results from the spring 2000 national college health assessment survey. *Suicide & Life-Threatening Behavior, 35*, 3–13.

Krieger, N., Rowley, D. L., Herman, A. A., Avery, B., & Phillips, M. T. (1993). Racism, sexism, and social class: Implications for studies of health, disease, and well-being. *American Journal of Preventive Medicine, 9*, 82–122.

LaFromboise, T., Coleman, H. L. K., & Gerton, J. (1993). Psychological impact of biculturalism: Evidence and theory. *Psychological Bulletin, 114*, 395–412.

Lau, A. S., Jernewall, N. M., Zane, N., & Myers, H. F. (2002). Correlates of suicidal behaviors among Asian American outpatient youths. *Cultural Diversity & Ethnic Minority Psychology, 8*, 199–213.

Le, T. N. (2002). Delinquency among Asian/Pacific Islanders: Review of literature and research. *Justice Professional, 15*, 57–70.

Le, T. N. (2005). Non-familial victimization among Asian Pacific Islander youth: The Oakland experience. *Journal of Ethnicity in Criminal Justice, 3*(3), 49–64.

Le, T. N., & Arifuku, I. (2005). Asian and Pacific Islander youth victimization and delinquency: A case for disaggregate data. *Amerasia Journal, 31*(3), 29–41.

Le, T. N., Monfared, G., & Stockdale, G. (2005). The relationship of school attachment, parent engagement, and peer delinquency with self-reported delinquency for Chinese, Cambodian, Lao/Mien, and Vietnamese youth. *Crime and Delinquency, 51*(2), 192–219.

Le, T. N., & Stockdale, G. (2005). Individualism, collectivism, and delinquency in Asian American adolescents. *Journal of Clinical Child and Adolescent Psychology, 34*, 681–691.

Le, T. N., & Stockdale, G. (2008). Acculturative dissonance, ethnic identity, and youth violence. *Cultural Diversity & Ethnic Minority Psychology, 14*, 1–9.

Le, T. N., & Wallen, J. (2009). Risks of non-familial violent physical and emotional victimization in four Asian ethnic groups. *Journal of Immigrant and Minority Health, 11*, 174–187.

Leadership Conference on Civil Rights Education Fund. (2009). *Confronting the new faces of hate: Hate crimes in America, 2009.* Washington, DC: Author.

Lee, J., Pomeroy, E. C., & Bohman, T. M. (2007). Intimate partner violence and psychological health in a sample of Asian and Caucasian women: The roles of social support and coping. *Journal of Family Violence, 22*(8), 709–720.

Leong Frederick, T. L., Leach, M. M., & Gupta, A. (2008). Suicide among Asian-Americans: A critical review with research recommendations. In M. M. Leach, F. T. L. Leong, & F. T. L. Leong (Eds.), *Suicide among racial and ethnic minority groups: Theory, research, and practice* (pp. 117–141). New York: Routledge/Taylor & Francis.

Leong, F., Leach, M. M., Yeh, C., & Chou, E. (2007a). Suicide among Asian Americans: What do we know? What do we need to know? *Death Studies, 31*, 417–434.

Leong, F. T. L., Leach, M. M., Yeh, C., & Chou, E. (2007b). Suicide among Asian Americans: What do we know? What do we need to know? *Death Studies, 31*, 417–434.

Lester, D. (1994). The epidemiology of suicide in Chinese populations in six regions of the world. *Chinese Journal of Mental Health, 7*, 25–36.

Liem, R., Lim, B. A., & Liem, J. H. (2000). Acculturation and emotion among Asian Americans. *Cultural Diversity and Ethnic Minority Psychology, 6*, 13–31.

Lin, K.-M., & Cheung, F. (1999). Mental health issues for Asian Americans. *Psychiatric Services, 50*, 774–780.

Lin, M. H., Kwan, V. S. Y., Cheung, A., & Fiske, S. T. (2005). Stereotype content model explains prejudice for an envied outgroup: Scale of anti-Asian American stereotypes. *Personality and Social Psychology Bulletin, 31*, 34–47.

Liu, W. M., Pope-Davis, D. B., Nevitt, J., & Toporek, R. L. (1999). Understanding the function of acculturation and prejudicial attitudes among Asian Americans. *Cultural Diversity and Ethnic Minority Psychology, 5*, 317–328.

Livengood, J. S., & Stodolska, M. (2004). The effects of discrimination and constraints negotiation on leisure behavior of American Muslims in the Post-September 11 America. *Journal of Leisure Research, 36*, 183–208.

Low, L.-F., & Anstey, K. J. (2009). Dementia literacy: recognition and beliefs on dementia of the Australian Public. *Alzheimer's & Dementia, 5*, 43–49.

Maddux, W. W., Galinsky, A. D., Cuddy, A. J. C., & Polifroni, M. (2008). When being a model minority is good…and bad: Realistic threat explains negativity toward Asian Americans. *Personality and Social Psychology Bulletin, 34*, 74–89.

Mayeda, D. T., Hishinuma, E. S., Nishimura, S. T., Garcia-Santiago, O., & Mark, G. Y. (2006). Asian/Pacific Islander youth violence prevention center: Interpersonal violence and deviant behaviors among youth in Hawai'i. *Journal of Adolescent Health, 39*, 276.e1–276.e11.

Mehta, S. (1998). Relationship between acculturation and mental health for Asian Indian immigrants in the United States. *Genetic, Social, and General Psychology Monographs, 124*, 61–78.

Menard, S. (2002). *Short- and long-term consequences of adolescent victimization: Office of Juvenile Justice and Delinquency Prevention (OJJDP) Juvenile Justice Bulletin*. Washington, DC: U.S. Department of Justice.

Molidor, C., & Tolman, R. M. (1998). Gender and contextual factors in adolescent dating violence. *Violence Against Women, 4*, 180–194.

Morrison, L., & Downey, D. L. (2000). Racial differences in self-disclosure of suicidal ideation and reasons for living: Implications for training. *Cultural Diversity and Ethnic Minority Psychology, 6*(4), 374–386.

Muehlenkamp, J. J., Gutierrez, P. M., Osman, A., & Barrios, F. X. (2005). Validation of the positive and negative suicide ideations (PANSI) inventory in a diverse sample of young adults. *Journal of Clinical Psychology, 61*, 431–445.

Nansel, T. R., Overpeck, M., Pilla, R. S., Ruan, W. J., Simons-Morton, B., & Scheidt, P. (2001). Bullying behavior among the U.S. youth: Prevalence and association with psychological adjustment. *Journal of the American Medical Association, 285*(16), 2094–2100.

National Asian American Pacific Legal Consortium. (2002). *Audit of violence against Asian Pacific Americans.* Retrieved January 23, 2011, from http://www.advancingequality.org/ files/2002_Audit.pdf

National Asian Women's Health Organization. (1998). *Expanding options: A reproductive and sexual health survey of Asian American women.* San Francisco: Author.

National Asian Women's Health Organization. (2002). *Silent epidemic: A survey of violence among young Asian American women*, available at http://www.nawho.org/pubs/NAWHOSilentEpidemic.pdf

Ngo, H. M., & Le, T. N. (2007). Stressful life events, culture, and violence. *Journal of Immigrant Health, 9*, 75–84.

Phinney, J. S., Cantu, C. L., & Kurtz, D. A. (1997). Ethnic and American identity as predictors of self-esteem among African-American, Latino, and White adolescents. *Journal of Youth and Adolescence, 26*, 165–185.

Phinney, J. S., Chavira, V., & Tate, J. D. (1995). Parental ethnic socialization and adolescent coping with problems related to ethnicity. *Journal of Research on Adolescence, 5*(1), 31–53.

Phinney, J. S., & Flores, J. (2002). "Unpackaging" acculturation: Aspects of acculturation as predictors of traditional sex role attitudes. *Journal of Cross-Cultural Psychology, 33*, 320–331.

Pippins, J. R., Alegría, M., & Haas, J. S. (2007). Association between language proficiency and the quality of primary care among a national sample of insured Latinos. *Medical Care, 45*(11), 1020–1025.

Purnell, L. D., & Kim, S. (2003). People of Korean heritage. In L. D. Purnell & B. J. Paulanka (Eds.), *Transcultural health care: A culturally competent approach* (pp. 249–378). Philadelphia: F.A. Davis.

Raj, A., & Silverman, J. G. (2002). Intimate partner violence against South-Asian women in Greater Boston. *Journal of the American Medical Women's Association, 57*(2), 111–114.

Raj, A., & Silverman, J. G. (2003). Immigrant South Asian women at greater risk for injury from intimate partner violence. *American Journal of Public Health, 93*(3), 435–437.

Range, L. M., Leach, M. M., McIntyre, D., Posey-Deters, P. B., Marion, M. S., Kovac, S. H., et al. (1999). Multicultural perspectives on suicide. *Aggression and Violent Behavior, 4*(4), 413–430.

Reeves, T. J., & Bennett, C. E. (2004). *We the people: Asians in the United States, Census 2000 Special Report (CENSR-17)*. Washington, DC: Bureau of the Census.

Rennison, C. (2001). *Violent victimization and race, 1993-1998.* Washington, D.C.: U.S. Department of Justice, Bureau of Justice Statistics Special Report.

Rodríguez, M., Valentine, J. M., Son, J. B., & Muhammad, M. (2009). Intimate partner violence and barriers to mental health care for ethnically diverse populations of women. *Trauma, Violence & Abuse, 10*, 358–374.

Rosenbloom, S. R., & Way, N. (2004). Experiences of discrimination among African American, Asian American, and Latino adolescents in an urban high school. *Youth and Society, 35*(4), 420–451.

Ryder, A. G., Alden, L. E., & Paulhus, D. L. (2000). Is acculturation unidimensional or bidimensional? A head-to-head comparison in the prediction of personality, self-identity, and adjustment. *Journal of Personality and Social Psychology, 79*, 49–65.

Sampson, R. J., & Lauritsen, J. L. (1997). Racial and ethnic disparities in crime and criminal justice in the United States. *Crime and Justice, 21*, 311–374.

Shrake, E. K., & Rhee, S. (2004). Ethnic identity as a predictor of problem behaviors among Korean American adolescents. *Adolescence, 39*(155), 601–622.

Silverman, J. G., Decker, M. R., & Raj, A. (2007). Immigration-based disparities in adolescent girls' vulnerability to dating violence. *Maternal and Child Health Journal, 11*(1), 37–43.

Silverman, J. G., Raj, A., Mucci, L. A., & Hathaway, J. E. (2001). Dating violence against adolescent girls and associated substance use, unhealthy weight control, sexual risk behavior, pregnancy, and suicidality. *Journal of the American Medical Association, 286*, 572–579.

Smokowski, P. R., David-Ferdon, C., & Stroupe, N. (2009). Acculturation and violence in minority adolescents: A review of the empirical literature. *Journal of Primary Prevention, 30*, 215–263.

Song-Kim, Y. I. (1992). Battered Korean women in urban United States. In S. M. Furuto, R. Biswas, D. K. Chung, K. Murase, & Y. F. Ross-Sheriff (Eds.), *Social work practice with Asian Americans* (pp. 213–226). Thousand Oaks, CA: Sage Publications, Incorporated.

Sorenson, S., & Shen, H. (1996). Homicide risk among immigrants in California, 1970 through 1992. *American Journal of Public Health, 86*, 97–100.

Southern Poverty Law Center. (2011). 2009 year of hate. Retrieved January 23, 2011, from http://www.splcenter.org/

Substance Abuse and Mental Health Services Administration. (2000). *United States Center for Mental Health Services: Cultural competence standards in managed care mental health services: Four underserved/underrepresented racial/ethnic groups* (Publication No. SMA00-3457). Washington, DC, Retrieved February 25, 2010, from http://mentalhealth.samhsa.gov/publications/allpubs/sma00-3457/default.asp

Sue, S., & Chu, J. Y. (2003). The mental health of ethnic minority groups: Challenges posed by the supplement to the Surgeon General's report on mental health. *Culture, Medicine and Psychiatry, 27*, 447–465.

Sun, W., & Starosta, W. J. (2006). Perceptions of minority invisibility among Asian American professionals. *Howard Journal of Communications, 17*, 119–142.

Takahashi, Y. (1989). Suicidal Asian patients: Recommendations for treatment. *Suicide and Life-Threatening Behavior, 19*, 305–313.

Tjaden, P., & Thoennes, N. (2000). *Extent, nature and consequences of intimate partner violence: Research report.* Washington, DC: National Institute of Justice and the Centers for Disease Control and Prevention.

Tran, C. G. (1997). *Domestic violence among Vietnamese refugee women: Prevalence, abuse characteristics, psychiatric symptoms, and psychosocial factors.* Unpublished dissertation, Boston University, Boston

Tseng, W.-S., Asai, M., Jieqiu, L., Wibulswasdi, P., Suryani, L. K., & Wen, J.-K. (1990). Multi-cultural study of minor psychiatric disorders in Asia: Symptom manifestations. *The International Journal of Social Psychiatry, 36*(4), 252–264.

Turner, M. A., Ross, S. L., Bednarz, B. A., Herbig, C., & Lee, S. J. (2003). *Discrimination in metropolitan housing markets: Phase 2 Asians and Pacific Islanders.* Retrieved http://www.huduser.org/publications/hsgfin/hds_phase2.htm

U.S. Census Bureau. (2003). *Language use and English-speaking ability: 2000.* Retrieved http://www.census.gov/prod/2003pubs/c2kbr-29.pdf

U.S. Conference of Catholic Bishops. (2002). Asian and Pacific Presence Harmony in Faith. Washington, D.C.: U.S. Conference of Catholic Bishops, Inc.

U.S. Department of Health and Human Services. (2007). *Health, United States, 2007.* Washington, DC: United States Department of Health and Human Services. Retrieved January 10, 2011, from http://www.cdc.gov/nchs/data/hus/hus07.pdf

U.S. Department of Health and Human Services [DHHS]. (2001). *Mental health: Culture, race, and ethnicity: A supplement to mental health. A Report of the Surgeon General.* Rockville, MD: U.S. Department of Health and Human Services, Public Health Service, Office of the Surgeon General.

Ward, C., & Kennedy, A. (1994). Acculturation strategies, psychological adjustment, and sociocultural competence during cross-cultural transitions. *International Journal of Intercultural Relations, 18*, 329–343.

Weil, J. M., & Lee, H. (2004). Cultural considerations in understanding family violence among Asian American Pacific Islander families. *Journal of Community Health Nursing, 21*, 217–227.

Whitaker, D. J., & Reese, L (Eds.). (2007). *Preventing intimate partner violence and sexual violence in racial/ethnic minority communities: CDC's demonstration projects.* Atlanta, GA: Centers for Disease Control and Prevention, National Center for Injury Prevention and Control.

Willgerodt, M. A., & Thompson, E. A. (2006). Ethnic and generational influences on emotional distress and risk behaviors among Chinese and Filipino American adolescents. *Research in Nursing & Health, 29*, 311–324.

Wolitzky-Taylor, K. B., Ruggiero, K. J., Danielson, C. K., Resnick, H. S., Hanson, R. F., & Smith, D. W. (2008). Prevalence and correlates of dating violence in a national sample of adolescents. *Journal of the American Academy of Child and Adolescent Psychiatry, 47*, 755–762.

Woloshin, S., Bickell, N. A., Schwartz, L. M., Gany, F., & Welch, H. G. (1995). Language barriers in medicine in the United States. *Journal of the American Medical Association, 273*(9), 724–728.

Woloshin, S., Schwartz, L. M., Katz, S. J., & Gilbert Welch, H. (1997). Is language a barrier to the use of preventive services? *Journal of General Internal Medicine, 12*(8), 472–477.

Wong, Y. J., Brownson, C., & Schwing, A. E. (2011). Risk and protective factors associated with Asian American students' suicidal ideation: A multi-campus, national study. *Journal of College Student Development, 52*, 396–408.

Wong, Y. J., Brownson, C., & Schwing, A. E. (in press). Predictors of Asian American students' suicidal ideation: A multi-campus, national study. *Journal of College Student Development.*

Wong, F. Y., DiGangi, J., Young, D., Huang, Z. J., Smith, B. D., & John, D. (2011). Intimate partner violence, depression, and alcohol use among a sample of foreign-born Southeast Asian women in an urban setting in the United States. *Journal of Interpersonal Violence, 26*, 211–229.

Wong, E., & Haglin, R. (2006). The "model minority": Bane or blessing for Asian Americans? *Journal of Multicultural Counseling and Development, 34*, 38–49.

Wong, E. C., Marshall, G. N., Shetty, V., Zhou, A., Belzberg, H., & Yamashita, D.-D. R. (2007a). Survivors of violence-related facial injury: Psychiatric needs and barriers to mental health care. *General Hospital Psychiatry, 29*(2), 117–122.

Wong, E. C., Marshall, G. N., Shetty, V., Zhou, A., Belzberg, H., & Yamashita, D. R. (2007b). Survivors of violence-related facial injury: Psychiatric needs and barriers to mental health care. *General Hospital Psychiatry, 29*, 117–122.

Wong-Stokem, N. A. E. (1998). Acculturation in relation to somatization and mental health attitudes among Asian-Americans. *Dissertation Abstracts International: Section B: Science & Engineering, 58*(8-B), 4530.

Yang, K. (2004). Southeast Asian American children: Not the "model minority". *The Future of Children, 14*, 127–133.

Yang, B., & Clum, G. A. (1994). Life stress, social support, and problem-solving skills predictive of depressive symptoms, hopelessness, and suicide ideation in an Asian student population: A test of a model. *Suicide & Life-Threatening Behavior, 24*, 127–139.

Yeh, C. J. (2003). Age, acculturation, cultural adjustment, and mental health symptoms of Chinese, Korean, and Japanese immigrant youths. *Cultural Diversity and Ethnic Minority Psychology, 9*, 34–48.

Ying, Y.-W., Lee, P. A., & Tsai, J. L. (2000). Cultural orientation and racial discrimination: Predictors of coherence in Chinese American young adults. *Journal of Community Psychology, 28*, 427–442.

Yoshihama, M. (1999). Domestic violence against women of Japanese descent in Los Angeles: Two methods of estimating prevalence. *Violence Against Women, 5*(8), 869–897.

Yoshioka, M. R., DiNoia, J., & Ullah, K. (2001). Attitudes toward marital violence. *Violence Against Women, 7*(8), 900–926.

Young, K. (1998). Help seeking for emotional/psychological problems among Chinese Americans in the Los Angeles area: An examination of the effects of acculturation. *Unpublished doctoral dissertation.* Los Angeles: University of California, Los Angeles.

Yu, S. M., Zhihuan, H., Schwalberg, R. H., Overpeck, M., & Kogan, M. D. (2003). Acculturation and the health and well-being of US immigrant adolescents. *Journal of Adolescent Health, 33*, 479–488.

Zane, N., & Mak, W. (2003). Major approaches to the measurement of acculturation among ethnic minority populations: A content analysis and an alternative empirical strategy. In K. Chun, P. Organista, & G. Marin (Eds.), *Acculturation: Advances in theory, measurement, and applied research* (pp. 39–60). Washington, DC: American Psychological Association.

Zhang, A. Y., Snowden, L. R., & Sue, S. (1998). Differences between Asian- and White-Americans' help-seeking and utilization patterns in the Los Angeles area. *Journal of Community Psychology, 26*, 317–326.

Zhou, M., & Bankston, C. L. (1994). Social capital and the adaptation of the second generation: The case of Vietnamese youth in New Orleans. *International Migration Review, 28*, 821–845.

Falling through the Cracks: Models, Barriers, and the Future of Health Care Access for Asian Americans

22

Stephen Vong and Ricky Y. Choi

Introduction

Access to health care is one of the greatest challenges for Asian Americans. As a largely new immigrant community, cultural barriers related to immigration status, language, and limited familiarity with the health care system negatively impact the ability to obtain needed health care. In the United States, health insurance is a necessity for affordable primary and specialty care. However, many Asian Americans face legal or economic challenges to getting health insurance, leaving 17% of Asian Americans uninsured (US Census Bureau, 2010a, 2010b). Consequently too often these patients fall through the cracks.

A few years ago a Korean American gentleman came to a community health center in Oakland because of a persistent cough. He was a small business owner, and because of the high cost, he did not purchase individual health insurance for himself. Without a regular doctor and fearful of the high cost of seeing a doctor out of pocket, he waited until his cough became so severe it interfered with his daily activity. When he finally saw a physician, he was told that he

may have lung cancer. Because he now had a preexisting condition, making him uninsurable, he went to South Korea with hopes for care in their universal health care system. There he was told his disease was too advanced for treatment. He returned home and died shortly afterwards. Responding to a similarly unfortunate situation, community health center patient Hye Yeong Cho states, "I believe that something must be done to make health care more affordable and easily accessible to everyone, regardless (Anonymous, Personal communication, n.d.)."

For Asian-American immigrants, the challenges to getting health care shake confidence in their new homeland. The threat of Medicaid cuts in California prompted a response from a patient: "My friend is very frustrated with this government that prides itself on its democracy and equality for all, and yet blindly takes away the most basic services from its most vulnerable people who cannot otherwise afford or have access to medical care. There are millions of others in the same situation and it gets worse for those with multiple chronic conditions (Anonymous, Personal communication, n.d.)."

S. Vong (✉)
San Francisco State University,
San Francisco, CA, USA
e-mail: svng926@gmail.com

R.Y. Choi
Asian Health Services Community Health Center,
Oakland, CA, USA

Health Care Access Definition and Models

Health care access is defined as the ease with which an individual receives health care (RAND Corporation, 2011). However, the variables that affect access, such as income level or availability of services, as well as how to actually measure the "ease" of receiving care, must also be considered.

Several health care access models have been proposed, providing a concrete way to view health care access and connect empirical research and theory. Karikari-Martin (2010) provided a comprehensive overview of three such models, each with different strengths in examining modern health policies. The need to understand and choose a model to evaluate policies are even more pertinent due to the effects of the recent Patient Protection and Affordable Care Act of 2010 (Karikari-Martin, 2010). The following is a brief summary of these three models.

Theoretical Models of Health Care Access

The Behavioral Model of Health Services Use (Andersen, 1968; David, Andersen, Wyn, & Brown, 2004) focused on both individual (e.g., demographic factors and income) and community (e.g., physician supply) characteristics in explaining access outcomes (e.g., doctor visits). The strength of the behavioral model lies in providing factors that can be used to explain utilization of services (Karikari-Martin, 2010).

Penchansky's Model (Penchansky & Thomas, 1981) referred to access in terms of how patients and their health care network matched with one another in five specific areas: availability, accessibility, accommodation, affordability, and acceptability. The overall outcome measured was client satisfaction. This model is well served to examine subjective experiences in health care access and can illustrate the effects of policies on particular populations (Karikari-Martin, 2010).

Lastly, the Institute of Medicine (IOM) Model of Access Monitoring (1993) considers the ability of individuals and/or groups to receive care. Access is defined through barriers (e.g., availability and insurance coverage), use of services, and mediators (e.g., quality of providers). The outcomes of access are measured through health status (e.g., mortality and morbidity) and equity of services. Contrasted with Penchansky's Model,

the IOM model focuses on the objective outcomes of access instead of the subjective (Karikari-Martin, 2010).

Models of Health Care Access and Asian Americans

To our knowledge, no models of health care access have been developed specifically for Asian Americans. The authors of the present review propose that the Behavioral Model (Andersen, 1968; David, Andersen, Wyn, & Brown, 2004) is most suited for guiding future research with Asian Americans for a variety of reasons. First, the model accommodates for factors that may differ from a Western perspective. For instance, Vietnamese culture often use coin rubbing to help treat a cold – no such belief exists in the majority of Western culture (Yeatman & Dang, 1980).

Second, Asian Americans are experiencing an increase in poverty rates along with an increased uninsured rate over the last decade from 14.4% (Algeria et al., 2006) to approximately 17.6% (US Census Bureau, 2010a, 2010b). Accordingly, it is extremely important to consider the relevant neighborhood characteristics specific to Asian Americans. Because there are dense pockets of Asian Americans within different regions, such as San Francisco and Los Angeles, there are relevant community characteristics which require evaluation. The local health care market and safety-net services are examples of such characteristics. The Behavioral Model addresses such variables, allowing possible interventions to tailor services specific to the needs of Asian American population and their subgroups.

Third, many studies have focused on the utilization of services by Asian American populations (e.g., Lee, Ju, Vang, & Lundquist, 2010; Mathur, Schaubel, Gong, Guidinger, & Merion, 2010; Pourat, Kagawa-Singer, Breen, & Sripipatana, 2010), which is gauged within the model. Comparison between these other and future studies using the same model will provide a strong baseline that may shed light into how to increase access for Asian Americans. Overall, the use of models provides a basis to study and better understand how to improve access – one aspect of this involves studying barriers to care.

Barriers to Health Care Access for Asian Americans

Though still limited, there has been an expansion of studies on health care access of Asian Americans over the last decade. The current review evaluates key topics on barriers that may affect access to care. Kim and Keefe (2010) noted the need to examine the specific ethnic groups under the blanketed term of Asian Americans when discussing health care needs. In their research, they discussed four major barriers (language and culture, health literacy, health insurance, and immigrant status) that may affect Asian American groups. Because these barriers often influence the lives of those receiving care, we provide a review of similar barriers with updated studies to further understand the differences between Asian Americans. However, it should be noted that there exists a myriad of other barriers that could adversely affect their health care access.

Insurance

Between 2002 and 2003, the National Latino and Asian American Survey (Algeria, Cao, McGuire, et al., 2006) reported that 71.8% of Asian Americans had private insurance, 8.3% had public insurance, 5.5% had other insurance, and 14.4% were uninsured. Similarly, the Kaiser Family Foundation (KFF, 2008) found that 65% of Asian Americans had employer health insurance coverage, 8% had private insurance, 11% had Medicaid or other public insurance, and 17% were uninsured for the period of 2004–2006. The latest data available, published in 2008 found that the uninsured rate for Asian Americans was 17.6% (US Census Bureau, 2010a, 2010b), similar to that of previous years.

There are also large variations in rates of uninsured between Asian American subgroups. The National Latino and Asian American Survey (Algeria, Cao, McGuire, et al., 2006) found that the Vietnamese had the highest uninsured rates (20.2%) while the "Other Asian" category had the lowest (13.3%). In contrast, the KFF data (2008) reported Koreans had the highest uninsured rate (31%) while Asian Indians had the lowest uninsured rate (12%).

Not surprisingly, Asian Americans with health insurance utilized more medical care than those without insurance. According to the KFF (2008), Asian Americans who are uninsured were less likely to have a regular source of care (52%), higher than non-Hispanic Whites (46%). Furthermore, uninsured Asian Americans were less likely to have been to the doctor in the last year compared to uninsured non-Hispanic Whites (51% versus 39%, respectively). Other studies have echoed similar findings, as uninsured older Chinese adults had lower physician utilization levels than those with insurance (Miltiades & Wu, 2008); this trend was also found for Koreans (Shin, Song, Kim, & Probst 2005). In addition, uninsured "Other Asian" (58%) and Chinese (55%) groups had the highest rate of not having visited a doctor in the past year, while Indians (42%) and Filipinos (36%) were comparable to non-Hispanic whites (KFF, 2008).

Kim and Keefe (2010) explained these findings by postulating that many Asian Americans are self-employed, with incomes too high for government assisted insurance but too low to afford private insurance. However, the ability to afford insurance is further complicated by how it affects access to care. A study by Shin, Song, Kim, & Probst (2005) reported that for Koreans, health insurance status only significantly affected access to care with low-income individuals. For higher income groups, no significant relationship existed between insurance and health service utilization.

Some key points can be ascertained from the data. The percent of uninsured Asian Americans have remained fairly steady over the years, though an increase was noted in 2003. Unfortunately, aggregate surveys of Asian Americans as a group do not provide enough information on how to decrease the number of individuals that are uninsured. Lastly, one factor that appears to affect health care access for Asian Americans is whether or not they possess insurance, which fits in with the Behavioral Model as an enabling individual characteristic. But, as mentioned previously, having insurance doesn't necessarily affect access to care.

Culture

Culture is an encompassing term that includes language, thoughts, beliefs, values, and religion. It often refers to shared human behavior patterns in such areas (Anderson, Scrimshaw, Fullilove, Fielding, & Normand, 2003). Not surprisingly, culture plays a vital role in health care access, particularly for Asian American immigrants.

Acculturation is defined as the exchange of cultural behaviors when two different cultures come into continuous contact (Kottak, 2005). It should be noted that acculturation is often studied from the perspective of a minority acculturating to the dominant majority culture in which they reside.

Previous studies have concluded that the level of acculturation does account for differences in use of health services within ethnic groups after controlling for age, gender, health status, and insurance (Anderson, Wood, & Sherbourne, 1997; Burnam, Hough, Karno, Escobar, & Telles, 1987). Still, the impact of acculturation on the decision to seek out health care is still unclear for Asian Americans. Jenkins, Le, McPhee, Stewart, and Ha (1996) found that many agreed that traditional beliefs such as coin rubbing, eating rice and soup, and deep breathing of herbal vapors, would treat a cold among the Vietnamese. Yet these beliefs did not interfere with their use of medical services. Interestingly, Fung and Wong (2007) found that greater acculturation in younger Vietnamese was associated with regular visits to their physician. In some studies, there was a positive relationship between acculturation and health service use for Koreans (e.g., Juon, Kim, Shankar, & Han, 2004) while another (Shin et al., 2005) found that it was not a critical factor. Finally, Yang, Corsini-Munt, Link, & Phelan, (2009) also found that the use of traditional Chinese medicine for psychiatric disorders decreased with acculturation.

The issue of acculturation is often complicated when recognizing that each Asian ethnic group is unique, complex, and constantly evolving. While greater acculturation is generally linked to increased use of health care services, the unidirectional relationship between the two for Asian Americans require further study.

Language and Health Literacy

Language can also be a major barrier for Asian Americans seeking access to health care. Sentell, Shumway, and Snowden (2007) found that Asian Americans who did not speak English had significantly lower odds of receiving services compared to their English speaking counterparts. Chinese and Vietnamese patients with low English skills who wanted to discuss uses of non-Western medical practices with their providers often met with significant language barriers (Ngo-Metzger et al., 2003). Those who had limited English proficiency (LEP) were also less likely to identify the need to use mental health services and use fewer services directed towards mental disorders (Bauer, Chen, & Algeria, 2010). In contrast, Chinese women with greater English proficiency were more likely to have received regular Pap testing (Ji, Chen, Sun, & Liang, 2010) and mammography screening (Liang et al., 2009).

Individuals with limited English proficiency often had difficulties making appointments and communicating with health care providers (Kim & Keefe, 2010). Understandably, language competency is also tied to health literacy, which is defined as an understanding of health-related content. It follows that English language skills would affect understanding health care material written in English.

Rudd & Kirsch (2004) developed the Health Activities Literacy Scale (HALS) as a means to measure health literacy. The instrument assigns a score between 0 and 500, with a higher score indicating higher literacy. Using data from the National Adult Literacy Survey, the average HALS score for foreign-born Asians was 228, compared to 286 for US-born whites. For foreign-born Asians with an education less than that of high school, the average score was 179.

Strategies for improving health literacy for Asian Americans are an ongoing issue that needs to be addressed. Moreover, documenting the link between health care literacy and health care access for Asian Americans is in need of further study. In addition to the numerous barriers affecting access, the changing climate in American health care appears to be drastically evolving due to the implementation of the new health care reform bill.

The Impact of Health Care Reform on Health Care Access

In March of 2010, President Obama signed the Patient Protection and Affordable Care Act (ACA) (US Government Printing Office, 2010). The primary impetus of this bill was to address the large number of Americans left out of the health care system due to a lack of health insurance.

For low income populations, the ACA expands the criteria to qualify for Medicaid to 133% of the federal poverty line (FPL) (US Government Printing Office, 2010). For those between 133% and 400% of the FPL, individuals will be able to get affordable health insurance through a health exchange, with financial assistance from the federal government. This law will enable 60% of uninsured Asian Americans to get affordable health insurance. Asian Americans will also benefit from insurance industry reforms and free preventative services stipulated in the ACA.

Medicaid is a federal-state program that serves low income families and people with certain disabilities. Adults without children and families who have incomes above the means tested limit do not qualify for Medicaid. The passage of the ACA elevates the income requirement to 133% FPL in 2014, allowing more low income families into the program. In addition, single childless adults will newly qualify as well. In total, it is estimated that 1.3 million non-elderly Asian Americans can now qualify for Medicaid (Families USA, 2010).

Those uninsured who do not qualify for Medicaid will be able to purchase affordable quality insurance through newly created state health insurance exchange. By 2014, the ACA stipulates that all states must establish an easy to use exchange where people can shop for a plan that meets their needs. All participating plans in the exchange must meet the minimum requirements for services and quality. Those between 133% and 400% of FPL can get federal subsidies so that premiums do not exceed 10% of their income. Also eligible to participate in the exchange and federal subsidies are legal immigrants who have resided in the U.S. for less than 5 years. One-and-a-half million Asian Americans are expected to be eligible for these federal subsidies (Families USA, 2010).

Another large group of uninsured is young adults. Under the ACA, children under the age of 26 can stay on their parents' health insurance plan. This is estimated to help 25% of uninsured Asian and Pacific Islander to get health insurance (Families USA, 2010).

The ACA is bringing significant reforms to the health insurance industry. Stories of patients rejected by their health insurance plan after developing a serious illness or denied coverage because of a preexisting condition are shockingly commonplace. By 2014, the ACA will prohibit health insurance companies from revoking coverage due to an illness or denying coverage due to a preexisting condition. There will no longer be annual or lifetime caps on spending for health care. In fact, the only criteria used to determine the premium will be age and smoking status. Asian Americans, who are the least likely to utilize preventative screenings, will substantially benefit from preventative care that will be free for all new private insurance plans. Medicare recipients will also get free annual physicals.

Tied to the expansion of access to health care and insurance reforms is the mandate for all Americans to carry health insurance. By 2014 every American will be required have health insurance or face a financial penalty. Health insurance is only economically viable when it includes a mix of people who are sick and healthy. The mandate is central to popular insurance reforms that prevent the exclusion of people with preexisting conditions and affordable premiums.

Otherwise people will get insurance only when they are sick, making the cost of insurance unfeasible.

While the ACA represents the biggest change in the health care system in the past 50 years, it does have significant shortcomings which can adversely affect the Asian American community. As a consequence of considerable debate and rancor in the country over the issue of illegal immigration, undocumented individuals are largely left out the ACA's reforms. Undocumented immigrants will not be allowed to buy health insurance through the newly formed health insurance exchange or receive subsidies for health insurance. Additionally, there will be no changes to current federal law that prohibits qualified new legal immigrants from enrolling into public insurance if they are newly eligible for subsidies to get private health insurance.

Those not covered by health care reform will still be able to go to community health centers which are mandated to serve patients regardless of insurance status. Community health centers, which are located in the community in which they serve, are highly regarded for providing high quality, low cost, culturally competent care. The substantial increases in community health center funding to the tune of $11 billion beginning in 2011 will significantly increase capacity and services for these groups (U.S. Government Printing Office, 2010).

Future Direction in Health Care Access for Asian Americans

Looking forward, researchers must determine whether the current models of health care access are applicable and viable for Asian Americans. Because each Asian ethnic group is unique, some variables may hold more importance than others. As cited previously, treatments for the common cold in the Vietnamese population (e.g., coin rubbing) may not affect use of services but will be important for providers to take into account when discussing possible treatment options with the patient.

In addition, the authors of this chapter endorse the use of the Behavioral Model of Health Services Use (Davidson et al., 2004) as a launching point for future researchers. We advocate for this model because it considers the characteristics of both the community and individual, and includes important and various objective outcomes of access. Furthermore, as Karikari-Martin (2010) noted, it has been utilized in various studies that has influenced health policy decisions throughout the world (Anderson, Bozzette, Shapiro et al., 2000; Hargraves & Hadley, 2003; Jang, Chirihoga, Allen, Kwak, & Haley, 2010; Smith & Kirking, 1999; Thind, Mohani, Banerjee, & Hagogo, 2008). The factors proposed by the model to influence access should be studied in-depth, especially aimed toward developing interventions for areas with concentrated Asian Americans populations.

Another factor, insurance, appears to play a role in whether Asian Americans use services and have access to care. However, it is unclear as to why some subgroups suffer disproportionately higher uninsured rates. Furthermore, the uninsured rates across Asian Americans as a whole continue to remain steady, indicating the possibility that current policies aimed at helping Asian Americans obtain health care need to be modified. Research should focus on the effectiveness of current policies and possible alternatives that would be aimed at increasing the insured rates for Asian Americans.

Unfortunately, the role of culture and acculturation for Asian Americans and health care access is also unclear. A meta-analysis of past studies to consolidate current understanding and examine the role in which alternative medicine plays in culture and access to care would be worthwhile. Similarly, language and health literacy are also important for future evaluation. Better language skills results in greater utilization of more services, though this is not necessarily true of the more acculturated. Increasing access may be based in helping individuals with language competency and improving health care literacy, and less so in acculturating to Western civilization. This dynamic remains unclear and warrants further study.

Conclusion

Access to health care is a significant concern for the Asian American community. The Affordable Care Act will provide substantial benefits as it makes health insurance available to 60% of uninsured Asian Americans and creates important protections from health insurance companies. Health care access for Asian Americans is a growing field of study as researchers continue to determine how to improve access and remove barriers to care. Asian Americans are a heterogeneous group of many ethnic groups. Future research should continue to focus on understanding why particular groups have lower rates of health care access compared to others. The expansion of knowledge in these areas will not only help develop interventions to circumvent obstacles, but also increase the knowledge base with which policy makers can change the health care system to better meet the needs of Asian Americans.

References

Algeria, M., Cao, Z., McGuire, T. G., Ojeda, V. D., Sribney, B., Woo, M., et al. (2006). Health insurance coverage for vulnerable populations: Contrasting Asian Americans and Latinos in the United States. *Inquiry, 43*(3), 231–254.

Andersen, R. M. (1968). Behavioral model of families' use of health services (Research series, Vol. 25). Chicago: Center for Health Administration Studies, University of Chicago.

Andersen, R., Bozzette, S., Shapiro, M., St. Clair, P., Morton, S., Crystal, S., et al. (2000). Access of vulnerable groups to antiretroviral therapy among persons in care for HIV disease in the United States. HCSUS consortium. HIV cost and services utilization study. *Health Services Research, 35*(2), 389–416.

Anderson, L. M., Scrimshaw, S. C., Fullilove, M. T., Fielding, J. E., & Normand, J. (2003). Culturally competent health care systems. A systematic review. *American Journal of Preventive Medicine, 24*(3 Suppl), 68–79.

Anderson, L. M., Wood, D. L., & Sherbourne, C. D. (1997). Maternal acculturation and childhood immunization levels among children in Latino families in Los Angeles. *American Journal of Public Health, 87*(12), 2018–2021.

Bauer, A. M., Chen, C. N., & Algeria, M. (2010). English language proficiency and mental health service use among Latino and Asian Americans with mental disorders. *Medical Care, 48*(12), 1097–1104.

Burnam, M. A., Hough, R. L., Karno, M., Escobar, J. I., & Telles, C. A. (1987). Acculturation and lifetime prevalence of psychiatric disorders among Mexican Americans in Los Angeles. *Journal of Health and Social Behavior, 28*(1), 89–102.

Davidson, P., Andersen, R., Wyn, R., & Brown, R. (2004). A framework for evaluating safety-net and other community-level factors on access for low-income populations. *Inquiry, 41*, 21–38.

Families USA. (2010, September). How health reform helps Asian Americans. Retrieved June 6, 2011, from http://www.familiesusa.org/assets/pdfs/health-reform/Help-for-Asian-Americans.pdf.

Fung, K., & Wong, Y. L. R. (2007). Factors influencing attitudes towards seeking professional help among East and Southeast Asian immigrant and refugee women. *The International Journal of Social Psychiatry, 53*(3), 216–231.

Hargraves, J., & Hadley, J. (2003). The contribution of insurance coverage and community resources to reducing racial/ethnic disparities in access to care. *Health Services Research, 38*, 809–829.

Institute of Medicine. (1993). *Access to health care in America*. In M. Milliman (Ed.), Committee on monitoring access to personal health care. Washington, DC: National Academy Press.

Jang, Y., Chirihoga, D., Allen, J., Kwak, J., & Haley, W. (2010). Willingness of older Korean-American adults to use hospice. *Journal of American Geriatrics Society, 58*, 352–356.

Jenkins, C. N., Le, T., McPhee, S. J., Stewart, S., & Ha, N. T. (1996). Health care access and preventive care among Vietnamese immigrants: Do traditional beliefs and practices pose barriers? *Social Science & Medicine, 43*(7), 1049–1056.

Ji, C. S., Chen, M. Y., Sun, J., & Liang, W. (2010). Cultural views, English proficiency and regular cervical cancer screening among older Chinese American women. *Women's Health Issues, 20*(4), 272–278.

Juon, H. S., Kim, M., Shankar, S., & Han, W. (2004). Predictors of adherence to screening mammography among Korean American women. *Preventive Medicine, 39*(3), 474–481.

Kaiser Family Foundation. (2008). Health insurance coverage and access to care among Asian Americans and Pacific Islanders. Retrieved April 5, 2011, from http://www.kff.org/minorityhealth/upload/7745.pdf.

Karikari-Martin, P. (2010). Use of health care access models to inform the patient protection and affordable care act. *Policy, Politics & Nursing Practice, 11*(4), 286–293.

Kim, W., & Keefe, R. H. (2010). Barriers to health care among Asian Americans. *Social Work in Public Health, 25*(3), 286–295.

Kottak, C. P. (2005). Windows on humanity (pp. 209–423). New York: McGraw Hill.

Lee, H. Y., Ju, E., Vang, P. D., & Lundquist, M. (2010). Breast and cervical cancer screening among Asian

American women and Latinas: Does race/ethnicity matter? *Journal of Women's Health (Larchmt), 19*(10), 1877–1884.

Liang, W., Wang, J., Chen, M. Y., Feng, S., Yi, B., & Mandelblatt, J. S. (2009). Cultural views, language ability, and mammography use in Chinese American women. *Health Education & Behavior, 36*(6), 1012–1025.

Mathur, A. K., Schaubel, D. E., Gong, Q., Guidinger, M. K., & Merion, R. M. (2010). Racial and ethnic disparities in access to liver transplantation. *Liver Transplantation, 16*(9), 1033–1040.

Miltiades, H. B., & Wu, B. (2008). Factors affecting physician visits in Chinese and Chinese immigrant samples. *Social Science & Medicine, 66*(3), 704–714.

Ngo-Metzger, Q., Massagli, M. P., Clarridge, B. R., Manocchia, M., Davis, R. B., Iezzoni, L. I., et al. (2003). Linguistic and cultural barriers to care. *Journal of General Internal Medicine, 18*(1), 44–52.

Penchansky, R., & Thomas, J. (1981). The concept of access: Definition and relationship to consumer satisfaction. *Medical Care, 19*, 127–140.

Pourat, N., Kagawa-Singer, M., Breen, N., & Sripipatana, A. (2010). Access versus acculturation: Identifying modifiable factors to promote cancer screening among Asian American women. *Medical Care, 48*(12), 1088–1096.

RAND Corporation. (n.d.). Health care access. Retrieved April 15, 2011, from http://www.rand.org/topics/health-care access.html.

Rudd, R. I., & Kirsch, K. Y. (2004). *Literacy and health in America*. Washington, DC: Educational Testing Service, Research and Development, Policy Information Center, Center for Global Assessment.

Sentell, T., Shumway, M., & Snowden, L. (2007). Access to mental health treatment by English language and proficiency and race/ethnicity. *Journal of General Internal Medicine, 22*(Suppl 2), 289–293.

Shin, H., Song, H., Kim, J., & Probst, J. (2005). Insurance, acculturation, and health service utilization among Korean-Americans. *Journal of Immigrant Health, 7*(2), 65–74.

Smith, S., & Kirking, D. (1999). Access and use of medications in HIV disease. *Health Services Research, 34*, 123–144.

Thind, A., Mohani, A., Banerjee, K., & Hagogo, F. (2008). Where to deliver? Analysis of choice of delivery location from a national survey in India. *BMC Public Health, 8*, 29.

United States Census Bureau. (2010a). Asian/Pacific American heritage month: May 2010. Retrieved June 6, 2011, from http://www.census.gov/newsroom/releases/pdf/cb10-ff07.pdf.

United States Census Bureau. (2010b). Income, poverty and health insurance coverage in the United States: 2009. Retrieved May 25, 2011, from https://www.census.gov/newsroom/releases/archives/income_wealth/cb10-144.html.

United States Government Printing Office. (2010). The patient protection and affordable care act. Retrieved June 6, 2011, from http://www.gpo.gov/fdsys/pkg/PLAW-111publ148/content-detail.html.

Yang, L. H., Corsini-Munt, S., Link, B. G., & Phelan, J. C. (2009). Beliefs in traditional Chinese medicine efficacy among Chinese Americans: Implications for mental health service utilization. *The Journal of Nervous and Mental Disease, 197*(3), 207–210.

Yeatman, G. W., & Dang, V. V. (1980). Cao Gio (coin rubbing). Vietnamese attitudes toward health care. *JAMA, 244*(24), 2748–9.

Quality of Health Care for Asian Americans*

23

Dara H. Sorkin, Heather Ngai,
and Quyen Ngo-Metzger

One of the main goals set out as a national health objective for 2010 was the elimination of racial and ethnic disparities in health care (U.S. Department of Health and Human Services, 2000). Severe and persistent racial and ethnic disparities have been documented across many illnesses and health care services (Institute of Medicine, 2003). Asian Americans (particularly those who speak little or no English) frequently stand out as being the least well-served by the health care system in the United States (Weech-Maldonado, Morales, Spritzer, Elliott, & Hays, 2004). Previous research has shown that Asian Americans report worse health care experiences than White, African-American, or Latino patients, are more likely to be dissatisfied with care, and rate primary care performance lower than other racial/ethnic groups

(Meredith & Siu, 1995; Murray-Garcia, Selby, Schmittdiel, Grumbach, & Quesenberry, 2000; Taira et al., 1997). This chapter focuses on whether these low ratings of satisfaction still persist after 10 years of efforts to address such disparities.

These racial/ethnic differences in patient satisfaction likely arise out of the experiences that Asian Americans have with the health care system. Asian patients experience lower-quality health care than other groups possibly due to linguistic, cultural, and economic barriers that limit their ability to obtain the type of care they need and desire (Haviland, Morales, Dial, & Pincus, 2005; Saha, Arbelaez, & Cooper, 2003; Woloshin, Schwartz, Katz, & Welch, 1997). For example, the Commonwealth Fund 2001 Health Care Quality survey (Collins et al., 2002) found that Asian Americans were the least likely of racial/ethnic groups to receive preventive health services, and nearly one in five Asian Americans had been without health insurance in the past year. Furthermore, one in four Asian Americans reported having problems communicating with their doctors. Asian Americans were the least likely to feel that their doctors understood their backgrounds, to have confidence in their doctors, and to be as involved in decision-making as they would have liked.

Understanding from where these disparities arise requires evaluating both the clinical and interpersonal components of health care quality. First we focus on current issues around barriers to receipt of high quality clinical care, including preventive care and screening, chronic disease care, and mental health management. We then discuss

*The views expressed in this publication are the opinions of the authors and do not necessarily reflect the official policies of the US Department of Health and Human Services or the Health Resources and Services Administration, nor does mention of the department or agency names imply endorsement by the US government.

D.H. Sorkin (✉)
Division of General Internal Medicine, Health Policy Research Institute, University of California,
Irvine, CA, USA
e-mail: dsorkin@uci.edu

H. Ngai • Q. Ngo-Metzger
Department of Health and Human Services, Data Branch, Office of Quality and Data, Bureau of Primary Health Care, Health Resources and Services Administration,
Rockville, MD, USA
e-mail: qngo-metzger@hrsa.gov

G.J. Yoo et al. (eds.), *Handbook of Asian American Health*,
DOI 10.1007/978-1-4614-2227-3_23, © Springer Science+Business Media, LLC 2013

current issues around barriers to receipt of high quality interpersonal care. Interpersonal care involves effective communication between patients and their medical providers. Effective communication may be hindered by linguistic and cultural barriers that limit the ability to build a relationship of mutual trust, respect, and shared decision-making. We discuss these barriers and the ability of interpreter services to overcome some of these barriers. Finally, we examine the role of Federally Qualified Health Centers (FQHCs) in providing care for Asian Americans. We describe the history of FQHCs in the United States and their role in improving access to care for the most vulnerable populations as a usual source of care. We then describe the unique services provided by a subset of FQHCs whose populations are comprised of more than 20% Asian American patients. We feature the unique services provided by these FQHCs, including the availability of enabling services such as case managers, health educators, outreach workers, and interpretation and transportation services. We conclude by describing the quality of care provided by this subset of clinics compared to other FQHCs.

It is important to acknowledge that Asian Americans comprise a heterogeneous group. Asian Americans represent over 20 ethnic subgroups, each with its distinct language, culture, educational level, and pre- and post-migration experience (Trinh-Shevrin, Islam, & Rey, 2009). When possible, we highlight whether the patterns found among Asian Americans varied across the various ethnic and demographic subgroups. We also suggest directions for further research of ways to improve medical care for Asian Americans.

Barriers to Receipt of High Quality Clinical Care

Having a regular care provider or having a specific place where care is provided has been shown to be strong predictors of access to care (Gentry, Longo, Housemann, Loiterstein, & Brownson, 1999; Okoro, Strine, Young, Balluz, & Mokdad, 2005). Furthermore, use of clinical

preventive services also can serve as an indicator of access to quality health care services. Barriers to access, whether financial (e.g., not having adequate health insurance), structural (e.g., lack of primary care providers), or personal (e.g., language), have been shown to limit access (Committee on Quality Health Care in America, 2001; Institute of Medicine, 2001).

Although there is marked heterogeneity among the Asian subgroups, many Asian Americans are immigrants to the United States. As such, many Asian Americans describe how they lack access to services simply because they are unaware of the available resources and how to obtain these services. This is especially true among older Asian Americans, who not only have the greatest need for health services, but also commonly report experiencing cultural and linguistic barriers that make it difficult to access and utilize the health care system. These barriers likely contribute to Asian Americans' generally low ratings of the quality of care received. Three areas in which Asian Americans consistently report low quality care warrant special attention: preventive screening, monitoring and control of chronic conditions, and the detection and treatment of mental health disorders.

Low Rates of Preventive Screening and Counseling Services

Asian Americans have some of the lowest rates of preventive screening compared to other racial/ethnic groups. Asian American and Hispanic adults receive preventive care services, including physical exams, cholesterol and blood pressure tests, and cancer screenings less frequently than non-Hispanic White adults. For example, findings from a cross-sectional study of access to health care and preventive services using data from Behavioral Risk Factor Surveillance System 2005–2007 revealed that compared to non-Hispanic Whites, Asian Americans were significantly less likely to have cervical, colon, or prostate cancer screening, cholesterol testing, or pneumococcal vaccination (McPhee et al., 1997; Nguyen, McPhee, Nguyen, Lam, & Mock, 2002; Wen &

Balluz, 2010). Receipt of counseling services, including those for smoking cessation and the importance of a healthy diet and regular exercise, is also lower among Asian Americans in general, and most profoundly among limited-English proficient Asians (Ngo-Metzger, Sorkin, & Phillips, 2009; Wong et al., 2008). For example, programs for smoking cessation are offered at much lower rates to Asian American (68%) and Hispanic (58%) smokers compared to non-Hispanic White and African American smokers (82% and 78%, respectively).

One of the greatest risks facing Asian Americans is the low rates of immunization (Daniels et al., 2010; Miller, 2010), particularly hepatitis B vaccinations (Chen et al., 2001). Liver cancer, one of the most frequently occurring malignancies among Asian Americans, is due to the high prevalence of chronic viral hepatitis, mainly chronic hepatitis B. A report in 1999 revealed that Asian Americans were 3–13 times more likely to die from liver cancer than non-Hispanic Whites, with Vietnamese Americans at 13 times higher risk, Korean Americans at 8 times higher risk, and Chinese Americans at 6 times higher risk (Lee, Hontz, Warner, & Park, 2005). Several community-based screening studies conducted in the U.S. consistently have confirmed these substantially higher hepatitis B virus (HBV) infection rates in many Asian communities compared with those reported in non-Asian communities (Hsu et al., 2007; Hsu, Zhang, Yan, Shang, & Le, 2010; Lin, Chang, & So, 2007). This malignancy is largely preventable by receipt of the hepatitis B vaccination; however, few Asians have been tested for HBV, and even fewer still have been vaccinated. Work by Wu, Lin, So, & Chang (2007) suggested that less than 60% of Asian Americans reported having been tested for HBV, and only 31% reported having been vaccinated against HBV. Only 44% of Asian Americans reported having had their children vaccinated.

Among access indicators, insurance coverage and having a usual source of care are two of the most important predictors of effective screening in general, and this is especially true among Asian Americans (Moy, Greenberg, & Borsky, 2008). Lack of health insurance and a usual source of care, which are barriers to all population groups, may act as significantly greater barriers for newer immigrants, often those from countries with different health care delivery systems. Asian Americans, specifically those from Korea, Vietnam, and South Asia, are less likely to have insurance compared to their non-Hispanic White counterparts (Shah et al., 2010; Sorkin, Ngo-Metzger, & De Alba, et al., 2010; Sorkin et al., 2011). For many immigrants, the process of selecting and purchasing private coverage can be a bewildering experience. Types of insurance coverage may influence screening rates differentially. Public insurers, especially Medicaid, have lower provider reimbursement, limited benefits, or have stricter service authorization requirements than private insurers. Likewise, identifying a usual source of care requires English proficiency and knowledge of how to compare providers and health insurance plans selectively.

Poor Monitoring and Control of Chronic Conditions

The literature is mixed as to whether Asian Americans are at higher risk for poor health than other people from various racial or ethnic backgrounds (Chen & Betty, 1995; Li, Liao, Fan, Zhang, & Balluz, 2010; Lin-Fu, 1993; Sorkin, Tan, Hays, Mangione, & Ngo-Metzger, 2008). Data generated from large national datasets that compare Asian Americans to Native Americans, African Americans, Whites, and Hispanics, generally suggests that Asian Americans report better or similar health status to non-Hispanic Whites (Centers for Disease Control and Prevention, 2010; McGee, Liao, Cao, & Cooper, 1999). However, the few studies that have examined subgroup differences in health status suggest that there is marked heterogeneity in physical health status across the various ethnic groups (Mui & Domanski, 1999; Mui, Kang, Kang, & Domanski, 2007; Shibusawa & Mui, 2010). One of the few studies deconstructing the health status of six subgroups of older Asian Americans (i.e. Chinese, Filipino, Indian, Japanese, Korean, Vietnamese) reported significant variations on health-related outcomes—especially chronic conditions and global self-rated health (Kim et al., 2010). This study found that older Vietnamese and Filipinos tended to have poorer physical health than older Chinese, Japanese, and Koreans. The poorest self-rated health and the highest disability rates were found in older Vietnamese adults. Filipino Americans also exhibited the greatest number of chronic diseases, including the highest rates of asthma, high blood pressure, and heart disease; however, older Korean Americans had the fewest self-reported chronic diseases and the least evidence of disease co-morbidity (Kim et al., 2010).

Asian Americans who have a chronic condition may be differentially at risk for suboptimal quality of care. Findings from the Commonwealth Fund 2001 Health Care Quality survey (Collins et al., 2002) suggest that among respondents with high blood pressure, heart disease, or diabetes, Hispanic and Asian Americans were least likely to receive clinical services important to monitoring and controlling these chronic conditions. For example, among patients with high blood pressure, Asian Americans (74%) and Hispanics (71%) were the least likely to have their blood pressure checked every six months, compared to African Americans (89%) and Whites (80%).

Among patients with diabetes, previous research, including our own studies (Ahrens, DuBois, Richardson, Fan, & Lozano, 2008; Ngo-Metzger, Massagli, Clarridge, Moorhead, & Phillips, 2003; Sorkin et al., 2011), suggests that some Asian Americans have more diabetes-related complications, higher diabetes-related mortality, more distrust of insulin therapy, greater preference for traditional remedies to manage diabetes, and poorer quality of diabetes care compared with non-Hispanic whites (Carter, Pugh, & Monterrosa, 1996; Garay-Sevilla, Malacara, Gonzalez-Parada, & Jordan-Gines, 1998; Haffner et al., 1993; Harris, 2001; Karter et al., 2002). In a small study of diabetics living in Orange County, CA, 78% had never received a single hemoglobin A1c (HbA1c) test, which measures blood glucose control, and 45% had poorly-controlled diabetes (hemoglobin A1c (HbA1c) >8%) (Mull, Nguyen, & Mull, 2001).

Furthermore, for people with diabetes, having regular blood pressure checks as well as eye and foot exams are vital for preventing complications and maintaining health. Yet diabetic care is often inadequate and varies by race and ethnicity. Asian American patients with diabetes were the least likely to have had their feet examined in the previous year, and the least likely to have had all three important exams within a given year (eye, foot, and blood pressure monitoring) compared to African American, White, and Hispanic patients (Collins et al., 2002).

Under-Detection and Under-Treatment of Mental Health Disorders

A third area of healthcare quality that warrants special attention concerns the treatment of mental health issues among Asian Americans. Mental health diagnosis and treatment is another specific area in which Asian Americans receive suboptimal quality of care.

Estimates of the lifetime experience with depression, anxiety disorders, or substance abuse-related disorders for Asian Americans have ranged from 13.95% to as high as 18.29% (Takeuchi et al., 1998, 2007), with mixed evidence for the presence of racial and ethnic disparities in prevalence rates. We found, for example, that Asian American older adults were more likely to report mental distress compared to non-Hispanic Whites, even after adjusting for multiple sociodemographic characteristics and health status (Sorkin, Pham, & Ngo-Metzger, 2009). There is evidence of significant subgroup heterogeneity in the prevalence of mental health symptoms. Shibusawa and Mui (2002) found that 20% of community-dwelling Japanese American elders were mildly depressed. Stokes, Thompson, Murphy, & Gallagher-Thompson (2002) observed an even higher prevalence of depression among Chinese older adults at a rate of 29%. In a representative cohort of California's non-institutionalized older adults, we (Sorkin et al., 2011) found more Filipino (20%), Korean (18%), Vietnamese (14%), Chinese and South Asian (each around 12%) older adults reported symptoms indicative of mental distress compared to non-Hispanic whites (9.7%).

Despite the documented need, studies also have consistently reported lower use of mental health services among Asian Americans compared with the general population (Abe-Kim et al., 2007; Leong & Lau, 2001; Sorkin et al., 2009). We found, for example, that Asian Americans of all subgroups (except South Asian) were less likely to see a primary care provider or take prescription medication for their mental health compared to non-Hispanic White older adults (Sorkin et al., 2011). Perhaps one reason for the lower use of mental health services among Asian Americans is due to the low rates of recognition and treatment by primary care providers. Primary care physicians serve as the initial point of contact for most patients with depression (Pignone et al., 2002). Although the U.S. Preventive Services Task Force (USPSTF) recommends routine depression screening of all adults in primary care (Pignone et al., 2002), usual care by primary care physicians recognizes only about *half* of the depressed patients who present for care (Borowsky et al., 2000; Chung et al., 2003; Schmaling & Hernandez, 2005). In a sample of patients with co-morbid diabetes, we found that Vietnamese patients with depressive symptoms were less likely to be diagnosed and treated compared to non-Hispanic Whites (Sorkin, Ngo-Metzger, et al., 2011).

Special challenges may exist in the primary care setting that compromise the effective recognition and diagnosis of depression, such as patients often presenting with multiple, ill-defined physical complaints (Klinkman, 1997). Furthermore, patients may not desire or expect psychosocial assistance when they present for medical care, and therefore do not acknowledge mental distress, but focus instead on other symptoms as their primary concern (Alegria et al., 2008). Because most primary care visits last only 10–15 minutes, physicians must prioritize according to patients' requests or demands, which often results in the treatment of only one or two "chief complaints." Competing demands, such as the treatment of an acute medical illness, chronic disease management, and preventive services often take up the allotted 15-minute encounter (Klinkman, 1997).

Asian Americans may face additional unique barriers to having their depression detected and treated adequately (Wells, Klap, Koike, & Sherbourne, 2001). Primary care physicians are generally poorer at recognizing depression among Asian American patients compared to white patients (Chung et al., 2003). First, symptom presentation for mental health disorders varies across racial and ethnic groups and can differ from the typical symptom constellation. For example, Asian American patients with depression may not report depressed mood or feeling sad, which are often considered to be the central symptoms of depression. Unless the physician asks about other symptoms, such as a lack of pleasure in usual activities (anhedonia) or low energy, the diagnosis may be missed (Chung et al., 2003).

Second, language and health literacy barriers can compromise treatment efforts by hindering effective doctor-patient communication (Fiscella, Franks, Doescher, & Saver, 2002; Leng, Jyotsna, Tseng, & Gany, 2009; Lewis-Fernandez, Das, Alfonso, Weissman, & Olfson, 2005; Schillinger et al., 2002). Among Asian Americans with mental disorders, limited-English proficiency (LEP) contributes to disparities in access to care and longer duration of untreated disorders (Bauer & Alegria, 2010; Bauer, Chen, & Alegria, 2010). Following an onset of a mental disorder, LEP Asian Americans are less likely to perceive a need for treatment or seek treatment, particularly specialty care, and experience longer durations of untreated illness compared to their English-proficient counterparts.

In many Asian cultures it is also considered a taboo to discuss mental health issues openly, and thus people tend to hide, neglect, or deny symptoms rather than seek help. Asian American individuals often report that they do not seek professional help even if they feel they need professional help for their mental health issues (Lee et al., 2009). They are more likely to rely on family members or trusted friends than to seek professional help. Moreover, in some Asian cultures, "clinical depression" is not always acknowledged as a medical disease. Thus, many individuals do not recognize their symptoms as mental health problems (Lee et al., 2009).

Asian Americans may also be less likely to receive mental health services due to decreased access and referrals (Sorkin, Ngo-Metzger, et al., 2011; Vega, Kolody, Aguilar-Gaxiola, & Catalano, 1999). Asian Americans may be more likely to have low paying-jobs that lack health insurance with mental health benefits (Abe-Kim et al., 2007; Alegria et al., 2008; Leong & Lau, 2001; Ojeda & McGuire, 2006). Furthermore, studies suggest that the lack of bilingual, bicultural mental health services may contribute to suboptimal care for minority patients with mental health needs (Gary, 2005; Van Ta, Holck, & Gee, 2010). Culturally responsive services that take into account the unique cultural and religious values of diverse patients, including the importance of the family and migration experience, are needed (Kinder et al., 2006; Lin & Cheung, 1999; Stockdale, Lagomasino, Siddique, McGuire, & Miranda, 2008).

Barriers to Receipt of High Quality Interpersonal Care

High quality interpersonal care, which involves effective communication between patients and their medical providers, is as important to an individual's health as the technical quality of care received (Campbell, Roland, & Buetow, 2000; Heisler, Bouknight, Hayward, Smith, & Kerr, 2002; Heisler et al., 2003). Yet, many of the same economic, cultural, and linguistic barriers that limit Asian Americans' receipt of high quality clinical care also impede their receipt of high quality interpersonal care.

Effective communication involves both verbal and non-verbal behaviors. It includes asking questions and exchanging information. However, effective communication also involves building a relationship of mutual trust and respect so that shared decision-making can occur. Medical providers cannot correctly diagnose disease or provide successful treatments without effective communication; and without effective communication, patients cannot make informed decisions or participate fully in their self-management regimens.

Asian Americans consistently report having poorer interpersonal care and poorer communication with their medical providers compared to Non-Hispanic White patients (Meredith & Siu, 1995; Murray-Garcia et al., 2000; Ngo-Metzger, Legedza, & Phillips, 2004; Saha, Arbelaez, & Cooper, 2003; Saha & Hickam, 2003; Taira et al., 1997). Asian Americans are more likely than Whites to report that their physicians did not listen to them, spend as much time with them, or involve them in decision-making (Ngo-Metzger et al., 2004). Less than one-half of Asian Americans reported that they felt their physicians listened to everything they had to say (49%) or that they understood everything their doctor said (48%) (Collins et al., 2002) Furthermore, only 54% of Asian Americans expressed a great deal of confidence in their doctors, compared with 72% of Whites (Collins et al., 2002). Ratings of confidence are even lower among Asian respondents from different ethnic backgrounds. Specifically, respondents of Korean or Vietnamese heritage were less likely than other Asian Americans to have a high level of confidence in their doctor (Collins et al., 2002).

Given the link between increased patient participation in care and improved health outcomes (Anderson, 1995; Bodenheimer, Lorig, Holman, & Grumbach, 2002; Bodenheimer, Wagner, & Grumbach, 2002; Lorig, 2002), it is likely that Asian Americans would benefit from greater participation in treatment decisions. However, there may be unique and non-trivial cultural and linguistic barriers to implementing such participation, including the presence of language barriers and the failure by providers to provide culturally competent care.

Language Barriers

Communication problems between providers and patients are exacerbated among Asian Americans who speak limited English (Doty, 2003; Morales, Elliott, Weech-Maldonado, Spritzer, & Hays, 2001; Ngo-Metzger, Massagli, Clarridge, Michael, et al., 2003; Weech-Maldonado, Morales, Spritzer, Elliott, & Hays, 2001). An estimated four million Asian Americans are LEP and encounter language barriers when obtaining health care (Trinh-Shevrin et al., 2009). Over half of Chinese, Vietnamese, and Korean Americans speak limited English (Barnes & Bennett, 2002).

Language barriers result in worse access to care (Weech-Maldonado et al., 2003) and less health information given to LEP patients (Ngo-Metzger et al., 2007). Furthermore, LEP patients experienced more medical errors (Divi, Koss, Schmaltz, & Loeb, 2007), received more medical tests (Hampers & McNulty, 2002), and stayed in the hospital longer (John-Baptiste et al., 2004) compared to English-speaking patients. This lack of communication resulted in more unmet health care needs among Asian Americans compared to Whites (Ngo-Metzger et al., 2003a). For example, Chinese and Vietnamese Americans reported problems obtaining both urgent and routine medical appointments when they needed them, and also reported problems getting referrals to specialty care (Ngo-Metzger et al., 2003a).

Having access to medical providers who speak one's native language can help patients overcome language barriers. Patients with chronic diseases such as diabetes and hypertension reported better outcomes when providers spoke their language (Perez-Stable, Napoles-Springer, & Miramontes, 1997). When patients and providers did not speak the same language, patients were less likely to understand medication instructions and were more likely to report medication errors (Gandhi et al., 2000). Patients with a provider who did not speak their language were also less likely to be satisfied with their care and less likely to return for follow-up care (Ngo-Metzger et al., 2007; Sarver & Baker, 2000).

Patients with language barriers often rely on family members to interpret for them. However, this reliance, especially upon children to interpret for their parents, alters the family dynamics and often creates discord (Ngo-Metzger et al., 2003a; Ngo-Metzger et al., 2003b). Respect for elders is an important Asian cultural value, and this value is undermined when parents have to rely on their children for interpreting support. Asian patients also reported that their family members were not adequately trained in medical terminology and were often not available to accompany them to medical visits (Ngo-Metzger et al., 2003a; Ngo-Metzger et al., 2003b). Thus, patients preferred having trained interpreters provided by the clinic rather than using family members as interpreters.

The use of interpreter services has been associated with more appropriate medical care and preventive services compared to not having an interpreter (Jacobs et al., 2001). Having access to interpreters may also be cost-saving overall, especially in the context of decreased amount of medical tests ordered during emergency room visits (Bernstein et al., 2002). Interpreters also enhance health education and facilitate communication during office visits (Ngo-Metzger et al., 2007).

The majority of LEP patients in the U.S., however, still lack access to interpreter services (Doty, 2003). The U.S. Department of Health and Human Services (HHS) recognized the lack of adequate interpreter services as a form of discrimination in medical care. Thus, HHS has developed a set of mandates and guidelines for culturally and linguistically appropriate services (CLAS) (Agency for Healthcare Research and Quality [AHRQ], 2008). The CLAS standards require that providers who receive federal funding must provide language assistance services to LEP patients, and exclude the use of family members as interpreters unless the patient specifically requests them. Unfortunately, as most LEP patients still do not have access to interpreters during their office visit, they have to attempt to communicate in English "as best as they can" (New California Media [NCM], 2003). A study conducted in California found that only 9% of LEP patients had access to professional interpreters, and the majority had to rely on family members for interpretation (New California Media [NCM], 2003). Health policy makers need to invest in the recruitment and training of more professional interpreters, as well as the provision of adequate reimbursement for interpreter services.

Failure to Provide Culturally Competent Care

Cultural competence in health care has been defined as the incorporation of an awareness of health beliefs and behaviors, disease prevalence and incidence, and treatment outcomes for different patient populations. It is a component of health care delivery that has been receiving greater attention within efforts to eliminate health care disparities and improve medical outcomes for racial/ethnic minorities.

Some racial/ethnic minorities may perceive unequal treatment in health care (Sorkin et al., 2010). Individuals who feel disconnected, disempowered, and mistreated in the medical care setting may be reluctant to openly discuss their individual situations. Furthermore, differences in the cultural backgrounds of patients and their medical providers may contribute to poor interpersonal quality of care. Medical providers in the United States often have a mechanistic view of biomedical diseases (e.g., disease is the result of malfunctioning organ systems or chemical pathways). In contrast, Asian patients may have various explanations for symptoms that may include the religious (e.g. God's will), supernatural (e.g. evil spirits), or metaphysical (bad airs or seasonal changes) (Kagawa-Singer & Kassim-Lakha, 2003). If the provider misunderstands or dismisses a patient's views of his or her own illness, frustration and distrust may occur.

Compared to non-Hispanic Whites, Asian Americans also are less likely to report that their doctor understood their health beliefs, backgrounds, and values (Ngo-Metzger et al., 2004). For example, one out of five Asian Americans reported that their doctor showed disrespect towards them (AHRQ, 2008). In a qualitative study of Chinese and Vietnamese immigrants, patients defined "being treated with respect" as "being treated as an equal" (Ngo-Metzger et al., 2003b). Asian culture emphasizes showing deference to authority and the avoidance of overt conflict. Asian Americans may be more likely to view the health care professional as the "expert," and may be less likely to acknowledge disagreement with a treatment plan directly, out of respect for authority (Kramer, Ivey, & Ying, 1999; Mull et al., 2001). Thus, Asian patients may be less likely to question medical professionals directly, even when they disagree or do not understand, and may be more likely to leave the office visits with unresolved questions and unmet expectations.

One area of the doctor-patient relationship plagued by a lack of communication between the provider and patient is the patient's use of herbal and traditional folk medicine (Ngo-Metzger

et al., 2003a, 2003b). For example, our own studies (Ngo-Metzger et al., 2003a, 2003b) and others (McPhee, 2002; Mull et al., 2001) have shown that Asian Americans often do not tell their providers when they stop their prescribed medications or use folk medicine or complementary and alternative medicine (CAM) to treat their diseases. In a national study of over 3,000 Chinese and Vietnamese patients, two-thirds reported that they used CAM while also receiving Western medical care (Ahn et al., 2006). Yet, less than 10% of patients reported that their doctors discussed CAM use with them. Medical providers who understood patients' health beliefs and discussed them were more likely to have satisfied patients (Ahn et al., 2006; Ngo-Metzger et al., 2003b). Furthermore, discouraging a patient from using herbal medicine concurrently with prescription medicine may prevent life-threatening medication interactions (Boullatta & Nace, 2000). Health care providers may need to receive more training to better understand and discuss patients' cultural beliefs, values, and behaviors. Providing culturally competent medical care is a worthwhile endeavor that ultimately will result in increased satisfaction for both patients and their providers.

Importance of Federally Qualified Health Centers (FQHCs) for Addressing Health Care Needs of Asian Americans

While Asian Americans face issues such as language barriers and a lack of culturally competent care, Federally Qualified Health Centers (FQHCs) provide a successful model of a system of care that has been shown to effectively reduce health disparities experienced by Asian Americans and other racial and ethnic minorities (Proser, 2005). FQHCs are community-based clinics that receive support from the Health Resources and Services Administration (HRSA) under the Health Center Program (Section 330 of the Public Health Service Act). HRSA is the primary federal agency of the U.S. Department of Health and Human Services responsible for improving access to health care services for people who are uninsured, isolated or medically vulnerable. Federally Qualified Health Centers are located in or serve high-need communities and provide comprehensive primary health care services to all, regardless of the ability to pay. For more than 40 years, these health centers have served low-income, uninsured, and geographically isolated populations, reaching across cultural and linguistic boundaries. In 2009, FQHCs served 18.8 million Americans, including 6.5 million children and 480,000 Asian Americans (Bureau of Primary Heath Care, 2009).

Federally Qualified Health Centers function under the direction of a community board consisting of the patients who are users of the health care system. The core of an FQHC (also referred to as a health center) that is distinct from many other health care providers is the focus on providing culturally competent, comprehensive health care to all eligible patients. One of the key features of the FQHC is its focus and ability to provide enabling services for high-risk patients, including services such as interpretation, case management, outreach, and transportation.

In addition to serving the uninsured and people of all ages, races, and ethnicities, FQHCs focus on special populations such as homeless, migrant and seasonal farm workers, and residents of public housing (Bureau of Primary Health Care, 2009). Today, over 1,100 FQHCs through 7,900+ service sites provide comprehensive primary care services, including pharmacy, mental health and substance abuse services, and dental care, as well as enabling services. The services provided by the FQHCs reach one in 16 Americans, one in 28 Asian Americans, one in four Americans at or below 100% of poverty, and one in seven uninsured Americans (U.S. Census Bureau, 2005).

Health centers serve a critical role in addressing barriers to accessing health care due to patients being uninsured or underinsured. The steady increase in uninsured Americans has placed great emphasis on health center services. Nationally, 50.7 million Americans were uninsured in 2009, up from 46.3 million in 2008 (DeNavas-Walt et al., 2010). Among Asian Americans, over

2.4 million were uninsured (DeNavas-Walt et al., 2010). The uninsured account for the highest proportion of health center patients (38%), exceeding patients with Medicaid (37%) and other public insurance (3%) (Bureau of Primary Health Care, 2009). Among the 18.8 million patients, 1,512,020 were uninsured children (ages 0–19) and 5,645,017 were uninsured adults.

Health centers, FQHCs are successful models of care not only because they provide services to the uninsured, but also because they focus on socioeconomic and other factors in the community that affect access to health care. Research has shown that enabling services are essential to accessing health care effectively (Chovan & Shin, 2002) and that users of enabling services are more likely to be racial/ethnic minorities (Weir et al., 2010). Patients need to navigate the health care system in order to access services. This includes finding transportation to a health care provider that may or may not be in the local community and steering through the enrollment and financial verification process. Asian Americans, especially those who are LEP, may encounter cultural and linguistic barriers to care. Health centers address these barriers by providing access to case management, eligibility assistance, outreach, transportation, and interpretation services. These enabling services are required services at FQHCs. Patients often cannot access medical care without the provision of these services.

Indicators of Quality of Care Among FQHCs Serving Asian Americans

Health centers provide culturally and linguistically competent care to nearly 12 million patients who are racial and ethnic minorities. Racial and ethnic minorities comprise approximately 63% of the health center patient population; approximately 35% are Hispanic, 27% are African American, and 3% are Asian American. Twenty eight out of 1,131 health centers nationally serve a patient population of 20% or more Asian Americans. While little research has been conducted on the Asian American health center population, a review of data collected from these 28

Table 23.1 Health center patient characteristics (U.S. Department of Health and Human Services. Health Resources and Services Administration. Bureau of Primary Health Care, 2009)

	All health centers (n=1,131) (%)	Health centers with 20% or more Asian American patients (n=28) (%)
100% poverty and below[a]	71.4	71.6
Uninsured	38.2	41.5
Medicaid	37.1	38.4
Other public insurance	2.9	6.4
Enabling services utilized (percent of total visits)	6.5	15.1
Patients best served in a language other than English (percent of total patients)	24.7	61.2

[a]% known

Table 23.2 Health center clinical quality measures (Uniform Data System, 2009)

	All health centers (n=1,131) (%)	Health centers with 20% or more Asian American patients (n=28) (%)
Childhood immunization rate, estimated % of patients immunized	68.8	82.5
First trimester of entry into prenatal care	67.3	74.1
Pap test rate, estimated % of patients tested	58.2	72.5
% Low and very low birth weight	7.3	7.0
Hypertension, estimated % of patients with controlled blood pressure	63.1	67.4
Diabetes, estimated % of patients with HbA1c < or =9%	70.7	77.0

health centers is important for gaining further understanding of the quality of care provided for this patient group.

Compared to all health centers, these 28 centers were localized in predominantly urban areas of nine states. These states include California, Massachusetts, New York, Washington, and Illinois. Patients seen at these health centers utilized more enabling services and were more likely to prefer receiving care in a non-English language.

Although most data from the 28 health centers were similar to national health center data, these 28 health centers were found to have provided over two times more enabling services than all 1,131 health centers nationally (Table 23.1). Furthermore, 61% of the patients seen at the 28 health centers were best served in a language other than English, compared to only 25% in all health centers. This suggests that more bilingual and interpretation staff were utilized in the 28 health centers than in all other health centers nationally.

FQHCs consistently provide high quality care, compared to other providers (Proser, 2005). For example, rates for low and very low birth weight babies for all health centers (7.3%), including the 28 health centers that serve a patient population of 20% or more Asian Americans (7.0%), are well below the national average (8.2%). In addition, while all health center patients receive care equivalent to or better than the quality of care received elsewhere (Proser, 2005), Asian American and other patients from these 28 health centers received even higher quality care, compared to all health centers nationally. As shown in Table 23.2, clinical quality at the 28 health centers for all measures (including childhood immunizations, first trimester of entry into prenatal care, pap test rates, low birth weight, controlled hypertension, and diabetes) met or exceeded the level seen at all health centers nationally.

The availability and greater utilization of enabling services (including case managers, patient/community education specialists, outreach workers, transportation staff, eligibility assistance workers, and interpretation staff) may have contributed to the high clinical quality of care that met or exceeded the level seen at all health centers nationally. These findings further support the conclusion that health centers provide overall high quality care to underserved and vulnerable populations by addressing many of the financial, linguistic, and cultural barriers they face related to health and access to health care. FQHCs provide access and a support structure to promote the receipt of high quality medical care through the availability of enabling services and an emphasis on providing culturally and linguistically competent care for underserved and vulnerable patients. As the number of Asian Americans who seek care at health centers continues to increase (12% increase from 2008 to 2009), more studies will be needed to illuminate the unique needs of this population and to find ways to address barriers that may exist.

Conclusions and Future Directions

Many of the challenges that Asian Americans face in having their health care needs met are similar to those barriers faced by individuals from other minority ethnic/racial backgrounds: being under or uninsured; delaying care which leads to more chronic disease and disability; feeling discriminated against; lacking a usual source of care; missing care coordination; and lacking providers with cultural or linguistic competency. Efforts to address these barriers must promote the best, promising, and evidence based practices that are culturally and linguistically appropriate. Furthermore, greater effort needs to be directed toward building a diverse, bilingual, culturally-competent workforce.

The national health objectives for 2020 have just been released (U.S. Department of Health and Human Services, 2011). Included among the many goals are improving the quality of the doctor-patient relationship, increasing the proportion of persons who report that their health care provider shows them respect, increasing the proportion of persons who report that their health care provider explains things so they can be understood, and increasing the proportion of persons who report that their health care providers have satisfactory communication skills. These are lofty goals, and certainly ones that, if achieved, will go a long way in improving both the clinical and interpersonal quality of care that Asian Americans receive. As a clinical and research community, how we undertake achieving these goals may best be addressed by looking to see how high quality FQHCs have attempted to meet the needs of their Asian American patients. Case studies and closer examination of all aspects of these high performing health centers (e.g., enabling and other services utilized, policies and procedures, staffing and financial characteristics) are needed to understand fully how systems of care can be improved and duplicated in all health care settings.

References

Abe-Kim, J., Takeuchi, D. T., Hong, S., Zane, N., Sue, S., Spencer, M. S., et al. (2007). Use of mental health-related services among immigrant and US-born Asian Americans: Results from the national Latino and Asian American study. *American Journal of Public Health, 97*(1), 91–98.

Ahn, A. C., Ngo-Metzger, Q., Legedza, A. T. R., Massagli, M. P., Clarridge, B. R., & Phillips, R. S. (2006). Complementary and alternative medical therapy use among Chinese and Vietnamese Americans: Prevalence, associated factors, and effects of patient-clinician communication. *American Journal of Public Health, 96*(4), 647–653.

Ahrens, K. R., DuBois, D. L., Richardson, L. P., Fan, M.-Y., & Lozano, P. (2008). Youth in foster care with adult mentors during adolescence have improved adult outcomes. *Pediatrics, 121*(2), 246–252.

Agency for Healthcare Research and Quality (AHRQ). (2008). *2007 National Healthcare Disparities Report* (No. AHRQ Pub. No. 08–0041). Rockville, MD: U.S. Department of Health and Human Services, Agency for Healthcare Research and Quality.

Alegria, M., Chatterji, P., Wells, K., Cao, Z., Chen, C.-N., Takeuchi, D., et al. (2008). Disparity in depression treatment among racial and ethnic minority populations in the United States. *Psychiatric Services, 59*(11), 1264–1272.

Anderson, R. M. (1995). Patient empowerment and the traditional medical model. A case of irreconcilable differences? *Diabetes Care, 18*(3), 412–415.

Barnes, J. S., & Bennett, C. E. (2002). *The Asian population: 2000* (No. C2KBR/01-16). Washington, DC: U.S. Census Bureau.

Bauer, A. M., & Alegria, M. (2010). Impact of patient language proficiency and interpreter service use on the quality of psychiatric care: A systematic review. *Psychiatric Services, 61*(8), 765–773.

Bauer, A. M., Chen, C.-N., & Alegria, M. (2010). English language proficiency and mental health service use among Latino and Asian Americans with mental disorders. *Medical Care, 48*(12), 1097–1104.

Bernstein, J., Bernstein, E., Dave, A., Hardt, E., James, T., Linden, J., et al. (2002). Trained medical interpreters in the emergency department: Effects on services, subsequent charges, and follow-up. *Journal of Immigrant Health, 4*(4), 171–176.

Bodenheimer, T., Lorig, K., Holman, H., & Grumbach, K. (2002). Patient self-management of chronic disease in primary care. *The Journal of the American Medical Association, 288*(19), 2469–2475.

Bodenheimer, T., Wagner, E. H., & Grumbach, K. (2002). Improving primary care for patients with chronic illness. *The Journal of the American Medical Association, 288*(14), 1775–1779.

Borowsky, S. J., Rubenstein, L. V., Meredith, L. S., Camp, P., Jackson-Triche, M., & Wells, K. B. (2000). Who is at risk of nondetection of mental health problems in primary care? *Journal of General Internal Medicine, 15*(6), 381–388.

Boullatta, J. I., & Nace, A. M. (2000). Safety issues with herbal medicine. *Pharmacotherapy, 20*(3), 257–269.

Bureau of Primary Health Care, Health Resources and Services Administration. (2009). 2009 Uniform Data System.

Campbell, S. M., Roland, M. O., & Buetow, S. A. (2000). Defining quality of care. *Social Science and Medicine, 51*(11), 1611–1625.

Carter, J. S., Pugh, J. A., & Monterrosa, A. (1996). Non-insulin-dependent diabetes mellitus in minorities in the United States. *Annals of Internal Medicine, 125*, 221–232.

Centers for Disease Control and Prevention. (2010). Racial/ethnic disparities and geographic differences in lung cancer incidence—38 states and the district of Columbia, 1998–2006. *MMWR Morbidity and Mortality Weekly Report, 59*(44), 1434–1438.

Chen, M. S., Jr., & Betty, L. H. (1995). A debunking of the myth of healthy Asian Americans and Pacific Islanders. *American Journal of Health Promotion, 9*(4), 261–268.

Chen, Q. S., Ngo-Metzger, Q., Tran, L. Q., Sugrue-McElearney, E., Levy, E. R., Williams, G., et al. (2001). Hepatitis B vaccination among Vietnamese-American children in a Boston community clinic. *Asian American Pacific Islander Journal of Health, 9*(2), 179–187.

Chovan, T., & Shin, P. (2002). NACHC REACH 2000 Survey. Retrieved July 23, 2012, from http://www.nachc.com/hcdir.cfm.

Chung, H., Teresi, J., Guarnaccia, P., Meyers, B. S., Holmes, D., Bobrowitz, T., et al. (2003). Depressive symptoms and psychiatric distress in low income Asian and Latino primary care patients: Prevalence and recognition. *Community Mental Health Journal, 39*(1), 33–46.

Collins, K. S., Hughes, D. L., Doty, M. M., Ives, B. L., Edwards, J. N., & Tenney, K. (2002). *Diverse communities, common concerns: Assessing health care quality for minority Americans*. New York: The Commonwealth Fund.

Committee on Quality Health Care in America. (2001). *Crossing the quality chasm*. Washington, DC: National Academy Press.

Daniels, N. A., Gildengorin, G., Nguyen, T. T., Liao, Y., Luong, T.-N., & McPhee, S. J. (2010). Influenza and pneumococcal vaccination rates among Vietnamese, Asian, and non-Hispanic white Americans. *Journal of Immigrant and Minority Health, 12*(3), 370–376.

DeNavas-Walt, C., Proctor, B. D., & Smith, J. C. (2010). *Income, poverty, and health insurance coverage in the United States: 2009*. Washington, DC: U.S. Government Printing Office.

Divi, C., Koss, R. G., Schmaltz, S. P., & Loeb, J. M. (2007). Language proficiency and adverse events in US hospitals: A pilot study. *International Journal for Quality in Health Care, 19*(2), 60–67.

Doty, M. (2003, February). Hispanic patients' double burden: Lack of health care insurance and limited English. *The Commonwealth Fund*, Pub. #592.

Fiscella, K., Franks, P., Doescher, M. P., & Saver, B. G. (2002). Disparities in health care by race, ethnicity, and language among the insured: Findings from a national sample. *Medical Care, 40*(1), 52–59.

Gandhi, T. K., Burstin, H. R., Cook, E. F., Puopolo, A. L., Haas, J. S., Brennan, T. A., et al. (2000). Drug complications in outpatients. *Journal of General Internal Medicine, 15*(3), 149–154.

Garay-Sevilla, M. E., Malacara, J. M. H., Gonzalez-Parada, F., & Jordan-Gines, L. (1998). The belief in conventional medicine and adherence to treatment in non-insulin-dependent diabetes mellitus patients. *Journal of Diabetes and Its Complications, 12*(5), 239–245.

Gary, F. A. (2005). Stigma: Barrier to mental health care among ethnic minorities. *Issues in Mental Health Nursing, 26*, 979–999.

Gentry, D., Longo, D. R., Housemann, R. A., Loiterstein, D., & Brownson, R. C. (1999). Prevalence and correlates of physician advice for prevention: Impact of type of insurance and regular source of care. *Journal of Health Care Finance, 26*(1), 78–97.

Haffner, S. M., Mitchell, B. D., Moss, S. E., Stern, M. P., Hazuda, H. P., Patterson, J., et al. (1993). Is there an ethnic difference in the effect of risk factors for diabetic retinopathy? *Annals of Epidemiology, 3*(1), 2–8.

Hampers, L. C., & McNulty, J. E. (2002). Professional interpreters and bilingual physicians in a pediatric emergency department: Effect on resource utilization. *Archives of Pediatrics and Adolescent Medicine, 156*(11), 1108–1113.

Harris, M. I. (2001). Racial and ethnic differences in health care access and health outcomes for adults with type 2 diabetes. *Diabetes Care, 24*(3), 454–459.

Haviland, M. G., Morales, L. S., Dial, T. H., & Pincus, H. A. (2005). Race/ethnicity, socioeconomic status, and satisfaction with health care. *American Journal of Medical Quality, 20*(4), 195–203.

Heisler, M., Bouknight, R. R., Hayward, R. A., Smith, D. M., & Kerr, E. A. (2002). The relative importance of physician communication, participatory decision making, and patient understanding in diabetes self-management. *Journal of General Internal Medicine, 17*(4), 243–252.

Heisler, M., Vijan, S., Anderson, R. M., Ubel, P. A., Bernstein, S. J., & Hofer, T. P. (2003). When do patients and their physicians agree on diabetes treatment goals and strategies, and what difference does it make? *Journal of General Internal Medicine, 18*(11), 893–902.

Hsu, C. E., Liu, L. C.-H., Juon, H.-S., Chiu, Y.-W., Bawa, J., Tillman, U., et al. (2007). Reducing liver cancer disparities: A community-based hepatitis-B prevention program for Asian-American communities. *Journal of the National Medical Association, 99*(8), 900–907.

Hsu, C. E., Zhang, G., Yan, F. A., Shang, N., & Le, T. (2010). What made a successful hepatitis B program for reducing liver cancer disparities: An examination of baseline characteristics and educational intervention, infection status, and missing responses of at-risk Asian Americans. *Journal of Community Health, 35*(3), 325–335.

Institute of Medicine. (2001). *Coverage matters: Insurance and health care*. Washington, DC: National Academies Press.

Institute of Medicine. (2003). *Unequal treatment: Confronting racial and ethnic disparities in health care*. Washington, DC: National Academy Press.

Jacobs, E. A., Lauderdale, D. S., Meltzer, D., Shorey, J. M., Levinson, W., & Thisted, R. A. (2001). Impact of interpreter services on delivery of health care to limited-English-proficient patients. *Journal of General Internal Medicine, 16*(7), 468–474.

John-Baptiste, A., Naglie, G., Tomlinson, G., Alibhai, S. M. H., Etchells, E., Cheung, A., et al. (2004). The effect of English language proficiency on length of stay and in-hospital mortality. *Journal of General Internal Medicine, 19*(3), 221–228.

Kagawa-Singer, M., & Kassim-Lakha, S. (2003). A strategy to reduce cross-cultural miscommunication and increase the likelihood of improving health outcomes. *Academic Medicine, 78*(6), 577–587.

Karter, A. J., Ferrara, A., Liu, J. Y., Moffet, H. H., Ackerson, L. M., & Selby, J. V. (2002). Ethnic disparities in diabetic complication in an insured population. *The Journal of the American Medical Association, 287*(19), 2519–2527.

Kim, G., Chiriboga, D. A., Jang, Y., Lee, S., Huang, C.-H., & Parmelee, P. (2010). Health status of older Asian Americans in California. *Journal of the American Geriatric Society, 58*(10), 2003–2008.

Kinder, L. S., Katon, W. J., Ludman, E., Russo, J., Simon, G., Lin, E. H. B., et al. (2006). Improving depression care in patients with diabetes and multiple complications. *Journal of General Internal Medicine, 21*(10), 1036–1041.

Klinkman, M. S. (1997). Competing demands in psychosocial care. A model for the identification and treatment of depressive disorders in primary care. *General Hospital Psychiatry, 19*(2), 98–111.

Kramer, E. J., Ivey, S. L., & Ying, Y.-W. (Eds.). (1999). *Immigrant women's health: Problems and solutions*. San Francisco: Jossey-Bass.

Lee, H., Hontz, I., Warner, A., & Park, S. J. (2005). Hepatitis B infection among Asian American Pacific Islanders in the rocky mountain area. *Applied Nursing Research, 18*(1), 2–6.

Lee, S., Ma, G. X., Juon, H.-S., Martinez, G., Hsu, C. E., & Bawa, J. (2009). Assessing the needs and guiding the future: Findings from the health needs assessment in 13 Asian American communities of Maryland in the United States. *Journal of Immigrant and Minority Health, 13*(2), 395–401.

Leng, J. C. F., Jyotsna C., Tseng C.-H., & F Gany. (2009). Detection of depression with different interpreting methods among Chinese and Latino primary care patients: A randomized controlled trial. *Journal of Immigrant Minority Health, 12*(2), 234–241.

Leong, F. T., & Lau, A. S. (2001). Barriers to providing effective mental health services to Asian Americans. *Mental Health Services Research, 3*(4), 201–214.

Lewis-Fernandez, R., Das, A. K., Alfonso, C., Weissman, M. M., & Olfson, M. (2005). Depression in US Hispanics: Diagnostic and management considerations in family practice. *Journal of the American Board of Family Practice, 18*(4), 282–296.

Li, Y., Liao, Y., Fan, A., Zhang, X., & Balluz, L. (2010). Asian American/Pacific Islander paradox in diabetic retinopathy: Findings from the behavioral risk factor surveillance system, 2006–2008. *Ethnicity and Disease, 20*(2), 111–117.

Lin, S. Y., Chang, E. T., & So, S. K. (2007). Why we should routinely screen Asian American adults for hepatitis B: A cross-sectional study of Asians in California. *Hepatology, 46*(4), 1034–1040.

Lin, K.-M., & Cheung, F. (1999). Mental health issues for Asian Americans. *Psychiatric Services, 50*(6), 774–780.

Lin-Fu, J. S. (1993). Asian and Pacific Islander Americans: An overview of demographic characteristics and health care issues. *Asian American Pacific Islander Journal of Health, 1*(1), 20–36.

Lorig, K. (2002). Partnerships between expert patients and physicians. *Lancet, 359*(9309), 814–815.

McGee, D. L., Liao, Y., Cao, G., & Cooper, R. S. (1999). Self-reported health status and mortality in a multiethnic US cohort. *American Journal of Epidemiology, 149*(1), 41–46.

McPhee, S. J. (2002). Caring for a 70-year-old Vietnamese woman. *The Journal of the American Medical Association, 287*(4), 495–504.

McPhee, S. J., Bird, J. A., Davis, T., Ha, N. T., Jenkins, C. N. H., & Le, B. (1997). Barriers to breast and cervical cancer screening among Vietnamese-American women. *American Journal of Preventive Medicine, 13*(3), 205–213.

Meredith, L. S., & Siu, A. L. (1995). Variation and quality of self-report health data. Asians and Pacific Islanders compared with other ethnic groups. *Medical Care, 33*(11), 1120–1131.

Miller, S. (2010). Health promotion in Asian-Americans. *The Journal of Practical Nursing, 60*(2), 2–4.

Morales, L. S., Elliott, M. N., Weech-Maldonado, R., Spritzer, K. L., & Hays, R. D. (2001). Differences in CAHPS adult survey reports and ratings by race and ethnicity: An analysis of the national CAHPS benchmarking data 1.0. *Health Services Research, 36*(3), 595–617.

Moy, E., Greenberg, L. G., & Borsky, A. E. (2008). Community variation: Disparities in health care quality between Asian and white Medicare beneficiaries. *Health Affairs (Millwood), 27*(2), 538–549.

Mui, A. C., & Domanski, M. D. (1999). A community needs assessment among Asian American elders. *Journal of Cross-Cultural Gerontology, 14*(1), 77–90.

Mui, A. C., Kang, S.-Y., Kang, D., & Domanski, M. D. (2007). English language proficiency and health-related quality of life among Chinese and Korean immigrant elders. *Health and Social Work, 32*(2), 119–127.

Mull, D. S., Nguyen, N., & Mull, J. D. (2001). Vietnamese diabetic patients and their physicians: What ethnography can teach us. *Western Journal of Medicine, 175*(5), 307–311.

Murray-Garcia, J. L., Selby, J. V., Schmittdiel, J., Grumbach, K., & Quesenberry, C. P., Jr. (2000). Racial and ethnic differences in a patient survey: patients' values, ratings, and reports regarding physician primary care performance in a large health maintenance organization. *Medical Care, 38*(3), 300–310.

New California Media (NCM). (2003). Bridging language barriers in health care: Public opinion survey of California immigrants from Latin America, Asia and the Middle East. Woodland Hills, CA: The California Endowment.

Ngo-Metzger, Q., Legedza, A. T. R., & Phillips, R. S. (2004). Asian Americans' reports of their health care experiences: Results of a national survey. *Journal of General Internal Medicine, 19*, 111–119.

Ngo-Metzger, Q., Massagli, M. P., Clarridge, B. R., Michael, M., Davis, R. B., Iezzoni, L. I., et al. (2003a). Linguistic and cultural barriers to care: Perspectives of Chinese and Vietnamese immigrants. *Journal of General Internal Medicine, 18*, 44–52.

Ngo-Metzger, Q., Massagli, M. P., Clarridge, B. R., Moorhead, J., & Phillips, R. S. (2003b). Health care experiences of limited-English proficient Chinese and Vietnamese Americans. *Journal of General Internal Medicine, 18*(S), 184.

Ngo-Metzger, Q., Sorkin, D. H., & Phillips, R. S. (2009). Health care experiences of limited-English proficient Asian Americans. *The Patient: Patient-centered Outcomes Research, 2*(2), 113–120.

Ngo-Metzger, Q., Sorkin, D. H., Phillips, R. S., Greenfield, S., Massagli, M. P., Clarridge, B., et al. (2007).

Providing high-quality care for limited English proficient patients: The importance of language concordance and interpreter use. *Journal of General Internal Medicine, 22*, 324–330.

Nguyen, T. T., McPhee, S. J., Nguyen, T., Lam, T., & Mock, J. (2002). Predictors of cervical Pap smear screening awareness, intention, and receipt among Vietnamese-American women. *American Journal of Preventive Medicine, 23*(3), 207–214.

Ojeda, V. D., & McGuire, T. G. (2006). Gender and racial/ethnic differences in use of outpatient mental health and substance use services by depressed adults. *The Psychiatric Quarterly, 77*(3), 211–222.

Okoro, C. A., Strine, T. W., Young, S. L., Balluz, L. S., & Mokdad, A. H. (2005). Access to health care among older adults and receipt of preventive services. Results from the behavioral risk factor surveillance system, 2002. *Preventive Medicine, 40*(3), 337–343.

Perez-Stable, E. J., Napoles-Springer, A., & Miramontes, J. M. (1997). The effects of ethnicity and language on medical outcomes of patients with hypertension or diabetes. *Medical Care, 35*(12), 1212–1219.

Pignone, M. P., Gaynes, B. N., Rushton, J. L., Burchell, C. M., Orleans, C. T., Mulrow, C. D., et al. (2002). Screening for depression in adults: A summary of the evidence for the U.S. Preventive Services Task Force. *Annals of Internal Medicine, 136*(10), 765–776.

Proser, M. (2005). Deserving the spotlight: Health centers provide high-quality and cost-effective care. *Journal of Ambulatory Care Management, 28*(4), 321–330.

Saha, S., Arbelaez, J. J., & Cooper, L. A. (2003). Patient-physician relationships and racial disparities in the quality of health care. *American Journal of Public Health, 93*(10), 1713–1719.

Saha, S., & Hickam, D. H. (2003). Explaining low ratings of patient satisfaction among Asian-Americans. *American Journal of Medical Quality, 18*(6), 256–264.

Sarver, J., & Baker, D. W. (2000). Effect of language barriers on follow-up appointments after an emergency department visit. *Journal of General Internal Medicine, 15*(4), 256–264.

Schillinger, D., Grumbach, K., Piette, J., Wang, F., Osmond, D., Daher, C., et al. (2002). Association of health literacy with diabetes outcomes. *The Journal of the American Medical Association, 288*(4), 475–482.

Schmaling, K. B., & Hernandez, D. V. (2005). Detection of depression among low-income Mexican Americans in primary care. *Journal of Health Care for the Poor and Underserved, 16*(4), 780–790.

Shah, A. M., Guo, L., Magee, M., Cheung, W., Simon, M., LaBreche, A., et al. (2010). Comparing selected measures of health outcomes and health-seeking behaviors in Chinese, Cambodian, and Vietnamese communities of Chicago: Results from local health surveys. *Journal of Urban Health, 87*(5), 813–826.

Shibusawa, T., & Mui, A. C. (2002). Stress, coping and depression among Japanese American elders. *Journal of Gerontological Social Work, 26*(1/2), 63–82.

Shibusawa, T., & Mui, A. C. (2010). Health status and health services utilization among older Asian Indian immigrants. *Journal of Immigrant and Minority Health, 12*(4), 527–533.

Sorkin, D. H., Ngo-Metzger, Q., & De Alba, I. (2010). Racial/ethnic discrimination in health care: Impact on perceived quality of care. *Journal of General Internal Medicine, 25*(5), 390–396.

Sorkin, D. H., Ngo-Metzger, Q., Billimek, J., August, K. J., Greenfield, S., & Kaplan, S. H. (2011). Under-identified and under-treated depression among racially/ethnically diverse patients with type 2 diabetes. *Diabetes Care, 34*(3), 598–600.

Sorkin, D. H., Nguyen, H., & Ngo-Metzger, Q. (2011). Assessing the mental health needs and barriers to care among a diverse sample of Asian American older adults. *Journal of General Internal Medicine, 26*(6), 595–602.

Sorkin, D. H., Pham, E., & Ngo-Metzger, Q. (2009). Racial and ethnic differences in the mental health needs and access to care of older adults in California. *Journal of the American Geriatrics Society, 57*, 2311–2317.

Sorkin, D. H., Tan, A. L., Hays, R. D., Mangione, C. M., & Ngo-Metzger, Q. (2008). Self-reported health status of older Vietnamese and non-Hispanic whites in California. *Journal of the American Geriatrics Society, 56*, 1543–1548.

Stockdale, S. E., Lagomasino, I. T., Siddique, J., McGuire, T., & Miranda, J. (2008). Racial and ethnic disparities in detection and treatment of depression and anxiety among psychiatric and primary health care visits, 1995–2005. *Medical Care, 46*(7), 668–677.

Stokes, S. C., Thompson, L. W., Murphy, S., & Gallagher-Thompson, D. (2002). Screening for depression in immigrant Chinese-American elders: Results of a pilot study. *Journal of Gerontological Social Work, 36*(1/2), 27–44.

Taira, D. A., Safran, D. G., Seto, T. B., Rogers, W. H., Kosinski, M., Ware, J. E., et al. (1997). Asian-American patient ratings of physician primary care performance. *Journal of General Internal Medicine, 12*(4), 237–242.

Takeuchi, D. T., Chung, R. C.-Y., Lin, K.-M., Shen, H., Kurasaki, K., Chun, C.-A., et al. (1998). Lifetime and twelve-month prevalence rates of major depressive episodes and dysthymia among Chinese Americans in Los Angeles. *American Journal of Psychiatry, 155*(10), 1407–1414.

Takeuchi, D. T., Zane, N., Hong, S., Chae, D. H., Gong, F., Gee, G. C., et al. (2007). Immigration-related factors and mental disorders among Asian Americans. *American Journal of Public Health, 97*(1), 84–90.

Trinh-Shevrin, C., Islam, N. S., & Rey, M. J. (2009). *Asian American communities and health: Context, research, policy, and action.* San Francisco: Jossey-Bass/Wiley.

U.S. Census Bureau. (2005). American Community Survey, 2006. Retrieved July 23, 2012, from http://www.census.gov/acs/www/.

U.S. Department of Health and Human Services. Health Resources and Services Administration. Bureau of Primary Health Care. (2009). *Uniform Data System (UDS).* Rockville, MD.

U.S. Department of Health and Human Services. (2000). Healthy people 2010. Diabetes. Retrieved February 20, 2011, from http://www.healthypeople. gov/2010/.

U.S. Department of Health and Human Services. (2011). Healthy people, 2020. Retrieved April 1, 2011, from http://www.healthypeople.gov/2020/default.aspx.

Van Ta, M., Holck, P., & Gee, G. C. (2010). Generational status and family cohesion effects on the receipt of mental health services among Asian Americans: Findings from the national Latino and Asian American study. *American Journal of Public Health, 100*(1), 115–121.

Vega, W. A., Kolody, B., Aguilar-Gaxiola, S., & Catalano, R. (1999). Gaps in service utilization by Mexican Americans with mental health problems. *American Journal of Psychiatry, 156*(6), 928–934.

Weech-Maldonado, R., Elliott, M. N., Morales, L. S., Spritzer, K., Marshall, G. N., & Hays, R. D. (2004). Health plan effects on patient assessments of Medicaid managed care among racial/ethnic minorities. *Journal of General Internal Medicine, 19*(2), 136–145.

Weech-Maldonado, R., Morales, L. S., Elliott, M. N., Spritzer, K., Marshall, G. N., & Hays, R. D. (2003). Race/ethnicity, language, and patients' assessments of care in Medicaid managed care. *Health Services Research, 38*(3), 789–808.

Weech-Maldonado, R., Morales, L. S., Spritzer, K., Elliott, M. N., & Hays, R. D. (2001). Racial and ethnic differences in parents' assessments of pediatric care in Medicaid managed care. *Health Services Research, 36*(3), 575–594.

Weir, Rosy C., Emerson, H. P., Tseng, W., Chin, M. H., Caballero, J., Song, H., et al. (2010). Use of enabling services by Asian American, native Hawaiian, and other Pacific Islander patients at 4 community health centers. *American Journal of Public Health, 100*(11), 2199–2205.

Wells, K., Klap, R., Koike, A., & Sherbourne, C. (2001). Ethnic disparities in unmet need for alcoholism, drug abuse, and mental health care. *American Journal of Psychiatry, 158*(12), 2027–2032.

Wen, X. J., & Balluz, L. (2010). Racial disparities in access to health care and preventive services between Asian Americans/Pacific Islanders and non-Hispanic whites. *Ethnicity and Disease, 20*(3), 290–295.

Woloshin, S., Schwartz, L. M., Katz, S. J., & Welch, H. G. (1997). Is language a barrier to the use of preventive services? *Journal of General Internal Medicine, 12*(8), 472–477.

Wong, C. C., Tsoh, J. Y., Tong, E. K., Hom, F. B., Cooper, B., & Chow, E. A. (2008). The Chinese community smoking cessation project: A community sensitive intervention trial. *Journal of Community Health, 33*(6), 363–373.

Wu, C. A., Lin, S. Y., So, S. K., & Chang, E. T. (2007). Hepatitis B and liver cancer knowledge and preventive practices among Asian Americans in the San Francisco Bay area, California. *Asian Pacific Journal of Cancer Prevention, 8*(1), 127–134.

Complementary and Alternative Medicine Use in Asian Americans: Is Integrative Medicine the Ticket into the US Healthcare System?

24

Isha Weerasinghe, Lixin Zhang, Simona C. Kwon, and Serena Chen

Cao gio, literally translated as "rubbing out the wind," is a therapy used by Vietnamese and other Asian immigrant groups to treat cold and flu-like ailments (Purnell, 2008, p. 66). A hot ointment is rubbed onto the skin using the edge of a coin in order to release afflicting winds from the body. During the process, red marks are left on the skin (Purnell, 2008). Some conventional healthcare providers in the US, unfamiliar with cao gio, have accused parents of abuse or reported them to Child Protective Services upon discovering red marks on their children (Davis, 2000).

Cao gio is one of many forms of complementary and alternative medicine (CAM). While several definitions exist for CAM, they are all based on the same principles. Bonnie O'Connor, a leading researcher in CAM, defined CAM as:

> A broad domain of healing resources that encompasses all health systems, modalities, and practices and their accompanying theories and beliefs, other than those intrinsic to the politically dominant health system of a particular society or culture in a given historical period. "CAM" includes all such practices and ideas self-defined by their users as preventing or treating illness or promoting health and well-being. Boundaries within CAM and between the CAM domain and that of the dominant system are not always sharp or fixed (O'Connor, 1995).

This definition of CAM was later adopted by both the Cochrane Collaboration, an international health research organization known for their database of clinical trials of CAM therapies, as well as the National Institutes of Health.

The National Center for Complementary and Alternative Medicine (NCCAM), the main federal agency researching the myriad of medical practices outside of conventional medicine, defines "complementary medicine" as the use of therapies identified as "CAM" with conventional medicine to help alleviate pain. "Alternative medicine" is defined as the use of CAM therapies in place of conventional medicine (Barnes, Bloom, & Nahin, 2008; National Center for Complementary and Alternative Medicine, 2010). This definition assumes that conventional medicine is the "dominant health system," but this dichotomy may be changing slowly (Cohen, Ruggie, & Micozzi, 2006), with higher use of CAM and changing philosophies of how to better approach one's health.

I. Weerasinghe
NYU Institute of Community Health and Research,
Center of the Study of Asian American Health,
New York University School of Medicine,
New York, NY, USA
e-mail: isha.weerasinghe@nyumc.org

L. Zhang
San Francisco State University, CA, USA

S.C. Kwon (✉)
NYU Institute of Community Health and Research
and Department of Medicine, Division of General,
Internal Medicine, New York University School
of Medicine, New York, NY, USA
e-mail: simona.kwon@nyumc.org

S. Chen
Department of Sociomedical Sciences, Columbia
University Mailman School of Public Health,
New York, NY, USA

G.J. Yoo et al. (eds.), *Handbook of Asian American Health*,
DOI 10.1007/978-1-4614-2227-3_24, © Springer Science+Business Media, LLC 2013

According to the World Health Organization (WHO), traditional medicine is the "sum total of knowledge, skills and practices based on the theories, beliefs and experiences indigenous to different cultures that are used to maintain health, as well as to prevent, diagnose, improve or treat physical and mental illnesses" (World Health Organization, 2008). Considered complementary and alternative forms of treatment in the United States, these therapies are often the first line of treatment/healing methods for people in their countries of origin. In many countries outside of the US, CAM has been practiced for decades or centuries. CAM often serves as an indispensable and integrated primary care modality along with conventional health care services in many parts of the world.

Gradually, as CAM usage increases and becomes more prominent in the medical infrastructure, government agencies are relaxing restrictions against CAM. The Department of Health and Human Services (DHHS) now recognizes cao gio as a cultural healing practice and acknowledges its distinction from physical abuse in its manual on child abuse and neglect. However, in describing CAM, the DHHS also leaves room for interpretation, citing a researcher in the field who stated that "while cultural practices are generally respected, if the injury or harm is significant, professionals typically work with parents to discourage harmful behavior and suggest preferable alternatives" (Goldman, Salus, Wolcott, & Kennedy, 2003, p. 16).

The relationship between CAM and conventional medicine continues to progress and evolve as patients, healthcare providers, and policymakers negotiate the tensions and ambiguities of their interactions in an increasingly diverse US healthcare system. This chapter is meant to provide an overview of CAM use in the United States with a focus on Asian American communities, and explore its relationship and potential integration with conventional medicine.

CAM Popularity and Prevalence in the US

More than two-thirds of adults in the US have used CAM therapies in their lifetimes (Kessler et al., 2001). Interest and use of CAM in the US is increasing. Information about specific therapies is becoming more prevalent as more communities utilize CAM modalities and praise their efficacy (Maizes, Rakel, & Niemiec, 2009; Wu, Burke, & LeBaron, 2007).

Greater consumer use of CAM therapies over the past decades led to the creation of the National Center of Complementary and Alternative Medicine (NCCAM) as part of the National Institutes of Health (NIH), in 1998. The aim of NCCAM is to fund CAM research, train researchers, disseminate information about CAM, and help to integrate current CAM therapies into Western practice (National Center for Complementary and Alternative Medicine, 2011).

According to the 2007 National Health Interview Survey (NHIS), a nationwide survey on a broad range of health topics administered by the U.S. Census Bureau (Centers for Disease Control and Prevention, 2011), adults in the United States make more than 300 million visits to CAM providers every year. Although the population of Asian Americans has increased significantly from 2002 to 2007, usage rates of CAM for non-Hispanic Whites were higher than all racial and ethnic minorities (Su & Li, 2011). These trends are continuing to change for both Asian Americans and the general population.

Levels of use of CAM therapies are not homogenous throughout the US, and vary by population, geographic region, Asian subgroup, and immigrant status. For example, in the West and Northeast of the United States, the prevalence of acupuncture use among the general population is much higher than in other regions, especially with Asian women (Burke, Upchurch, Dye, & Chyu, 2006). This may be due to greater consumer demand in these areas (Burke et al., 2006) and/or because these regions have higher numbers of immigrant communities that welcome a more holistic approach to health.

The link between these and other sociodemographic factors and CAM therapy use is tenuous (Conboy et al., 2005), signifying the need for more research. Some studies on the general population have not found a link between demographic and social factors (e.g. job status, country of origin, age, gender) and use of CAM in the US (Krauss, Godfrey, Kirk, & Eisenberg,

1998), although some have found an association between higher education levels and income strata with greater use of alternative therapies (Eisenberg et al., 1993, 1998; Mehta, Phillips, Davis, & McCarthy, 2007).

How and Why Is CAM Used?

CAM's Patient-Centered Holistic Approach

CAM encompasses entire systems of medicine (e.g. Traditional Chinese Medicine [TCM], Ayurvedic medicine, homeopathy), and includes specific modalities or treatments (e.g. massage therapy) (see Table 24.2) (Maizes et al., 2009). Ayurvedic medicine, which has evolved over thousands of years in India, include breathing exercises, massages, and herbal remedies. These treatments do not exist in isolation, but rather within Ayurvedic wellness beliefs that center upon ideas of universal interconnectedness and harmony, a person's unique constitution (prakritti), and the balance of three life forces (doshas) (National Center for Complementary and Alternative Medicine, 2005). Many TCM therapies aim to restore balance in the body, reflecting the influence of Taoist philosophy and the worldview that complementary but opposing "yin" and "yang" forces shape the universe (National Center for Complementary and Alternative Medicine, 2009). The Chinese belief of a circulating vital energy called "qi" is reflected in the practices of acupuncture and mind-body exercises such as qi gong and tai chi, which promote wellness by encouraging the healthy flow of qi (Birdee, Wayne, Davis, Phillips, & Yeh, 2009; National Center for Complementary and Alternative Medicine, 2007, 2009). These traditional medical practices are based on centuries-old traditional health systems with fundamental cultural and spiritual ideologies (Bodeker, Kronenberg, & Burford, 2007).

TCM and Ayurveda are examples of healing systems that focus on balance, such as between the self and the community or between the self/community and the environment. Treatments stemming from these healing philosophies do not only address isolated diseases, but also the

Table 24.1 Categories of complementary and alternative medicine from the NCCAM and OCCAM (National Center for Complementary and Alternative Medicine & National Institutes of Health, 2010; Office of Cancer Complementary and Alternative Medicine, 2011)

Category	Examples
Natural products	Herbal medicines (e.g. dietary supplements, probiotics)
Mind–body medicine	Meditation, yoga, acupuncture, other aspects of Traditional Chinese Medicine, deep-breathing exercises, guided imagery, hypnotherapy, progressive relaxation, support groups, art/music therapy, qi gong, tai chi
Manipulative and body-based practices	Acupuncture, massage therapy, osteopathic manipulation
Other CAM practices	Movement therapies (e.g. Feldenkrais method, Alexander technique, pilates), traditional healing practices (e.g. Native American healers), energy field manipulation (e.g. qi gong, Reiki, acupuncture, electromagnetic-based therapies), Ayurveda, homeopathy, naturopathy

greater balance between entities (Bodeker, Kabatesi, Homsy, & King, 2000).

Commonalities in CAM systems and therapies exist in the fact that they are all "patient-centered care... [allowing the patient to] address the mind, body, and spiritual aspects of health" (Maizes et al., 2009, p. 278). The NHIS and NCCAM have their own system of categorizing CAM therapies: natural products/energy medicine, manipulative and body-based practices, mind-body interventions, alternative medical systems, and biologically based therapies (see Table 24.1) (Maizes et al., 2009).

As the DHHS states in the National Health Statistics Reports, practitioners of CAM therapies hold a holistic view of treating illness, treating the "physical, and biochemical manifestations of illness, but also the nutritional, emotional, social, and spiritual context in which the illness arises" (Barnes et al., 2008, p. 1). In some circumstances, the line between medical systems is not clearly defined; certain medical practices, particularly in categories like mind-body medicine, may be considered either or both CAM and/or conventional medicine (Cohen et al., 2006), showing some grey areas between both systems. Often, CAM practitioners will use a variety of therapies to treat a patient. For example,

TCM doctors will often recommend that patients integrate therapies like acupuncture with herbal medicine, balancing the 'yin and yang' (Wong, 2009). These philosophies are the foundation of the holistic approach – the use of a number of techniques to approach an illness or ailment, as well as addressing the patient's overall condition.

Utilization of CAM over Conventional Medicine

Some populations prefer alternative medicine over conventional medicine for minor illnesses, using homemade remedies first and then progressing to other therapies such as acupuncture, acupressure, meditation, and Reiki when homemade remedies are ineffective (Rao, 2006). In the US, more people are using CAM therapies for various severe and chronic illnesses, including asthma, cancer, arthritis, back pain, irritable bowel syndrome, autism, and HIV (Cherkin & MacCornack, 1989; Conboy et al., 2005; Cronan, Kaplan, Posner, Blumberg, & Kozin, 1989; Smart, Mayberry, & Atkinson, 1986; Wong, 2009). Treatments are often used in complement with conventional therapies. However, CAM is increasingly being used as an alternative form of care when conventional treatments are ineffective or when a patient experiences harrowing side effects from conventional medicine (Burke et al., 2006; Chao, Wade, Kronenberg, Kalmuss, & Cushman, 2006; Maizes et al., 2009; Rao, 2006; Wong et al., 1998; Wong, 2009), when conventional medicine cannot provide an explanation for the medical problem (Rao, 2006), an illness has reached a late stage (Lee, Lin, Wrensch, Adler, & Eisenberg, 2000).

The Appeal of CAM

Americans use CAM for several reasons, a few of which are described throughout this chapter: (1) to alleviate minor illnesses or maintain health/wellbeing, (2) to counteract severe side effects from other medications, (3) to avoid the conventional system with illnesses that are normally stigmatized, and (4) for spiritual reasons. Many, regardless of

race/ethnicity, use CAM therapies as a result of personal beliefs, rather than being dissatisfied with conventional medicine (Chao et al., 2006). Many ascribe using CAM therapies as being synonymous with spiritual and personal growth (Lee et al., 2000). Some studies show that Asian Americans use CAM therapies to maintain health and wellbeing as opposed to curing a particular illness (Mehta et al., 2007). On the other hand, individuals may also pursue CAM therapies for stigmatizing issues such as mental illnesses in order to avoid the conventional medical system. For example, practicing meditation and other therapies like Reiki provides an outlet for therapy and an avoidance of acknowledging the onset of mental illness in the conventional US health system (Rao, 2006).

Growing Asian American Populations and Their Influence on CAM

The 2010 Census reported an increase in population in all racial groups from 2000 to 2010, with the proportion of Asian Americans increasing by the greatest percentage (United States Census, 2010). Asian Americans, an extremely diverse racial category defined by the U.S. Census Bureau as people with origins from the Far East, Southeast Asia, or the Indian subcontinent, increased by 43.3% between 2000 and 2010, with a population of over 14.5 million nationally in 2010 (United States Census, 2010). Many of these communities have ideas and practices of health and healing that are different from the standards of the American healthcare system, based on conventional medicine. When the racial makeup of the population changes, the needs of the general population change, especially in areas such as healthcare. In order to maintain the health and wellness of the changing population, it becomes increasingly necessary to understand CAM and its use.

Prevalence of CAM Use in Asian American Communities

Asian Americans in the US use a number of CAM therapies, with 40% of the Asian American population using at least one form of therapy according to the 2007 NHIS (Bloom et al., 2008; Mehta et al., 2007). In the general population, Su, Li, and Pagan found, after comparing the 2003 and 2007 NHIS CAM supplements, that US-born Americans use CAM more than US immigrants (2008). However, the 2007 NHIS does not report a difference in CAM use between US-born and foreign-born Asian Americans (Mehta et al., 2007). Manipulative, body-based therapies and herbal medicines (natural products) are commonly used among Asian American populations, while the use of alternative systems and biologically based therapies is rare (Mehta et al., 2007). The Chinese population, for example, often uses herbal therapies for many acute and chronic illnesses, including influenza, persistent cough, rheumatologic problems, arthritis, and breast cancer (Lee et al., 2000; Wong et al., 1998). A study of Chinese and Vietnamese Americans with limited English proficiency (LEP), i.e. speaking English less than "very well," found that 60% of the population surveyed used TCM-related CAM therapies (Ahn et al., 2006). Certain Asian American populations use TCM and other alternative therapies to alleviate symptoms such as a cold, cough, headache, fever, and dizziness (Wu et al., 2007). As the Asian American population is diverse, CAM use also varies in scope.

Integration of Care in Asian American Communities

CAM modalities practiced in Asian cultures arise from diverse and deeply rooted belief systems, and must be contextualized within their broader worldviews in order to be properly understood. As conventional Western medicine gained prominence in Asia, countries like China and India developed integrated medical systems which incorporate both traditional and Western medical philosophies and treatments. These philosophies are slowly migrating to the United States, generally in areas with greater Chinese immigrant populations (Chao et al., 2006). Integrated care is a preferred option for Indian communities who ascribe to alternative practices, as it gives patients

the option to choose treatments according to their preferences (Kaptchuk & Eisenberg, 2001). In an integrated system, physicians may be more apt to discuss a patient's beliefs about alternative therapies, and suggest multimodal treatments depending on a practice's culture and geography (Chen, Kramer, & Chen, 2003).

Gaps in Research on CAM and Asian Americans

There is a severe lack of data of Asian Americans and their CAM use in the US. As Asian Americans share distinct cultural and social backgrounds, many studies looking at CAM and/or integrative medicine as a whole may oversimplify use within the population and among populations (Ruy, Young, & Kwak, 2002). It is difficult to fully ascertain usage of CAM therapies in the Asian American population with the national survey data currently available. The NHIS, for example, did not include open-ended questions to list CAM therapies not listed on the survey, and therefore did not capture many of the alternative treatments inherent in Asian cultures. While Asian Americans were oversampled, the total sample of Asian-Americans was small and limited as the survey was offered only in English and Spanish, thus failing to capture individuals with limited English proficiency (Mehta et al., 2007).

Surveys like the NHIS need to be revised to reflect the trends in medical care with regards to CAM therapies and integrative medicine (Deng, Weber, Sood, & Kemper, 2010). Furthermore, as the NHIS is currently the only national survey that has data on the use of CAM therapies by Asian Americans, more open-ended questions need to be added to capture accurate data and the myriad of therapies that Asian American populations use in the US.

Research and Empirical Validation

In the recent past, researchers have complained of a lack of randomized controlled trials (RCTs) that show efficacy of alternative therapies (US Department of Health and Human Services, 1994). Since the safety and efficacy of many CAM therapies are not regulated or clearly stated, average physicians face difficulties when attempting to consult with patients to accurately assess and discuss a treatment plan involving complementary therapies (Adler & Fosket, 1999; Eisenberg, 1997; Gray et al., 1997).

The *Cochrane Database Systematic Review*, which reviews human health-related primary research, houses over 500 reviews as of March 2012, based on randomized and clinical controlled trials, as well as observational studies of complementary medicine (The Cochrane CAM Field, 2012). Clinical trials are showing benefits of CAM therapies (e.g. Traditional Chinese Medicine (TCM), acupuncture, and herbalism) for pain management and treating ailments such as irritable bowel syndrome, cardiovascular disease, and dermatologic issues (Bedi & Shenefelt, 2002; Bensoussan et al., 1998; Berman et al., 2004; Ernst & White, 1998; Mashour, Lin, & Frishman, 1998; Wu et al., 2007). Positive results from studies investigating CAM using various experimental research designs (e.g. RCT, single-blind trials) will help to give credence to the integration of CAM practices into Western medicine (Deng et al., 2010). However, certain CAM therapies such as herbal treatments may lack uniformity in consistency, methodology of administration, and indications for use depending on the treatment's cultural origin. This makes it difficult for clinical trials to address the majority of therapies and uses for which each therapy is attributed, stinting progress in clinical trials and the accreditation of CAM therapies (Deng et al., 2010).

CAM and the U.S. Health Care System

As the US healthcare system is dominated by conventional medicine, practitioners of CAM have often been regarded with suspicion, with concerns raised about the lack of regulation, scarce rigorous scientific research, and perceived incomparability with conventional therapies. CAM practitioners have had to struggle to legitimize their therapies and theoretical frameworks to be equitable choices as conventional

medicine. After seeking accreditation of CAM schools and pushing for more empirical research, CAM practitioners and advocates are gradually becoming more accepted in the US.

Conventional Provider Communication

In a large survey of Americans done in 1997, the majority of individuals (97%) received alternative therapies and conventional therapies for the same ailment, but only one-third of patients discussed the alternative treatments with their conventional physician (Eisenberg et al., 1998). Physicians may not believe that alternative therapies are beneficial to the patient, precluding them from having a discussion about other therapies with their patients (Lee et al., 2000). Patients also may not be sharing information about CAM therapies because they do not feel that their physicians have the knowledge to understand the therapies (Wu et al., 2007). Conventional providers need to learn more about therapies used by their patients in order to increase trust in the doctor-patient relationship and have the capacity to discuss all possible therapies with their patients (Wong, 2009).

Miscommunication may exist in the doctor-patient relationship; physicians make assumptions that patients tell them about all possible medications they use, including alternative therapies, and patients assume that physicians do not believe CAM treatments are viable therapies and will not approve of them (2001; Adler & Fosket, 1999; Sibinga, Ottolini, Duggan, & Wilson, 2004; Sikand & Laken, 1998).

Studies show reduced communication between patients and physicians about CAM use as a result of a heightened sense of stigma surrounding alternative therapies. Many communities do not discuss CAM therapies with their providers (Mehta et al., 2007; Wu et al., 2007), especially in non-English speaking immigrant populations (Ahn et al., 2006) that may have greater barriers to health care and may be using alternative therapies in place of conventional ones (Mehta et al., 2007).

As a result of the lack of communication, many patients may not be aware of potential drug interactions between Western and alternative therapies. Physicians may not have adequate information to determine how safe medications are. Those that manufacture herbal medications are not mandated to include dosages, side effects, and toxicity (Wong, 2009). This limits patients from receiving adequate information about therapies, and leads to a lack of informed consent (Cohen et al., 2006).

Cost and Insurance Coverage of CAM Therapies

As mentioned earlier, it is debatable whether reduced financial resources lead to lower utilization of CAM therapies (Burke et al., 2006; Conboy et al., 2005). Patients have been reported to seek conventional medical care when CAM therapies are not covered by insurance (Rao, 2006). However, for populations insured by Medicaid and Medicare, there are some challenges with coverage. As Medicaid plans depend on the state, CAM coverage differs. Medicare covers biofeedback, acupuncture, and intravenous histamine therapy, but only for certain illnesses and the person covered must provide notice of use. According to a study done in 2002, reimbursements were commonly given for chiropractic, biofeedback, acupuncture, hypnotherapy, and naturopathy. For Medicare, coverage depends on the type of treatment required for a particular ailment or illness. Furthermore, the number of covered visits to a CAM practitioner is limited, and a patient must get a referral to see their CAM practitioner from their primary physician (Steyer, Freed, & Lantz, 2002).

As CAM becomes more accepted in the US, more 'alternative providers' are being recognized as primary care providers by insurance companies (Steyer et al., 2002). According to the NHIS, in the 12 months prior to the study in 2009, adults spent $33.9 billion on CAM therapies and products, classes, and materials; $11.9 billion were spent on practitioner visits alone. Out of all out-of-pocket costs for CAM, 44% (14.8 billion) were spent on non-vitamin, non-mineral, natural products (Nahin et al., 2009). About three-quarters of visits made to CAM practitioners and out-of-pocket costs attributed to CAM practitioners were related to manipulative and body-based therapies (Nahin et al., 2009). These costs contribute to a significant proportion of the total out-of-pocket healthcare costs in the US.

The Introduction of Integrative Medicine

The use of acupuncture and other alternative therapies has brought forth ideas to integrate conventional and complementary therapies (Burke et al., 2006). For some illnesses (e.g. autism), alternative therapies are considered equivalent to conventional therapies. Consequently, a paradigm shift is starting to occur from 'conventional/alternative' to a multimodal or multi-tiered treatment approach (Wong, 2009), partly attributed to the incorporation of CAM practitioners in Western medicine. Philosophies between the two streams of medicine (alternative and conventional) amalgamate to what is known in the US as integrative medicine.

What is Integrative Medicine (IM)?

NCCAM states that 'integrative medicine' is a practice that "combines both conventional and CAM treatments for which there is evidence of safety and effectiveness" (National Center for Complementary and Alternative Medicine, 2010). Integrative medicine is defined by the Consortium of Academic Health Centers for Integrative Medicine (CAHCIM) as the practice of medicine that "reaffirms the importance of the relationship between practitioner and patient, focuses on the whole person, is informed by evidence, and makes use of all appropriate therapeutic approaches, healthcare professionals and disciplines to achieve optimal health and healing" (The Consortium of Academic Health Centers for Integrative Medicine, 2009). A key principle of integrative medicine is that it is a "holistic approach to health care that integrates the physical, mental-emotional, and spiritual sides of the health of the individual and the community" and "[trains] health care practitioners to be role models for health and well being, to be open to new concepts of health, and to be aware of cultural nuances in patient communities" (Cook, 2008, pp. 1023–1024). It includes an "immense range of ideas, including whole systems of medicine (e.g. TCM, Ayurveda, homeopathy), modalities (e.g. massage, botanical medicine, manipulation practices), and therapies (e.g. Reiki, healing touch). Patient-centered care and patient empowerment are primary components of these fields, as is the commitment to address the mind, body, and spiritual aspects of health" (Maizes et al., 2009, p. 278). Integrative medicine utilizes the holistic approach implicit in CAM therapies, and incorporates conventional therapies.

The Relationship Between Patient and Provider

Studies with Asian Americans using CAM therapies have shown that there is a high correlation between a positive discussion about CAM use between patient and provider and a patient's reported perception of the visit (Ahn et al., 2006). Eisenberg (1997) suggests that providers discuss the use of CAM with their patients by asking them their treatment preferences, asking them to fill symptom diaries, and scheduling regular patient visits to ensure that symptoms and side effects are managed. Utilizing an integrative medicine approach may also help to increase communication between doctor and patient, as both sides already may feel more amenable to alternative therapies. Common terminology should be adopted in order for providers of these paradigms to communicate easily (Maizes et al., 2009).

Growth of IM in the US and National Initiatives

In 2000, the White House Commission on Complementary and Alternative Medicine Policy

was created in response to consumer need. They released a final report in 2002, with a number of recommendations to identify and lower the barriers to integrating CAM practices into conventional US medicine (White House Commission on Complementary and Alternative Medicine Policy, 2002). As integrative medicine has gained popularity, more providers and institutions are accepting of CAM practices (Maizes et al., 2009). This has resulted in the need for more integrative medicine centers and a call to action through workshops such as the Summit on Integrative Medicine and the Health of the Public, held in 2009 by the Institute of Medicine (IOM) (IOM, 2009).

It is difficult to determine the patterns of integrative care or consumer-driven integrated care because of a lack of historical and longitudinal data (Burke et al., 2006). Knowing more about integrative medicine and its impact in the United States among Asian Americans and the general population will help to direct research and policy (Burke et al., 2006).

Incorporation of IM in Medical Education

As many CAM practitioners have not been accredited, patients may not trust CAM practitioners (Rao, 2006), leading individuals to seek conventional care. More medical schools are offering courses in CAM medicine (Wetzel, Eisenberg, & Kaptchuk, 1998), with accreditation offered for schools providing training in chiropractic, naturopathic, acupuncture, Traditional Chinese Medicine (TCM), midwifery, and massage therapy (Maizes et al., 2009). The first homeopathic medical college was licensed in 2008, and Ayurvedic and Tibetan medical programs (see Table 24.2) have been recently introduced in the US (Maizes et al., 2009). The nursing certification exam includes content about CAM, and holistic nursing is recognized as a specialty with standards of practice (Denner, 2007). An increase in educational courses about CAM and integrative medicine will increase health professionals' knowledge about alternative therapies so that they are more willing to talk about all possible

Table 24.2 Common CAM modalities

CAM modalities	Description
Acupuncture	A TCM practice that seeks to unblock and facilitate the flow of "qi," or life energy along the body's meridians, by stimulating strategic points on the body with thin metal needles. Used for a wide variety of conditions, and very popular for pain relief (National Center for Complementary and Alternative Medicine, 2007).
Ayurveda	A medical system originating in India, which promotes healing through balancing the body, mind, and spirit. Involves multiple modalities such as herbs, massage, and oils (National Center for Complementary and Alternative Medicine, 2005).
Coin rubbing and spooning (e.g. cao gio in Vietnamese, gua sha in Chinese, kerikan in Indonesia)	Practice cultures in which a smooth hard edge such as a coin or spoon is firmly stroked on the skin, usually with oil, in order to scrape away or draw out a fever or cold. Often leaves red marks on the skin (Ravanfar & Dinulos, 2010).
Moxibustion	A TCM therapy in which a mugwort herb is placed on an acupuncture point and burned on or near the skin (Ravanfar & Dinulos, 2010).
Reflexology	Modality with origins in TCM, usually in the form of applying pressure and massaging feet or hands to impact other parts of the body, often to relieve pain and stress (Stephenson et al., 2007).
Tai chi	Mind–body martial arts and health practices rooted in TCM, intended to regulate the balance of the body's qi through regulated movements, breathing, and relaxation (Birdee et al., 2009).
Tibetan medicine	Highly associated with Tibetan Buddhism. Philosophies are similar to this form of Buddhism (disease as a form of suffering, life is impermanent, diseases are caused by karma). Anatomy, pathology, and pharmacology are based on the five basic energies: earth, water, fire, air, and space. When these energies are disturbed, disease occurs (Fan & Holliday, 2007).

therapies (Wong et al., 1998; Wong, 2009; Wu et al., 2007). This will hopefully foster awareness, respect, and relationships between conventional and CAM providers, to the benefit of their patients.

Patient Protection and Affordable Care Act of 2010

The healthcare reform debates preceding the passage of the Patient Protection and Affordable Care Act in 2010 (PPACA) touched upon a plethora of health and access related topics, but barely mentioned CAM or IM. Some leaders in the field of CAM have speculate that it was largely absent in the national discourse because it does not contribute much to burgeoning healthcare costs, is perceived as an extra benefit supplementing conventional medicine and therefore less of a priority than giving basic coverage to the millions of uninsured, and because CAM professionals failed

to organize themselves (Majette, 2010). Three major problems at the forefront of the recent 2009–2010 national healthcare reform debates included healthcare access for millions of uninsured, skyrocketing healthcare costs, as well as the neglect of disease prevention in the healthcare system. If given the opportunity, CAM may have the potential to address all three of these issues.

While the role of CAM was not explicitly stated in the bill (Majette, 2010), integrative medicine is mentioned, by way of the creation of an Advisory Group to the President on integrative medicine. It is yet to be determined, however, whether integrative medicine will be a priority, or even addressed at all.

Some believe that the health reform bill's clauses on prevention, chronic disease management, and patient-centered care present the opportunity for inclusion of IM (Horrigan, 2010). These appear mainly in Subtitles A, C, and D of Title IV, which cover the modernization of disease prevention and public health systems, community health initiatives, and patient-centered outcomes research (Horrigan, 2010). For example, subtitle A, section 4001 designates a Council and an Advisory Group of 25 non-Federal members on "Prevention, Health Promotion, and Integrative and Public Health" within the DHHS. The Council will be responsible for developing wellness strategies, suggesting federal health policy changes, and making recommendations to the President and Congress. The Advisory Group will inform the Council, and its president-appointed membership is recommended to be "a diverse group of licensed health professionals, including integrative health practitioners who have expertise in worksite health promotion…" giving integrative medicine providers the chance to share expertise and influence policy at the federal level (Horrigan, 2010, p. 221). IM may figure more prominently in health promotion initiatives in the future if the opportunities for the inclusion of IM experts and initiatives are taken advantage of in the PPACA (Horrigan).

Others, who are skeptical towards CAM, believe that health reform neglected to seize the opportunity to better regulate CAM products and practitioners (Jibrin, 2010).

Future Directions: Finding a Place for CAM in the US Medical System

Legitimacy and Inclusion Through Research and Reimbursement

Legitimacy and inclusion into the mainstream medical system continue to be major challenges for CAM practitioners. An American Hospital Association survey found that the major barrier to successful integration of CAM therapies in hospitals was physician resistance. Mainstream healthcare providers must learn about CAM therapies as part of their education in order to be better informed and more familiar with them, in light of its widespread use (Denner, 2007). A 2005 survey of both conventional and CAM practitioners revealed agreement that collaboration and cooperation must be established in

professional education in order to successfully incorporate integrative medicine in American health care reform (Riley, 2009).

Rigorous scientific studies are key to proving the safety and efficacy of CAM therapies, and to gain acceptance into the healthcare marketplace (Ruggie & Cohen, 2005). The White House Commission on Complementary and Alternative Medicine Policy recommended increased coverage of CAM therapies by insurance companies, increasing legitimacy, viability of running IM centers, and accessibility of CAM therapies for patients. Actual expansions of this nature, however, are not considered likely (Ruggie & Cohen, 2005) unless policy changes are made. In the case of Medicaid, several states prohibit usage of funds for "experimental treatments" by physicians, which further underscores the need for solid CAM efficacy studies (Steyer et al., 2002). Positive efficacy studies in CAM would help to initiate policy changes to integrate CAM and conventional medicine.

Others fear that CAM therapies will lose their individualized and holistic nature and will take on flaws of the mainstream conventional system if they become covered under insurance (Denner, 2007). Studies often focus on the efficacy of individual modalities in isolation, contradicting the holistic nature of many CAM therapies and ignoring the complex systems from which they arose. There is also a need for more research examining the process of healing, qualitative experiences of those using CAM, and the impact of integrating CAM modalities with conventional therapies (Denner, 2007).

Professionalization, Licensure, and Legal Issues of CAM Practitioners

In a healthcare system dominated by conventional medicine, practitioners of CAM have often been regarded with suspicion, with concerns raised regarding lack of regulation, lack of scientific research, and perceived incompatibility with conventional therapies. CAM practitioners have struggled to legitimize their therapies, but are now experiencing increasing acknowledgment from insurers, hospitals, and conventional providers (Barrett et al., 2003; Hirschkorn, 2006).

The regulation of medical practitioners, including licensure and definition of scope of practice, is typically done at the state level and is influenced by the judgment of the medical community. More recently, some states such as Alaska and Colorado have enacted statutes that protect physicians practicing CAM therapies from judgment of professional incompetence if no physical harm was done to the patient. The Federation of State Medical Boards has suggested guidelines for physician practice of CAM therapies in the context of safety and efficacy, but the language of actual statutes varies from state to state. The issue of malpractice standards is also significant, as evidenced by the court case Charell v. Gonzalez, where physician practice of non-conventional therapies is at risk of being considered negligence or substandard care (Cohen et al., 2006). In this case, the law has not been able to make a differentiation between these illegitimate practices and standard CAM therapies, signifying the need for more empirical research, licensure, and regulation.

Laws at the state level also have the ability to regulate patients' access to CAM. As of 2007, health freedom laws were active in 18 states, which allow patients to access CAM services from licensed physicians. Currently, health freedom laws that incorporate CAM treatments are consistently debated in many states. Unlicensed provision of CAM services is also legal in other states, such as California. However, the Food and Drug Administration (FDA) restricts certain supplements and therapies at the federal level (Denner, 2007). The FDA also regulates certain materials used by CAM practitioners, such as acupuncture needles, which are required to be sterile, single-use only, and used only by licensed acupuncture providers (National Center for Complementary and Alternative Medicine, 2007). There have been efforts to introduce legislation at the federal level to make it possible for individuals to receive their care of choice from any healthcare providers who are licensed, but such efforts have not been successful (Denner, 2007). As stated before, more regulation must be in place to legitimize therapies by funding empirical research and regulating the licensure of practitioners to practice CAM.

Access to Healthcare

Although CAM therapies may be making strides in the US health system, it is unknown whether Asian Americans, particularly Asian immigrants, are able to access available services within integrated systems housed by conventional medical centers. Linguistic concerns, cultural barriers, and the prevalence of stigma between patient and conventional care provider come into play. Without more rigorous data concerning Asian Americans and CAM use, it is difficult to determine whether continuing to integrate these therapies will open the doors for Asian American patients who are outside of the conventional medical system, and help to relieve the cost-burden on the healthcare system.

Lowering Healthcare Costs

Despite the overall lack of data on CAM, some studies show that CAM therapies and integrative medicine have proven to be cost-effective methods in care (Maizes et al., 2009; Block, 2010). A review article by Block cites numerous studies where use of IM (e.g. relaxation tapes before surgery) was associated with shorter hospital stays, fewer complications, and therefore lower overall costs (Block, 2010). However, others believe that cost-effectiveness research in CAM is still in its nascent stages and data is lacking to convincingly argue a cost-saving benefit of CAM (Majette, 2010). According to the American Hospital Association, US hospitals are gradually adding more CAM therapies to their services, some of which offer more than one CAM therapy (Maizes et al., 2009).

Encouraging Health Promotion and Disease Prevention

Growing awareness and interest in preventative health on Capitol Hill may be beneficial to the integration of CAM into mainstream systems. Many CAM therapies have a focus on holism and maintaining wellness, and could experience the most acceptance and success in integration with the field of preventative medicine. For example, the Healthy Workforce Act of 2007 (which was proposed but never signed into law) would have created incentives for companies to spend money on prevention and wellness initiatives for their employees (2007). These wellness initiatives were required to be evidence-based, but no language in the legislation excluded CAM modalities, which would have opened a door for its role in health promotion at the workplace (Majette, 2010). Given the high prevalence of chronic disease in the US, prevention and lifestyle approaches have become exceedingly important. IM has the potential to empower individuals to manage their own health and wellness (Riley, 2009). It is imperative that the Patient Protection and Affordable Care Act, with its focus on prevention, highlights and stresses the importance of integrative medicine in the US medical system.

References

Adler, S. R., & Fosket, J. R. (1999). Disclosing complementary and alternative medicine use in the medical encounter: A qualitative study in women with breast cancer. *The Journal of Family Practice, 48*, 453–458.

Ahn, A. C., Ngo-Metzger, Q., Legedza, A. T. R., Massagli, M. P., Clarridge, B. R., & Phillips, R. S. (2006). Complementary and alternative medical therapy use among Chinese and Vietnamese Americans: Prevalence, associated factors, and effects of patient – clinician communication. *American Journal of Public Health, 96*(4), 647–653.

Barnes, P. M., Bloom, B., & Nahin, R. L. (2008). Complementary and alternative medicine use among adults and children: United States, 2007. *National Health Statistics Reports, 12*, 1–23.

Barrett, B., Marchand, L., Scheder, J., Plane, M. B., Maberry, R., Appelbaum, D., et al. (2003). Themes of holism, empowerment, access, and legitimacy define complementary, alternative, and integrative medicine in relation to conventional biomedicine. *Journal of Alternative and Complementary Medicine, 9*, 937–947.

Bedi, M. K., & Shenefelt, P. D. (2002). Herbal therapy in dermatology. *Archives of Dermatology, 138*, 232–242.

Bensoussan, A., Talley, N. J., Hing, M., Menzies, R., Guo, A., & Ngu, M. (1998). Treatment of irritable bowel syndrome with Chinese herbal medicine: A randomized controlled trial. *The Journal of the American Medical Association, 280*, 1585–1589.

Berman, B. M., Lao, L., Langenberg, P., Lee, W. L., Gilpin, A. M., & Hochberg, M. C. (2004). Effectiveness of acupuncture as adjunctive therapy in osteoarthritis of the knee: A randomized, controlled trial. *Annals of Internal Medicine, 141*, 901–910.

Birdee, G. S., Wayne, P. M., Davis, R. B., Phillips, R. S., & Yeh, G. Y. (2009). T'ai chi and qigong for health: Patterns of use in the United States. *Journal of Alternative and Complementary Medicine, 15*, 969–973.

Bodeker, G., Kabatesi, D., Homsy, J., & King, R. (2000). A regional task force on traditional medicine and AIDS in East and Southern Africa. *Lancet, 355*, 1284.

Bodeker, G., Kronenberg, F., & Burford, G. (2007). Policy and public health perspectives on traditional, complementary, and alternative medicine: An overview. In G. Bodeker & G. Burford (Eds.), *Traditional, complementary, and alternative medicine: policy and public health perspectives*. Oxford: Imperial College Press.

Block, K. I. (2010). Cost savings with clinical solutions: The impact of reforming health and health care economics with integrative therapies. *Integrative Cancer Therapies, 9*, 129–135.

Burke, A., Upchurch, D. M., Dye, C., & Chyu, L. (2006). Acupuncture use in the United States: Findings from the national health interview survey. *Journal of Alternative and Complementary Medicine, 12*, 639–648.

Centers for Disease Control and Prevention. (2011). National health interview survey (Vol. 2011).

Chao, M. T., Wade, C., Kronenberg, F., Kalmuss, D., & Cushman, L. F. (2006). Women's reasons for complementary and alternative medicine use: Racial/ethnic differences. *Journal of Alternative and Complementary Medicine, 12*(8), 719–722.

Chen, H., Kramer, E. J., & Chen, T. (2003). The bridge program: A model for reaching Asian Americans. *Psychiatric Services, 54*, 1411–1412.

Cherkin, D. C., & MacCornack, F. A. (1989). Patient evaluations of low back pain care from family physicians and chiropractors. *The Western Journal of Medicine, 150*, 351–355.

Cohen, M. H., Ruggie, M., & Micozzi, M. S. (2006). *The practice of integrative medicine: A legal and operational guide*. New York: Springer.

Conboy, L., Patel, S., Kaptchuk, T. J., Gottlieb, B., Eisenberg, D., & Acevedo-Garcia, D. (2005). Sociodemographic determinants of the utilization of specific types of complementary and alternative medicine: An analysis based on a nationally representative survey sample. *Journal of Alternative and Complementary Medicine, 11*, 977–994.

Cook, A. (2008). Integrative medicine for the poor and underserved: A win-win situation. *Journal of Health Care for the Poor and Underserved, 19*, 1023–1028.

Cronan, T. A., Kaplan, R. M., Posner, L., Blumberg, E., & Kozin, F. (1989). Prevalence of the use of unconventional remedies for arthritis in a metropolitan community. *Arthritis and Rheumatism, 32*, 1604–1607.

Davis, R. E. (2000). Cultural health care or child abuse? The Southeast Asian practice of cao gio. *Journal of the American Academy of Nurse Practitioners, 12*, 89–95.

Deng, G., Weber, W., Sood, A., & Kemper, K. J. (2010). Research on integrative healthcare: Context and priorities. *Explore (NY), 6*, 143–158.

Denner, S. S. (2007). The advanced practice nurse and integration of complementary and alternative medicine: Emerging policy issues. *Holistic Nursing Practice, 21*, 152–159.

Eisenberg, D. M. (1997). Advising patients who seek alternative medical therapies. *Annals of Internal Medicine, 127*, 61–69.

Eisenberg, D. M., Davis, R. B., Ettner, S. L., Appel, S., Wilkey, S., Van Rompay, M., et al. (1998). Trends in alternative medicine use in the United States, 1990–1997: Results of a follow-up national survey. *The Journal of the American Medical Association, 280*, 1569–1575.

Eisenberg, D. M., Kessler, R. C., Foster, C., Norlock, F. E., Calkins, D. R., & Delbanco, T. L. (1993). Unconventional medicine in the united States. Prevalence, costs, and patterns of use. *The New England Journal of Medicine, 328*, 246–252.

Ernst, E., & White, A. R. (1998). Acupuncture for back pain: A meta-analysis of randomized controlled trials. *Archives of Internal Medicine, 158*, 2235–2241.

Goldman, J., Salus, M. K., Wolcott, D., & Kennedy, K. Y. (2003). *A coordinated response to child abuse and neglect: The foundation for practice.* Washington, DC: U.S. Department of Health and Human Services.

Gray, R. E., Fitch, M., Greenberg, M., Voros, P., Douglas, M. S., Labrecque, M., et al. (1997). Physician perspectives on unconventional cancer therapies. *Journal of Palliative Care, 13*, 14–21.

Hirschkorn, K. A. (2006). Exclusive versus everyday forms of professional knowledge: Legitimacy claims in conventional and alternative medicine. *Sociology of Health & Illness, 28*, 533–557.

Horrigan, B. J. (2010). Health care reform bill contains opportunities for integrative medicine. *Explore: The Journal of Science and Healing, 6*, 221–224.

IOM (Institute of Medicine). (2009). Summit on integrative medicine and the health of the public: A summary of the February 2009 summit. In A. M. Schultz, S. M. Chao, & J. M. McGinnis (Eds.), *Summit on integrative medicine and the health of the public.* Washington, DC: The National Academies Press.

Jibrin, I. (2010). Complementary and alternative medicine: The other healthcare reform. *Southern Medical Journal, 103*, 605–606.

Kaptchuk, T. J., & Eisenberg, D. M. (2001). Varieties of healing. 1: Medical pluralism in the United States. *Annals of Internal Medicine, 135*, 189–195.

Kessler, R. C., Davis, R. B., Foster, D. F., Van Rompay, M. I., Walters, E. E., Wilkey, S. A., et al. (2001). Long-term trends in the use of complementary and alternative medical therapies in the United States. *Annals of Internal Medicine, 135*, 262–268.

Krauss, H. H., Godfrey, C., Kirk, J., & Eisenberg, D. M. (1998). Alternative health care: Its use by individuals with physical disabilities. *Archives of Physical Medicine and Rehabilitation, 79*, 1440–1447.

Lee, M. M., Lin, S. S., Wrensch, M. R., Adler, S. R., & Eisenberg, D. (2000). Alternative therapies used by women with breast cancer in four ethnic populations. *Journal of the National Cancer Institute, 92*, 42–47.

Maizes, V., Rakel, D., & Niemiec, C. (2009). Integrative medicine and patient-centered care. *Explore: The Journal of Science and Healing, 5*, 277–289.

Majette, G. R. (2010). Healthcare reform & the missing voice of complementary and alternative medicine. *Houston Journal of Health Law & Policy,* pp. 35–62.

Mashour, N. H., Lin, G. I., & Frishman, W. H. (1998). Herbal medicine for the treatment of cardiovascular disease: Clinical considerations. *Archives of Internal Medicine, 158*, 2225–2234.

Medicare National Coverage Determinations Manual. (2001). American academy of pediatrics: Counseling families who choose complementary and alternative medicine for their child with chronic illness or disability. Committee on children with disabilities. *Pediatrics, 107*, 598–601.

Medicare National Coverage Determinations Manual. (2007). Healthy Workforce Act of 2007. In *S.1753.* United States: GovTrack.US.

Medicare National Coverage Determinations Manual. (2010). Patient Protection and Affordable Care Act. In *H.R. 3590,* Title IV: Prevention of chronic disease and improving public health. United States.

Mehta, D. H., Phillips, R. S., Davis, R. B., & McCarthy, E. P. (2007). Use of complementary and alternative therapies by Asian Americans. Results from the national health interview survey. *Journal of General Internal Medicine, 22*(6), 762–767.

Nahin, R. L., Barnes P. M., Stussman B. J., & Bloom, B. (2009). Costs of complementary and alternative medicine (CAM) and frequency of visits to CAM practitioners: United States, 2007. *National Health Statistics Reports,* pp. 1–14.

National Center for Complementary and Alternative Medicine. (2005). *Ayurvedic medicine: An introduction* (Vol. 2011). Bethesda, MD: Author.

National Center for Complementary and Alternative Medicine. (2007). *Acupuncture: An introduction* (Vol. 2011). Bethesda, MD: Author.

National Center for Complementary and Alternative Medicine. (2009). *Traditional Chinese medicine: An introduction* (Vol. 2011). Bethesda, MD: Author.

National Center for Complementary and Alternative Medicine. (2011). *NCCAM facts-at-a-glance and mission* (Vol. 2011). Bethesda, MD: National Institutes of Health.

National Center for Complementary and Alternative Medicine, National Institutes of Health. (2010). What is complementary and alternative medicine? (Vol. 2011). Bethesda, MD: Author.

O'Connor, B. B. (1995). Defining and describing complementary and alternative medicine. Panel on definition and description (pp. 49–57). In CAM Research Methodology Conference, Vol. 3: Alternative therapies in health and medicine.

Purnell, L. D. (2008). Traditional Vietnamese health and healing. *Urologic Nursing, 28*, 63–67.

Rao, D. (2006). Choice of medicine and hierarchy of resort to different health alternatives among Asian

Indian migrants in a metropolitan city in the USA. *Ethnicity and Health, 11*, 153–167.

Riley, D. (2009). The doctor's dilemma: Healthcare reform and integrative medicine. *Alternative Therapies in Health and Medicine, 15*, 10–11.

Ruggie, M., & Cohen, M. H. (2005). Integrative medicine centers: Moving health care in a new direction. *Seminars in Integrative Medicine, 3*, 9–16.

Ruy, H., Young, W. B., & Kwak, H. (2002). Differences in health insurance and health service utilization among Asian Americans: Method for using the NHIS to identify unique patterns between ethnic groups. *The International Journal of Health Planning and Management, 17*, 55–68.

Sibinga, E. M. S., Ottolini, M. C., Duggan, A. K., & Wilson, M. H. (2004). Parent-pediatrician communication about complementary and alternative medicine use for children. *Clinical Pediatrics, 43*, 367–373.

Sikand, A., & Laken, M. (1998). Pediatricians' experience with and attitudes toward complementary/alternative medicine. *Archives of Pediatrics & Adolescent Medicine, 152*, 1059–1064.

Smart, H. L., Mayberry, J. F., & Atkinson, M. (1986). Alternative medicine consultations and remedies in patients with the irritable bowel syndrome. *Gut, 27*, 826–828.

Steyer, T., Freed, G., & Lantz, P. (2002). Medicaid reimbursement for alternative therapies. *InnoVision Communications, 8*, 84–88.

Su, D., & Li, L. (2011). Trends in the use of complementary and alternative medicine in the United States: 2002–2007. *Journal of Health Care for the Poor and Underserved, 22*, 296–310.

Su, D., Li, L., & Pagan, J. A. (2008). Acculturation and the use of complementary and alternative medicine. *Social Science & Medicine, 66*, 439–453.

The Cochrane CAM Field. (2012). Complementary medicine field. In T. C. Collaboration (Ed.), *The Cochrane Library*.

The Consortium of Academic Health Centers for Integrative Medicine. (2009, January). Definition of integrative medicine.

United States Census. (2010). 2010 census results. In *2010 census data* (Vol. 2011).

US Department of Health and Human Services. (1994). *Alternative medicine: Expanding medical horizons: A report to the national institutes of health on alternative medical systems and practices in the United States*. Bethesda, MD: Public Health Service, National Institutes of Health.

Wetzel, M. S., Eisenberg, D. M., & Kaptchuk, T. J. (1998). Courses involving complementary and alternative medicine at US medical schools. *The Journal of the American Medical Association, 280*, 784–787.

White House Commission on Complementary and Alternative Medicine Policy. (2002). White House Commission on Complementary and Alternative Medicine Policy FINAL REPORT.

Wong, V. (2009). Use of complementary and alternative medicine (CAM) in autism spectrum disorder (ASD): Comparison of Chinese and western culture (part A). *Journal of Autism and Developmental Disorders, 39*, 454–463.

Wong, L. K., Jue, P., Lam, A., Yeung, W., Cham-Wah, Y., & Birtwhistle, R. (1998). Chinese herbal medicine and acupuncture. How do patients who consult family physicians use these therapies? *Canadian Family Physician, 44*, 1009–1015.

World Health Organization. (2008). Traditional medicine (Vol. 134). Geneva: Author.

Wu, A. P. W., Burke, A., & LeBaron, S. (2007). Use of traditional medicine by immigrant Chinese patients. *Family Medicine, 39*, 195–200.

A Passage to a Good Death: End of Life Care for Asian Americans

25

Evaon Wong-Kim and Nancy J. Burke

Mrs. Yee was an elderly Chinese immigrant woman diagnosed with end stage lung cancer. Her family was considering transferring Mrs. Yee to a nursing home for hospice care. To qualify for hospice care, a Do Not Resuscitate (DNR) order had to be obtained. The physician handling her case realized, after speaking with her through an interpreter, that Mrs. Yee did not understand the meaning of a DNR order. When he brought the issue of the DNR up with her family via an interpreter, Ms. Yee's son and husband responded angrily. Later, when interviewing Mrs. Yee again using a different interpreter, the social worker realized that Mrs. Yee was fully aware of her prognosis and the possibility of death within months or even weeks. Soon after, Mrs. Yee suffered cardiac arrest and was put on a respirator in the Intensive Care Unit. Since both her lungs and liver failed to function due to the spread of the cancer, the Intensive Care Team discussed withdrawing the life support system that was artificially sustaining her with Mrs. Yee's family. After seeing all of the machines that had maintained Mrs. Yee's vital signs, her husband could not give up on the medi-cal technology that he felt might still save her life. When their son, Wai, was approached regarding withdrawing life support, he responded to the team, "I cannot tell you to kill my mother."

Two weeks later, after intense counseling and reassurance, the family agreed to turn off the machines. Mrs. Yee died three hours after life support was withdrawn. After giving consent to withdraw Mrs. Yee's life support, the son and husband told the social worker that they felt the medical team acted in an unethical manner when they told Mrs. Yee directly that she had a poor prognosis. They believed that this knowledge caused her to give up the will to live. The family also believed that the discussion of death in front of her evoked an evil spirit that eventually took over her body. The father and son felt that if they had been allowed to protect Mrs. Yee as was their responsibility, she would not have suffered such a tragic end.

Mrs. Yee's family's experience highlights the unique rifts family dynamics, quality of life perceptions, culturally-based philosophies about caring for the terminally ill, language barriers, and decision-making expectations can cause between Asian American patients and health care providers. The Yee family, for example, did not understand the concept of hospice care, informed consent, meanings of a DNR, and the need for Mrs. Yee to be transferred to a long-term care facility. They had witnessed the deaths of many close relatives in hospitals in China, and assumed the same would not happen in America. It was shocking to them to learn that there were limitations in the medical system, and that the withdrawal

E. Wong-Kim (✉)
Department of Social Work, California State University, East Bay, Hayward, CA, USA
e-mail: evaon@csueastbay.edu

N.J. Burke
Department of Anthropology, History, and Social Medicine, Helen Diller Comprehensive Cancer Center, University of California, San Francisco, CA, USA

G.J. Yoo et al. (eds.), *Handbook of Asian American Health*,
DOI 10.1007/978-1-4614-2227-3_25, © Springer Science+Business Media, LLC 2013

of life support was a decision to be made by the family, not physicians. They did not trust this process and were left feeling mistreated, isolated and discriminated against by health care providers during the time Mrs. Yee was hospitalized.

On the other hand, providers who took care of Mrs. Yee felt that the family was being unreasonable and that family members were not communicating openly with the medical team. As a result, the health care team felt inhibited in their attempts to provide comfort care and to help Mrs. Yee die peacefully. Issues relating to decision-making and pain control raised in Mrs. Yee's case are particularly pertinent problems that may create difficulties for caregivers, families, as well as health care providers in caring for patients.

The present chapter discusses end of life care issues that are important to Asian Americans. While there is great ethnic diversity within the group "Asian American" and a breadth of difference in end of life preferences within each subgroup, this chapter takes on the challenge of identifying some cross-cutting themes in the growing scholarship addressing death and end of life care among Asian Americans. First, we set the context for the discussion of end of life among Asian Americans by recognizing that this occurs within American hospitals subject to the constraints and benefits of the highly technological US healthcare system. Second, we identify key concepts mobilized in end of life care (e.g. comfort care, palliative care, hospice) and review recent research on these topics in Asian American populations. Third, we address disclosure practices and pain management. Last, we suggest areas for future research and implications for Asian American end of life care.

American Healthcare

American health care spending reached $2.5 trillion in 2009 which translates to $8,086 per person or 17.6% of the nation's Gross Domestic Product (Wilson, 2011), yet the United States is not the healthiest nation in the world as indicated by a shorter life expectancy, higher infant mortality rate and chronic diseases as compared to other industrialized countries (WHO, 2000). The United States also ranked last overall with poor scores on all three major indicators of long, healthy, and productive lives (Davis, Schoen, & Stremikis, 2010). Parallel to this issue we also spend a good amount of resources to care for people during the last 6 months of their life. The population 65 years and over increased at a faster rate (15.1 percent) than the total U.S population (9.7 percent) between 2000 and 2010 (US Census, 2010). As a result, more people will be diagnosed and living with terminal illnesses such as cancer. One eighth of Medicare total expenditures are spent on patients in their last month of life (Smith et al., 2003). This high cost of keeping people alive during the last stage of life has created a great deal of discussion and introduced difficult choices. One would expect that with this kind of expense, people should be able to choose a "good death," but in reality dying free of pain, dying with dignity, and dying surrounded by family and loved ones hardly describes the American experience of death and dying.

Anthropologist Sharon Kaufman's work on dying in American hospitals (2006) chronicles the painful and seemingly impossible processes families experience when faced with the "decision" to end life-sustaining technologies. Recent work in Japan illustrates the difficulty physicians face in managing family expectations and their own ethical responsibilities at the end of life. A qualitative study of physician withdrawal of life support suggests that, unlike the families in Kaufman's ethnography, or Mrs. Yee's husband and son, families in Japan were not asked to make the decision to withdraw life support (Aita & Kai, 2009). Rather, it was the physician's decision and many were reluctant to do so if withdrawal would cause immediate death. Physicians reported that they would feel the death was their responsibility in these cases, rather than the fault of the underlying illness (Aita & Kai, 2009). Physicians also reported a preference for a "soft landing" (a slow and gradual death without drastic and immediate changes) as a way to help the family accept the patient's death and to facilitate the family's involvement in the dying process and the death itself, elements of a 'good death' in Japan (Aita & Kai, 2009). This family-oriented end of life care, however, was observed to not always occur with the family's informed consent. Rather the authors describe the "soft landing" as a "well-intentioned paternalist approach so that the moral responsibility for the patient's death is not shared with the family members" (Aita & Kai, 2009). Such an approach contrasts sharply with the family-based decision making in which the Yee family, and all families in American hospitals, were asked to engage.

The ambiguity faced by Japanese physicians in Aita and Kai's 2009 study raises two important concerns when thinking about Asian American end of life care in American hospitals. First, clinical practices in countries of origin that differ from those in the United States may strongly influence immigrant patient and family expectations of end of life care. As exemplified in Mrs. Yee's family's experience, being faced with the responsibility of the decision to end life support was unexpected and perceived as inappropriate. Second, the concept of a 'good death' is multivocalic and complex. In Aita and Kai's study, physicians often performed seemingly unnecessary cardiopulmonary resuscitation (CPR) on dying patients to enable family to reach the hospital due to the belief that having family and loved ones share in the dying process were important aspects of "good death" (Aita & Kai, 2009). A study of Chinese seniors' perspectives on end of life decisions (Bowman & Singer, 2001) revealed that a "good death" was perceived as when a person had completed his or her contribution to society through obligations such as work and family. Anthropologist Scott Stonington (Aita & Kai, 2009) describes a good death in Northern Thailand as being preceded by children giving "heart power" or encouragement (emotional support that fills the heart and prevents a worrying mind from harming the body), and ending with the dying elder taking his or her last breath at home. The key, Stonington found, was that death was conceived as taking place in a moment – the last breath – and not as a period of time in which death could be considered and planned ("end of life"). Stonington's article traces how this perception of death has undergone change in the last 20 years as the concept of "end of life" and the practice of palliative care has been introduced in Thai hospitals.

In American hospitals, more likely than not, lack of planning, complicated medical intervention and the medical system's greater focus on treating – than not treating – those who have terminal illnesses prevents the ideal from being the reality. Because of the tendency to treat, many patients receive acute care intervention and as a result are kept alive artificially, whether they want to be kept alive via technology or not (Kagawa-Singer & Blackhall, 2001). Therefore, rather than experiencing the dying process and death *with* patients, family members are faced with an array of decisions about DNRs, hospice care, and ending life support.

Understanding End of Life Care

When discussing end of life care, there are several different terminologies used in medicine that can be confusing to those less familiar with medical terminology. Three of these terms are *comfort care*, *palliative care*, and *hospice care*. Each term reflects a different level of care offered to people with very limited chances of getting well, for which medical treatment is no longer considered productive. One common theme across these three terms is that they usually imply that the patient is dying. However, some medical treatments may still be appropriate during this period of time to keep the patient comfortable. Health care providers also use these terms to differentiate the type of care a person may receive during the end stages of life.

Comfort Care

Comfort care is focused on relieving symptoms and optimizing patient comfort. Comfort care does not seek to aggressively treat illness or disease, especially when these treatments are not going to cure the person (Kolcaba, 1995). Comfort care can be given at home, at nursing facilities, or in a hospital. When comfort care is mentioned, it indicates the beginning of discussions with health care providers that treatments are no longer available to stop the progression of the disease(s).

Comfort care infers pain management, a complex area for Asian American patients as indicated in a needs assessment conducted with Chinese elders in Northern California (Chow, Auh, Scharlach, Lehning, & Goldstein, 2010). Interviews discussed: (1) lack of information in Chinese on pain management; (2) poor communication between patients and providers due to linguistic and cultural differences; and (3) deep fear of addiction to pain medication, even in the last stage of illness. We discuss pain management, and the use of complementary and alternative medicine (CAM) for these purposes, in more depth below.

Palliative Care

Palliative Care (from Latin *palliare*, to cloak) is any form of medical care or treatment that focuses on reducing the severity of disease symptoms, in contrast to treatments attempting to delay or reverse progression of an illness disease in order to provide a cure (Jordhoy et al., 2007). It is designed as a comprehensive approach to treating patients and families living with a life-threatening or severe advanced illness expected to progress toward dying, focusing on alleviating suffering and promoting quality of life (Liao & Arnold, 2006). The psychological and spiritual well-being of the patient is a priority in addition to the patient's physical status.

A recent study of the experiences of Chinese American and Mexican American immigrant families requiring pediatric palliative care, however, found that language and cultural differences created barriers to the kinds of information sharing necessary to promote the psychological and spiritual well-being of patients and families (Davies, Contro, Larson, & Widger, 2010). Instead, the authors found that communication problems contributed to frustration, anger, and sadness for parents, feelings that continued long after the child's death (Davies et al., 2010). The persistence of anger and guilt was also present in the experience of Mr. Yee and his son, who, despite giving 'informed consent', were left feeling mistreated and isolated after Mrs. Yee's death. While the goal of palliative care is to assist

patients to achieve the best possible quality of life by relieving suffering and controlling pain and symptoms (Kirk & Margaret, 2010), communication problems between the interdisciplinary health care teams offering care and immigrant families may inhibit success. These challenges extend to the next stage of end of life care, hospice.

Hospice Care

Hospice is a philosophy and type of care that provides comprehensive, loving support for people with terminal illnesses that have progressed beyond a physician's expectation of cure (Smith, Earle, & McCarthy, 2009). Hospice care is designed to help patients and their families with the end-of-life transition. The care model provides a choice for patients who do not want aggressive interventions for an otherwise terminal condition (Chilton, Wong-Kim, Guidry, Gor, & Jones, 2008; Vig, Starks, Taylor, Hopley, & Fryer-Edwards, 2010). Hospice care includes the same effective pain management techniques as used in palliative care or comfort care. Hospice care is designed to help people live and die with dignity, in comfort, and in peace as they approach the end of their lives (American Academy of Hospice and Palliative Medicine, 2011).

Unlike comfort care and palliative care, there are set criteria for receiving hospice services. They include (1) physician's documentation to indicate the patient's prognosis is 6 months or less, (2) willingness to forego active medical treatment, and (3) a "Do Not Resuscitate" (DNR) order on file (Casarett, 2011). In other words, receipt of hospice care requires open discussion, communication, and documentation of impending death, something often avoided in Asian American families. Recent research, however, has called in to question the assumption that Asian American elders do not want to know about their diagnosis. A study of decision-making at the end of life in Japanese American families, for example, unexpectedly found that a high proportion of deceased relatives (72.7%) had had advance care directives (ACDs) in place prior to death (Colclough & Young, 2007). The deceased family member made decisions when he or she was healthier, or before the decision was required, which the authors argue provides evidence for the value of explicit discussion about ACDs and apparent willingness of Japanese American families to talk about death and dying (Colclough & Young, 2007). A study of what and when Korean American older adults want to know about serious illness recently found that participants were more likely to prefer complete disclosure if there was very little chance of survival (Berkman & Ko, 2010). The same study found that Korean American physicians tended toward less disclosure, likely due to their cultural beliefs or assumption that this was expected of them (Berkman & Ko, 2010). As Kagawa-Singer and Blackhall argued in 2001, "assuming a Chinese woman would not want to be told her diagnosis because she is Chinese is stereotyping. Insisting that she must be told, even at the risk of violating her rights, is a form of cultural imperialism. The challenge is to navigate between these poles" (p. 2993). The requirements for hospice necessitate such navigation.

While previous research found that Asians rarely utilize hospice services (Ngo-Metzger, Phillips, & McCarthy, 2008), a recent study of home-based palliative care services for underserved populations found hospice care to be acceptable and appropriate to both patients and caregivers in an Asian American population (Fernandes et al., 2010). Whether hospice care is provided at home or in nursing home or in-patient hospice setting some argue that this may influence utilization of services (Kagawa-Singer & Blackhall, 2001). Filial piety (expectation that children will care for their parents), an important concept in many parts of Asia including Korea, China, and Japan, may partially account for this preference (Berkman & Ko, 2010). Hospice constitutes acceptance of care from outsiders, and may potentially dishonor the parents by suggesting to the family and community that the family is unable to provide adequate care (Kagawa-Singer & Blackhall, 2001). Accepting hospice care in the home allows for more direct oversight and control, thus enabling family members to feel they are the primary caregivers and are fulfilling filial obligations (Kagawa-Singer & Blackhall). Concepts of filial piety are not static, however, and are undergoing modification in the United States. As Frank and colleagues argue in their study of Korean immigrant elders' end of life expectations, "changing gender roles and economic stresses that result in women's fuller participation in the labor force make it difficult for wives, daughters-in-law, and other female kin to provide the same level of support for parents that was expected of them traditionally" (Frank et al., p. 414). In the context of changing family structures and subsequent modifications of concepts such as filial piety in the United States, effective communication of the value and availability of hospice services is essential (Jang, Chiriboga, Allen, Kwak, & Haley, 2010).

Informed Consent and Disclosure: To Tell or Not to Tell

Independence, individual rights, and the value of personal autonomy underlie the quest for informed consent in the United States (Widdershoven & Verheggen, 1999). Such values are not inherent in other cultures. In Japan, for example, it is not uncommon for physicians not to disclose a grim prognosis to the patient. Very often the family is informed of the poor prognosis instead of the patient because it is perceived as the family's responsibility to take care of the dying patient (Gabbay et al., 2005). Disclosing information such as a poor prognosis is sometimes considered unethical because it may cause patients to feel abandoned and speed up the dying process (Bito & Asai, 2007).

Similar to disclosure practices in Japan, forcing Chinese families to tell patients about their poor prognoses or insisting on disclosing poor prognosis related to treatment outcomes is to make death a reality, like a self-fulfilling prophecy, and many Chinese families believe it will cause the death of the patient (Hsu, O'Connor, & Lee, 2009). As evidenced in Mrs. Yee's son's and father's reaction to the health care team's communication of prognosis, speaking openly of death may be seen as equal to inviting death and thus considered extremely rude and disrespectful. Instead, withholding information may be equated with maintaining hope and keeping the patient alive. Informed decision making, valued in Western medicine, can conflict with the family's perception of their duty to protect the patient from knowing about his/her immanent death and to make the remaining time comfortable and free of distress.

At the same time, recent research suggests great diversity in attitudes toward diagnosis and prognosis disclosure among Asians. Studies in Japan (Miyata, Takahashi, Saito, Tachimori, & Kai, 2005) and Taiwan (Tang & Lee, 2004) indicate that the majority preferred to know the complete truth about cancer diagnosis. Studies with older patients in Korea (Noone, Crowe, Pillay, & O'Keefe, 2000; Yun, Lee, Kim, Heo, Kim, & Lee, 2004) and cancer patients in Taiwan (Tang et al., 2006) found that participants wanted more information than their relatives recommended. A cross-sectional study of 26 Korean Amerian elders found that most thought doctors should tell patients (n = 23) and relatives (n = 25) if they had cancer, and should tell patients (n = 22) and relatives if they were likely to die from the disease (Berkman & Ko, 2009). Less than half (n = 9) felt that doctors should not discuss death and dying with patients. Those who agreed that a doctor should disclose a cancer diagnosis to the patient were younger and had lived in the United States longer than those who disagreed (Berkman & Ko, 2009). As a result, researchers recommend against health care professionals making assumptions regarding preferences for disclosure about diagnosis, prognosis or treatment options on the basis of culture or age of patient (Berkman & Ko, 2009, 2010; Kagawa-Singer & Blackhall, 2001).

Who Makes the Decisions?

Disclosure preferences are complicated by the value placed on non-verbal or indirect communication in many Asian societies as an important means of interpersonal connection. *Zhih Yi*, the Chinese term for nonverbal communication, is translated as "just knowing what the other thinks and feels" (Kagawa-Singer & Blackhall, 2001). The Japanese *inshin denshin* holds a similar meaning (knowing without being told), and the Korean *nunchi* communicates knowing through social, nonverbal cues (Kagawa-Singer & Blackhall, 2001). In their study of Korean American older adults' disclosure preferences, Berkman & Ko, (2010) found that the ambiguity of *nunchi* (nonverbal communication) allowed participants to save face by not having their feelings hurt and "minimizing the burden" of knowledge (p. 252). One effect of these communication processes is that older Asian American patients may assume that their children know their end of life preferences, and therefore perceive direct discussion, such as that needed to develop an advance care directive (ACD), as unnecessary.

If a person is not able to make his or her own health care decision due to a sudden loss of cognitive function or a long term progression of diseases, an ACD can be created before this loss and decisions of end of life care can be made in advance. ACD is a document intended to maximize the decision-making power of a person in terms of his or her end-of-life treatment. It is a combination of two documents, the Natural Death Act Declaration (known as living will) and the Durable Power of Attorney for Health Care (or DPAHC). It contains two parts, the instructional directives, which allow a person to indicate his or her health care preference in terminal conditions, and the appointment of a proxy to make such decisions (Pearlman, Cole, Patrick, Starks, & Cain, 1995). These two parts are independent from each other – a person can choose to fill out either part or both sections. A 2001 study designed to develop a culturally appropriate Chinese advance directive document found the endeavor to be fruitless (Bowman & Singer, 2001). The main problem was the proxy decision-making feature of the document. Participants did not value this as to identify a proxy or proxies was seen to limit the opinions of other family members not named. By doing so, participants felt the document could inhibit family decision-making (Bowman & Singer, 2001).

Pain Control

Pain is a very important aspect in end of life care because it can greatly affect a person's quality of life when coping with terminal diseases. (Herr et al., 2010). However, very few research studies have been conducted among Asian Americans to ascertain how cultural beliefs and orientations affect acceptance and use of pain medication. Two other significant issues include communicating with medical and support services regarding pain management and the use of Complimentary and Alternative Medicine (CAM) for pain control. While there is a dearth of research conducted in the area of pain control and end of life care among the Asian American populations, some observations can be extrapolated from Chinese American breast cancer patients who reported a decrease in quality of life due to pain and treatment side effects (Bloom, Stewart, Johnston, & Banks, 1998). Another study compared Chinese born and American born breast cancer patients and their use of CAM for pain control (Wong-Kim & Merighi, 2007). Women from both groups experienced pain during active treatment for their cancer, as well as after treatments were completed. However, when compared with the foreign-born research participants, U.S.-born participants reported a lower level of pain medication and described a smaller range of pain.

The use of herbs and other traditional and culturally accepted medication for pain is very common among Asian American subgroups. For many Asian immigrants, number of years residing in the U.S. and the age they migrated to the US as well as the level of acculturation may explain attitudes about CAM and the concept of healing in Chinese culture. Affordability can be a barrier to using CAM to control pain (Wong-Kim & Merighi, 2007), as most CAM treatments are not covered by medical insurance such as Medicare and Medicaid (National Center for Complementary and Alternative Medicine, 2008). Given that many Asian immigrants have limited monetary resources this greatly reduces the opportunities for the use of CAM for pain control. In addition to affordability, doubts about quality assurance are also identified as a barrier to utilizing CAM for pain management.

Being able to use CAM appropriately and how to identify a skilled and knowledgeable CAM practitioner are also important determinants of CAM use for pain control. In order to support Asian Americans who are receiving end of life care, quality assurance must be addressed at the practitioner level, reimbursement for third party payment, and integration of Western and CAM approaches to healing. Given the cultural acceptance of using CAM (especially herbs and acupuncture) in the Asian Americans community, health care practitioners and health insurance providers should make additional efforts to improve access to the full range of CAM therapies. Conventional pain medications are often prescribed by physicians, despite the fact that some patients express concern about the side effects of these medications, as well as the potential for long-term issues including kidney or liver damage. One advantage of using CAM for pain control is minimizing such adverse side effects.

Although studies indicate an increase in CAM use in the U.S. general population (Ndao-Brumblay & Green, 2010) and in people diagnosed with cancer, end of life care and the use of CAM for pain control are two distinct and often separate disciplines. For instance, there can be little communication or coordination between practitioners in these two disciplines and patients may be faced with getting information about CAM through a variety of sources and not from their physician. Bringing Western medical providers and CAM practitioners together can increase the likelihood that patients who are receiving care at their end of life can also benefit from coordinated and culturally appropriate and sensitive pain management. They will have improved access to a variety of treatment and pain management options. These options can help achieve good quality of life for dying patients. Future medical research should look at the possibility of a more comprehensive approach to end of life care that includes a combination of Western medicine and CAM for pain control. A more holistic approach to pain control will maximize quality of life for all dying patients.

Future Directions

During this special season of the life cycle, the roles of health care professionals are to work creatively and sensitively with the patients and their families to meet their needs, and help them create an environment in which they feel supported and comfortable during their final stages of life. While it is important for health care professionals to provide ongoing and open communication with patients, and their families or decision-makers, the research reviewed in this chapter illuminates the challenges to effective communication and the need for further training. Preventing and treating pain, supporting families and caregivers, ensuring continuity of care, making informed decisions, attending to emotional and spiritual well-being, sustaining function, and improving quality of life are some of the important goals for health care professionals during this important passage of life.

Future directions in addressing end of life issues that are important to Asian Americans include how cultural practices can be used to enhance a "good death." Harnessing community resources to help address communication and linguistic barriers during this vulnerable time is an important area for further exploration. The Chinese American Coalition for Compassionate Care (CACCC) provides one model for possible emulation. The CACCC is the only community-based organization in the United States devoted solely to end of life education and services for Chinese Americans. The CACCC aims to consolidate the most relevant and reliable information on end of life and to provide a centralized information resource for Chinese American families (Chou, Stokes, Citko, & Davies, 2008). Their collection of bilingual materials has been adopted by the National Hospice and Palliative Care Organization (2010) for their bilingual archive and is publically available (www.caccc-usa.org). In addition the organization has developed a speaker's bureau and held trainings for lay health workers to address end of life issues at the community level (Chou et al., 2008). Such mobilization of community assets bodes well for the advancement of more culturally informed care for both patients and families at the end of life.

References

Aita, K., & Kai, I. (2010). Physician's psychosocial barriers to different modes of withdrawal of life support in critical care: A qualitative study in Japan. *Social Science & Medicine, 70*, 616–622.

American Academy of Hospice and Palliative Medicine. (2011). Retrieved June 15, 2011, from www.aahpm.org.

Berkman, C. S., & Ko, E. (2009). Preferences for disclosure of information about serious illness among older Korean American immigrants in New York city. *Journal of Palliative Medicine, 12*(4), 351–357.

Berkman, C. S., & Ko, E. (2010). What and when Korean American older adults want to know about serious illness. *Journal of Psychosocial Oncology, 28*(3), 244–259.

Bito, S., & Asai, A. (2007). Attitudes and behaviors of Japanese physicians concerning withholding and withdrawal of life-sustaining treatment for end-of-life patients: Results from an internet survey. *BMC Medical Ethics, 8*, 7.

Bloom, J. R., Stewart, S. L., Johnston, M., & Banks, P. (1998). Intrusiveness of illness and quality of life in young women with breast cancer. *Psycho-Oncology, 7*(2), 89–100.

Bowman, K. W., & Singer, P. A. (2001). Chinese seniors' perspectives on end-of-life decisions. *Social Science & Medicine, 53*, 455–464.

Casarett, D. J. (2011). Rethinking hospice eligibility criteria. *Journal of the American Medical Association, 305*(10), 1031–1032.

Chilton, J. A., Wong-Kim, E. C., Guidry, J. J., Gor, B. J., & Jones, L. A. (2008). The utility of a connecting framework to facilitate understanding of and reduce the disparities in hospice care experienced by racial and ethnic minorities. *Primary Psychiatry, 15*(10), 38–44.

Chou, W.-Y., Stokes, S. C., Citko, J., & Davies, B. (2008). Improving end of life care through community-based grassroot collaboration: development of the Chinese American coalition of compassionate care. *Journal of Palliative Care, 24*(1), 31–40.

Chow, J. C.-C., Auh, E. Y., Scharlach, A. E., Lehning, A. J., & Goldstein, C. (2010). Types and sources of support received by family caregivers of older adults from diverse racial and ethnic groups. *Journal of Ethnic & Cultural Diversity in Social Work: Innovation in Theory, Research & Practice, 19*(3), 175–194.

Colclough, Y. Y., & Young, H. M. (2007). Decision making at end of life among Japanese American families. *Journal of Family Nursing, 13*, 201–224.

Davies, B., Contro, N., Larson, J., & Widger, K. (2010). Culturally-sensitive information-sharing in pediatric palliative care. *Pediatrics, 125*, e859–e865.

Davis, K., Schoen, C., & Stremikis, K. (2010). *Mirror mirror on the wall, how the performance of the U.S. health care system compares internationally, 2010 update*. New York: The Commonwealth Fund.

Fernandes, R., Braun, K. L., Ozawa, J., Compton, M., Guzman, C., & Somogyi-Zalud, E. (2010).

Home-based palliative care services for underserved populations. *Journal of Palliative Medicine, 13*(4), 413–419.

Frank, G., Blackhall, L. J., Michel, V., Murphy, S. T., Azen, S. P., & Park, K. (1998). A discourse of relationships in bioethics: Patient autonomy and end-of-life decision making among elderly Korean Americans. *Medical Anthropology Quarterly, 12*(4), 403–423.

Gabbay, B. B., Matsumura, S., Etzioni, S., Asch, S. M., Rosenfeld, K. E., Shiojiri, T., et al. (2005). Negotiating end-of-life decision making: A comparison of Japanese and U.S. residents' approaches. *Academic Medicine, 80*(7), 617–621.

Green, J. W. (2008). *Beyond the good death. The anthropology of modern dying*. Philadelphia: University of Pennsylvania Press.

Herr, K., Titler, M., Fine, P., Sanders, S., Cavanaugh, J., Swegle, J., et al. (2010). Assessing and treating pain in hospices: Current state of evidence-based practices. *Journal of Pain and Symptom Management, 39*(5), 803–819.

Hsu, C. Y., O'Connor, M., & Lee, S. (2009). Understandings of death and dying for people of Chinese origin. *Death Studies, 33*(2), 153–174.

Jang, Y., Chiriboga, D. A., Allen, J. Y., Kwak, J., & Haley, W. E. (2010). Willingness of older Korean-American adults to use hospice. *Journal of the American Geriatrics Society, 58*(2), 352–356.

Jordhoy, M. S., Ringdal, G. I., Helbostad, J. L., Oldervoll, L., Loge, J. H., & Kaasa, S. (2007). Assessing physical functioning: A systematic review of quality of life measures developed for use in palliative care. *Palliative Medicine, 21*(8), 673–682.

Kagawa-Singer, M., & Blackhall, L. J. (2001). Negotiating cross-cultural issues at the end of life: "You got to go where he lives". *Journal of the American Medical Association, 286*(23), 2993–3001.

Kaufman, S. R. (2006). *And a time to die: How American hospitals shape the end of life* (1st ed.). Chicago: University of Chicago Press.

Kirk, T. W., & Margaret, M. M. (2010). National Hospice and Palliative Care Organization (NHPCO) position statement and commentary on the use of palliative sedation in imminently dying terminally ill patients. *Journal of Pain and Symptom Management, 39*(5), 914–923.

Kolcaba, K. Y. (1995). The art of comfort care. *Journal of Nursing Scholarship, 27*(4), 287–289.

Liao, S., & Arnold, R. M. (2006). Caring for caregivers: The essence of palliative care. *Journal of Palliative Medicine, 9*(5), 1172–1173.

Miyata, H., Takahashi, M., Saito, T., Tachimori, H., & Kai, I. (2005). Disclosure preferences regarding cancer diagnosis and prognosis: To tell or not to tell? *Journal of Medical Ethics, 31*(8), 447–451.

National Center for Complementary and Alternative Medicine, National Institutes of Health. (2008). Paying for complementary and alternative medicine treatment: Information for patient. *Journal of Pain & Palliative Care Pharmacotherapy, 22*(2), 153–157.

National Hospice and Palliative Care Organization. (2010). *NHPCO facts and figures: Hospice care in America*. Retrieved June 12, 2011, from http://www.nhpco.org/files/public/Statistics_Research/Hospice_Facts_Figures_Oct-2010.pdf.

Ndao-Brumblay, S. K., & Green, C. R. (2010). Predictors of complementary and alternative medicine use in chronic pain patients. *Pain Medicine, 11*(1), 16–24.

Ngo-Metzger, Q., Phillips, R. S., & McCarthy, E. P. (2008). Ethnic disparities in hospice use among Asian-American and Pacific Islander patients dying with cancer. *Journal of the American Geriatrics Society, 56*(1), 139–144.

Noone, I., Crowe, M., Pillay, I., & O'Keefe, S. T. (2000). Telling the truth about cancer: Views of elderly patients and their relatives. *Irish Medical Journal, 93*(4), 104–105.

Pearlman, R. A., Cole, W. G., Patrick, D. L., Starks, H. E., & Cain, K. C. (1995). Advance care planning: Eliciting patient preferences for life-sustaining treatment. *Patient Education and Counseling, 26*(1–3), 353–361.

Smith, T. J., Coyne, P., Cassel, B., Penberthy, L., Hopson, A., & Hager, M. A. (2003). A high-volume specialist palliative care unit and team May reduce in-hospital end-of-life care costs. *Journal of Palliative Medicine, 6*(5), 699–705.

Smith, A. K., Earle, C. C., & McCarthy, E. P. (2009). Racial and ethnic differences in end-of-life care in fee-for-service Medicare beneficiaries with advanced cancer. *Journal of the American Geriatric Society, 57*, 153–158.

Stonington, S. (2011). Facing death, gazing inward: End-of-life and the transformation of clinical subjectivity in Thailand. *Culture, Medicine and Psychiatry, 35*, 113–133. online first 15 May.

Tang, S. T., & Lee, S. Y. C. (2004). Cancer diagnosis and prognosis and prognosis in Taiwan: Patient preferences versus experiences. *Psycho-Oncology, 13*, 1–13.

Tang, S., Liu, T., Lai, M., Liu, L., Chen, C., & Koong, S. (2006). Congruence of knowledge, experiences and preferences for disclosure of diagnosis and prognosis between terminally ill cancer patients and their family caregivers in Taiwan. *Cancer Investigation, 24*(4), 360–366.

United States Census. (2010). Retrieved June 1, 2011, from http://2010.census.gov/2010census/.

Vig, E. K., Starks, H., Taylor, J. S., Hopley, E. K., & Fryer-Edwards, K. (2010). Why don't patients enroll in hospice? Can we do anything about it? *Journal of General Internal Medicine, 25*(10), 1009–1019.

Weijer, C. (2005). A death in the family: Reflections on the Terri Schiavo case. *Canadian Medical Association Journal, 172*(9), 1197–1198.

Widdershoven, G. A. M., & Verheggen, F. W. S. M. (1999). Improving informed consent by implementing shared decision making in health care. *IRB: A Review of Human Subjects Research, 21*(4), 1–4.

Wilson, K. B. (2011). California Health Care Almanac, health care costs 101. *California HealthCare Foundation, Oakland CA*. Retrieved June 9, 2011, from http://www.chcf.org/publications/2011/05/health-care-costs-101.

Wong-Kim, E., & Merighi, J. R. (2007). Complementary and alternative medicine for pain management in U.S.- and foreign-born Chinese women with breast cancer. *Journal of Health Care for the Poor and Underserved, 18*, 118–129.

World Health Organization. (2000). *World health report 2000*. Geneva: WHO.

Yun, Y. H., Lee, G. G., Kim, S. Y., Heo, D. S., Kim, J. S., Lee, K. S., Hong, Y. S., et al. (2004). The attitudes of cancer patients and their families toward the disclosure of terminal illness. *Journal of Clinical Oncology, 22*, 307–314.

Early Chinese Immigrants Organizing for Healthcare: The Establishment of the Chinese Hospital in San Francisco

26

Laureen D. Hom

The Chinese Hospital of San Francisco is the first independent hospital in the United States with the mission to provide accessible health care to the Chinese American community. The Hospital was founded in 1925 and was one of the few modern American hospitals of the early twentieth century to provide modern Western care to the first Asian immigrants. Despite access to limited resources and finances, the Chinese community leaders were able to establish and sustain this hospital to help improve the health of the Chinatown community when the government and mainstream society refused to do so. The history of its establishment is one of the earliest moments of the Chinese American community mobilizing in response to the discrimination they faced and working together to build the San Francisco Chinatown community.

The Early Chinese Immigrants

The first Chinese to immigrate to San Francisco was recorded in the year 1848. Only three Chinese were documented in California in that year, and by 1852, approximately 20,000 Chinese had resided in California. San Francisco was the port of entry for many of the Chinese who were immigrating to the U.S.

Most of these early immigrants came as laborers who were hoping for better financial opportunities. China was facing much social and political upheaval towards the turn of the century, and local financial opportunities were difficult to find. Many Chinese had heard of stories about the Gold Rush in California and came with dreams that they too would strike gold in California. While some came to San Francisco to seek a new life, most of the early immigrants were family men who came with the intention to return to China after they had sent enough money back home. Common work industries for Chinese immigrants included the laundry, agriculture, and restaurant businesses. Some arrived as independent merchants, but many came seeking employment, and American businesses took advantage of the Chinese immigrants as a source of cheap labor. In particular, the Chinese were a major source of labor for the construction of the Central Pacific Railroad. Many Chinese were injured and died during construction, and those who worked on the railroad were out of jobs as soon as construction was done.

This mass migration of Chinese to the U.S. did not mean that they were welcomed by American society. On the contrary, since the Chinese were being hired for work at lower wages, resentment towards Chinese immigrants only increased. Not many recognized that the lower wages were an indication that the Chinese were actually being exploited and had practically no rights to argue for higher wages. The common sentiment was that the Chinese were competition and stealing jobs away from white citizens.

L.D. Hom (✉)
Independent Scholar, New York, NY, USA
e-mail: laureen.hom@gmail.com

G.J. Yoo et al. (eds.), *Handbook of Asian American Health*,
DOI 10.1007/978-1-4614-2227-3_26, © Springer Science+Business Media, LLC 2013

353

As a result of this "yellow peril" fear, laws were put in place that restricted Chinese immigration and the rights of the Chinese who currently resided in the U.S. Some laws strictly prohibited Chinese from a number of rights that citizens had, including testifying in court, purchasing and owning land, and using civic services, such as public schools and local hospitals. Other laws were meant to harm Chinese businesses, including penalties for laundrymen who did not haul laundry using a horse drawn cart. Chinese immigrants were also unfairly taxed for services upon arrival to San Francisco, including police and hospital taxes. Many of these civic services were generally not even used by the Chinese because of other discriminatory laws and simple prejudice from mainstream society.

The Exclusion Act of 1882 arguably had the greatest impact on Chinese immigration and for Chinese living in the U.S. This law banned future Chinese laborers from entering the U.S. for 10 years and prohibited the Chinese currently living in the U.S. to apply for citizenship. The Exclusion Act would continually be renewed and was not repealed until 1943. The Immigration Act of 1924 further restricted immigration to the U.S. by setting preferences for immigrants who have at least one relative who was a naturalized citizen or for immigrants who were merchants or skilled in a certain trade or industry, such as agriculture. Since citizenship was denied to the Chinese, those who could immigrate to the U.S. were not able to vote and have any political influence over many of the discriminatory taxes and laws placed against them. These laws were successful in slowing down the influx of Chinese immigrants and severely limiting the rights of the Chinese residing in the U.S.

In response to the prejudices and social isolation from mainstream society, community associations formed to build some type of local infrastructure that provided services to the Chinese community (Lai, 2003). Life in the U.S. for these early immigrants was not easy, as many were separated from their family and residing in an unfamiliar place that they initially had no intention of moving to permanently. The men in these "bachelor societies" naturally turned to each other for support, especially among those who came from the same villages and shared ethnic and dialectal similarities. In San Francisco, six distinct benevolent associations quickly emerged formed during the first years of Chinese immigration as the key fraternal organizations in Chinatown: the Sam Yup Company, Yeong Wo Company, Kong Chow Company, Ning Yung Company, Hop Wo Company, and Yan Wo Company. For the most part, each of these six companies operated independently and provided services that the Chinese were either banned from or had great difficulty in receiving, including housing and sending remittances to China. These associations had the same mission to provide protection and services to their members, but the relationship between and within the associations could be tense, often due to territorial issues. Despite these differences, the increasing anti-Chinese sentiment in San Francisco and the U.S. helped to unite the associations together for a common cause: to fight against the discrimination the Chinese faced. The companies formally came together in 1882 to establish the first Chinese Consolidated Benevolent Association in the U.S., also known as the Chinese Six Companies. The Chinese Six Companies would become a leader in ensuring that basic services and rights were given to the Chinatown community.

Chinatown as the Source of Disease

The late nineteenth century not only marked the first major influx of Chinese immigrants to the U.S., but it also was the time of major epidemics, such as the Bubonic Plague, small pox, and cholera. These infectious diseases tended to be most prevalent amongst the poor and working class areas of cities because of the dense populations and poor upkeep of the neighborhoods. However, the popular sentiment of the time was that these diseases were embodied by the individuals who lived in these neighborhoods. Germ theory was not the predominant theory for spreading sickness at the time. The prevailing belief was miasma theory: by breathing "sick air," one will become sick. Many felt that by going to many of the working class ethnic neighborhoods, such as Chinatown, they would breathe this sick air. These beliefs helped to promote classist and racist beliefs that individuals of ethnic minority or poor and working class backgrounds were inferior and sickly.

Because of these beliefs, as well as the general racist attitudes towards Chinese immigrants, the Chinatown neighborhood became a scapegoat for many of the public health problems and epidemics. The original Chinatown encompassed a 15 square block region around Portsmouth Square in Downtown San Francisco. Chinatown did not receive general sanitary services, and many Chinese were forced to live in squalid and over-crowded conditions. Because of the poor physical conditions of Chinatown, the Chinese were accused of spreading almost every urban epidemic in San Francisco. During the smallpox epidemic in 1876, the Chinese were blamed as the source of the disease because of the unsanitary conditions of Chinatown. In 1900, a recently deceased Chinese laborer was falsely identified to have passed away due to the plague, causing a 3 month quarantine of Chinatown (Loo, 1991). The Chinese community was dehumanized during this time and was popularly depicted in the media as rats and pigs – animals that were associated with spreading diseases and living in filth. Fear of the Chinese was not just that they were competition for jobs, but also harbingers of disease and death.

However, instead of supporting efforts to improve the conditions of Chinatown, the Board of Health and Board of Supervisors subjected Chinatown and its residents to multiple health inspections. These health reports did not find any evidence supporting the claim that the Chinese were spreading diseases. However the government still concluded the area as unsanitary, and thus a danger to neighboring communities and the city itself (Loo, 1991; Shah, 2001).

The government continued its discriminatory efforts to further punish and quarantine the Chinese that was said to be done for the public health good of San Francisco. In 1870, the Cubic Air Ordinance required that each tenant have at least 500 cubic feet of air. This law was a passive way to address overcrowding, but in actuality it allowed the police to harass the Chinese in their homes as most were living in overcrowded tenements in Chinatown and improving their conditions on their own was virtually impossible. Furthermore, the overcrowding in Chinatown was often dismissed by health officials as an innate behavior of Chinese to seek out and live in crowded conditions. As a part of the quarantines, Chinese residents were prohibited from leaving the city out of fear that they would spread diseases beyond the confines of Chinatown. The Board of Supervisors supported efforts to shut down many Chinese businesses. Many places in Chinatown were condemned and destroyed because they were considered sources of sickness, particularly underground stores and residences.

Along with the lack of services within Chinatown, the Chinese could not access hospitals outside the neighborhood. City and county hospital medical records indicate that only 34 Chinese individuals were admitted to the city hospitals between 1870 and 1897. The Chinese represented less than 1% of the total hospital admission rate (Chow, Lau, Leung, Loos, & Yee, 2007). The low hospital utilization rate of the Chinese reflects the barriers that they faced in trying to receive services and care from the city hospitals. Most hospitals were far away from Chinatown, and making the trek to the other parts of the city meant an increased risk for harassment and beatings. There were also linguistic barriers because the physicians and staff working at the city hospitals did not speak any dialect of Chinese. If a hospital was willing to serve them, Chinese individuals had to pay higher hospital fees than other residents which was in addition to the hospital tax that they were required to pay when they arrived in San Francisco. Even the free charity hospitals and public health clinics that served the European immigrant communities discriminated against the Chinese and rarely served them. In addition to these institutional barriers, the Chinese were also well aware of the high mortality rates of the San Francisco hospital and thus were hesitant to go to hospitals. They associated Western medicine and hospitals with the current epidemics and death (Shah, 2001). Most of the Chinese relied on folk healers in Chinatown who had established shops that provided traditional Chinese medicine. Because of these reasons the Chinese in San Francisco could not and did not go to a hospital unless completely necessary.

Because of the general racism against the community, the early Chinese immigrants faced many challenges in receiving basic services that would help their health and quality of life. This systematic exclusion only perpetuated the prevailing beliefs that Chinese were spreading diseases and were a "sickly race" because they had limited access to services that would help to improve their conditions. The push for fixing the health problems of Chinatown thus had to come from within the community.

The Tung Wah Dispensary: The First Place for Medical Care in Chinatown

The Chinese Six Companies took the lead in establishing a health care facility that would finally serve the Chinese community. Since the first major wave of Chinese immigration, the community associations had repeatedly attempted to establish a neighborhood health care facility, but were met with resistance from various Downtown neighborhood lobby groups and denied each time by the Board of Supervisors. Even a plan that proposed to build a hospital outside of Chinatown, in the outskirts of the city, to provide traditional Chinese health care was vetoed by the Board of Supervisors who were weary of the validity of using Chinese medicine and worried that the Chinese would spread diseases if they left Chinatown (Shah, 2001). The Board of Supervisors also vetoed plans to build a hospital in Chinatown because it would be a "nuisance to the surrounding neighborhoods" and did not want to support a hospital that would be managed and operated by Chinese individuals (Loo, 1991). While the Board of Supervisors was

concerned about the health of the city, they felt no sympathy or responsibility for helping the Chinese community. Their focus was not to support initiatives that helped improve the health of the Chinese, but instead to support initiatives that would get rid of the Chinese because they were considered the source of disease. However, despite constant barriers to establishing a hospital in Chinatown, the Chinese Six Companies was still determined to create a place for the Chinese to receive health services. They decided to set plans in motion without the support or approval of the Board of Supervisors and instead with the help of other community organizations and community members.

The Chinese Six Companies opened the Tung Wah Dispensary in 1900 in Chinatown at 828 Sacramento Street. They were able to establish the Dispensary through major fundraising efforts led by the Chinese consulate officials in San Francisco (Chen, 2000; Loo, 1991). The Tung Wah Dispensary was named after the Tung Wah Hospital in Hong Kong and was the first official Chinese operated medical facility in the U.S. The Dispensary housed 25 beds and provided both Western and traditional Chinese medicine. The staff who worked at the Dispensary were volunteers from the community as well as physicians from outside the community, including three White physicians who provided Western care through the assistance of interpreters. The Chinese physicians provided traditional Chinese care, as at that time no Chinese Americans had been trained in Western medicine. Following the model of the free public health clinics and charity hospitals, the Tung Wah Dispensary did not turn away any patients and provided free or low cost care to the patients who could not afford health care.

Despite having a new, more easily accessible place to receive health care, many people in Chinatown did not see the Tung Wah Dispensary as their primary source for health care. This attitude towards hospitals and health care facilities reflected how the majority of Chinese still believed that these places were associated with disease and death rather than a place to improve one's health. Receiving advice and herbal remedies from traditional medical practitioners was still the primary source of health care for most

Chinese immigrants. It was both more familiar and cheaper than using Western medicine. Only after these methods failed was an individual willing to go to the Dispensary. However, at this point most individuals were close to death and used the Tung Wah Dispensary as a final resting place for them. Records show that most of the patients of the Dispensary died. Thus it was nicknamed "Death House" by the community (Quock, 1978).

In 1906, San Francisco experienced the Great Earthquake that devastated most of Chinatown, including the Tung Wah Dispensary. However, it was quickly rebuilt in Trenton Alley as there was a growing need for a health care facility that could provide care to the sick and injured in Chinatown. Within less than 10 years of its establishment, the Tung Wah Dispensary was beginning to outgrow their current space and capacity (Chinese Hospital, 1965). This initial rebuilding after the 1906 earthquake was not enough and efforts to expand the Dispensary into a modern hospital were set in motion in 1918.

The Building of a Modern Hospital in Chinatown

The plan to expand the Tung Wah Dispensary to a modern hospital relied on the capacity and connections of the major organizations and associations operating in Chinatown. While the Chinese Six Companies spearheaded the campaign, additional organizations became more actively involved with the expansion. The organizations leading the campaign were:
- Chee Kung Tong
- Chinese-American Citizens Alliance
- Chinese Chamber of Commerce
- Chinese Christian Union
- Chinese Constitution Party Headquarters
- Chinese Six Companies
- Chinese Y.M.C.A.
- Hoy-Sun Ning Young Benevolent Association
- Hop Wo Benevolent Association
- Kong Chow Benevolent Association
- Kuomintang Headquarters
- Ning Yung Benevolent Association

- Sam Yup Association
- Sue Hing Benevolent Association
- Yen Wo Benevolent Association
- Young Wo Benevolent Association

These groups were the most well-known and trusted institutions and had much political, social, and financial capital in Chinatown. This was also a diverse group of community stakeholders that represented fraternal, financial, political, and religious interests. As noted previously, these community organizations already had a history of providing services to the community and acting as a voice for the Chinese community. But this marked one of the first times that the key stakeholders of San Francisco Chinatown united to build a major community facility that everyone could use, regardless of group membership. These community groups felt it was necessary to build a hospital because the Chinese were discriminated against and could not access health services. However, there were also other reasons why there was a push to build a modern hospital.

While almost all the groups promoted and maintained aspects of traditional Chinese culture in the U.S., some groups, especially the YMCA and other Christian based groups, were also community leaders in facilitating Chinese assimilation to modern American values, which included health and hygiene (Shah, 2001). There were also some Chinese Americans who were beginning to embrace Western medicine since the establishment of the original Dispensary. In fact, in the early 1900s, Chinese Americans were beginning to be formally trained in Western medicine and graduating from American medical schools. However, these Chinese American physicians could only practice within Chinatown due to discriminatory practices and prejudices. While many had started up private practices in the community, a Chinese Hospital would provide a setting for them to expand their services to more people and promote Western health care in the community.

A modern hospital that focused on providing Western care in Chinatown also had many potential long term benefits for the building of a modern Chinatown. The Hospital would help establish important infrastructure for the rebuilding of Chinatown after the earthquake, as at that point Chinatown had no major infrastructure that provided social services other than the current system of services that were offered through the various associations and community groups. The rebuilding of Chinatown was a stressful process as the community leaders had to fight off groups and associations from neighboring communities that were lobbying for Chinatown to be physically relocated to the outskirts of the city. The hospital would show that the Chinese were beginning to assimilate and adopt the Western model of health care and hygiene and help combat some of the racist beliefs that the Chinese were charged with during the epidemics. However, by building the hospital themselves, this adoption of Western culture could be from within the community and done on their own terms, rather than being dictated from outside the community. Western practices were difficult for the larger community to embrace, but there was a better chance that the community would be more receptive if it came from trusted community groups and not from the government or outside institutions. Lastly, it was important that the Chinese had access to a community hospital with more capacity than the Dispensary and was just as modern as the others in San Francisco. Chinatown residents deserved to have access to care that was equivalent to what was already available to all San Franciscans.

Creating a modern hospital was a larger project than establishing the Tung Wah Dispensary. The fundraising goal was $200,000, double what was originally decided when the plan was just to remodel the Dispensary. In 1922, fundraising efforts officially began, headed by Reverend Lok Sang Chan (Ng & Wilson, 1995). The fundraising efforts reached out to every level of the community, from Chinatown residents to Chinese-owned businesses. Efforts were diverse and included charity shows, sales, and door-to-door solicitations. Donations not only came from local benefactors, but also from donors from other cities in the U.S. and abroad. The Miss Chinatown Pageants originated from one of the original fundraising activities for the

Chinese Hospital. The pageants were able to attract donations from both Chinatown and non-Chinatown residents (Chen, 2000). By the end of 1923, enough money had been raised to purchase a lot on Jackson Street. Originally a plot of land that was adjacent to the Dispensary was purchased in 1920 (Quock, 1978) but because the original expansion plan was abandoned, a new larger plot of land was sought out. Three Chinese American citizens, T.J. Gintjee, M.S. Jung, and Yituan Tan, purchased the Jackson Street lot and construction permit and later transferred ownership of the Chinese Hospital. These three community members did this on behalf of the Hospital to bypass the Alien Land Laws that prohibited non-citizens from purchasing land (Ng & Wilson, 1995). In many ways, the fundraising efforts showed how connected and united the Chinese were locally and internationally. It also was an indication of how invested the early Chinese were in their San Francisco community; San Francisco was now as much as their home as China was to them.

The Board of Supervisors approved this project, which marked a major stepping stone because less than 50 years earlier, the Board had denied every type of plan to build a health facility that would help bring services and care to the Chinese. Racist and xenophobic sentiments still existed, but the approval indicated that there was growing recognition that the Chinese community in San Francisco had rights to services that every San Francisco citizen had. With the $200,000 goal met, the purchase of the Jackson Street lot, and the approval of the Board, construction for the hospital was underway for the next 2 years. Soon after the construction of the Chinese Hospital, the Chinatown leaders also lobbied for government support for establishing other important neighborhood infrastructure within the next few decades, including the Chinese Health Center, the Chinatown Playground, and the Ping Yuen housing projects (Shah, 2001). After many decades of rejection and struggle, the Chinatown community was finally victorious and beginning to receive the services they needed.

The Chinese Hospital's Early Years: Securing Financial and Community Support

On April 18, 1925 the Chinese Hospital officially opened its doors to the public. The grand opening of the Chinese Hospital was a huge celebration in Chinatown and lasted for several days. This new hospital was 5 stories tall with 55 beds. Thirty six licensed physicians and one dentist were employed by the hospital. Similar to the Dispensary, both Western and traditional medicine was offered in order to cater to the community wants and needs. Even the hospital's architecture was symbolic of the co-existence of Eastern and Western culture; the hospital had a similar façade and layout as other modern community hospitals with the exception of the traditional Chinese pagoda style awnings. Many of the physicians providing Western care in the Hospital were White. However, unlike the Dispensary, the first generation of medical staff also included four Chinese American physicians trained in Western medicine who presided over the major clinical departments, Dr. James Hall, Dr. Joseph Lee, Dr. Wong Him, and Dr. Margaret Chung. The Chinese Hospital was not only founded by Chinese Americans, but the clinical operations were being managed by some of the very first Chinese Americans who were practicing Western medicine in the U.S.

The Chinese Hospital found it difficult to secure consistent financial support during the early years. It was established as the U.S. was beginning to face the Great Depression and as China was facing both a civil war and an impending war with the Japanese. As the country went deeper into a depression, many individuals, including the Chinese were losing their jobs and could not afford health care. Furthermore, Chinese individuals and organizations were using what money they could spare to help send remittances back home as well as to fund the wars in China. The Chinese Hospital, which did not deny patients, found an increasing number of patients asking for free treatments, as well as those who could not pay their hospital debts. Within the first

4 years, the hospital had already treated over 700 patients, but was quickly running out of money as most of the care was provided free of charge. The Chinese Hospital faced on average a $1,000 debt each month during its first 5 years (Chinese Hospital, 1965). Even after the opening of the Chinese Hospital, it continued to depend on financial support from local and international groups, including major donations and loans from the Chinese Six Companies, the Tung Wah Hospital in Hong Kong, and the Bank of Canton in Hong Kong (Chinese Hospital, 1965). Every effort was made to keep the hospital running.

Another major problem that the Hospital continued to face was the community's indifference and distrust towards Western medicine, especially among the older generation. Even though the hospital was constantly in debt because it was providing free services to the community, the management and staff struggled in convincing the community to use the hospital for primary care. For the most part, the Hospital was under-utilized during the Depression that was largely due to resistance from most of the community to use Western medicine unless it was absolutely necessary (Loo, 1991; Shah, 2001). The attitude that hospitals are a last resort for health care was still strong in the community and difficult to change. As previously noted, the founders of the Chinese Hospital recognized these attitudes as a barrier and despite the mission of the hospital to primarily provide Western care, they did offer traditional care and herbal remedies. In particular, Dr. Lee and Dr. Him practiced homeopathy in addition to the Western care they provided for their patients. However, for the most part, providing traditional Chinese and Western medicine under one roof provided mixed results. An account with one of the physicians, Dr. Collin Dong, indicated that he felt that patients did not entirely adapt the Western practices and instead went back and forth between the Western and herbal remedies according to their own liking (Loo, 1991). These attitudes still permeate today as many Chinese Americans, especially older patients, rely on traditional herbal remedies as their primary source of health care.

Many of the first generation of Chinese American physicians at the Hospital had already established private practices and were important figures in the Chinatown community. The involvement of these physicians with the Chinese Hospital was just as important as the involvement of the community groups in helping to build trust and buy-in with the community. In particular, both Dr. Hall and Dr. Lee were already well-known community physician and were the first Chinese Americans to practice Western medicine in San Francisco and the U.S. Dr. Hall was also active outside the Chinese Hospital, as he was the president of the Chinese American Citizens Alliance and Chairman of the Board of the Bank of Canton, which had helped provide much financial support during the construction and early years of the hospital (Chinn, 1989; Quock, 1978). Dr. Chung, the head of the Obstetrics and Gynecology Department, was also very active in the community in promoting Western medicine and did outreach and education in local schools (Wu, 2005). Dr. Rose Goong Wong who also practiced women's health was a strong advocate of providing free care and was one of the first physicians to provide free postnatal care for Chinese women and their newborns (Shah, 2001). The Chinese Hospital benefitted from having these well known Chinese American community physicians working to outreach and build connections in the community.

However, not all physicians had the ability to outreach as passionately as others during these early years. In fact, many physicians began to question the Hospital's ability to provide free and low cost care to the community, especially given the constant debt the Hospital had. Understandably, many physicians were also worried about their own financial situation and constraints during this time. Because of these concerns many of the Hospital physicians grew reluctant to provide free and low cost care to the community. Some doctors resigned within the first few years, and others had brought up the idea to close the hospital during the Depression Era. These sentiments led to tension among the Chinese American physicians

as Dr. Hall openly criticized those doctors who were reluctant to provide free care for being selfish and not thinking of the greater good of the community (Wu, 2005).

Despite these struggles, the Chinese Hospital was able to survive the first few decades after its opening. After World War II, the Chinese Hospital slowly gained its financial footing and was finally no longer in debt. Since then, the hospital has been able to receive a steady stream of donations through local community organizations and foundations, as well as continuing fundraising efforts (Chinese Hospital, 1965). Also during this time, the Chinese Hospital stopped providing traditional medicine as a part of the routine care and focused on only providing Western medical care. By the mid-1970s, the Chinese Hospital expanded to an additional, larger building that was built in the adjacent lot to provide more Western medical services. The original building was converted to administrative offices. In 2013, the Chinese Hospital will once again expand to keep up with the increasing demand of the Chinese residents of San Francisco. The original building will be demolished and a modern facility will be built to provide more beds and services in addition to the newer building constructed in the 1970s.

The Chinese Hospital is still active today and continues to evolve according to the needs of the community. The Hospital's Board of Directors still includes representatives from the original 15 organizations that spearheaded the initial fundraising efforts, along with one community member. The mission of the hospital remains the same; to provide health care that responds to the needs of the San Francisco Chinatown community. The current mission is as follows: *The Chinese Hospital, a general acute care community-owned, not-for-profit organization, provides quality health care in a cost effective way. It is responsive to the community's ethnic and cultural uniqueness and is accessible to all socioeconomic levels. Chinese Hospital is governed by a voluntary Board of Trustees, broadly representative of the community, and strives to assume a leadership role in all health matters.*

The Impact of the Chinese Hospital: Local and Beyond

The Chinese Hospital of San Francisco not only is the first health care facility in the U.S. to provide Western medical services to the Chinese community, but also provides health education and supports advocacy efforts to improve the health of the community. In the 1970s, the Chinese Hospital received a Hill-Burton grant for the hospital to become a comprehensive health care center (Chinn, 1989). From this initial grant, the Chinese Hospital quickly expanded to provide services beyond clinical care to include services that improved community education and access to care.

The Chinese Hospital helped to establish the Chinese Community Health Care Association (CCHCA) in 1982, a non-profit entity with the goal to increase access to health care in the Chinese community. CCHA includes members of the Chinese Hospital staff as well as other physicians and health care professionals working with the Chinese community in San Francisco. Through CCHCA, the Hospital has helped to facilitate the establishment of many important programs and organizations. The Chinese Community Health Resource Center was established by the Hospital and CCHA to provide community and patient education on important Asian American health issues including cancer, preventative care, and osteoporosis. The Chinese Community Health Plan (CCHP) was founded in 1986 to help increase the availability of managed care programs for the Chinese community (Chow, Lau, Leung, Loos, & Yee, 2007). The Chinese Hospital's involvement with this program shows how the Hospital is tackling the problem of health care access beyond the provision of services by also addressing the community need for easier access to health insurance. CCHCA was fundamental in helping to establish advocacy and research centers that advance the Asian American health agenda. The NICOS Chinese Health Coalition in San Francisco provides research, training, advocacy, coalition-building

and programs to help enhance the health of the Chinese community in San Francisco. It also helped to establish the Asian Pacific Islander American Health Forum (APIAHF), a national health organization that works to influence policy, mobilizes communities, and strengthens programs and organizations to improve the health of Asian Americans, Native Hawaiians, and Pacific Islanders. The Hospital's involvement with programs and organizations that go beyond clinical services helps to ensure that all health care concerns of the community are comprehensively addressed.

The Chinese Hospital was created in response to the systematic discrimination that the Chinese faced in trying to receive appropriate health care and services. In many ways, the Chinese Hospital was a predecessor for the establishment of neighborhood health centers to serve underprivileged communities. In the 1970s, health centers, such as the Charles B. Wang Community Health Center in New York City, South Cove Community Health Center in Boston, and the Chinatown Service Center in Los Angeles, were established to provide accessible, affordable, and culturally and linguistically appropriate care to the Asian American communities in those respective cities. In the 1980s, during the rise of the HIV/AIDS, clinics such as the Asian Pacific Islander Wellness Center in San Francisco and the Asian Pacific Islander Coalition on HIV/AIDS in New York City, were established to provide culturally competent HIV/AIDS care to Asian Americans, who were ignored in the larger HIV/AIDS discourse. While these health centers and clinics were established over half a century later and drew from inspiration and opportunities provided through the activism of the Civil Rights Era, their origins and mission are remarkably similar to the Chinese Hospital. They also started at a grassroots level with community stakeholders who recognized the need for health services and worked together to create a place in the community to address this need. While major strides have been made since the Chinese Hospital, it is clear that the struggle for providing accessible and appropriate care for Asian Americans continues.

The Chinese Hospital of San Francisco is an important part of San Francisco Chinatown, as well as Asian American history. The origin of the Hospital marks one of the earliest moments of the early Chinese immigrant leaders successfully coming together to advocate and provide services that would help build their community on their own terms. The Hospital was the first major institution to be built in San Francisco Chinatown and helped to establish Chinatown as an important community in San Francisco. The Hospital is still the only Chinese operated and governed health care facility in the U.S., as well as the last independently operated hospital in San Francisco. Because of this distinction, it continues to be locally and internationally recognized as one of the most trusted place for new and old Chinese immigrants to receive culturally and linguistically appropriate Western medical care in the U.S.

Acknowledgements The author would like to acknowledge the following individuals in their assistance in providing relevant resources for the development of the text: Phillip Choy, Lorraine Dong, Stuart Fong, Marlon Hom, Rolland Lowe, and Collin Quock.

References

Chen, Y. (2000). *Chinese San Francisco, 1850–1943: A trans-Pacific community.* Stanford, CA: Stanford University Press.

Chinese Hospital. (1965). *Chinese hospital 40th anniversary.* San Francisco: Chinese Hospital.

Chinn, T. W. (1989). *Bridging the Pacific: San Francisco Chinatown and its people.* San Francisco: Chinese Historical Society of America.

Chow, E.A., Lau, B., Leung, L.E., Loos, R., & Yee, B. (2007). The development of a community-based integrated health care system for the San Francisco Chinese community. *Chinese America: History and Perspectives 21.*

Lai, H. M. (2003). *Becoming Chinese American: A history of communities and institutions.* Walnut Creek, CA: Alta Mira Press.

Loo, C. M. (1991). *Chinatown: Most time, hard time.* New York: Praeger.

Ng, F., & Wilson, J. D. (Eds.). (1995). *The Asian American encyclopedia* (Vol. 1). New York: Marshall Cavendish.

Quock, C. P. (1978). *The dawning.* San Francisco: Chinese Hospital Medical Staff Archives.

Shah, N. (2001). *Contagious divides: Epidemics and race in San Francisco's Chinatown.* Berkeley, CA: University of California Press.

Wu, J. T.-C. (2005). *Doctor Mom Chung of the fair-haired bastards: The life of a wartime celebrity.* Berkeley, CA: University of California Press.

Lives Were Saved: The Asian American Donor Program

27

Jonathan Leong, Kira Donnell, and Emily Avera

"Miracles happened where there was seemingly no hope. Dreams were realized. Friends were made. Lives were saved."

Carolyn Tam

Introduction

For over 20 years, the Asian American Donor Program (AADP) has registered thousands of Asian American bone marrow donors as well as other ethnic minorities for the National Marrow Donor Program. Using unique donor recruitment strategies, public education, and community organizing, AADP has made ground-breaking strides in Asian American public health and saved countless lives along the way.

Each year, more than 30,000 people in the United States are diagnosed with life threatening blood diseases (Asians for Miracle Marrow Matches, 2011). For many, the only treatment option is a bone marrow transplant. With a high probability of success, the new bone marrow can treat several types of cancers such as leukemia, lymphoma, myeloma and breast cancer. Transplants can also help patients who suffer from blood disorders such as thalassemia and sickle cell anemia as well as certain immune-deficiency diseases like congenital neutropenia or chronic granulomatous disease.

Because bone marrow needs to be matched by genetic traits, patients have the best chance of finding a donor who is of the same racial background. For Caucasian patients, finding an unrelated bone marrow donor match through the National Marrow Donor Program registry has a success rate of 80%. For Asian and other ethnic minority patients, the odds of finding a donor match are only about 30% successful (Asian American Donor Program, 2011).

Addressing the needs of minority patients, the Asian American Donor Program (AADP) is a community non-profit (501c3) organization dedicated to increasing the availability of potential stem cell donors for patients with life-threatening diseases curable by a stem cell transplant. AADP has specialized in conducting outreach and donor registration drives in the Asian American, Pacific Islander, and multi-racial communities throughout the United States. Although AADP's name includes the word "Asian," AADP, first and foremost, focuses on the client's needs and the necessity of finding a match, regardless of ethnicity. AADP treats each client who seeks their help individually with compassion and care. AADP works with individuals who share cultural, generational, and most importantly, genetic similarities, which has led AADP to approach each patient and potential donor as an individual even as it reaches out to the national and international level:

> To increase the opportunities of saving as many lives as possible, AADP works to recruit from various Asian groups, Chinese, Japanese, Korean, Vietnamese, East Indians, Mongolians, Filipinos, and other Asian ethnic groups, and works with

J. Leong (✉) • E. Avera
Asian American Donor Program, Alameda, CA, USA
e-mail: jonathan.leong9@gmail.com

K. Donnell
Department of Ethnic Studies, University of California Berkeley, Berkeley, CA, USA

G.J. Yoo et al. (eds.), *Handbook of Asian American Health*,
DOI 10.1007/978-1-4614-2227-3_27, © Springer Science+Business Media, LLC 2013

individuals with mixed races. With a simple cotton swab, miracles can happen for cancer patients. The difficulty comes in matching DNA of the donor with the patient. This has been the long standing goal and mission of AADP - to increase the number of transplants in the Asian community," states (J. Leong, Personal Communication, May 25, 2011).

Becoming a bone marrow donor is a simple process. Upon registering with the National Marrow Donor Program, individuals fill out a short health history form and provide a DNA sample from a painless swab of the inner cheek. From the DNA sample, the individual's HLA type (Human Leukocyte Antigen) is determined. HLA are inherited "markers" on the white blood cells. In a tissue transplant, the closer the match in HLA type between the donor and the recipient, the greater the chance that the transplant will be successful. When a registry member is found to be a match, the donor undergoes one of two out-patient donation processes depending upon the needs of the patient.

They include marrow extraction which is used in 30% of donations. It entails taking out hemato-poeitic (blood-producing) stem cells from the back of the pelvic bone. The other procedure, apheresis, occurs in 70% of donations and requires the use of medication to increase pro-duction of hematpoeitic stem cells. On the fourth or fifth day, the donor's blood is drawn. The stem cells are separated out and the remaining blood components are returned to the donor's body.

The Birth of a Movement

The National Marrow Donor Program (NMDP) was established in September 1987 with fewer than 10,000 donors for the purpose of recruiting and registering more potential volunteer donors in the United States (McCullough, Perkins, & Hansen, 2006, p. 1252). Since then, the registry has grown to nine million donors and has facili-tated over 43,000 transplants to patients with matching tissue types (NMDP, 2011). But in its early days, NMDP had developed tissue typing with Caucasian types and overlooked the urgency of ethnic diversity in donor recruitment numbers

and the corresponding limited accessibility of transplants for minority patients. In an effort to minimize the disparities of resources available for all patients, the Asian American community began a donor recruitment campaign that evolved into the first major health care movement in Asian America.

The Asian American Donor Program began in 1989 when two Bay Area Asian leukemia patients, Amanda Chiang (nine months old) and Judith Jang Berkoltz (32 years old), who were in desperate need of bone marrow transplants. Both patients were unable to find a match within their own families and turned to the National Marrow Donor Program Registry hoping to find unrelated marrow donors. In 1989, there were only 123 Asian donors listed on the National Registry, and Amanda and Judith's families were told that the prospects of finding compatible donors were vir-tually impossible. Determined family and friends of the two patients made a statewide appeal to recruit more Asians onto the Registry.

Spearheading this effort was Jonathan Leong, a long-standing community advocate and leader in Bay Area, who used his many ties to various local Asian groups to respond to this vital need. "It wasn't an emotional thing – I just saw there was a need," Leong said in a 1995 interview. "If I didn't get involved, maybe nobody else would, or maybe they would, but not today" (Nakao, 1995, p. A). A graduate of San Francisco State University, Leong is an active community partici-pant and successful businessman.

In 1989, encouraged by his friends, Leong called upon his local business associates, com-munity advocates and political contacts to step up and step forward to get involved and save lives. Leong recalls, Leong saw the need as a commu-nity issue rather than an individual one and decided to get involved. Through the collective efforts of Leong, Art Louie, Herb Chiu and Ted Kao, AADP has become an important resource for the Asian communities. After witnessing fam-ily and friends face the need for a marrow donor, they came together to found an organization that would provide ongoing education and recruitment of potential donors from the Asian American community.

This small group of concerned citizens, running the program out of Leong's insurance office on a shoestring budget would become the founders of one of the first and most successful public health movements in Asian America. Using their entrepreneurial experience and community connections, the organizational founders strove to recruit Asian American marrow donors and find matches for patients. Additionally, they were able to find generous funders for the financial costs of conducting the scientific tests required to determine the tissue typing for each of the potential donors enrolled in the registry.

Initially, outreach was largely done through ethnic media along with the efforts of patient-based campaigns and public recruitment drives led through family and friends. The snowball effect of these actions led to robust fundraising, and the recruitment and typing of several thousand donors in the space of a few years. As the community awareness of bone marrow donation grew, so did the recruitment and fundraising campaigning, which led to the formation of an assembly of a Board of Directors, then-Executive Director Mabel Teng, and staff treasurer/accountant Carol Gillespie – who later became Executive Director, and the establishment of the organization's non-profit status.

Officially acting as a subcontractor of the NMDP, AADP became the first program in the U.S. to conduct bone marrow donor outreach and recruitment targeting the Asian Pacific Islander community. AADP was a key player in bringing awareness to the national organization about the importance of ethnic tracking and outreach in minority communities. Supported by scientific research linking ethnicity and tissue types important to stem cell transplantation, and the unrelenting advocacy of AADP and patient families, the NMDP approached the Department of Defense in 1990 to allocate funding specifically for the typing of minority donors (McCullough, Perkins, & Hansen, 2006). This greatly expanded the recruitment abilities of the AADP and enabled the organization to focus more funding on effective outreach (Fig. 27.1).

Outreach Strategies: Model for Community Engagement

Fueled by a dedicated staff of outreach coordinators, AADP's recruitment efforts and community engagement have grown from inception to present day. Utilizing a community network system of recruitment and outreach, AADP has galvanized the Asian American community to take action and save lives. In addition to understanding the sensitivities and sensibilities of culture, race and religion, AADP collaborates with community leaders in churches, neighborhood centers and other venues where Asian Americans congregate to educate and to dispel the fallacies that many potential donors believe. In turn, these respected community leaders are encouraged to take the lead in informing their group of the essential message and mission that AADP advocates. Heeding Leong's mantra of "there's no such thing as an Asian," outreach coordinators strove to customize and individualize their entreaties, taking different approaches to recruiting and educating the varying demographics within the Asian American community. Rather than attempting to cast a wide net with large holes across the vast Asian American population, AADP recruits specific ethnic populations using specific cultural recruitment strategies. Through information and demonstration, AADP has respected their differences and formed bridges with these communities, addressing potential donors' concerns and dispelling misinformation.

One example is the unease in some cultures of even giving blood. Heddy Chiang, who was previously introduced as the mother of leukemia patient Amanda Chiang, elaborated on this concern:

> In Chinese culture, people are hesitant about giving blood, let alone bone marrow. They are not only superstitious about giving up part of their bodies, but also very fearful about the risks...The way they think, if something bad happened to me, I must have done something wrong. If they give their blood, they think the bad will go to them (Yabu & Yee, 1990, p. 4).

Comparably, Kingman Kan, director of the Asian outreach project for the National Marrow

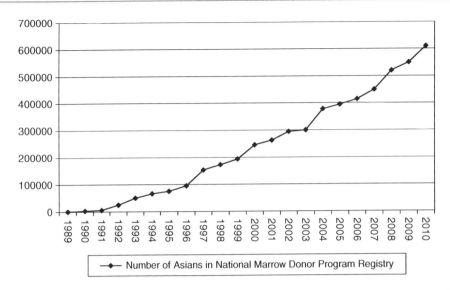

Fig. 27.1 Number of Asians registered in the National Marrow Donor Program (*Source*: National Marrow Donor Program)

Donor Registry program, makes a similar observation:

> Part of the old, old Chinese superstitious belief is when you die and are buried, you must be buried as a whole. The idea of a transplant bothers people. What we need to do is change the term to transfusion, so older Chinese don't misunderstand and think they are losing part of their soul (Lee, 1989, para. 16).

Through mutual understanding and reverence of individual Asian identities, AADP developed collaborative outreach programs and meaningful partnerships with each Asian subgroup to fulfill the goal of saving lives.

Recruitment efforts most often took the form of donor registration drives. These drives were set up in a variety of ways. Most commonly they were initiated by families and friends of patients who wanted to organize a community drive and contacted AADP for assistance. Through those family and friends, community groups or a combination of both, a site is selected and a drive is sponsored. For patients like Alan Kuo, this meant taking advantage of multiple media outlets and reaching as many people as possible. After a long search for a donor, Kuo agreed to go public about his need for a bone marrow. His story was publicized in radio and news stories. His friends and families had set up a webpage, and distributed flyers and posters (Sawano, 1998).

Within five years of its establishment, AADP was already holding drives in community spaces as varied as temples, churches, universities and colleges, and Asian American community fairs, conferences, and festivals.

In addition to literature and registration forms in multiple languages, AADP outreach coordinators over the years have had linguistic skills, speaking to ethnic media outlets and potential donors at drives including Cantonese, Vietnamese and Tagalog. The ethnic communities that coordinators have focused on most certainly facilitated greater outreach in those communities. AADP has often relied on the creativity of these coordinators and their understanding of socio-cultural specificities to formulate different recruitment strategies. In the Filipino American community, for example, recruiters have found that the best appeal to potential donors is in a one-on-one setting or at a small community event, rather than a mass recruitment. Different forms of media have proved more effective in different sectors as well. In the South Asian community, using respected public figures like leaders and doctors, recognizing the important role of educating both the donor and their family, and negotiating religious principles with regard to stem cell donation all factor into the outreach efforts.

By having outreach coordinators who are themselves members of such communities, who are equipped to understand the resistances and doubts, and represent someone a potential donor can identify with, is a key tenet of AADP's outreach philosophy. It is also an approach that can change and renegotiate the way certain ethnicities view themselves in biocitizenry (Rose & Novas, 2004). Currently, the frictions between more traditional notions of citizenship and a new biocitizenship is particularly relevant to recruitment in both Asian and Latino immigrant populations and how AADP navigates this issue is key. Articulating that long-term residency is more critical than citizenship and that being available to donate when called are key factors. All media efforts must include a sentence about residency and that AADP does not report to any government agency.

Mainstream, but most especially ethnic media (TV, print, and radio) have been crucial in providing accurate health education about marrow transplantation and attracting Asian American donors to drives. In multilingual coverage, hundreds of articles have been written, often focusing on a particular patient of a certain ethnic background. Not only does the story of a patient from a specific community become a face for the cause, it is a compelling way to educate and mobilize that community into action. As one Asian donor stated:

> "Community is such an important part of our culture and to think you would be helping someone from your own community. They may not live down the road from you but they are still from your own community" (Nolan, 2011, para. 5).

The plight of patients in these communities also, shows the larger imperative of increasing donor registration in these communities as a matter of survival. An individual patient's story becomes a way for people to connect to their communities in an act of biosociality; reconfiguring of social groupings based on genetic and biological relationships linked to ethnic or racial solidarity (Rabinow, 1996).

Donor retention is also an important endeavor that AADP has worked to make more community-oriented. Retention, simply put, is whether a donor who has registered is available if they are identified as a match, and still have a willingness to donate. Only 30–40% of Asians contacted as matches agree to donate compared to 70–80% for other ethnic groups (Project Michelle Fact Sheet, 2008a). AADP has advocated for the adoption of certain practices to improve retention. One of the most important advocacy breakthroughs in AADP's practice was calling back matching donors. Previously, when a match for a patient was found, the transplant center would call the potential donor informing them that they are a match. But with feedback from community members and significantly lower retention rates among minority donors in general, AADP began to encourage NMDP to adopt the practice of having the recruitment organization contact the donor instead. Since AADP has started calling donors, retention rates have increased this is likely due to the greater connection a donor feels to the community-based initiative and recruitment group that first approached them. Again, the trust and representational connection to one's community are crucial in willingness to donate.

Furthermore, AADP has been working toward improving retention by recognizing that education of the whole family is just as important as educating the individual donors. Research in minority organ donation patterns show that culturally sensitive education centered on family communication is crucial in the process of organ donation and transplantation (Spigner, Weaver, Cardenas, & Allen 2002). Generationally speaking, this is an opportunity for the younger generation to engage in open communication with the older generations. This also highlights how many in ethnic communities view decision-making (even about the uses of their own biological tissue) to be a family decision. At the time a donor is called as a match, AADP encourages the potential donor to discuss this with their family and encourage the family to call AADP separately if need be, to answer any questions. AADP also includes brochures in mailings to potential donors to be shared with the family, in their native language and in English. Thus, the relationship between family and individual, and cultural differences in kinship are crucial to donor consent.

Project Michelle: A Nationwide Community

Michelle Maykin's story demonstrates how one person's plight can be the catalyst for social change for thousands as they unite as a community for the single purpose of aiding one of their own. A Bay Area resident of Vietnamese and Chinese/Thai heritage, Michelle was an active community member who grew up in the close-knit community of the Fremont Thai community. In February 2007, 27-year old Michelle was diagnosed with acute myeloid leukemia. After undergoing five rounds of chemotherapy, Michelle reached a state of remission and slowly began to reclaim her life. However, in April of 2008, two months after returning to work, Michelle began to feel symptoms similar to those she had felt prior to her original diagnosis. Her oncologist confirmed that she had relapsed. Michelle began another rigorous treatment plan that included even more intensive chemotherapy and radiation. Her best chance of survival was to receive a bone marrow transplant.

Project Michelle was started in 2008 as a local recruitment effort by Michelle's friends and family with the help of AADP to find a marrow match. Relying on community ties and social media networking, friends, acquaintances, and friends of friends got involved, and Project Michelle soon flourished into a nationwide grassroots initiative dedicated to increasing the deficient numbers of minority bone marrow donor registrants in the national registry. Within five weeks of the initiative's launch, Project Michelle had secured support from major corporations such as Google, Amazon, Nokia, and Microsoft, and held over 250 donor registration drives across 12 cities coast to coast, registering over 9,000 potential minority bone marrow donors and receiving over 3,000 online requests

for at-home registration kits (Project Michelle, 2008, para. 5). Commenting on the outpouring of support, Michelle's mother, Hoang Mong Thu stated:

> The reception we've had from the communities who have heard Michelle's story has been unbelievable, and the hard work put in by every volunteer has been an inspiration to Michelle and all of us in her family. The efforts to date have paid off as we watch the number of new donor registrants climb daily, and we are enthusiastic about Project Michelle's momentum (Project Michelle, 2008, para. 4).

Most who registered probably would never meet Michelle, but they were spurred to action because in her story, something connected with them. Michelle represented a classmate, a coworker, a neighbor, a friend, a family member who had been or could someday be in a similar situation. Thousands followed her online blog and shared the hope and the heartbreak as Michelle went through round after round of treatment.

While it was hoped that Project Michelle's efforts would result in a bone marrow match for Michelle Maykin, the larger goals of the initiative were for the improved health of the Asian American community as a whole through outreach and education. In a press release, the coordinators of Project Michelle stated, "One of Project Michelle's main goals is to bring attention to the dire shortage of minority bone marrow donors, an avoidable problem that could be eliminated by educating and reaching out to the over ten million unregistered Asians in America" (Project Michelle, 2008, para. 5). Sadly, despite a cord blood transfusion, Michelle's leukemia proved to be extremely resistant to treatment, and she passed away in July 2009. However, this remarkable woman's legacy lives on and continues to saves lives. To date, Project Michelle has registered 18,157 potential donors. Four patients have found donor matches through AADP from Project Michelle donor registration drives, and several others have been identified as possible matches and are awaiting further testing (Maykin, 2009).

Being the Match: The Movement Gains Momentum

The Asian American Donor Program has seen excellent capacity building over its two decades of existence. The organizational structure is a successful mix of long term experienced leadership invigorated and supported by youthful personnel. The Board of Directors, advisory board members and staff management has changed very little over the years. In contrast, the outreach staff has slowly increased from a few volunteers to nearly ten full time employees working on education, awareness, recruitment, and retention. Along with its wider Asian American and multiethnic scope, the staff has also focused on the particular ethnic communities that the organization has been able to reach. Some staff members are individually dedicated to South Asian, Vietnamese, Chinese, Filipino, and even Latino/Hispanic populations. Through the years, AADP has managed to stay relevant, maintaining donor recruitment numbers and increasing retention rates through a balance of breadth and specificity, using a meet-the-need ad hoc approach to campaign strategies and services.

The expansion to the Latino/Hispanic community in 2008 was a watershed moment in AADP's evolving inclusivity. This coalition was initiated by a Latino patient whose unmitigated passion for donor outreach in his community convinced AADP to help in these efforts. Twenty-four year old Jorge Ochoa was diagnosed in 2008 with acute lymphoblastic leukemia and chronic myelogenous leukemia. With only 5.3% of the national marrow registry classified as Latino/Hispanic, finding a match and receiving support was a daunting task (Avila, 2008). "We're here to ask the community to open up their minds and open up their hearts so that together as a community not only can we find a donor for my brother, but find donors for thousands of other people," pleaded Laura, Jorge Ochoa's sister, in a 2008 youtube press conference (Ochoa, 2008). There was no local organization that was established to focus on the Latino community, so AADP answered Ochoa's call for help. "When we heard about Jorge's situation, we just decided we have to do it," stated AADP's executive director, Carol Gillespie. "No one is focusing on this community. We feel it's the right time" (Gomez, 2009, para. 4). Now AADP's website and outreach materials are also available in Spanish, adding the slogan "Serving multi-ethic communities" to their logo. AADP recognizes that ethnic identities and community engagement are in constant redefinition and renegotiation, and that sensitivity to this ongoing process is proved by their effective outreach. It simultaneously encompasses the umbrellas of the Asian American, Latino, and multi-racial/ethnic, while also disaggregating its outreach efforts by ethnic communities.

In addition to the flexibility AADP has demonstrated in the populations it serves, the organization has also changed with the times in regards to its campaigning strategies. Registering young potential donors ensures that they remain eligible for donation for decades. A major source of AADP's donors comes from registration drives held on college campuses. Lambda Phi Epsilon, the nation's first and only internationally-recognized Asian-interest fraternity has made AADP its national philanthropy, and holds registration drives each year on its chapters' campuses. The fraternity was spurred to action in 1995 when Evan Chen, a member of Lambda Phi Epsilon's Theta Chapter at Stanford University, was diagnosed with leukemia.

Family, friends, and fraternity members worked tirelessly to find a donor for Evan. In a matter of days, they registered thousands with AADP. At that time, it was the largest recruitment effort that AADP had seen. Although a match was found, Evan shortly passed away from his disease in 1996. In his honor Lambda Phi Epsilon has steadfastly led education and recruitment campaigns on college campuses across the country and registered thousands of minority donors.

Yul Kwon, a reality television personality, has also been integral in AADP's efforts to target younger donors. Kwon was Evan Chen's college roommate and best friend since childhood. Kwon at the time devoted his energy towards finding a match for Chen, even at the expense of his schoolwork and grades. "It doesn't really matter to me. It does not compare to Evan's life (Chan, 1995, p. 1)." Kwon has remained passionate about creating awareness for the need for more minority bone marrow donors. Kwon gained popularity in 2006 when he won the reality television show, *Survivor: Cook Islands*. Kwon used his new fame as an opportunity to advocate for community change:

> In the years since Evan died, I've tried to stay active in the effort to register more bone marrow donors and to encourage more Asian Americans to get involved in politics or community service. When I was recruited to be on *Survivor*, I thought it was an opportunity to have a megaphone through which I could speak to these issues both within and outside our community... I've since tried to use the platform I've been given to get more people thinking about making a difference, doing something beyond the limits of self-interest, and volunteering for a cause, whether it's bone marrow, politics, or domestic violence (Kwon, 2009, para. 4).

In 2007, Kwon become a spokesperson for AADP, and donated $50,000 of his *Survivor* winnings to the organization, to ensure that Asian Americans could be continually educated on the importance of bone marrow donation (Examiner 2007). With the passion and celebrity Kwon brings as the face of AADP's recruitment campaign, AADP hopes to attract a new generation of Asian Americans to the cause.

The injection of new, energetic staff and volunteers, mostly under age 30, has also been advantageous in AADP's mobilization of young Asian American and Latino communities. This is most evident in their ability to utilize social networking sites, leading AADP to become less reliant on traditional ethnic media for publicity. The 2007 campaign, HelpVinayandSameer.Org, exemplifies how AADP is utilizing social media to save lives. In 2007, when two young South Asian Americans were diagnosed with acute myelogenous leukemia a massive recruitment campaign was launched to find bone marrow matches for Vinay Chakravarthy and Sameer Bhatia. Sameer's friend, Robert Chatwani reflects:

> We all knew we needed to do something. And we realized our choices were between doing something, anything, and doing something seismic. When framed in this way, the answer became simple:

> If the odds were 1 in 20,000, all we needed to do was hold bone marrow drives and register 20,000 South Asians (Chang, 2009, p. 3).

In what some academics are now calling "The Dragonfly Effect," Team Vinay and Sameer developed a four prong approach that would utilize the internet and engage the South Asian American community to take action. In the first stage, the campaign organizers focused their efforts on reaching out to strategic community members who could in turn pass the word around to other networks. They had a clear goal of recruiting 20,000 South Asians to register with AADP as potential bone marrow donors. The second wing of the strategy entails grabbing the attention of the public. The team used a chain email approach to increase awareness and call people to action and made HelpVinayandSameer.Org a recognizable brand through traditional media sources as well as online social media sources (Akers & Smith, 2011).

Stage three of the Dragonfly Effect worked to engage others, forging a personal connection to compel individuals to become involved. Vinay and Sameer relied on blogs to personalize their call to action and keep participants updated on the campaign's progress as well as the individual medical treatment progresses of Vinay and Sameer. In one post, Sameer blogged, "Can you ever imagine the fear that most cancer patients must experience? . . . As a donor, hopefully the path to being free of fear is a simpler one. Please think about this, discuss it with South Asians you know, and spread the word that life's too short to live in fear . . . Tell them that I'm the patient and I'm not afraid – are you?" (Chang, 2009, p. 8).

The fourth wing of the Dragonfly Effect enables and empowers others to take action. Robert Chatwani commented, "A contributing factor to the success of Team Vinay and Team Sameer was the fact that people felt the call to action to pick up an carry out on their own. We built a campaign that others could build upon" (Chang, 2009, p. 10). Help Vinayand Sameer. Org made all of their campaign content and recruiting materials open-source and available to the public. They provided how-to instructions and campaign templates that individuals could download and customize to organize and promote their own registration drives. "We knew we were doing something right when people we didn't even know started to self-organize, and the campaign began to grow faster than we, as organizers, could architect the growth," said Chatwani (Chang, 2009, p. 10).

With this model, HelpVinayandSameer.Org held 480 bone marrow drives and registered 23,611 new potential donors in just 12 weeks. AADP's Recruitment Director, Asia Blume, commented, "This is the biggest campaign I've ever been involved with. . . We never imagined that this campaign would blow up to this extent" (Chang, 2009, p. 12). Both Vinay Chakravarty and Sameer Bhati found donor matches and received transplants, though sadly, both relapsed and passed away in 2008. However, their campaign has left lasting effects with a clear replicable model for future campaigns and 24,000 potential donors added to the national registry that could be matches for other South Asian cancer patients.

In addition to digital social networking, AADP has also launched fundraising/awareness events and drives that appeal to young people. Hip Hop for Hope (HH4H), a contest for Bay Area dance crews, involved local hip hop/R &B stations, corporate sponsors, and dance and music luminaries. Using dance as a medium to communicate the need for more multi-ethnic bone marrow donors, the competition gave participants and attendants a wonderful opportunity to make a difference in the lives of many patients, donors, survivors, and the many friends and families touched by leukemia and other life-threatening blood diseases (Doan, 2010).

Recent years have also seen Laugh for Lives, a variety show that features Asian American stand-up comedians, targeting a college-age and young professional audience. A recent apparel design contest not only offered a showcase connecting aspiring artists and designers to the organization, but also provided good publicity through merchandise that was designed with a contemporary aesthetic.

AADP has continuously grown from a small cause run out of an insurance office to a smooth operating nonprofit organization that outreaches to thousands nationally and even internationally. To date, AADP holds over 300 registration drives annually, registering around 15,000 new potential donors each year (Leong, 2011). AADP is directly responsible for registering over 130,000 donors in the San Francisco Bay Area, accounting for over 20% of the national registry's Asian identified registrants, an incredible boost from the mere 123 listed prior to AADP's existence (de Lara, 2010).

Looking Forward: Advocacy Issues and Public Policy

Transplantation, along with the ethnically-specified HLA tissue types required for a match, creates social relationships amongst, donor, recipient, families, friends, and communities. Transplantation challenges the boundaries of the body, the boundaries between self and other, and by proxy, the boundaries of biocitizenship. Invoking Asian Americans, Latinos, and a range of ethnic identities, add an extra layer of complexity to these relationships. And the way AADP's advocacy efforts are informed by these social identities and inter-linkages with one another have great consequence. These are definitely broader concerns that AADP must consider as it moves forward. There is a global (or perhaps even "glocal") narrative that deeply entwines ethnic identities, community activism, and the deft navigation of the connection between biology and ethnicity implicated in the history and continued work of AADP.

AADP is at the forefront of advocating for the continuing urgency of providing the resources to facilitate transplants and equal access to these life-saving treatments. Biological differences (as reflected in the incredible diversity of immune system-based tissue types) require a change in how we mobilize around ethnicity and race. This, in turn, changes how we successfully use ethnicity and race to mobilize around important ethnic minority health issues confronting us today. In practice and in organizational values, AADP shows the delicate balance between community-widening multiethnic coalitions and grassroots outreach that is sensitive to local and ethnically-specific mores. This is the standpoint from which AADP strives for health equity.

Additionally, AADP promotes public policy that promotes donor motivation. Living donors, primarily for bone marrow/stem cell transplants and kidneys, make a commitment that has an enormous impact. Not only does this often save the life of another, it can also affect the donor's life and their loved ones. Anything that may be a disincentive for the donor, preventing them from making the commitment, can also have a devastating impact on a patient. There are many pressures a donor may already be concerned with, including being a targeted minority, the only hope for a someone else's survival, the concerns of their own family, as well as what they may lose in the process. Ideally speaking, donation should be an altruistic act. To maintain this altruism and encourage donors, eliminating disincentives to donation is essential.

Wage loss from time of donation and recovery is one of the most concrete donor disincentives that can be addressed. One of the most recent and compelling developments in eliminating this donor disincentive was the passage in 2010 of Senate Bill 1304, the Michelle Maykin Memorial Donation Protection Act. This bill was initiated by the mother of Michelle Maykin, and introduced by Senator Mark DeSaulnier. Summarized, the act provides employees that donate bone marrow or organs paid, protected leave from their employment. The passage of the bill, especially in difficult economic times, is a major recognition that transplantation and the act of donation is valued by the state government, politicians, health organizations, medical practitioners, patients, and labor interests. With its roots in a local focus patient's campaign for donors affiliated with AADP, the mobilizing effects transferred readily to enacting this landmark bill.

Bone marrow/stem cell transplantation is a globally-connected issue as well. Patients in different countries can also search the U.S. registry and registries in other countries if they cannot find a suitable match locally. As a result, international transplants are quite common. In fact, 54% of all transplants facilitated by the NMDP Registry involve an international donor or recipi-

ent (Be the Match, 2011). AADP is committed to connecting with international registries, acting as a broker. This additional organizational function stems from staff language competencies as well as the diasporic connections. The World Marrow Donor Association (WMDA) has been a hallmark of cooperation among registries around the world (including NMDP), and there has been some work on identifying global recruitment strategies. "TransplantInformers," a new AADP blog project has started to engage this. Using a bottom-up approach, the sharing of locally-based practices on an international scale can hopefully help create a larger global conversation around the interrelationships between social identity, genetic tissue typing and bone marrow/stem cell transplantation.

Conclusion

For over 20 years, the Asian American Donor Program has worked tirelessly to maintain the health of the Asian American community. Using unique recruiting strategies that include social networking, grassroots word-of-mouth organizing, and culture-specific campaigns, AADP has educated thousands on the importance of registering as a minority bone marrow donor, has been integral in bringing the number of Asians in the National Marrow Donor Program's registry from 123 to over 600,000, and has been a lifeline for hundreds of cancer patients and their families.

As the first public health movement to mobilize the Asian American community, AADP has left a lasting legacy of an effective community organizing model. The organization has blazed the trail for other minority health movements to follow. From Asians for Miracle Marrow Matches, to the Hep B Free campaign, to Stanford scholars touting the success of the Dragonfly Effect, all were influenced by the passion and effectiveness of AADP.

Although the Asian American Donor Program is classified as an "Asian" organization, its philosophy and goals are universal and reject classification. It exists because there was a need for people from Asia or with an Asian background who had nowhere to go when a loved one needed a bone marrow match. In terms of bone marrow, there is no such thing as an Asian because AADP does not view their clients as being Asian. The organization sees no color, no race, or continent. For AADP, there is a match or a potential match for another patient. The Asian American Donor Program is singular in its focus – saving lives.

References

Akers, J., & Smith, A. (2011). The dragonfly effect. *Stanford Social Innovation Review*, 31–35.

Asian American Donor Program. (1996). *Minority marrow donor recruitment subcontract #5025 proposal for continuation of subcontract*. Unpublished report, Asian American Donor Program, Alameda.

Asian American Donor Program. (2011). AADP. Retrieved May 3, 2011, from http://aadp.org/.

Asian American Net. (2006). Jonathan R. Leong. *Who's who of Asian Americans*. Retrieved April 30, 2011, from http://www.asianamerican.net/bios/Leong-Jonathan.html.

Asians for Miracle Marrow Matches. (2011). Donor resources: Why we need you. *A3M*. Retrieved May 3, 2011, from http://www.a3mhope.org/index.php/donor.

Avila, A. (2008). A call out for Jorge. *De-Bug: The online magazine of the South Bay. Silicone Valley De-Bug*. Retrieved May 18, 2011, from http://www.siliconvalleydebug.com/story/110208/120108/storys/ACallOutforJorge.html.

Be the Match. (2011). *Words to live by: Report to the community 2010*. Annual report. Minneapolis, MN: National Marrow Donor Program.

Cacas, S. (1998, January 7). Doing well by doing good: Jonathan Leong brings business savvy to community nonprofits. *AsianWeek*, 21.

Chan, C. K. H. (1995, June 16). Leukemia patient refuses to die young: Desperate call to Asian Americans to sign up on bone-marrow registry. *AsianWeek*, 1.

Chang, V. (2009). *Using social media to save lives: HelpVinayandSameer.Org*. Case study. Stanford Graduate School of Business, Leland Stanford Junior University, Stanford.

Chin, S. A. (1995, April 11). Asian marrow donors sought: Pacific Islanders, other minorities rare in registries that save leukemia patients' lives. *San Francisco Examiner*, pp. A.

de Lara, J. (2010). *Volunteer manual*. Alameda, CA: Asian American Donor Program.

Doan, A. (2010). Hip hop 4 hope dance competition. *Hip-Hop-Dance.Net*. Retrieved May 20, 2011, from http://www.hip-hop-dance.net/hip-hop-4-hope-dance-competition.html.

Gomez, M. (2009, February 7). Bay area effort under way to register more Latino bone marrow donors. *Oakland Tribune*.

Kwon, Y. (2009). Why do Asian Americans have such poor odds of surviving leukemia and other blood-related disorders? Asian Pacific Americans for Progress. Retrieved May 18, 2011, from http://www.apaforprogress.org/blogs/yulkwon.

Lambda Phi Epsilon. (2011). Programs: National philanthropies. Lambda Phi Epsilon National Fraternity. Retrieved May 18, 2011, from http://lambdaphiepsilon.com/programs/#national-philanthropies.

Lee, J. H. (1989). Parents race against time, superstition to help baby: Leukemia: Some Asians, who are most likely to match her marrow type, are afraid to be donors. *The Los Angeles Times*. Retrieved May 11, 2011, from (http://articles.latimes.com/1989-11-04/news/mn-226_1_marrow-donor.

Leong, J. (2011, May 25). Personal interview.

Maykin, M. (2008). About Michelle. *Project Michelle*. Retrieved October May, 2011, from http://projectmichelle.com/project-michelle-about-michelle/.

Maykin, M. (2009). *Project Michelle blog*. Retrieved April 30, 2011, from http://projectmichelle.com/blog/.

McCullough, J., Perkins, H. A., & Hansen, J. (2006). The national marrow donor program with emphasis on the early years. *Transfusions, 46*, 1248–1255.

Mei, M. (2008). *The maykazine*. Retrieved May 10, 2011, from http://themaykazine.com.

Nakao, A. (1995, May 1). Marrow donor registry saving bay area Asian lives. *San Francisco Examiner*, pp. A.

National Marrow Donor Program. (2011). Who we are-about the national marrow donor program. *Be the Match*. Retrieved May 3, 2011, from http://www.marrow.org/ABOUT/Who_We_Are/index.html.

Nolan, A. (2011). Donor: Sabina Raza. *The Anthony Nolan trust*. Retrieved May 12, 2011, from http://www.anthonynolan.org/What-we-do/Real-Stories/Donor–Sabina-Raza.aspx.

Ochoa, L. (2008). Matching marrow/stem cell donors can save lives. *YouTube*. Silicon Valley: DeBugTV.

Project Michelle. (2008). Project Michelle fact sheet. *Project Michelle*. San Francisco. Retrieved May 10, 2011, from http://projectmichelle.com/for-the-media/.

Project Michelle. (2010). Letter of support for SB 1304. *Project Michelle*. Retrieved May 15, 2011, from http://www.projectmichelle.org.

Rabinow, P. (1996). *Essays on the anthropology of reason*. Princeton: Princeton University Press.

Rose, N., & Novas, C. (2004). Biological citizenship. In A. Ong & S. Collier (Eds.), *Global assemblages: Technology, politics, and ethics as anthropological problems* (pp. 439–465). Oxford: Blackwell.

San Francisco Examiner. (2007). *Local 'survivor' puts winnings to good use*. Retrieved May 19, 2011, from http://www.sfexaminer.com/local/local-survivor-puts-winnings-good-use?page=0%2C0%2C0%2C1.

Sawano, N. (1998, January 16). Marrow donor saves Alan Kuo. *The Harvard Crimson*. Retrieved April 30, 2011, from http://www.thecrimson.com/article/1998/1/16/marrow-donor-saves-alan-kuo.html.

Spigner, C., Weaver, M., Cardenas, V., & Allen, M. D. (2002). Organ donation and transplantation: Ethnic differences in knowledge and opinions among urban high school students. *Ethnicity and Health, 7*(2), 87–101.

Yabu, E. M., & Yee, K. L. (1990, February 8). Asian bone marrow recipients face great odds. *Synapse*, 1 & 4.

HIV/AIDS in Asian and Pacific Islanders in the United States

Don Operario, Judy Tan, and Caroline Kuo

Introduction

The HIV/AIDS epidemic is currently one of the nation's most urgent and challenging public health issues. HIV/AIDS affects every population and region in the United States, and has become increasingly represented among people of color, women, and young people under the age of 25 (Centers for Disease Control and Prevention [CDC], 2011). The CDC recently estimated that nearly 60,000 new HIV infections occurred in the United States every year between 2003 and 2006 (Hall et al., 2008). Although there are now highly effective treatments to prolong the lives of people living with HIV, access to treatment is limited and there exists no known cure for HIV infection.

Prevention remains the best strategy for reducing the number of new HIV infections. As we shall see, however, HIV prevention priorities are often shortsighted, especially for communities with emerging but not yet pronounced HIV epidemics. HIV prevention programs, which aim to reduce risk behaviors associated with HIV transmission and avert new infections, are generally targeted toward populations that have already been disproportionately burdened by HIV infection and AIDS illness. Epidemiology reports in the United States have thus urged for the prioritization of African American and Hispanic populations due to the high numbers of infected individuals in these groups. Because Asian and Pacific Islanders (APIs) in the United States have experienced a relatively lower burden of HIV infection and illness compared with other racial/ethnic groups, they have received far fewer resources and prioritization for HIV prevention. Community-based efforts to advocate for the HIV prevention needs in API populations have been vital for mobilizing attention from public health professionals, in the absence of a strong response from the policy sector.

In this chapter we review the state of HIV/AIDS prevention research in APIs. This chapter is organized into four sections: (1) the role of community-based organizations and social movements in responding to HIV/AIDS in APIs; (2) epidemiological trends suggesting an emerging risk for HIV among APIs; (3) social factors that increase HIV risk among APIs; and (4) existing HIV prevention interventions for APIs. Throughout each section, we will consider and critique how APIs have been represented and targeted, or overlooked and excluded, in research and prevention. We will also offer suggestions for

D. Operario (✉)
Program in Public Health, Brown University,
Providence, RI, USA
e-mail: Don_Operario@brown.edu

J. Tan
Center for AIDS Prevention Studies, University of
California San Francisco, San Francisco, CA, USA

C. Kuo
Department of Psychiatry, Rhode Island Hospital
and Alpert Medical School, Brown University,
Providence, RI, USA

G.J. Yoo et al. (eds.), *Handbook of Asian American Health*,
DOI 10.1007/978-1-4614-2227-3_28, © Springer Science+Business Media, LLC 2013

future research, intervention, and community mobilization strategies to respond to the growing HIV/AIDS epidemic among APIs.

Community-Based Organizations and Social Movements Addressing HIV/AIDS in Asian and Pacific Islanders

The HIV epidemic in the United States began at a pivotal time in the nation's history of racial/ethnic and sexual minority community development. The first HIV infections were identified among gay men in Los Angeles, New York, and San Francisco in 1981 – not long after the historic "Stonewall riots" of 1969 which marked the beginning of the gay liberation movement and on the heels of the civil rights movements for racial/ethnic equality in the United States. At the time the first HIV/AIDS cases were reported, community-based health and social organizations for racial/ethnic minority groups were just beginning to emerge in many cities. Community health organizations specifically targeting API populations were few in number, although some early prominent organizations included Chinatown Service Center-Community Health Center in Los Angeles, South Cove Community Health Center in Boston, Asian Health Services in Oakland, North East Medical Services in San Francisco, and the Charles B. Wang Community Health Center in New York – all of which were founded in the 1970s. Chin, Neilands, Weiss, and Mantell, (2008) characterize these as *community sentinel* health organizations, which are highly influential and historic mainstream agencies servicing the API population but with a mission to provide general health services rather than HIV/AIDS-specific services. None of the agencies was founded for the purpose of promoting sexual health or addressing sexually transmitted infections, and none was equipped with specific resources for gay men who represented the highest HIV risk group at the time.

As the epidemic expanded in the early 1980s, several community-based HIV/AIDS service organizations arose to advocate for improving the quality of health services for people living with HIV/AIDS, to fight against AIDS stigma and homophobia, and to promote safer sex in high-risk populations, especially gay men. These organizations included the Gay Men's Health Crisis in New York City, ACT Up in New York City, AIDS Project Los Angeles, AIDS Foundation of Chicago, and the San Francisco AIDS Foundation. Although their specific HIV/AIDS focus corresponded to the emerging public health needs, these organizations lacked early capacity to provide linguistic and culturally appropriate services for APIs.

API communities and API gay men in particular experienced a difficult tension with regard to the availability of community services for HIV/AIDS. Whereas many of the API community sentinel health organizations (named earlier) possessed linguistic, cultural, and professional competence for addressing general health concerns facing API clients, they lacked specific expertise related to HIV/AIDS illness, sexual risk reduction, gay men's health, and social issues including AIDS stigma and homophobia. API gay men also expressed discomfort in the large HIV/AIDS service organizations; some API men reported feeling isolated, excluded, or discriminated against in these mostly White organizational settings. API activists contested the concentration of power over HIV/AIDS prevention and public health resources in these powerful organizations that lacked capacity for serving people of diverse cultural and linguistic backgrounds, such as APIs (Reyes, 2000).

Consequently, API women and men sought to establish their own community-based organizations (CBOs) which addressed the intersection between HIV/AIDS and the racial/ethnic, cultural, and societal factors that underpin effective public health practices for APIs. Among the most established of these organizations are the Asian Pacific Islander Wellness Center (APIWC) in San Francisco, Asian Pacific Islander AIDS Intervention Team (APIAIT) in Los Angeles, and Asian and Pacific Islander Coalition on HIV/AIDS (APICHA) in New York City. Reyes (2000) described how these and other API HIV/AIDS organizations clearly demonstrated the effectiveness of grassroots advocacy for challenging the early dominant voices and representations of

HIV/AIDS as a white, gay male disease. Indeed, as the epidemic has unfolded since the 1980s, the faces of HIV/AIDS have increasingly become those of people of color and women, and the necessity of API HIV/AIDS organizations (as well as other race/ethnic-specific organizations) has increased over time.

The majority of the known CBOs that serve API populations offer linguistically sensitive programs, possess awareness into the ethnic/ cultural diversity and diverse needs of API populations, and have API professionals and paraprofessionals on staff. Notably, many of these organizations are attuned to the sexual and gender diversity in API communities, and have specific HIV prevention programs and support groups for gay or bisexual men and women, transgendered individuals, sex workers, youth, as well as heterosexual couples. In an analysis of 22 organizations servicing API communities in New York City, Chin et al. (2008) identified a specific subgroup of CBOs known as paradigm shifters, which are the most progressive, innovative, and often the youngest CBOs serving the API community. In addition to serving their health and social service missions, paradigm shifter CBOs are also strong advocates for social justice and for challenging the status quo, especially with regard to homosexuality and gender norms in the API community. These CBOs aimed to question the legitimacy of traditional cultural views and provoked change in favor of equality for marginalized API subgroups, such as HIV-positive APIs.

Arguably, the most effective and far-reaching API HIV/AIDS service organizations embody these paradigm-shifting characteristics. Researchers who have studied the experiences of front-line CBO professionals who work in API HIV/AIDS service organizations have illuminated the necessary practices for fighting the epidemic – practices that expand far beyond providing general HIV educational information. These studies suggest that the basic "safer sex" approach to HIV prevention, which focuses on encouraging condom use and safer sex practices, might be insufficient for reducing risks in API communities. Work by Yoshikawa et al. (2003) highlighted the theoretical limitations of many HIV prevention

frameworks – which tend to focus exclusively on improving sexual behaviors among individuals as the primary unit of change – when applied to API populations. Findings from interviews of peer educators working in a API-focused CBO highlighted the need for interventions to address API social networks, environmental contexts of risk behavior, and cultural preferences and attitudes of API clients; these factors are absent in many traditional theories that guide HIV prevention research (Yoshikawa et al., 2003). Research by Han (2009) further broadens the scope of CBO-based HIV prevention services for APIs, by stressing the need for programs to address homophobia in the API community, racism in the general and gay communities, low self-esteem among many APIs, and the absence of positive role models for APIs, especially API "men who have sex with men" (MSM).

It is clear from the body of literature that the work of grassroots activists, and the organizations they developed, was central to developing an aggressive response to HIV/AIDS in API communities. Paradigm shifting CBOs have not only promoted HIV awareness, safer sex, condom use, and HIV testing, but have also challenged dominant power structures based on race/ethnicity, gender, sexuality, immigration status, language, and income. These CBOs provided alternative spaces (which, in some cases, have become mainstream over time) for providing culturally and linguistically sensitive services for APIs. Studies of the development and current practices of these CBOs have highlighted the need for community-academic collaborative partnerships at every stage of HIV prevention program planning, research, and policy – beginning from the earliest phases of problem definition, to the hands-on phases of program implementation and oversight, until the final phases of program evaluation and dissemination of findings (Operario, Nemoto, Ng, Syed, & Mazarei, 2005). Partnerships and alliances between activists, CBOs, researchers, and policy-makers will continue to be essential for improving and sustaining HIV prevention efforts in API communities (Takahashi, Magalong, Debell, & Fasudhani, 2006).

HIV/AIDS Epidemiological Trends Among Asian and Pacific Islanders

APIs experience a curious tension in the scientific HIV/AIDS literature: although APIs currently show low HIV prevalence and incidence relative to other racial/ethnic groups, studies reveal startling high levels of sexual risk behavior in APIs. What accounts for this disconnect between the number of infections and the levels of behavioral risk? And how does this influence the prioritization of APIs in HIV/AIDS policies? These are difficult questions that must be examined by applying a critical lens to the data.

According to data from the CDC, APIs accounted for 1% of all people living with HIV in the United States (CDC, 2011). From the beginning of the epidemic to 2008, an estimated 9,184 APIs were diagnosed with AIDS, of which 85% were males and 15% were females (Adih, Campsmith, Williams, Hardnett, & Hughes, 2011). Between 2001 and 2008, approximately 2,870 APIs were diagnosed with HIV infection in states reporting name-based HIV data to the federal government. For males, same-sex behavior accounted for most HIV infections (78% overall), whereas for females, heterosexual contact accounted for most HIV infections (86% overall).

Multiple epidemiological studies have indicated high rates of unprotected anal sex among API men who have sex with men (MSM) (Choi, Han, Hudes, & Kegeles, 2002; McFarland, Chen, Weide, Kohn, & Klausner, 2004). As mentioned, one of the striking contradictions in HIV research is the relatively low prevalence of HIV infection but high levels of sexual risk behavior among API MSM (Wei et al., 2011). Studies have documented that API MSM are equally or more likely to have unprotected sex and multiple sex partners compared with White, African American, and Hispanic MSM (Brooks, Lee, Newman, & Leibowitz, 2008; CDC, 2002; Rosser et al., 2009; Xia et al., 2006). Studies of API MSM have also reported high prevalence of other factors associated with HIV risk, including heavy alcohol use and non-injection drug use (Choi et al., 2005; Operario et al., 2006;

Peterson, Bakeman, & Stokes, 2001), other sexually transmitted infections (STIs) (McFarland et al., 2004; Raymond et al., 2006), and depression (Chae & Yoshikawa, 2008). These co-occurring risk factors highlight a propensity for increased HIV prevalence in this population.

Although heterosexual contact plays a significant role in HIV infection among API women, few studies have addressed this group. Heterosexual contact accounts for a greater proportion of HIV infections among API women than it does for African American and Hispanic women (CDC, 2011). A recent study of API women found that only 51% reported condom use during their last sexual episode and 63% used condoms inconsistently (Hahm, Lee, Rough, & Strathdee, 2011). Analysis of a national representative sample of young APIs found that "13% of API women had ever had a STI" – roughly four times the likelihood of API men having a STI – with chlamydia being the most commonly reported infection (Hahm, Lee, Ozonoff, & Amodeo, 2007). Recent studies have brought attention to high rates of unprotected sex, risk for HIV and other STIs, and violence among API female sex workers, particularly those working in massage parlors in the United States (Nemoto, Operario, Takenaka, Iwamoto, & Le, 2003). Among API women who engage in compensated sex, economic pressures and violence play a significant role in HIV risk (Nemoto, Iwamoto, Wong, Le, & Operario, 2004; Nemoto, Iwamoto, Oh, Wong, & Nguyen, 2005). Studies among API transgender women also documented high rates of HIV risk due to frequency of unprotected sex and commercial sex work (Operario & Nemoto, 2005).

Analysis of a national youth risk surveillance dataset found that, compared to their peers, API high school students were less likely to have had sex or be sexually active (Lowry, Eaton, Brener, & Kann, 2011). However, once they become sexually active, APIs are equally or more likely as other racial/ethnic peer groups to have sex under the influence of alcohol or drugs and to have unprotected sex (Lowry, Eaton, Brener, & Kann, 2011). A study among high school students in San Diego from 1993 to 2005 showed that API students reported consistently lower condom use at last sexual intercourse compared to their racial/ethnic peers (Lee & Rotheram-Borus, 2009).

Although estimated HIV prevalence in APIs has historically been lower compared to other racial/ethnic groups in the United States, there are reasons for concern about the growing and unrecognized epidemic in APIs. First, within the past decade, APIs face alarmingly high numbers of new HIV infections and one of the most rapidly increasing epidemics among the racial/ethnic groups in the United States. According to research by Chin, Leung, Sheth, & Rodriguez, (2007) and Adih et al. (2011), APIs experienced the greatest annual percentage increase in new HIV/AIDS diagnoses between 2000 and 2008. Second, APIs are frequently underrepresented in national surveillance, likely leading to an under-estimation of HIV among APIs. For example, many national HIV prevalence estimates are based on data from states that conduct name-based HIV case reporting and provide HIV incidence surveillance to the CDC. These estimates do not include data from California, Hawaii, and Massachusetts – states that contain some of the largest API populations in the nation – because these states only recently have provided name-based HIV data to the CDC (Hall et al., 2008). Third, many community surveys have low samples of API respondents resulting in a limited understanding of the challenges faced by APIs at risk for HIV or living with HIV. A 2010 CDC report estimated HIV prevalence among MSM based on data from 8,153 participants recruited from 21 cities, but included only 185 APIs (CDC, 2010); a 2009 CDC report of HIV prevalence in injection drug users recruited from 23 cities did not report data for APIs due to a negligible sample size (CDC, 2009a). A 2009 CDC report of HIV testing from 12,120 high school students also did not report data for APIs (CDC, 2009b). Fourth, HIV prevalence estimates are affected by low rates of testing in API communities (Zaidi et al., 2005), even among those who perceived themselves as being at risk for HIV (Kahle, Freedman, & Buskin, 2009). A study of API MSM in San Francisco found that one-quarter of respondents had never been tested for HIV (Do et al., 2005),

and analysis of data from a national survey of young adult women found that API women had the lowest proportion of HIV testing (17.2%) compared to women in other racial/ethnic groups (Hahm, Song, Ozonoff, & Sassani, 2009). Alarmingly, APIs who test positive for HIV are likely to do so later in the course of infection. Of 2,395 APIs who tested HIV-positive between 2001 and 2007, 37% progressed to AIDS within 12 months of their initial HIV test (Adih et al., 2011). The brief interval between HIV diagnosis and AIDS status indicates delayed HIV testing and missed opportunities for HIV treatment for many APIs.

Owing to these acknowledged limitations, the existing epidemiological data on HIV among APIs must be interpreted with caution. Our knowledge of HIV risk and prevention among APIs would be greatly increased with improved epidemiology, community recruitment, and rates of testing. This entails building improved systems of surveillance and extending outreach efforts for this underrepresented and understudied population. In the context of current national policy priorities for HIV/AIDS funding, APIs are relegated to the bottom of the list of prioritized groups or absent altogether. Prevention policies tend to de-prioritize those groups that have not yet shown heavy burden of illness, which is precisely where prevention efforts might have the strongest impact.

Social Factors Associated with HIV Risk Among Asian and Pacific Islanders

A number of social factors contributing to HIV risk among API populations have been reported in the literature. Among the most frequently mentioned social factors related to HIV risk are homophobic stigma toward same-sex behavior within API communities, racial/ethnic stereotypes about APIs in the general population and in predominantly White gay communities, sexual silence and discomfort of sexuality in traditional API cultures, and the lack of culturally competent HIV prevention and care services.

Homophobia and stigmatizing attitudes toward same-sex behavior have been repeatedly shown to be determinants of sexual risk behavior among API gay men. Many API gay men experience tensions between their identity as both gay and API, and risk rejection by either or both communities (Han, 2009; Operario, Han, & Choi, 2008). Many API men who engage in same-gender sex do not identify as gay, which they perceive as a "White" construct that is inconsistent with cultural norms and identity formulations. Researchers have consequently adopted the terminology "men who have sex with men" (MSM) to refer to the population of all men who have same-gender sex regardless of their sexual identity.

In qualitative studies, API MSM described rejection from family and peers, feelings of social isolation, and internalization of negative attitudes toward homosexuality (Nemoto, Operario, & Soma et al., 2003). Because many traditional cultural values place emphasis on family obligation, masculine roles, and continuing the family name through having children, API MSM frequently feel that they violate family and cultural expectations. Consequently, many API MSM keep their sexual identity and same-sex behaviors hidden from family, and might not utilize HIV prevention and health education programs that require disclosing their sexual behavior to others. The internalization of stigma, discomfort, and guilt around sexual identity and sexual desire may contribute to API MSM having poor skills and making suboptimal decisions regarding condom use, partner selection, and co-occurring behaviors such as substance use.

Research has also shown that HIV risk behavior is influenced by racial/ethnic stereotypes about APIs held in the general population and in the White gay community in particular. Studies of API MSM have reported experiences of subtle yet pervasive forms of racism in the gay community, including being perceived as sexually undesirable, emasculated, or sexually objectified by White MSM. The idea of "rice queens" and Asian "boys" as fetishized accessories of White MSM is a theme that many of API MSM report experiencing, in addition to feeling rejected or excluded in the gay community (Nemoto, Operario, &

Soma et al., 2003). This constellation of stereotypes can compromise API MSM's feelings of self-efficacy to select partners, discuss safer sex, and use condoms (Han, 2008). Studies have also indicated that API women might be perceived as passive, weak, exotic, and subservient, and that these negative racial/ethnic stereotypes can influence their ability to engage in safer sex practices and make reproductive health choices (Chin, 1999). Moreover, these stereotypes of API women might also contribute to intimate partner violence and sexual coercion (Nemoto et al., 2005).

Cultural norms of sexual silence in API communities can affect individuals' self-efficacy and abilities to practice safer sex behaviors. Issues such as premarital sex, homosexuality, and sexual health are considered taboo topics in many API cultures, and API individuals may develop feelings of discomfort or avoidance toward these topics (Chin et al., 2007). Avoidance of these issues might have particular consequences for the sexual decision-making and behaviors of API youth. Studies have highlighted strong cultural barriers that prevent API parents and adolescents from talking about sex (Chung et al., 2007; Kim & Ward, 2007). As mentioned, although API youth generally experience sexual debut later than other racial/ethnic groups, once they become sexually active their sexual behaviors are just as risky, or sometimes more risky, compared to other racial/ethnic groups (Lee & Rotheram-Borus, 2009; Lowry et al., 2011).

Lack of culturally competent prevention and care services also contributes to HIV risk in API communities. Often, prevention and care services rely on superficial strategies to address cultural competence, such as placing pictures of API individuals on health education materials; however, as Han (2009) astutely remarked, "Chopstocks don't make it culturally competent." On a deeper level, cultural competent HIV prevention and care services must address structural, demographic, familial, and psychosocial issues and values that reflect the determinants of HIV risk for API individuals. A notable challenge to providing culturally competent HIV services is the diversity among APIs. The API category encapsulates multiple languages, cultures, socioeconomic groups, and immigration histories, and this diversity is likely to impact HIV risk and prevention needs in different ways. Risk behavior may be related to cultural or language barriers that contribute to discomfort in engaging with medical professionals in discussions related to HIV and sexual health (Takahashi et al., 2006).

HIV Prevention Programs and Interventions for Asian and Pacific Islanders

To date, there has been only one empirically validated HIV prevention intervention developed specifically for APIs. This prevention program, conducted by Choi et al. (1996) in San Francisco between 1992 and 1994, involved a randomized controlled trial to test the efficacy of a brief group counseling program to reduce HIV risk behaviors among 329 API MSM. The participants were predominantly ethnic Chinese (37%), Filipino (34%), Japanese (10%) or Vietnamese (8%); immigrants to the United States (67%); college graduates (66%); and openly gay to their friends (98%). Participants were randomly assigned to either small counseling groups or to a wait-list control group. The counseling groups involved a single 3-h interactive discussion session addressing four topics: developing positive ethnic and sexual identities; safer sex education; eroticizing safer sex; and building safer sex negotiation skills. Three months following enrollment in the study, participants in the counseling groups reported significantly fewer sex partners and greater AIDS knowledge and AIDS-related anxiety compared to those in the control group. In addition, Chinese and Filipino participants in the counseling groups reported significantly less unprotected anal sex at 3-month follow-up compared to those in the control group. It was unclear as to why unprotected anal sex declined in only certain ethnic groups. One explanation offered by the authors was that Chinese and Filipino MSM in San Francisco may have larger peer networks than other MSM of other API ethnicities, which ostensibly provided them

with more opportunities for behavioral reinforcement and social support for engaging in safer sex. Although this program was notable in being the first HIV prevention program targeting API MSM (or any API population), it is disappointing to note that no other HIV prevention interventions for APIs have since been evaluated in a randomized controlled trial.

Several other HIV prevention programs and interventions targeting APIs have been identified (see Table 28.1). However, these programs were not rigorously tested in randomized controlled trials, thereby limiting their scientific validity. Among the more rigorous studies, Siegel, DiClemente, Durbin, and Krasnovsky, (1995) evaluated a school-based AIDS education program targeting mostly Asian and African American junior high students in Northern California, and found that students reported greater AIDS knowledge and increased tolerance towards AIDS-affected people compared with students in schools that did not receive the program. Six studies have described the potential for increasing the capacity of community-based organizations (CBOs) by establishing inter-agency partnerships and formalizing collaborations between community stakeholders and academic researchers (Chin, Kang, Kim, Martinez, & Eckholdt, 2006; Loue, Lloyd, & Phoombour, 1996; Operario et al., 2005; Sheth, Operario, Latham, & Sheoran, 2007; Takahashi, Candelario, Young, & Mediano, 2007; Wong et al., 2011).

Research studies by Sheth et al. (2007) and Wong et al. (2011) are particularly notable for developing national-level networks and community-research partnerships in multiple sites in the United States to improve HIV education and testing in API populations. A study by Nemoto, Iwamoto, Kamitani, Morris, and Sakata (2011) described an aggressive strategy of providing targeted outreach and referrals to high-risk API subpopulations – MSM, substance users, and incarcerated individuals.

The current body of empirical HIV prevention and intervention research targeting API populations is limited. To our knowledge, only one intervention has been validated in a rigorous

Table 28.1 Summary of published HIV prevention programs and interventions targeting API populations in the United States

Citation	Project title; community organizations[a]	Aims	Location	Methods	Outcome measures
Chin et al., (2006)	The Bridges Project; APICHA	To improve the ability of API who are HIV+ to utilize HIV-related health services by bridging language and cultural barriers through language interpretation, client escort, advocacy and case management	NYC	Established referral ties with identified hospital and community-based clinics; annual cultural competence training of staff at participating sites; training of services available through the program; providing language translation (12 API languages/dialects) and escort services; peer advocating and case management of services outside of program	Service use: needing and receiving primary care services; number of reported barriers per service overall, and between documented and undocumented participants, and between Asian-primary-language and English-primary language participants
Choi et al. (1996)	Brief group counseling using culturally appropriate HIV risk reduction; the Living Well Project (APIWC)	To reduce HIV risk behaviors among API MSM: to address the context of being both gay and API (i.e., to acknowledge community stigma, racism, homophobia), present positive images of gay API, to increase knowledge, enhance safer sex attitudes and skills	San Francisco Bay Area, CA	Randomized controlled trial. Participants randomly assigned to either intervention or control group; trained co-facilitators delivered 3-h interventions to groups of 8 using piloted intervention materials; issues such as stigma, dual identity, media representation were discussed; safer sex education (discussing attitudes, identifying risks, providing facts about HIV transmission); eroticizing safer sex; building safer sex behavioral skills	3-Month assessment of HIV-related knowledge, attitudes, skills; perceived risk; AIDS-related anxiety; condom enjoyment; sexual communication; sexual negotiation with new partners; HIV risk behaviors (i.e., # of sexual partners within last 3 months, # of UAI within last 3 months)

Loue et al., (1996)	Case study of API community organizing; Project Health for Asian Pacific Islanders (HAPI) and Asian Pacific Islander Community AIDS Project (ADICAP)	To reduce HIV transmission risk via community organization	San Diego, CA	Focus groups (private citizens, community leaders, social service providers, educators, legislators, religious leaders, HIV-infected individuals, health care providers); questionnaires developed based on focus groups were administered to convenience sample assessing HIV knowledge, attitudes, and risk behaviors; development of community organization/program providing technical assistance to CBOs serving HIV-infected individuals with materials developed from community focus groups, questionnaires; community outreach and serving as coordinator of efforts between HIV CBOs, projects	Community participation (Network density analysis of "connectedness" with other organizations) of 20 CBOs involved with Project HAPI/ADICAP
Nemoto et al., (2011)	Targeted Expansion Project for Outreach and Treatment (TEPOT) for substance use and HIV risk behaviors in API Communities; Public Health Institute, Oakland	To conduct outreach and referrals to substance use and HIV prevention services in targeted API communities; distribute culturally sensitive safer sex materials; assess HIV and substance use prevention needs of API subgroups – MSM, substance users, and incarcerated individuals	San Francisco, San Mateo, and Santa Clara counties, CA	Ethnographic mapping to identify areas for targeted outreach; collaboration with culturally appropriate substance use and HIV prevention organizations; cross-sectional survey to API individuals	Sexual risk and substance use behaviors, mental and physical health issues, criminal history, HIV knowledge, attitudes toward drug use, attitudes toward condom use

(continued)

Table 28.1 (continued)

Citation	Project title; community organizations[a]	Aims	Location	Methods	Outcome measures
Operario et al. (2005)	Case study of a community collaborative research project – API/X (HIV prevention intervention for uninfected API MSM) and API/PLUS (HIV prevention intervention for HIV-positive API MSM); APIWC	To foster partnership between researchers and community-based HIV service organizations as a mechanism for improving the quality of HIV prevention services for HIV uninfected (API/X program) and HIV-positive (API/PLUS program) MSM; program evaluation	San Francisco Bay Area, CA	Formative research/pilot testing for developing intervention and evaluation curriculum; implementation; dissemination	Lessons learned: acknowledgment of differences in respective organizational culture; defining project roles and responsibilities; hiring, training, and support of front-line staff
Sheth et al. (2007)	API National Capacity-Building Assistance (CBA) Program; APIWC & APIAHF	To increase HIV testing and enrolment in HIV services, to increase acceptance of and destigmatize HIV/AIDS in API families and communities, to increase data collection and reporting of API HIV/AIDS data, increase API community's commitment to HIV services and organizations, and to build capacity in the Pacific Island jurisdictions	Nation-wide (NY, MA, Illinois, CA, and Hawaii)	One-on-one CBA (i.e., tailored technical consultation, training, coaching, and referrals to other CBOs and health departments), national and regional skills building training, and culturally competent information and technology transfer (e.g., program replication toolkits, fact sheets, best practice guides)	First-order effects (direct impact on clients of CBA), and system-level effects (at the community and policy levels) – only baseline data and results collected from trainings have been collected and analyzed thus far
Siegel et al. (1995)	AIDS-prevention education program for junior high schools with predominantly API and African American students; UCSF	To deliver a school-based intervention to junior high school students covering sex education, HIV biology, drug use, behavioral skills (decision-making and refusal)	Inner-city junior high school, Northern CA	Pretest–posttest control design involving 2 intervention and 1 control schools; a 7-unit, pretested curriculum focusing on information and behavioral skills was delivered didactically and interactively in 12 lessons over a 3-week period; teachers attended a 2-day training	AIDS-related knowledge, Attitudes towards people with AIDS, sexual risk-taking behavior

			Location		
Takahashi et al. (2007)	Case study – capacity building for HIV prevention in API organizations; APAIT	To build and strengthen a network of community-based social services and LGBTQ social organizations targeting API to increase culturally competent HIV prevention and treatment	Southern CA	Subcontracted organizations committed to HIV/AIDS issues in API communities; Provided technical assistance to organization stability and viability (i.e., organizational coaching, workshops, symposia, leading to building partnerships with other community agencies); technical assistant for HIV knowledge environments (i.e., workshops, meetings on HIV prevention and diverse populations)	Survey assessments at 3 timepoints over 2 years (baseline, mid-, and end-program) on organizational stability and viability (i.e., human resources, finance, service delivery, external relations, partnerships, strategic planning), and HIV knowledge
Wong et al. (2011)	Men of Asian Testing for HIV (MATH) Study; Georgetown University, George Washington University, APIAHF, ASIAC, AHS, APAIT, APICHA, APIWC, AACI, MAPS	To develop a national research and practice model for HIV prevention and testing for API MSM	Five cities: Boston, Los Angeles, New York Philadelphia, San Francisco Bay Area	Community-based participatory research; developed consortium of 7 community-based organizations to build partnerships; describe and enhance institutional capacity for HIV prevention programs for API MSM	Enhancing community-based infrastructure to conduct research; build/improve HIV testing capacity; increase outreach to hard-to-reach subpopulations; develop partnerships between researchers and community stakeholders; collect data to inform policies that affect API MSM

aOrganization acronyms: *AACI* Asian Americans for Community Involvement, *AHS* Asian Health Services, *APAIT* Asian Pacific AIDS Intervention Team, *APIAHF* Asian and Pacific Islander American Health Forum, *APICHA* Asian and Pacific Islander Coalition on HIV/AIDS, *APIWC* Asian Pacific Islander Wellness Center, *ASIAC* AIDS Services in Asian Communities, *MAPS* Massachusetts Asians and Pacific Islanders for Health experimental design (Choi et al., 1996) and one other intervention has been evaluated in a quasi-experimental design (Siegel et al., 1995). Other identified studies demonstrate potentially promising results, but warrant more rigorous evaluation. The few evaluations of HIV programs targeting APIs highlight the importance of cultural considerations, including meeting the diverse language needs of this population (Chin et al., 2006), strengthening inter-agency collaboration (Wong et al., 2011) and addressing multiple layers of racial and HIV-related stigma (Sheth et al., 2007; Takahashi et al., 2007).

The research on HIV/AIDS interventions for APIs is limited by the paucity of existing studies. This may be linked to larger structural issues regarding lack of funding, a limited number of researchers focusing on HIV in API communities (Yanagihara, Chang, & Ernst, 2009), and the limited capacity of CBOs to design and scale up culturally relevant HIV programs for APIs (Operario et al., 2005; Sheth et al., 2007; Takahashi et al., 2007). Clearly, much more work needs to be done to understand how HIV prevention and care services can optimize the provision of culturally competent programs to APIs.

Conclusion

In this chapter we have described current research on the community movements, epidemiology, social risk factors, and prevention programs addressing HIV/AIDS in API communities. Although the research to date is commendable for identifying and advocating for the unique HIV prevention and care needs among APIs, this chapter highlights the limitations to the body of research. Not only are the number of studies limited, but the methodologies for recruitment, measurement, and intervention with APIs remain in a stage of infancy.

The scientific literature continues to describe APIs as a low-risk group, based on comparisons with African American and Hispanic populations. As a consequence, there continues to be limited research and programmatic attention to HIV among APIs, and APIs continue to be

perceived as the "model minority" in comparison with other communities of color. This tension highlights a paradox in public health: prevention programs tend to focus exclusively and reactively on populations that have already been affected, and consequently neglect populations that may have an emerging HIV epidemic but that do not yet show high rates of morbidity and mortality. Due to constraints in funding, time, and human and technical capacities, HIV resources tend to be rationed and restricted for APIs. As this chapter has reviewed, research on the growing risk for HIV transmission in API communities, especially in MSM but also among heterosexual women and youth, should provide us with a sense of urgency and indicate a need to reconsider HIV prevention priorities.

A new generation of researchers, health professionals, and activist community members is needed to improve on our understanding of HIV/AIDS in API communities. This new cadre of professionals will hopefully contribute strategies for engaging, researching, and responding to API communities and their needs for HIV prevention and care. Innovations produced by the next generation of professionals studying HIV in API communities can also offer valuable insights for developing public health responses in other emerging epidemics.

Acknowledgement Preparation of this chapter was supported by a National Institute of Mental Health traineeship (T32-MH074387) and a National Science Foundation Doctoral Dissertation Award to Judy Tan, and by a National Institute of Mental Health training grant (T32-MH078788) to Caroline Kuo.

References

Adih, W. K., Campsmith, M., Williams, C. L., Hardnett, F. P., & Hughes, D. (2011). Epidemiology of HIV among Asians and Pacific Islanders in the United States, 2001–2008. *Journal of the International Association of Physicians in AIDS Care* Apr 20 [Epub ahead of print].

Brooks, R. A., Lee, S.-J., Newman, P. A., & Leibowitz, A. A. (2008). Sexual risk behavior has decreased among men who have sex with men in Los Angeles but remains greater than that among heterosexual men and women. *AIDS Education and Prevention, 20*(4), 312–324.

Centers for Disease Control and Prevention. (2002). *HIV testing survey, 2002*. Atlanta, GA: Author.

Centers for Disease Control and Prevention. (2009a). HIV-associated behaviors among injection-drug users – 23 cities, United States, May 2005–February 2006. *Morbidity and Mortality Weekly Report, 58*(13), 329–332.

Centers for Disease Control and Prevention. (2009b). HIV Testing among high school students – United States, 2007. *Morbidity and Mortality Weekly Report, 58*(24), 665–668.

Centers for Disease Control and Prevention. (2010). Prevalence and awareness of HIV infection among men who have sex with men – 21 Cities, United States, 2008. *Morbidity and Mortality Weekly Report, 59*(37), 1201–1207.

Centers for Disease Control and Prevention. (2011). *Epidemiology of HIV infection through 2009*. Atlanta, GA: Division of HIV/AIDS Prevention/National Center for HIV/AIDS/Viral Hepatitis/STD/TB Prevention.

Chae, D. H., & Yoshikawa, H. (2008). Perceived group devaluation, depression, and HIV-risk behavior among Asian gay men. *Health Psychology, 27*(2), 140–148.

Chin, D. (1999). HIV-related sexual risk assessment among Asian/Pacific Islander American women: An inductive model. *Social Science & Medicine, 49*(2), 241–251.

Chin, J. J., Kang, E., Kim, J. J., Martinez, J., & Eckholdt, H. (2006). Serving Asians and Pacific Islanders with HIV/AIDS: Challenges and lessons learned. *Journal of Health Care for the Poor and Underserved, 17*(4), 910–927.

Chin, J. J., Leung, M., Sheth, L., & Rodriguez, T. R. (2007). Let's not ignore a growing HIV problem for Asian and Pacific Islanders in the U.S. *Journal of Urban Health, 84*(5), 642–647.

Chin, J. J., Neilands, T. B., Weiss, L., & Mantell, J. E. (2008). Paradigm shifters, professionals and community sentinels: Immigrant community institutions' roles in shaping places and implications for stigmatized public health initiatives. *Health & Place, 14*(4), 866–882.

Choi, K.-H., Han, C.-S., Hudes, E. S., & Kegeles, S. (2002). Unprotected sex and associated risk factors among young Asian and Pacific Islander men who have sex with men. *AIDS Education and Prevention, 14*(6), 472–481.

Choi, K.-H., Lew, S., Vittinghoff, E., Catania, J. A., Barrett, D. C., & Coates, T. J. (1996). The efficacy of brief group counseling in HIV risk reduction among homosexual Asian and Pacific Islander men. *AIDS, 10*(1), 81–87.

Choi, K.-H., Operario, D., Gregorich, S. E., McFarland, W., MacKellar, D., & Valleroy, L. (2005). Substance use, substance choice, and unprotected anal intercourse among young Asian American and Pacific Islander men who have sex with men. *AIDS Education and Prevention, 17*(5), 418–429.

Chung, P. J., Travis, R., Kilpatrick, S. D., Elliot, M. N., Lui, C., Khandwala, S. B., et al. (2007). Acculturation and parent-adolescent communication about sex in Filipino-American families: A community-based participatory research study. *Journal of Adolescent Health, 40*(6), 543–550.

Do, T. D., Chen, S., McFarland, W., Secura, G. M., Behel, S. K., MacKellar, D. A., et al. (2005). HIV testing patterns and unrecognized HIV infection among young Asian and Pacific Islander men who have sex with men in San Francisco. *AIDS Education and Prevention, 17*(6), 540–554.

Hahm, H. C., Lee, J., Ozonoff, A., & Amodeo, M. (2007). Predictors of STDs among Asian and Pacific Islander young adults. *Perspectives on Sexual and Reproductive Health, 39*(4), 231–239.

Hahm, H. C., Lee, J., Rough, K., & Strathdee, S. A. (2011). Gender power control, sexual experiences, safer sex practices, and potential HIV risk behaviors among young Asian-American women. *AIDS and Behavior* Jan 23 [Epub ahead of print].

Hahm, H. C., Song, I. H., Ozonoff, A., & Sassani, J. (2009). HIV testing among sexually experienced Asian and Pacific Islander young women: Association with routine gynecologic care. *Women's Health Issues, 19*(5), 279–288.

Hall, H. I., Song, R., Rhodes, P., Prejean, J., An, Q., Lee, L. M., et al. (2008). Estimation of HIV incidence in the United States. *Journal of the American Medical Association, 300*(5), 520–529.

Han, C.-S. (2008). A qualitative exploration of the relationship between racism and unsafe sex among Asian Pacific Islander gay men. *Archives of Sexual Behavior, 37*(5), 827–837.

Han, C.-S. (2009). Chopsticks don't make it culturally competent: Addressing larger issues for HIV prevention among gay, bisexual, and queer Asian Pacific Islander men. *Health and Social Work, 34*(4), 273–281.

Kahle, E. M., Freedman, M. S., & Buskin, S. E. (2009). HIV risks and testing behavior among Asians and Pacific Islanders: Results of the HIV testing survey, 2002–2003. *Journal of the National Medical Association, 97*(Suppl. 7), 13S–18S.

Kim, J. L., & Ward, L. M. (2007). Silence speaks volumes: Parental sexual communication among Asian American emerging adults. *Journal of Adolescent Research, 22*(1), 3–31.

Lee, S.-J., & Rotheram-Borus, M. J. (2009). Beyond the "model minority" stereotype: Trends in health risk behaviors among Asian/Pacific Islander high school students. *Journal of School Health, 79*(8), 347–354.

Loue, S., Lloyd, L. S., & Phoombour, E. (1996). Organizing Asian Pacific Islanders in an urban community to reduce HIV Risk: A case study. *AIDS Education and Prevention, 8*(5), 381–393.

Lowry, R., Eaton, D., Brener, N. D., & Kann, L. (2011). Prevalence of health-risk behaviors among Asian American and Pacific Islander high school students in the US, 2001–2007. *Public Health Reports, 126*(1), 39–49.

McFarland, W., Chen, S., Weide, D., Kohn, R., & Klausner, J. (2004). Gay Asian men in San Francisco follow the international trend: Increases in rates of unprotected anal intercourse and sexually transmitted diseases, 1999–2002. *AIDS Education and Prevention, 16*(1), 13–18.

Nemoto, T., Iwamoto, M., Kamitani, E., Morris, A., & Sakata, M. (2011). Targeted expansion project for outreach and treatment for substance abuse and HIV risk behaviors in Asian and Pacific Islander communities. *AIDS Education and Prevention, 23*(2), 175–191.

Nemoto, T., Iwamoto, M., Oh, H. J., Wong, S., & Nguyen, H. (2005). Risk behaviors among Asian women who work at massage parlors in San Francisco: Perspectives from masseuses and owners/managers. *AIDS Education and Prevention, 17*(5), 444–456.

Nemoto, T., Iwamoto, M., Wong, S., Le, M. N., & Operario, D. (2004). Social factors related to risk for violence and sexually transmitted infections/HIV among Asian massage parlor workers in San Francisco. *AIDS and Behavior, 8*(4), 475–483.

Nemoto, T., Operario, D., Soma, T., Bao, D., Vajrabukka, A., & Crisostomo, V. (2003). HIV risk and prevention among Asian/Pacific Islander men who have sex with men: Listen to our stories. *AIDS Education and Prevention, 15*(1), 7–20.

Nemoto, T., Operario, D., Takenaka, M., Iwamoto, M., & Le, M. N. (2003). HIV risk among Asian women working at massage parlors in San Francisco. *AIDS Education and Prevention, 15*(3), 245–256.

Operario, D., Choi, K.-H., Chu, P. L., McFarland, W., Secura, G., Behel, S., et al. (2006). Prevalence and correlates of substance use among young Asian Pacific Islander men who have sex with men. *Prevention Science, 7*(1), 19–29.

Operario, D., Han, C.-S., & Choi, K.-H. (2008). Dual identity among gay Asian Pacific Islander men. *Culture, Health and Sexuality, 10*(5), 447–461.

Operario, D., & Nemoto, T. (2005). Sexual risk behavior and substance use among a sample of Asian Pacific Islander transgender women. *AIDS Education and Prevention, 17*, 430–443.

Operario, D., Nemoto, T., Ng, T., Syed, J., & Mazarei, M. (2005). Conducting HIV interventions for Asian Pacific Islander men who have sex with men: Challenges and compromises in community collaborative research. *AIDS Education and Prevention, 17*(5), 334–346.

Peterson, J. L., Bakeman, R., & Stokes, J. (2001). Racial/ethnic patterns of HIV sexual risk behaviors among young men who have sex with men. *Journal of the Gay and Lesbian Medical Association, 5*(4), 155–162.

Raymond, H. F., Chen, S., Truong, H.-H. M., Knapper, K. B., Klausner, J. D., Choi, K.-H., et al. (2006). Trends in sexually transmitted diseases, sexual risk behavior, and HIV infection among Asian/Pacific Islander men who have sex with men, San Francisco, 1999–2005. *Sexually Transmitted Diseases, 33*(10), 262–264.

Reyes, E. E. (2000). Profiles of API HIV/AIDS community-based organizations. *Journal of Asian American Studies, 3*(2), 241–250.

Rosser, B. R. S., Oakes, J. M., Horvath, K. J., Konstan, J. A., Danilenko, G. P., & Peterson, J. L. (2009). HIV sexual risk behavior by men who use the internet to seek sex with men: Results of the Men's INTernet Sex Study-II (MINTS-II). *AIDS and Behavior, 13*(3), 488–498.

Sheth, L., Operario, D., Latham, N., & Sheoran, B. (2007). National-level capacity-building assistance model to enhance HIV prevention for Asian & Pacific Islander communities. *Journal of Public Health Management and Practice, 13*, S40–S48.

Siegel, D., DiClemente, R., Durbin, M., & Krasnovsky, F. (1995). Change in junior high school students' AIDS-related knowledge, misconceptions, attitudes, and HIV-preventive behaviors: Effects of a school-based intervention. *AIDS Education and Prevention, 7*(6), 534–543.

Takahashi, L. M., Candelario, J., Young, T., & Mediano, E. (2007). Building capacity for HIV/AIDS prevention among Asian Pacific Islander organizations: The experience of a culturally appropriate capacity-building program in Southern California. *Journal of Public Health Management and Practice, 13*, S55–S63.

Takahashi, L. M., Magalong, M. G., Debell, P., & Fasudhani, A. (2006). HIV and AIDS in suburban Asian and Pacific Islander communities: Factors influencing self-efficacy in HIV risk reduction. *AIDS Education and Prevention, 18*(6), 529–545.

Wei, C., Raymond, H. F., Wong, F. Y., Silvestre, A. J., Friedman, M. S., Documet, P., et al. (2011). Lower HIV prevalence among Asian/Pacific Islander men who have sex with men: A critical review for possible reasons. *AIDS and Behavior, 15*(3), 535–549.

Wong, F. Y., Crisostomo, V. A., Bao, D., Smith, B. D., Young, D., Huang, J., et al. (2011). Development and implementation of a collaborative, multistakeholder research and practice model on HIV prevention targeting Asian/Pacific Islander men in the United States who have sex with men. *American Journal of Public Health, 101*(4), 623–631.

Xia, Q., Osmond, D. H., Tholandi, M., Pollack, L. M., Zhou, W., Ruiz, J. D., et al. (2006). HIV prevalence and sexual risk behaviors among men who have sex with men: Results from a statewide population-based survey in California. *Journal of Acquired Immune Deficiency Syndromes, 41*(2), 238–245.

Yanagihara, R., Chang, L., & Ernst, T. (2009). Building infrastructure for HIV/AIDS and mental health research at institutions serving minorities. *American Journal of Public Health, 99*, S82–S86.

Yoshikawa, H., Wilson, P. A., Hsueh, J., Rosman, E. A., Chin, J., & Kim, J. H. (2003). What front-line CBO staff can tell us about culturally anchored theories of behavior change in HIV prevention for Asian/Pacific Islanders. *American Journal of Community Psychology, 32*(1/2), 143–158.

Zaidi, I. F., Crepaz, N., Song, R., Wan, C. K., Lin, L. S., Hu, D. J., et al. (2005). Epidemiology of HIV/AIDS among Asians and Pacific Islanders in the United States. *AIDS Education and Prevention, 17*(5), 405–417.

Evolution of an Asian American, Native Hawaiian and Pacific Islander Cancer Advocacy Movement: Heroes Among Us

29

Susan Matsuko Shinagawa and Alan Y. Oda

On July 22, 2008, I stood on stage in front of 250 (primarily) Asian American, Native Hawaiian and Pacific Islander cancer survivors, family members and caregivers, along with cancer advocates, health professionals, academic researchers, public health educators, students, representatives from governmental and nongovernmental agencies and community-based organizations, to welcome them to the first-ever national "Asian American, Native Hawaiian & Pacific Islander Cancer Survivorship Conference: Dispelling Myths, Reducing Disparities & Providing Hope." Conferees from 14 U.S. states, the District of Columbia, and all six U.S.-associated Pacific Island jurisdictions – many clad in traditional ethnic attire – were about to embark on a unique journey of interactive plenary sessions and capacity building workshops. The room was alive with anticipatory excitement! (Shinagawa, 2011).

This chapter chronicles the story of our first author, Susan Matsuko Shinagawa Matsuko Shinagawa, co-founder and past chair of the Asian and Pacific Islander National Cancer Survivors Network and past chair of the Intercultural Cancer Council. She powerfully demonstrates the importance and value of *cancer advocacy* – an individual or group's active support of cancer patients, survivors and/or families, or proactive support, challenge or promotion of activities and/or issues related to the cancer care continuum in order to affect positive changes and improved patient outcomes. Our first author's story further illustrates how her advocacy efforts led directly to her contributions towards setting cancer health policy and cancer research agenda at the local, state and national levels, leading to important discoveries on both treating cancer and how the disease impacts diverse populations across the U.S., its associated territories, and American Indian nations and tribal organizations.

For many, a diagnosis of cancer continues to elicit fear, dread, and trepidation as it has throughout history. The course of treatment and therapy can be difficult, taxing, and challenging, both physically and emotionally. Fear and misinformation often complicate an already tough diagnosis for patients and their families.

The idea of cancer advocacy is reported as early as the 1970s. The Candlelighter Foundation brought together parents of children who were stricken with the disease. The American Cancer Society established I Can Cope, the organization's first support/advocacy group, developed by Judy Johnson in 1977 to provide education and support for recently diagnosed cancer patients. Perhaps one of the best known organizations is

S.M. Shinagawa (✉)
Asian and Pacific Islander National Cancer Survivors Network (Asian & Pacific Islander American Health Forum, San Francisco, CA), Intercultural Cancer Council (Baylor College of Medicine, Houston, TX), Spring Valley, CA, USA
e-mail: smsadvocacy.cancer@gmail.com

A.Y. Oda
Department of Undergraduate Psychology, Azusa Pacific University, Azusa, CA, USA
e-mail: aoda@apu.edu

Susan G. Komen For The Cure,[1] founded by Nancy Brinker in 1982 as a promise to her sister who died of the disease (Braun, 2003; Hoffman & Stovall, 2006).

Today, the idea of long-term survivorship and advocacy for cancer patients is more often the norm rather than the exception, both within the medical community and with the public at large, yet this was largely unheard of prior to 1986. Hoffman and Stovall (2006), in their review of the history of cancer advocacy, stated that the creation of the National Coalition for Cancer Survivorship (NCCS) helped redefine support for patients and their families:

> The founders of NCCS concluded that persons diagnosed with cancer should be allowed to call themselves cancer survivors from the moment of diagnosis and for the balance of their lives…NCCS embraced this broader definition to recognize that the impact of a person's cancer did not begin and end within a rigid 5-year period.
>
> (Hoffman & Stovall, 2006, p. 5154)

Sociologists have written about the role of cancer survivors as key activists in breast cancer social movements. In *The Biopolitics of Breast Cancer: Changing Cultures of Disease and Activism*, author Maren Klawiter (2008) provides an understanding of how everyday breast cancer survivors-turned-activists have changed the course of breast cancer care and treatment, including challenging screening guidelines, treatment availability, and pushing for more support options. All of these changes are a result of breast cancer survivors coming together to demand change for a more patient-centered form of care. Artists have helped inspire advocates in the ongoing movement. Images such as *RavenLight* and books like, *Winged Victory: Altered Images, Transcending Breast Cancer* (Myers, 1996), portraying breast cancer survivors whose openly displayed surgically-altered chests proved to be pivotal in organizing and educating breast cancer survivors to take social action and to ask questions of the medical establishment, as well as raising awareness among women *and* men personally impacted by breast cancer.

Although the breast cancer activist movement has been successful in achieving many gains, mostly absent from mainstream cancer movements prior to the new millennium had been Asian American, Native Hawaiian and Pacific Islander (AA and NHPI) voices and faces. The first author's role has proved to be pivotal in raising awareness and putting a face to cancer. Her story presents a tale of patient-turned-activist, bringing the disease and women living with breast cancer into the consciousness of AA and NHPI communities.

In 1991, five months after taking a breast self-examination workshop, Shinagawa discovered a prominent and painful lump in her right breast. After monitoring it for two months, she sought clinical evaluation. Though unconcerned, her physician ordered a mammogram, which was negative. However, the diagnostic radiologist decided to perform a sonogram, which revealed the breast lump to be a solid mass, leading to a referral:

> (The radiologist) sent me to see a surgical oncologist, who took my family history, reviewed the mammogram and sonogram, and performed a clinical breast exam. His response was immediate and unequivocal. *"You're too young to have breast cancer; you have no family history of cancer; and, besides, Asian women don't get breast cancer".*

The surgeon's response was not atypical, as Asian Americans were generally assumed not to be at risk for the disease. The "model minority" stereotype, often associated with the purported economic and educational success of Asian Americans, has also been erroneously used in health issues, including cancer. Specifically, it was widely believed that Asians did not get cancer very often, a belief that was also accepted by Asians themselves (Nguyen & Bellamy, 2006). In reality, cancer has been the leading cause of death among AA and NHPI women across several different demographics since 1986 (Chen, 2005). This is dissimilar to other U.S. population groups, for whom cardiac disease is the number one killer (National Center for Health Statistics [NCHS], 2010). Marked underutilization of screening programs (Kagawa-Singer et al., 2007; McCracken et al., 2007; Schleicher, 2007; Pourat, Kagawa-Singer, Breen, & Sripipatana, 2010) may

---

[1] Formerly, the Susan G. Komen Breast Cancer Foundation. Recently, this major international non-profit breast cancer education and research granting organization has come under fire for controversial changes to its grants program.

have contributed to lower reported rates of cancer in the past, while marked elevation of breast cancer risk within the first 10 years of immigrating to the U.S. among foreign-born Asian women (Ziegler et al., 1993; Ziegler et al., 1995), as well as rising rates associated with longer time in the U.S. (Gomez et al., 2010) may be contributing to increasing Asian American breast cancer rates. This does not, however, account for the rapid rise in breast cancer rates among some Asian American groups, such as Japanese Americans (Deapen, Liu, Perkins, Bernstein, & Ross, 2002).

Shinagawa's frustration with the medical system was just beginning:

> Despite my pleas, the surgeon refused to do a biopsy. Fortunately for me, the pain I felt each time my husband hugged me or as I rolled over in bed kept the breast lump in the forefront of my mind. Six weeks later, I sought a second opinion, and finally underwent an excisional biopsy. The following day I received a phone message to call the surgeon who had performed the biopsy. Upon reaching him, he pronounced, "I'm sorry, Susan, but you have breast cancer." It was the first, though not the last time I would hear those words. I felt like I had crashed head-on into a brick wall traveling 60 miles per hour. I was only 34 years old, I was scared, and I had no idea what lay ahead.

> (Shinagawa, 2011)

Because her surgeon did not expect to find breast cancer during the excisional biopsy, it was necessary for Shinagawa to undergo a second surgery to ensure removal of all the cancer. She elected to have a modified radical mastectomy with axillary node dissection, followed by adjuvant chemotherapy. As she had become more knowledgeable about the disease, Shinagawa was able to make informed decisions about her treatment. She tolerated eight cycles of combination chemotherapy, administered over a period of six months, relatively well. Even before Shinagawa had completed her chemotherapy regimen, she was already speaking publicly about her cancer experience, determined to educate other women about their (then) one-in-nine chance of being diagnosed with breast cancer sometime during their life (American Cancer Society [ACS], 1991; Feuer et al., 1993).

Raised by parents who were active volunteers in multiple community and civic organizations, advocacy came easy to Shinagawa. She was fortunate

that her *Nisei*[2] father unashamedly shared his experiences as one of 120,000 U.S. citizens and legal residents imprisoned in U.S. "internment camps" during World War II – guilty of nothing more than being of Japanese ancestry. Shinagawa developed a deep sense of civil rights and wrongs, and concern about the unequal application of civil liberties and social justice in the U.S. At the age of 11, Shinagawa was part of a community coalition that petitioned the local school district to include Asian American history lessons in all U.S. history classes, and was later appointed to the curriculum development team of teachers, students and community leaders that wrote the district's first Asian American history teaching curriculum (Richmond Unified School District [RUSD], 1972).

Much of cancer advocacy has emerged from the study and care of breast cancer survivors. From the advocacy of the National Breast Cancer Coalition[3] to having seats on decision-making panels of the National Cancer Institute (NCI) and other breast cancer research entities, breast cancer advocacy has been far-reaching and transformative (McNeil, 2001). One area of advocacy involves screening programs and policies. To state that such advocacy is controversial is a diplomatic description at best. Fletcher (1997, 2011) decried how scientific data was being ignored in favor of emotional debates in determining guidelines for screening, particularly for women ages 40 through 49. Specifically, the National Institutes of Health (NIH), citing the available research demonstrated little benefit to survival in screening women before the age of 50, recommended against a policy of early screening. The heated reaction from those favoring screening for women between the ages of 40 and 49 produced inflammatory statements accusing the panel of "condemning American women to death" (Fletcher, 1997, p. 1181).

---

[2] *Nisei* (Japanese) "second-generation"; a native-born citizen of the United States whose parents emigrated to the U.S. from Japan.

[3] Founded in 1991, NBCC is the nation's leading coalition of breast cancer advocacy organizations, scientists and activists fighting to increase breast cancer research funding, access and influence. In 1992, NBCC successfully fought for federal appropriations to the Department of Defense, establishing the DOD Breast Cancer Research Program, which continues today.

Subsequent reviews have revealed contradictory evidence and suppositions. The Canadian National Breast Screening Study conducted in 1985 did not show any diminution in mortality rates for women who received earlier (i.e. between 40 and 49 years) mammography screenings (Fletcher, 1997; Miller, Baines, To, & Wall, 1992, 2002). In contrast, a meta-analysis of previous studies concluded that are benefits with earlier screening (Humphrey, Helfand, Chan, & Woolf, 2002). With release of the U.S. Preventive Services Task Force's updated breast cancer screening recommendations against mammographic screening of women under age 50 (2009a, 2009b) and release of the results of the 30-year Swedish study (Tabár et al., 2011) reporting a marked benefit for women in this age group, the controversy continues.

As a young survivor and new cancer advocate, Shinagawa initially focused on reaching and teaching young women about breast health, including the proper method of performing breast self-examination, and encouraging women to become informed healthcare consumers and form true partnerships with their medical providers. After completing chemotherapy, Shinagawa became active with the American Cancer Society (ACS) as a Special Touch Breast Health Facilitator and Reach to Recovery (RtR) volunteer. The experience provided her with important insights as to differences in how women of diverse ages, communities, cultures, nativity, language use and English proficiency (as well as their spouses/partners and caregivers) react to cancer diagnoses, interact with providers, make decisions regarding diagnosis and treatment, view their self-image and self-worth, and the extent to which they will accept help from others. Her breast health workshops, conducted with fellow breast cancer survivor, Dani Grady, infused music, dance and humor to help their audiences overcome any pre-conceived fears while addressing the very serious (and admittedly frightening) issue of breast cancer. Their later efforts included a county-wide National Cancer Survivorship Day (NCSD) celebration, a multi-faceted extravaganza designed, planned and presented by the 350+ volunteer pool of cancer survivors, families, friends, caregivers, healthcare providers, students, and other community advocates across all racial and ethnic communities, socioeconomic status, age, gender, sexual orientation, ability/disability status and cancer type, and representing every cancer center, hospital, community clinic, and many private oncology practices in San Diego County. The two-day event, which attracted more than 3,000 attendees, was the start of a county-wide cancer advocacy movement, resulting in the establishment of San Diego's Cancer Survivorship Park,[4] and *Cancer Survivorship: San Diego!*, an annual education and advocacy conference and celebration presented by the non-profit community-based organization of the same name.

Advocacy, Breast Cancer Research, and "Asian/Pacific Islanders"

It was not until 1973 that the National Cancer Institute (NCI) started identifying cancer cases by the first of four Asian American or Pacific Islander subpopulation groups (Chinese, Filipino, Japanese and Hawaiian), reporting these "Asian/Pacific Islander" (API)[5] rates in the aggregate. Fifteen years

---

[4] Richard and Annette Bloch conceived the concept of and provided funding for Cancer Survivorship Parks across the U.S. San Diego's Cancer Survivorship Park was initiated by the local cancer survivorship community and dedicated on March 2, 2002.

[5] The acronym "API" appears in this chapter to reflect two different uses, though both uses refer to the terminology, "Asian and Pacific Islander," "Asian & Pacific Islander," "Asian/Pacific Islander" or their plural in the U.S. Here, "API" refers to the rubric for the aggregate racial category, "Asians/Pacific Islanders," used in reporting cancer surveillance data by the NCI and Centers for Disease Control and Prevention (CDC). The U.S. Bureau of the Census used "API" in the aggregate reporting of population and demographic data prior to Census 2000. U.S. race and ethnicity categories are set by the Office of Management and Budget (OMB). In 1997, in preparation for Census 2000, OMB revised the race and ethnicity categories by replacing the "API" race category with two separate race identifiers: (1) Asian and (2) Native Hawaiian and Other Pacific Islander (NHOPI). All Federal agencies reporting data on U.S. populations received a directive from OMB to begin modifying their data reporting to be in compliance with the new OMB race and ethnicity categories by 2000. CDC and NCI have yet to fully comply with the directive, and continue to primarily use "API" in the aggregate reporting of cancer data for all AA and NHPI populations. "API" is used in this section in specific reference to its use by NCI, CDC and OMB prior to 1997. (Explanation of the second use of "API" appears later in this chapter on page 29-10.).

passed before NCI identified cancer cases by additional Asian American subgroups[6] in 1988, while identification of cancer cases by other Pacific Islander subgroups[7] began in 1991 (Chu, 1998). Collection and reporting of "Asian/Pacific Islander" (API) data were first mandated under OMB's Race and Ethnic Standards for Federal Statistics and Administrative Reporting, as adopted May 12, 1977 (Office of Management and Budget [OMB], 1994). As with many studies of APIs, NCI's initial cancer surveillance data were collected and reported under the aggregate API category, making information about individual Asian American or Pacific Islander ethnic subgroups all but impossible to discern. Nonetheless, during that time period (1988–1992), it was reported that APIs exhibited the lowest breast cancer incidence and mortality rates among all U.S. race and ethnic populations (Centers for Disease Control and Prevention [CDC], 1994; Vainshtein, 2008). Physicians who informed their patients that "Asian women don't get breast cancer" were possibly relying on the information and conclusions associated with these aggregate NCI and/or CDC data.

However, subsequent studies reporting (then) available, disaggregated API data for Native Hawaiian and selected Asian American populations revealed Native Hawaiians had the second highest breast cancer incidence rate among all U.S. women (after non-Hispanic Whites) and that Japanese American breast cancer incidence rates were higher than rates for American Indian, Alaska Native and Hispanic/Latina women (Miller et al., 1996; Parker, Davis, Wingo, Ries, & Heath, 1998). Of those ethnic subgroups within the API rubric, Native Hawaiian and Japanese American breast cancer incidence rates were 3.7 and nearly 2.9 times higher, respectively, than for Korean American women (Miller et al., 1996; Parker et al., 1998). Additionally, Native Hawaiian women had the third highest breast cancer mortality rate of all U.S. population groups.

Yet these high breast cancer rates were completely obscured within the API rubric, where Native Hawaiians and Pacific Islanders (combined) made up only 5% of all APIs, with Native Hawaiians comprising <3% of the total API population in 1990 (U.S. Bureau of the Censis, 1993a). Of the 95% of immigrant APIs in 1990, their overall median age was 30.1 years (ranging from 12.5 years in the Hmong population to 36.3 years among Japanese), and greater than 66% were foreign-born (U.S. Bureau of the Census, 1993b), having emigrated from Asian countries with the lowest global breast cancer rates, less than half the U.S. rate in 1990 (Notani, 2001; Althuis, Dozier, Anderson, Devesa, & Brinton, 2005). Together, these factors also obscure higher breast cancer rates for some American-born Asian females, particularly among those Asian American communities in their third, fourth and fifth generations (and beyond) in which breast cancer rates are increasing with each successive generation (Deapen et al., 2002). These data both fascinated and concerned Shinagawa; disaggregating API cancer (and other health) data soon became her mantra, motivation, and the fuel that rocketed Shinagawa's advocacy activities to the next level.

In the early 1990s, mainstream breast cancer advocates began to reap successes at the legislative level. Passage of California's Breast Cancer Act of 1993,[8] which imposed a two-cents-per-pack cigarette tax, established two statewide breast cancer programs. One program was the Breast Cancer Early Detection Program (BCEDP) [later combined with the state's cervical cancer control program as "Cancer Detection Programs: Every Woman Counts" (CDP: EWC)], administered under California's Department of Health Services (DHS)[9] to provide no-cost and low-cost breast and cervical cancer screening services for the state's

---

[6] Asian Indian, Korean, Vietnamese, Hmong, Laotian, Kampuchean (Cambodian).

[7] Chamorran, Figi Islander, Guamanian, Melanesian, Micronesian, New Guinean, Polynesian, Tahitian, Samoan, Tongan, Other Asian [including Asian not otherwise specified (NOS), Oriental NOS, and Pacific Islander NOS].

[8] 1993 Breast Cancer Act (i.e., AB 2055 (B. Friedman) [Chapter 661, Statutes of 1993] and AB 478 (B. Friedman) [AB 478, Statutes of 1993].

[9] As of 2007, the California DHS was reorganized as two separate entities: the Department of Health Care Services (DHCS) and the California Department of Public Health (CDPH), under which CDP: EWC continues to operate (www.cdph.ca.gov/programs/CancerDetection/Pages/CancerDetectionProgramsEveryWomanCounts.aspx).

uninsured and underinsured women. Another newly created resource was the California Breast Cancer Research Program (CBCRP), "to eliminate breast cancer by leading innovation in research, communication, and collaboration within and between California's scientific and lay communities,"[10] administered under the University of California Office of the President. Additionally, the 1993 Breast Cancer Act mandated the establishment of the Breast Cancer Research Council (BCRC), delineating Council membership to ensure representation not only by cancer researchers and clinicians, but also from California's pharmaceutical and medical technology industries, non-profit and community based organizations (CBOs), and breast cancer survivor/advocates, as well.

In 1994, the concept of cancer professionals in academia and industry and community survivor/advocates working together was new and fraught with challenges. Today such partnerships are both common and successful in developing research priorities, determining funding mechanisms and award amounts, as well as participating in the scientific and programmatic review of applications for cancer research funding in many settings. Less common, though gaining in popularity, is Community-Based Participatory Research (CBPR) – in which investigators from academia (and/or industry) and communities (of the target population of study) serve as equal partners and collaborators in defining research questions, designing and conducting research methodologies, and reporting and disseminating research outcomes, is increasingly being recognized for its successful (or far-reaching potential for success), evidence-based interventions as "good science" (Tucker & Taylor, 2011).

Shinagawa was the first Asian American to serve on California's BCRC, elected in 1995 as the Research Council's second Chair, and was also tapped to serve on the inaugural Breast & Cervical Cancer Advisory Council (BCCAC), California DHS. She was concerned at being

selected as the "token API" representative for both bodies, though she later learned her appointments resulted from multiple nominations, as well as her willingness to speak openly about her cancer—a rarity among AA and NHPI individuals and communities at that time."

Speaking out about her disease was clearly a great opportunity, but there were consequences:

> I felt my comfort in speaking publicly about my cancer experience was a gift, but there were times, especially in the early years, it was also a burden. It was striking how I was (nearly always) the lone Asian appointed to serve on cancer advisory boards, programmatic committees, and research councils, and I soon came to realize that I was expected to represent and advocate on behalf of all AA and NHPI communities by both the mainstream entities that appointed me, and the AA and NHPI communities that came to rely upon me. My burden was trying to effectively represent the interests and concerns of the many diverse AA and NHPI communities, while the reality was that (as a monolingual, U.S.-born Sansei [third generation] woman) I knew little about all the respective traditions and cultures and felt ill-prepared to adequately – and respectfully – address their unique experiences and needs.
>
> As conscientious as I tried to be, I often felt like an imposter able to pass muster for those in the mainstream who knew even less than I about the diversity of AA and NHPI communities. I expressed my feelings of inadequacies with a few friends and colleagues, who felt I was being too self-critical and opined that for the first time, AA and NHPI communities had a seat and advocate (in me) at the table. That I was not (nor could never be) an expert for each AA and NHPI community was less important than my ability and willingness to advocate on their behalf.

Slowly, cancer advocacy efforts on behalf of AAs and NHPIs began to materialize. Funding became available for national, regional and/or community-based organizations to develop pilot programs for outreach, education, screening and early detection of breast and/or cervical cancers for ethnic minorities, the poor, and other underserved communities. Many AA-and/or NHPI-serving agencies applied for and received grant awards to design and implement services previously unavailable to low-income, non-English-speaking (NES) and limited English proficient (LEP) AA and NHPI communities.

[10] California Breast Cancer Research Program (http://cbcrp.org/).

Community advisory boards were established, either multiethnic, multicultural and/or multilingual (e.g., the "Promoting Early Detection of Breast and Cervical Cancer among Asian American and Pacific Islander Women Advisory Committee" convened by the Association of Asian Pacific Community Health Organizations (AAPCHO) as the precursor to its CARE Program (Association of Asian Pacific Community Health Organizations [AAPCHO], 2002), and Komen's Asian and Pacific Islander Advisory Group, Breast Cancer Education Materials Assessment and Development Project (Susan G. Komen for the Cure, 2007)), or ethnic-specific, culture-specific, and/or language-specific (e.g., Chinese Community Health Resource Center).[11] These advisory groups, drawing from multigenerational resources, are comprised of AA and/or NHPI clinicians, academicians, behavioral researchers, public health practitioners/educators, and community health advocates (including cancer survivors), enabling these organizations to tap into community expertise from diverse perspectives and disciplines to develop community-focused, culturally competent, and language appropriate strategies for outreach, education and intervention to increase breast and/or cervical cancer screening knowledge and behaviors among AA and NHPI women.

The work of breast cancer advocates continues to shift and expand in supporting both care and research about the disease. As previously noted, Fletcher (1997, 2011) rebuked advocacy efforts backing mammography for women in their 40s, citing those studies demonstrated little to no benefit compared to the overwhelming evidence of benefit to mammography for women ages 50 and older. The author expressed concern that policies encouraging earlier breast cancer screening were the result of emotional and political interests, rather than scientific research. Kolker (2004), in comparison, stated that health social movements – including breast cancer advocacy – had expanded to encourage both better patient care and greater research efforts focusing on the disease. Advocacy has also been key to

greatly increasing overall funding dedicated to breast cancer research (Radley & Bell, 2007).

Establishment of the California Breast Cancer Early Detection Program's Asian Pacific Islander Advisory Committee (API-AC)[12] in 1995 resulted in the immediate authorship of a position paper/report detailing the critical need to disaggregate cancer data for "Asian/Pacific Islander" populations and to factor in demographically-based projections of the state's rapidly growing AA and NHPI populations in developing and implementing statewide public health policies and programs addressing breast cancer, the nation's first such advocates-initiated report to any state health department. The ability to inform and advise governmental programs and public health policy at the state level (Asian Pacific Islander Advisory Committee, 1996), as well as local, regional (Sobero, Giraldo, Strode, Rosa, & Gail DeLuca, 2003) and federal (Islam, Trinh-Shevrin, & Rey, 2009) levels in a meaningful way, coupled with new funding opportunities for community-focused programs (Mandell & Mussuto, 2004; California Breast Cancer Research Program [CBCRP], 2008) signaled that public health strategies for AA and NHPI women were finally catching up with what communities had long known, that the one-size-fits all cancer control strategies for all Asian Americans, Native Hawaiians and Pacific Islanders must give way to culture-, ethnic- and language-specific strategies designed by community experts with specific AA, NH or PI communities. Shinagawa realized that it was important to incorporate more people from diverse AA and NHPI population groups into future cancer advocacy activities.

---

[11] Refer to http://www.cchrchealth.org/en/programs/cccic.html.

[12] The API-AC was advisory to the Breast and Cervical Cancer Advisory Council (BCCAC) for the Breast Cancer Early Detection Program (BCEDP) established under the 1993 California Breast Cancer Act (described previously). The BCEDP was later combined with the state's cervical cancer programs that was then renamed Cancer Detection Programs: Every Woman Counts (CDP: EWC). There was no formal ending to the API-AC; it simply faded during the early years of California's fiscal crises. Still, the API-AC changed the way women's cancer programs were conducted in California from the early years of the program and beyond.

The critical question for me was no longer how I could become better informed about other AA and NHPI communities in order to be a more effective (advisory board) advocate on their behalf. Rather, the key issues were: (1) how to best identify and recruit individuals from various AA and NHPI communities interested in serving on advisory bodies; (2) how to best train and prepare those individuals to ensure they meet the criteria for such appointments; (3) how to best facilitate and promote their nominations to these advisory bodies; and (4) once appointed, how to best support these individuals to ensure their success.

Shinagawa found it would take "a few more years" before more survivors from different AA and NHPI communities would be willing to share their personal cancer stories. Still, progress was beginning to be made in helping others understand that important subgroup distinctions under the umbrella of "Asian American" required further study and action. Similarly, there was greater effort to recognize diversity among and between AA and NHPI communities, as well as commonalities across minority and poor populations, which were critical to address as the overall U.S. cancer advocacy movement continued to expand.

Key to this progress was the Intercultural Cancer Council (ICC; http://iccnetwork.org). The ICC promotes policies, programs, partnerships, education and research to address the unequal burden of cancer experienced by U.S. racial and ethnic minorities and medically underserved populations. It operates with the conviction that communities of color and poverty share a greater cancer burden, as well as cross-cutting issues and concerns (e.g., barriers to accessing the cancer care continuum), than their higher socioeconomic White counterparts. Among the common concerns identified are high rates of medically uninsured individuals, provider and systems barriers (including institutional racism), and language and cultural barriers (Shinagawa, 2000). These factors, linked with the rapidly evolving U.S. cultural and demographic milieu that will result in a combined-minority majority by 2050 (President's Cancer Panel, 2011), give rise to the concern of ICC and others that minority, poor and other disenfranchised communities will continue to experience difficulties accessing the timely and

quality cancer care that all persons in the U.S. (i.e., Americans)[13] should be afforded. A critical tenant to ICC's culture is its Core Concept, set forth in its By Laws[14]:

> (ICC members) speak for the common needs of all racial and ethnic minorities and medically underserved populations, as well as those issues that address inequalities in the cancer burden of any or all of these populations. Individual ICC members agree that, when conducting ICC business, they will set aside personal, as well as organizational interests in favor of addressing the common needs of all ICC constituencies. In recognition of this core concept, the ICC has adopted as its motto, *"Speaking with One Voice."*[15]

ICC has directly addressed disparities pertaining to AA and NHPI communities through its Biennial Symposium Series on Minorities, the Medically Underserved and Cancer, resulting in important contributions to the biomedical and behavioral science literature, as well as recommendations addressing significant cancer concerns. Ishida, Toomata-Mayer, and Braginsky (2001) documented cultural challenges of breast self-examination and other preventative issues for Samoan women. Jenkins, Buu, Berger, and Son (2001) estimated the number of Asian and Pacific Islander children who will contract Hepatitis B at some time in the future to be 13,000, leading to more than 600 deaths due to the resulting liver cancers if (then) U.S. Hepatitis B immunization practices remain unchanged. Kagawa-Singer et al. (2006) reported on the effectiveness of a participatory action research approach to surveying Southeast Asian and Pacific Islander women about their breast and cervical cancer screening practices, for which no such previous data existed, while maintaining scientific rigor and a community survey participation rate of nearly 100%. In association with ICC's 11th Biennial Symposium, the Intercultural Cancer Council Caucus (ICC Caucus) issued a report (2008) citing multiple studies clearly delineating the existence of cancer

---

[13] For the purpose of this chapter, "American" is defined as [*noun*] "someone from the U.S." (Cambridge Dictionaries Online 2011).

[14] ICC ByLaws, Article I, Section 1.1 (draft revision), Oct 2010.

health disparities among U.S. racial minorities, the poor, and other medically underserved populations. Building upon its 2004 report, the ICC Caucus issued an update on the state of the nation's growing public health crisis with a call to the nation to address cancer health disparities through achievable steps to attenuate and ultimately eliminate inequalities in cancer control and health access (ICC Caucus, 2008).

Having successfully completed surgery and chemotherapy in her battle against cancer and on her way to becoming the most recognized Asian American cancer survivor/advocate in the U.S., Shinagawa forged ahead, continuing to experience successes in her professional and personal life.

> Nineteen ninety-six was a milestone year for me. I was promoted to Executive Administrator of the Bone & Marrow Transplantation Program at the University of California, San Diego (UCSD) Cancer Center, and was surprised later that year to be honored as UCSD's 1995–1996 Outstanding Staff Employee of the Year. With my growing volunteer activities, I was also honored with the first of many awards for my cancer advocacy work. But the pinnacle of 1996 was my April marriage to Rob Norberg with the full support and acceptance of his 12- and 19-year-old daughters, who served as my Maids of Honor.

Life could not have been better for Shinagawa, but new challenges ahead caught her completely off guard.

> Seven months after our wedding, I was abruptly stricken with multiple unexplained, concurrent and painful symptoms, including total left-sided weakness, landing me in a wheelchair. Following an aggressive 8-week diagnostic workup, in January 1997 I was given an exclusionary,[15] presumptive[16] diagnosis of carcinomatous meningitis (CM), then a rare, but increasingly more frequent type of cancer recurrence in the cerebrospinal fluid (CSF). According to the neuro-oncologist who made the

---

[15] An exclusionary diagnosis is made when a medical condition cannot be confirmed by cytologic or radiographic evidence; rather the diagnosis is made through systematic exclusion of all other possible diagnoses.

[16] A presumptive diagnosis is made when a medical condition cannot be confirmed by cytologic or radiographic evidence, all differential diagnoses have been eliminated, and there are reasonable grounds to presume a diagnosis is correct based upon the patient's.

diagnosis, 50% of CM cases are confirmed at autopsy, and, having given me a 10-month prognosis, he believed he would have such confirmation within the year.

Shinagawa readily admits that treatment with daily radiation and intrathecal chemotherapy (medication administered directly into the brain), severe side effects, and a subsequent excruciating bout with chemical meningitis led her to think, "lacking all quality of life, I wanted to stop treatment... then I wanted to stop living." But her introduction to a competent and compassionate pain management specialist – as well as the encouragement and support of her husband – provided needed relief. "While my neuro-oncologist focused only on my disease, my pain management physician's concerns were for my physical, mental, *and* emotional well-being." Shinagawa had experienced first-hand what far too many cancer (and other) patients experience, physicians who either under-appreciate or too easily dismiss the distress of pain before, during or after treatment. Unfortunately, this is particularly true for minority and female patients in pain who more often receive inadequate pain control (California State Legislature, 2004; Intercultural Cancer Caucus, 2008; Green, Hart-Johnson, & Loeffler, 2010; Institute of Medicine, 2011). Fortunately for Shinagawa, she was referred to a pain specialist who understood the importance of a comprehensive approach to pain management.

Though she continued to suffer with intractable pain and a multitude of health problems secondary to her treatments for recurrent cancer and pain, by late 1997 Shinagawa (now on permanent disability) was ready to resume some of her advocacy activities. She was invited to be a plenary session panelist on critical issues for healthy AA and NHPI communities, and to co-facilitate a strategy discussion session, entitled "Involving Consumers as Advocates" as part of the conference, "VOICES From the Community: A Call to Action for Asian and Pacific Islander Health in the New Millennium," sponsored by the Asian & Pacific Islander American Health Forum (APIAHF), based in San Francisco, California. From the time of her entrée into cancer advocacy through the 1997 VOICES conference, Shinagawa witnessed appreciable movement within AA and NHPI cancer survivorship communities towards a more open, vocal and public stance regarding cancer and individual survivorship status. Such a tangible demonstration informed Shinagawa that the community might be ready for the establishment of a national API[17] cancer survivorship and advocacy network. Following up on the VOICES conference, Shinagawa developed a proposal for APIAHF to establish the Asian & Pacific Islander National Cancer Survivors Network (APINCSN; see Appendix 1), which APIAHF accepted, and for which she would later serve as co-chair.

Over the decade that followed, AA and NHPI cancer survivorship advocacy and programs exploded. With one-on-one peer support and survivor-initiated support groups and programs, community-based participatory research (CBPR), and legislative/policy advocacy in city councils, state legislatures and the U.S. Congress, the landscape of AA and NHPI cancer survivorship advocacy was changing across the U.S. and Pacific. From ethnic- and language-specific support services to multicultural AA and NHPI cancer advocacy programs in English, the rapid rise of cancer survivorship advocacy in AA and NHPI communities – after a long and challenging beginning – pushed the APINCSN into the circle of mainstream cancer advocacy groups, all the while retaining and nurturing necessary and close ties to our diverse constituency communities.

Speaking Power to Truth: The Role of Patient Advocates

Avery and Bashir (2003) describe patients who become public health advocates as "speaking power to truth." The authors identified these patients as being driven by a deep-seeded desire to improve the patient experience, make the diagnosis and treatment process less traumatic, and improve the quality of life for others with similar diagnoses. These patient advocates are determined

to bring social justice to the voiceless within health disparity communities. Generally unfettered by powerful interests, these advocates are viewed as individuals challenging the status quo, pushing the envelope, and speaking out "creatively where others cannot because of political or economic conflicts" (Avery & Bashir, 2003).

In 1950, a young newlywed, Helene Brown, visited her doctor to determine whether she was pregnant. During that visit, she experienced her first pap smear, a procedure about which she had no prior knowledge. Inquiring with her doctor, the young bride learned that pap smears enabled doctors to detect the presence of human papillomaviruses (HPV), the earliest signs of cervical cancer, which can be easily be removed. Curious as to why this life-saving procedure against cervical cancer was not being offered to all women, Brown set out to learn all she could about pap smears and cervical cancer, and quickly became the driving force behind a national media campaign (in conjunction with the American Cancer Society) to educate women about the life-saving potential of pap smears against cervical cancer (Beyette, 1997). In 1950, few women received pap smears(Beyette, 1997). Nearly 85,000 U.S. White women[18] died from cervical cancer in the decade that followed (Devesa et al., 1999). By 1960, half of all U.S. women had had at least one pap smear (Beyette, 1997). By the end of that decade, cervical cancer death rates in the U.S. Southern region (with the highest rates in 1950) declined from a high of 15.87% to a low of 6.97%[19] among this population group (National Cancer Institute, 2011). In 2007, U.S. White cervical cancer mortality rates had decreased to 2.2% with 3,037 deaths among white U.S. women, and 4,021 deaths due to cervical can-

---

[17] In 1998, the phrase, "Asian & Pacific Islander" or "API," (as opposed to "AA and NHPI") was still the commonly used vernacular by many in AA and NHPI communities.

[18] From 1950 to 1969, cancer mortality rates in NCI's Atlas of Cancer Mortality in the United States, from which these data were gleaned, were available only for White Americans. This is because the Atlas reported cancer mortality rates at the county level, and census based on race during that 20-year period were unavailable for non-White populations. Cancer mortality rates for African Americans became available beginning in 1970, while such census and cancer mortality data for other minority populations were not available until 1988.

[19] Per 100,000 person-years.

cer among all U.S. women (U.S. Cancer Statistics Working Group, 2010).

Breast cancer advocacy can trace its roots to other movements demanding attention to critical health issues. More than a decade before HIV/AIDS[20] activists established ACT UP,[21] focusing fear and anger in New York City's Gay community into activism (Manganiello & Anderson, 2011), Rose Kushner was the singular face of the nation's earliest patient-initiated breast cancer advocacy movement (Lerner, 2001a). Diagnosed with breast cancer in 1974 at the age of 45, Kushner was determined to end the practice of the "one-step" biopsy-to-radical mastectomy procedure that had been the standard of care for women with breast cancer since its introduction in the 1890s by Johns Hopkins surgeon, Dr. William Halstead (Lerner, 2001a; Lerner, 2001b). Balancing her advocacy between being an agitator and conciliator, Kushner was successful in bringing about the change she sought, improving the medical protocol for breast cancer surgery that existed virtually unchanged for nearly a century (Lerner, 2001a; Lerner, 2001b).

These earliest examples of consumer-initiated cancer advocacy and patient-initiated cancer activism inform us on two key fronts. First, that significant impact on health policy and public health can result from the dedicated efforts of an individual or small group of individuals. Second, such advocacy efforts and the successes resulting from these efforts have had only minimal impact on increasing cancer screening (Kagawa-Singer et al., 2007; Pourat et al., 2010; Schleicher, 2007), or lowering cancer incidence and mortality among many AA and NHPI sub-population groups in the U.S. and its U.S. Associated Pacific Islands (Ho, Muraoka,

Cuaresma, Guerrero, & Agbayani, 2010; Lin et al., 2002; McCracken et al., 2007; Miller, Chu, Hankey, & Ries, 2008).

The modern era of cancer advocacy exists on a continuum between brightly colored ribbons and cause marketing on one end, and building upon HIV/AIDS activism with new attempts to force a paradigm shift in policy and research to bring about substantive progress in the nation's 40-year old war against cancer on the other end.

Then there's everything in between. Where individual AA or NHPI cancer advocates/activists and various AA and NHPI ethnic cancer advocacy communities fall along this continuum – or whether they land on the continuum at all – is dependent upon multiple factors, including (but not limited to) the individuals' or community's ethnicity, nativity, length of time in the U.S., acculturation level (Gomez et al., 2010), educational attainment, socioeconomic status, language proficiency, health care access, and cancer site. The existence of cancer advocates from AA and NHPI ethnic subpopulations who can serve as role models, mentors and provide leadership within the various cancer advocacy communities is key to the strength and sustainability of cancer advocacy movements within and across these respective communities at any point along the national cancer care/cancer advocacy continuum. Appendix 2 provides brief vignettes of selected key cancer survivor advocates/activists from several AA and NHPI ethnic communities.

Enduring Challenges, Continuing Journey and Abiding Appreciation

In 1997, the U.S. Office of Management and Budget revised Directive 15, creating separate race categories for "Asians" and "Native Hawaiians and Other Pacific Islanders" (OMB, 1997), and subsequently issuing Provisional Guidance on implementing the new standards to all Federal agencies and organizational units that "maintain, collect or present data for Federal statistical purposes" (OMB, 2000). The deleterious effects of reporting cancer

---

[20] HIV is the acronym for human immunodeficiency virus that can lead to acquired immune deficiency syndrome (AIDS), the late stage of HIV infection, when the patient is severely immunosuppressed.

[21] ACT UP (AIDS Coalition To Unleash Power) was established in 1987 to protest the federal government's apathy in addressing the growing AIDS crises. ACT UP helped to focus community fear and anger into activism, and played a major role in advancing research and health policy on HIV and AIDS (Manganiello & Anderson, 2011).

(and other) health data for all Asian Americans, Native Hawaiians and Pacific Islanders (AAs and NHPIs) in the aggregate as "APIs" has been exposed in numerous reports and articles (Shinagawa, 1999; Shinagawa et al., 1999; National Research Council, 2004). Yet more than a decade after the Provisional Guidance was released, several Federal agencies, including the NCI and CDC, have yet to fully implement the revised Directive (Papa Ola Lokahi, 2007). Shinagawa charges that this oversight can lead to deleterious results:

> Such inaction can manifest itself as physicians who fail to recommend regular cancer screening tests for their Asian American, Native Hawaiian and Pacific Islander patients, or fail to take AA and/or NHPI female patients seriously when they present with a suspicious breast lump. Two decades after I was denied a biopsy for this very reason, I still meet AA and NHPI women whose doctors told them they had nothing to worry about because *"API women don't get breast cancer"*. Until NCI, CDC and other cancer (and health) surveillance data are consistently disaggregated, I believe such fallacies will continue to be perpetuated by medical providers, endangering the lives of AA and NHPI women and the well-being of their families and communities. Those words *("API women don't get breast cancer")* set me on the path to cancer advocacy 20 years ago, and now these same words compel me to continue my cancer advocacy journey.

Recognizing that much work lay ahead for AA and NHPI cancer advocates, Shinagawa was able to experience a well-deserved sense of accomplishment as she appeared before the 2008 Asian American, Native Hawaiian & Pacific Islander Cancer Survivorship Conference audience.

> Looking out from the conference stage across the ballroom floor, I saw before me an amazing tapestry of diversity, passion, compassion and community that was our Asian American, Native Hawaiian and Pacific Islander cancer advocacy movement. I realized we had travelled a long, and, at times, treacherous journey of evolution from isolation and fear to a community of survivorship and advocacy. Though I know the road ahead is a long one, I want to always be mindful and appreciative of the progress we have made within our respective communities, and as diverse communities together in solidarity. Our work continues, but the road now travelled is one filled with many advocates, partners and friends – many more than I could have dreamed possible when I embarked upon this journey 20 years ago. All those who now walk beside me are the Heroes among us, and will forever be in my heart and a part of my journey.

Shinagawa closed the Conference with a song she wrote following completion of treatment for her first bout with cancer.[22]

> *Heroes, you're in my heart.*
> *Give me the will to carry on.*
> *Heroes, we'll never part.*
> *You make each day a brand new song.*
> *Dreams I dare to dream yet to unfold,*
> *life stories yet to be told.*
> *Memories, sweet, made of gold.*
> *No matter what my tomorrows may bring,*
> *I've got a song left to sing,*
> *For you, my Heroes.*
> *Thank you, my Heroes.*
> *You are my Heroes.*

She felt reinvigorated as she concluded her song. "Now, more than ever, I look forward to the next leg of our advocacy journey and all that lies ahead."

Appendix 1

An Original Proposal to Establish a National Asian & Pacific Islander Cancer Survivor and Advocacy Network

Presented by
Susan Matsuko Shinagawa to the Asian & Pacific Islander American Health Forum
April 1998

Proposal
Develop a national network for Asian and Pacific Islander (API) cancer survivors, family, friends, healthcare providers, educators and other advocates.

---

[22] Excerpt from "My Heroes," © 1993 Susan Matsuko Shinagawa.

Purpose

- To provide personal, empathetic support for API cancer survivors, their families and friends.
- To serve as a national clearinghouse for culturally sensitive and language appropriate API cancer related materials and resources.
- To serve as a national resource on cancer and its impact on API communities.
- To serve as a national coalition for API healthcare promotions, education, research, and service organizations.
- To empower API survivors and other advocates through advocacy education and training.
- To develop an API cancer survivor/advocate speakers bureau.
- To ensure API voices are represented on local, state, and national policy making bodies which impact upon the health and lives of our communities.

Background

The September 12-14, 1997 conference, "VOICES from the Community: A Call to Action for Asian and Pacific Islanders Health in the New Millennium," sponsored by the Asian Pacific Islander American Health Forum, was convened to "broaden and strengthen the voices of Asian and Pacific Islander communities in impacting local and national health policy." A number of the recommendations developed during the conference concerned advocacy and representation issues related to and impacting upon health in API communities. The development of a national API cancer survivors and advocacy network is a logical follow up to the conference.

Rationale

In the United States today, hundreds of organizations dealing with the special concerns and needs of cancer survivors are thriving. These organizations provide the necessary support for cancer patients, serve as educational resources for the general population, and advocate on issues germane to cancer survivors and their families at the local, state and national level.

In recent years, support programs for Chinese cancer patients and their families have developed on a local basis (e.g., Mandarin and Cantonese language women's cancer support groups in San Francisco, CA, and the Chinese Unit of the American Cancer Society in four metropolitan areas). However, for the vast majority of API cancer patients and their families, culturally sensitive and language appropriate support services and resources are non-existent.

In an era when most cancer survivors openly discuss their disease and are demanding (and getting) more monies for cancer research, many API cancer survivors are still reluctant to disclose their disease even to family members. Fewer still access traditional support group mechanisms. The development of an API cancer survivors and advocacy network would provide these survivors, their families and friends a safe haven to discuss their illness, their concerns, their fears and their needs with others who have a shared culture and socially-constructed history in the United States.

Sharing one's illness with others who have similar experiences is just the first step. The second step is to share one's illness and experience with others who have not had the experience themselves, but may at some time in the future, as well as those who seek to reach out and educate others about the disease, its risk, prevention (if possible), early detection, diagnosis, treatment, support, and the long-term concerns of survivors. Providing the necessary training and/or education of cancer survivors and advocates in order to develop a diverse and effective speakers bureau will serve not only to educate others, but will encourage those AA/PI cancer survivors who have been silent about their disease to speak out.

Numerous successful and respected regional and national API organizations (or organizational counterparts) focusing on healthcare promotions, education, research, and service exist. However, most conduct their activities autonomously. Accordingly, unnecessary and costly duplication of efforts may be occurring unchecked. This new Network could serve as the catalyst to bring these organizations together and to facilitate enhanced dialog and collaborations.

In the early 1990s, breast cancer survivors took a lead from AIDS activists and began demanding more federal research dollars. In just

5 short years, they were successful in increasing funding for breast cancer research from $90 million to over $500 million per year. More recently, prostate cancer patients have begun to successfully advocate for more research dollars. The programs developed from federal and state legislation crafted by and benefiting these cancer survivors are unique in that they legislatively mandate survivor participation on the bodies that both scientifically and programmatically review research grant applications, and which make the final funding recommendations. A few state health services programs also require survivor/advocate representation on their program advisory councils. Survivor advocates enjoy full voting status along with their scientist, physician, and health administrator counterparts on these councils. To date, however, only a handful of survivor/advocates from API communities have been appointed to these decision-making bodies.

In order for APIs to have a stronger voice in deciding on policy and research that may affect (and currently neglect) their communities, we must have a seat at the table. Through education and training, the API survivors and advocacy network can empower individuals and enhance community capacity so that our communities are well represented on these councils and committees. This purpose takes on an even stronger focus, since NCI Director Dr. Richard Klausner announced at a recent meeting that the NCI would utilize "consumer/advocates" on all study sections beginning this year.

Conclusion

The need for a national network of API cancer survivors, supporters, researchers, educators and other advocates has never been greater. At a time when other communities are openly discussing cancer, concerted efforts are being made to increase prevention and early detection behaviors, and advocates are demanding and getting increased funding for cancer control and research, APIs must have appropriate support mechanisms, a strong and united voice, and seat at the table in order to affect positive change for the health of our communities. We can be silent no longer. The time to act is now!

Appendix 2

Heroes Among Us

On the Shoulders of Giants
The phrase, "on the shoulder of giants," is attributed to Bernard of Chartres (circa 1130) by author and theologian, John Salisbury, who wrote in 1159:

> *...we are like dwarfs on the shoulders of giants, so that we can see more than they, and things at a greater distant, not by virtue of any sharpness on sight on our part, or any physical distinction, but because we are carried high and raised up by their giant size.* (NationMaster.com, 2011).

Advocacy movements achieve their success only through the help of pioneers who blaze the trails that make the journey easier for those who follow. Such is the case with the AA and NHPI cancer survivorship movement in the U.S. What follows are the stories of a few of those Heroes among us.

Cathy Masamitsu is a true pioneer. In 1989, while Cathy was working for ABC television's popular daytime program, *The Home Show*, she was diagnosed with breast cancer for the second time. Though few people knew about Cathy's first breast cancer, determined to share her story, she approached *The Home Show*'s producers about documenting and broadcasting her breast cancer experience through mastectomy and breast reconstruction for their national television audience. The resulting five-part series, entitled, *"Cathy Saved Her Life and You Can Too!,"* aired November 6–10, 1989, and received multiple awards, including the Susan G. Komen Breast Cancer Foundation's Award for Excellence in Media. Cathy has since travelled across the country and around the world, sharing her personal story of hope and inspiration to millions. She co-authored the 1997 book, *Breast Cancer? Let Me Check My Schedule!* (Harper Collins Westview Press) with nine other breast cancer survivors, and has been a speaker with the American Cancer Society and National Cancer Survivors Day Foundation. In August 2000, Cathy (a *Sansei*) was one of 500 breast cancer survivors from the U.S. and Japan who participated in a 2-day trek to the summit of Mt. Fuji, as part of U.S. Team for Climb Against The Odds, an international breast cancer outreach and fund-raising campaign of The Breast Cancer Fund. (Cathy and mutual friend and breast cancer survivor, Debra Oto-Kent, called Shinagawa at her home when they reached the summit!).

Cathy has enjoyed a long and distinguished career as a reporter and producer in mainstream media, and has conducted her cancer advocacy through primarily mainstream organizations. Perhaps for these reasons, Cathy seldom receives the credit she rightfully deserves from AA and NHPI communities, not only for being the first Asian American cancer survivor to share her story publicly, but also for being the first cancer survivor, anywhere, to share her real-time surgical experience – from mastectomy through breast reconstructive surgery – on television. You could say that Cathy's story broadcast on *The Home Show* in 1989 was the beginning of reality television! Although Shinagawa's cancer advocacy journey had already begun when she first learned of Cathy, the story of Cathy's courage and sustained commitment to helping others is one worthy of recognition and celebration!

Rev. Frank Chong, M.S.W., M.Div. was a young minister at age 28 in 1973 when he was diagnosed with metastatic nasopharyngeal cancer after discovering a lump on the side of his neck. Frank underwent surgery to remove the tumor, followed by radiation. Already an established community organizer, American Cancer Society volunteer, and a passionate advocate and champion on behalf of poor and disenfranchised communities, upon completing treatment, Frank became one of Hawai'i's most prolific and admired cancer health advocates. As a 25-year survivor of nasopharyngeal cancer in 1998, and member of the APIAHF's Board of Directors, Frank was the perfect partner to join Shinagawa in co-founding and co-chairing what would become known as the "Asian & Pacific Islander National Cancer Survivors Network" (APINCSN, "the Network"). From the beginning, Frank was the Network's "spiritual" leader in every sense of the word, instilling members with the feeling they belonged to a community much

larger than their own, and had embarked upon a mission far beyond what they had imagined." He taught these lessons with grace and humility. In 2003, Frank was diagnosed with squamous cell carcinoma (the second most common type of skin cancer). Then in late 2004, he began experiencing multiple late-effects from the radiation he received more than 30 years earlier, including losing all his teeth and suffering from Bell's palsy. Despite these set-backs, Frank continued in his role as a local, state (Hawai'i) and national health activist until his death on March 9, 2008, just months before the Network convened its first national conference in celebration of AA and NHPI cancer survivorship. To celebrate Frank's life and commemorate his life's work, the Network and APIAHF established the *Frank Atherton Hua Pei Chong Cancer Survivorship Champion Award*. The inaugural award was presented posthumously to Frank's family during the 2008 conference, and has since been presented as a biennial juried award to an AA or NHPI cancer survivor, family member or community cancer advocate who best exemplifies Frank's spirit of compassion, giving and hopefulness, and his dedication of service to community.

Lucy Young was born Young Wang Hei Chen in Taiwan in 1947. As a young girl, Lucy was passive and shy, but dreamed of becoming a teacher. She married Col. Rev. William Young in 1972, and in 1980 they emigrated to the U.S. with their 2-year-old daughter, Sharon, and infant son, Samuel. In 1987, Lucy was diagnosed with stage 2 breast cancer at the age of 40. Throughout her diagnosis, surgery and chemotherapy, Lucy was unable to find information or support services in her native Chinese language. Determined that no other Chinese American women should have to go through a similar experience alone, Lucy established the Chinese-American Cancer Association in Queens, New York; in 1993, her organization became the American Cancer Society's first-ever ethnic-specific unit, with Lucy serving as Executive Director. Lucy joined the APINCSN as an inaugural Steering Committee member in 1998, helping to set the Network's mission, vision and goals. In the early 2000s, William's ministry was transferred and the family moved to California, where Lucy established The Herald Cancer Association (HCA) in 2002 under the auspices of the Chinese Christian Herald Crusades in Los Angeles County, to educate and support Chinese-speaking cancer patients and their families of any religious background. In 1992 while still in New York, Lucy established the nation's first Mandarin-language Chinese breast cancer support group, affectionately named, "The Joy Luck Club," which now has over 500 members in the U.S. and abroad.

Jina Peiris was diagnosed with breast cancer in March 1993, after she discovered a lump during breast self-examination. A single mother and sole-bread winner for her family with two sons in college, Jina was desperate to speak with another Sri Lankan breast cancer survivor, but could find none, and often ran into resistance from community members who admonished her for talking about cancer. A chance meeting with Zul Surani,[23] a public health educator and advocate of Asian Indian descent, led to Jina's introduction to the South Asian Network, through which she conducted focus groups with cancer survivors and families from Los Angeles's diverse South Asian communities and shared her experiences as a cancer patient and survivor, becoming the first South Asian to speak publicly about her personal cancer story. Understanding the fear and stigma about cancer in South Asian communities, Jina became an American Cancer Society Reach to Recovery volunteer. Educating herself about breast cancer research issues, Jina began reviewing grant applications for the U.S. Department of Defense Breast Cancer Research Program, California Breast Cancer Research Program, Susan G. Komen For the Cure, LiveStrong (the Lance Armstrong Foundation) and other cancer research funders. In

1998, Jina became a founding Steering Committee member of the APINCSN. In 2004, Jina joined forces with Zul and other South Asian community health advocates to establish Saath USA, a CBO dedicated to addressing cancer survivorship and other health issues in Southern California's Asian Indian, Bangladeshi, Pakistani and Sri Lankan communities through outreach, education, support and community-based participatory research.

Thoa Nguyen recently retired from the University of California, San Francisco (UCSF) as Project Director of *Súc Khòe là Vàng* – Health is Gold!, the Vietnamese Community Health Promotion Project (VCHPP), following a distinguished 30-year career that earned her high praise from Vietnamese communities in the United States and abroad, as well as the greater national community of cancer control, health promotion and health education professionals across the U.S. Like many Vietnamese immigrants, Thoa (who arrived in the U.S. as an adult in the late 1970s) had difficulty understanding and adjusting to the Western medical system. Since graduating from college in the U.S., Thoa has worked tirelessly to help other Vietnamese immigrants understand and navigate through the U.S. medical system, and to advocate for better language access and culturally competent health services for themselves and their communities. She has served on numerous boards and advisory councils at the local, state and national levels, including the APINCSN as a founding Steering Committee member. Thoa has co-authored numerous community-tailored health education materials in Vietnamese, including the first-ever Asian language cancer education materials adopted by the NCI,[24] and four Vietnamese-language health education videos, for which she served as executive producer. In addition to her efforts on behalf of Vietnamese immigrants, Thoa dedicates her time as a volunteer teacher and principal at the Huong Viet Community Center Language School in Oakland, California, ensuring that young, U.S.-born Vietnamese American

[23] Zulfikarali H. R. Surani, MPH, (then) Manager of the University of California, Los Angeles Mobile Mammography Community Outreach Program, now Manager of the Patient Education and Community Outreach Center and the Jennifer Diamond Cancer Resource Library at the USC Norris Comprehensive Cancer Center, University of Southern California. Mr. Surani co-founded and serves as in-kind Director of Saath USA (http://saathusa.org/).

[24] *Cervical Cancer: What Vietnamese Women Should Know* (Sept 2005). National Cancer Institute Publication No. 05-5732 (http://www.cancer.gov/cancertopics/screeni ng/cervical-screening-vietnamese.pdf).

children understand their community's history, traditions and language, empowering them to best navigate through their blended cultures. In recognition of her dedicated community service, Thoa has been the recipient of numerous awards. After nearly a quarter century as a community leader in cancer control and health advocacy, Thoa was diagnosed with breast cancer in 2005, adding to her long list of roles the new title of "cancer survivor/advocate."

Victor Kaiwi Pang hails from Maui, Hawai'i, lives in the Southern California community of Huntington Beach, and is a long-time community activist, promoting traditional culture, language and arts in Native Hawaiian, as well as other Pacific Island communities. After Victor was diagnosed with non-Hodgkin's lymphoma (NHL) in 1990, he added cancer outreach, education and health promotion for NHPI communities to that list. At the time, Victor sought an NHPI men's cancer support group, but none existed. Undeterred, he sought the assistance of the Orange County Asian and Pacific Islanders Community Alliance (OCAPICA), establishing a men's health support group for AA and NHPI men. Eventually, Victor formed his own support group for Native Hawaiian men, and established "Ohana Retreat,"[25] an annual multi-generational family weekend retreat combining health education discussion groups (for men, women, teens and children), health-focused presentations, nutrition, and physical activity with traditional Hawaiian culture, language, arts and song.

Victor also founded the Pacific Islander Health Partnership (PIHP), a collaborative of NHPI community– and faith–based organizations dedicated to reducing NHPI health disparities "through education, training, advocacy, and building island community capacity for health," partnering with other CBOs and academic institutions to conduct outreach, education, screening, support and research programs in an effort to reduce health disparities among NHPI communities. In 2003, Victor was diagnosed with recurrent NHL, then breast cancer in 2009, undergoing a mastectomy

and chemotherapy. Only 1% of newly diagnosed breast cancer cases each year are in men; thus, Victor now advocates for the development and dissemination of more information about male breast cancer, and has started a support group for AA and NHPI male breast cancer survivors. Victor is married is Jane Ka'ala Pang (whom he refers to as his "co-survivor" and caregiver), and has two sons and three grandchildren.

Rosa D. Manglona (affectionately known as "Auntie Rose") is a Chamorro breast cancer survivor, diagnosed in January 2001 following routine mammogram. Rose was devastated when confronted with the heart-wrenching decision regarding the extent of her surgery. For medical reasons, she decided to undergo a modified radical mastectomy, but feared her husband would reject her since she was no longer a "whole" woman. Sensing his wife's sadness, when Fred Manglona asked Rose what was troubling her, with tears streaming down her face, she could hardly get the words out. To her surprise, Fred told her that he had not married her for her breasts; he married her, he explained, because he was in love with her. "And," he continued, "I still love you, Rose!" Bolstered by her husband's unwavering love and with support from their children, Rose soon began sharing her story with other Chamorro women in San Diego County – home to the largest Chamorro population in the United States (StatJump 2010) – and learned that quite a few Chamorro women had also been diagnosed with breast cancer. They began meeting informally to socialize and as a means of providing peer support. When a friend asked Rose to arrange entertainment for an upcoming Chamorro breast cancer survivors' luncheon, she penned a short play about an older Chamorro woman who had never had a mammogram, and the young niece who wanted her to get one. Storytelling is a deeply ingrained tradition in Chamorro culture, so Rose wrote "Nan Nena's Mammogram" as if she was telling a story, completely in the Chamorro language, with humor, and in the context of cultural relevance and meaning. It was a huge hit. At the time, there was little data and no cancer education materials reflecting breast can-

---

[25] *Ohana* (Hawaiian) "family"; also, "community."

cer in Chamorro women, and so "Nan Nena's Mammogram" not only became an important vehicle to provide much needed information about breast health and breast cancer screening to Chamorro women, it also encouraged them to obtain mammograms. The play was performed in Chamorro communities across California, and then travelled to Guam, where it was met with even greater enthusiasm. In 2008, "Nan Nena's Mammogram" was accepted as a poster presentation at the Intercultural Cancer Council's 10th Biennial Symposium on Minorities, the Medically Underserved & Cancer in Washington, D.C. Later that year, the NCI provided funding to capture the play on DVD with English subtitles for distribution to a much wider Chamorro- and English-speaking audience in the U.S. and across the Pacific (Manglona et al., 2010).

The success of Rose's play, coupled with the growing number of Chamorro women with breast cancer in Southern California lead to the establishment of the California Chamorro Breast Cancer Survivor Alliance (CCBCSA), and Rose's election as the group's first President from 2007 to 2009 (Manglona et al., 2010). Over the past decade, Rose has continued to share her personal cancer story both within and beyond Chamorro communities. As a WINCART (Weaving an Island Network for Cancer Awareness, Research and Training) member, she has presented at national conferences and co-authored peer-reviewed research articles. She is a member of WINCART's San Diego Community Advisory Group and a faculty speaker for the Minority Training Program for Cancer Control Research at the University of California, Los Angeles. Rose and Fred have two sons, one daughter, and six grandchildren. They celebrated their 40th wedding anniversary in 2011.

References

Althuis, M. D., Dozier, J. M., Anderson, W. F., Devesa, S. S., & Brinton, L. A. (2005). Global trends in breast cancer incidence and mortality 1973–1997. *International Journal of Epidemiology, 34*, 405–412.

American Cancer Society (ACS). (1991). *Cancer facts & figures – 1991*. Atlanta: ACS.

Asian Pacific Islander Advisory Committee, Breast Cancer Early Detection Program. (1996, May 31). *Breast cancer in Asian and Pacific American Women: Myths, realities and recommended solutions. Recommendations to the Breast and Cervical Cancer Advisory Council, California Department of Health Services by the Asian Pacific Islander Advisory Committee, Breast Cancer Early Detection Program.* Sacramento, CA.

Association of Asian Pacific Community Health Organizations (AAPCHO). (2002). *The CARE program: A case study monograph of breast and cervical cancer education and screening programs in six Asian American and Pacific Islander communities*. Oakland, CA: AAPCHO.

Avery, B. Y., & Bashir, S. A. (2003). The road to advocacy – Searching for the rainbow. *American Journal of Public Health, 93*(8), 1207–1210.

Beyette, B. (1997, February 23). Mission: Possible. *Los Angeles Times*. Retrieved September 20, 2011, from http://articles.latimes.com/1997-02-23/news/ls-31526_1_cancer-research.

Braun, S. (2003). The history of breast cancer advocacy. *The Breast Journal, 9*(2), S101–S103.

California Breast Cancer Research Program (CBCRP). (2008). *Community research collaboration awards: Funded by the California Breast Cancer Research Program, 1997–2007*. Oakland, CA: CBCRP.

California State Legislature. (2004, February 4). *Joint informational hearing of the SENATE COMMITTEE ON HEALTH AND HUMAN SERVICES, Senator Deborah Ortiz, Chair, and the LEGISLATIVE WOMEN'S CAUCUS, Senator Liz Figueroa, Chair; "Women in pain: trends and implications of under-diagnosis of chronic pain in female patients."* Hearing Transcript, Sacramento, CA. Retrieved September 19, 2011, from http://senweb03.senate.ca.gov/committee/standing/health/WOMEN_IN_PAIN_TRANSCRIPT.DOC.

Centers for Disease Control and Prevention (CDC). (1994). *Chronic disease in minority populations, African-Americans, American Indians and Alaska Natives, Asians and Pacific Islanders, Hispanic Americans*. Atlanta: CDC, Public Health Service, U.S. Department of Health and Human Services.

Chen, M. S., Jr. (2005). Cancer health disparities among Asian Americans: What we know and what we need to do. *Cancer, 104*(12 Suppl), 2895–2902.

Chu, K. C. (1998, November 18). *Cancer data for Asian Americans and Pacific Islanders*. Oral presentation at the 126th Annual Meeting of the American Public Health Association, Washington, D.C.

Deapen, D., Liu, L., Perkins, C., Bernstein, L., & Ross, R. K. (2002). Rapidly rising breast cancer incidence rates among Asian-American women. *International Journal of Cancer, 99*, 747–750.

Devesa, S. S., Grauman, D. J., Blot, W. J., Pennollo, G. A., Hoover, R. N., & Fraumeni, J. F., Jr. (1999). *Atlas of cancer mortality in the United States 1950-94 (NIH publication No. 99-4564)*. Bethesda, MD: National Cancer Institute.

Feuer, E. J., Wun, L.-M., Boring, C. C., Flanders, W. D., Timmel, M. J., & Tong, T. (1993). The lifetime risk of developing breast cancer. *Journal of the National Cancer Institute, 85*, 892–897.

Fletcher, S. W. (1997). Whither scientific deliberation in health policy recommendations? Alice in the wonderland of breast-cancer screening. *The New England Journal of Medicine, 336*(16), 1180–1183.

Fletcher, S. W. (2011). Breast cancer screening: A 35-year perspective. *Epidemiologic Reviews, 33*(1), 165–175.

Gomez, S. L., Quach, T., Horn-Ross, P. L., Pham, J. T., Cockburn, M., Chang, E. T., et al. (2010). Hidden breast cancer disparities in Asian women: Disaggregating incidence rates by ethnicity and migrant status. *American Journal of Public Health, 100*(4), S125–S131.

Green, C. R., Hart-Johnson, T., & Loeffler, D. R. (2010). Cancer-related chronic pain: Examining quality of life in diverse cancer survivors. *Cancer, 117*(9), 1994–2003.

Ho, R., Muraoka, M., Cuaresma, C., Guerrero, R., & Agbayani, A. (2010). Addressing the excess breast cancer mortality in Filipino women in Hawai'i through AANCART, an NCI community network program. *Hawai'i Medical Journal, 69*, 147–150.

Hoffman, B., & Stovall, E. (2006). Survivor perspectives and advocacy. *Journal of Clinical Oncology, 24*(32), 5154–5159.

Humphrey, L. L., Helfand, M., Chan, B. K. S., & Woolf, S. H. (2002). Breast cancer screening: A summary of the evidence for the U.S. Preventative Task Force. *Annals of Internal Medicine, 137*(1), 347–360.

Institute of Medicine. (2011). *Relieving pain in America: A blueprint for transforming prevention, care, education, and research*. Washington, D.C.: The National Academies Press.

Intercultural Cancer Council Caucus. (2004). *From awareness to action: The unequal burden of cancer*. Larkspur, CA: ICC Caucus.

Intercultural Cancer Council Caucus. (2008). *From awareness to action: A renewed call to eliminate the unequal burden of cancer*. Larkspur, CA: ICC Caucus. Retrieved September 19, 2011, from http://www.icc-caucus.org/ICC_Caucus_Action_Plan.pdf.

Ishida, D. N., Toomata-Mayer, T. F., & Braginsky, N. S. (2001). Beliefs and attitudes of Samoan women toward early detection of breast cancer and mammography utilization. *Cancer, 91*(Suppl 1), 262–266.

Islam, N. S., Trinh-Shevrin, C., & Rey, M. J. (2009). Toward a contextual understanding of Asian American health. In C. Trinh-Shevrin, N. S. Islam, & M. J. Rey (Eds.), *Asian American communities and health: Context, research, policy and action* (pp. 3–22). San Francisco: Jossey-Bass.

Jenkins, C. N. H., Buu, C., Berger, W., & Son, D. T. (2001). Liver carcinoma prevention among Asian Pacific Islanders. *Cancer, 91*(1 Suppl), 252–256.

Kagawa-Singer, M., Tanjasiri, S. P., Lee, S. W., Foo, M. A., Nguyen, T.-U. N., Tran, J. H., et al. (2006). Breast and cervical cancer control among Pacific Islander and Southeast Asian women: Participatory action research strategies for baseline data collection in California. *Journal of Cancer Education, 21*(1 Suppl), S53–S60.

Kagawa-Singer, M., Pourat, N., Coughlin, S., McLean, T. A., McNeel, T. S., & Ponce, N. A. (2007). Breast and cervical cancer screening rates of subgroups of Asian American women in California. *Medical Care Research and Review, 64*(6), 706–730.

Klawiter, M. (2008). *The Bio-politics of breast cancer*. Minneapolis: University of Minnesota Press.

Kolker, E. S. (2004). Framing as a cultural resource in health social movements: Funding activism and the breast cancer movement in the U.S. 1990–1993. *Sociology of Health & Illness, 26*(6), 820–844.

Lerner, B. H. (2001a). No shrinking violet: Rose Kushner and the rise of American breast cancer activism. *The Western Journal of Medicine, 174*, 362–365.

Lerner, B. H. (2001b). *The breast cancer wars: Hope, fear, and the pursuit of a cure in twentieth-century America* (p. 2001). New York: Oxford University Press.

Lin, S. S., Clarke, C. A., Prehn, A. W., Glaser, S. L., West, D. W., & O'Malley, C. D. (2002). Survival differences among Asian subpopulations in the United States after prostate, colorectal, breast, and cervical carcinomas. *Cancer, 94*(4), 1175–1182.

Mandell, E., & Mussuto, M. (2004). DHS' Cancer Detection Programs: Every Woman Counts uses innovative ethnic grocer promotion to reach out to California's Korean American community. *CBCRP Bulletin: News from the California Breast Cancer Research Program, 8*(2), 3.

Manganiello, M., & Anderson, M. (2011). *Back to basics: HIV/AIDS advocacy as a model for catalyzing change*. New York: FasterCures: The Center for Accelerating Medical Solutions, and Washington, D.C.: HCM Strategists.

Manglona, R. D., Robert, S., Isaacson, L. S. N., Garrido, M., Henrich, F. B., Santos, L. S., Le, D., & Peters, R. (2010). Promoting breast cancer screening through storytelling by Chamorro cancer survivors. *California Journal of Health Promotion, 8* (Special Issue) (Cancer Control), 90–95.

McCracken, M., Olsen, M., Chen, M. S., Jr. Jemal, A., Thun, M., Cokkinides, V., et al. (2007). Cancer incidence, mortality, and associated risk factors among Asian Americans of Chinese, Filipino, Vietnamese, Korean, and Japanese ethnicities. *CA: A Cancer Journal for Clinicians, 57*(4), 190–205.

McNeil, C. (2001). Cancer advocacy evolves as it gains seats on research panels. *Journal of the National Cancer Institute, 93*(4), 257–259.

Miller, A. B., Baines, C. J., To, T., & Wall, C. (1992). Canadian National Breast Screening Study: 1. Breast cancer detection and death rates among women aged 40 to 49 years. *Canadian Medical Association Journal, 147*(10), 1459–1476.

Miller, A. B., To, T., Baines, C. J., & Wall, C. (2002). The Canadian National Breast Screening Study-1: Breast cancer mortality after 11 to 16 years of follow-up. A randomized screening trial of mammography in women age 40 to 49 years. *Annals of Internal Medicine, 137*, 305–312.

Miller, B. A., Kolonel, L. N., Bernstein, L., Young, J. L., Jr., Swanson, M. G., West, D. W., et al. (1996). *Racial/ethnic patterns of cancer in the United States 1988–1992. (NIH Pub. No. 96-4104)*. Bethesda, MD: National Cancer Institute.

Miller, B. A., Chu, K. C., Hankey, B. F., & Ries, L. A. G. (2008). Cancer incidence and mortality patterns among specific Asian and Pacific Islander populations in the U.S. *Cancer Causes & Control, 19*, 227–256.

Myers, A. (1996). *Winged victory: Altered images, transcending breast cancer*. San Diego, CA: Photographic Gallery of Fine Art Books.

National Cancer Institute. (2011). *Cancer mortality maps webpage*. Retrieved September 26, 2011, from http://ratecalc.cancer.gov/ratecalc/.

National Center for Health Statistics (NCHS). (2010). *Health, United States, 2010: With special feature on death and dying*. Hyattsville, MD: NCHS.

National Research Council. (2004). Eliminating health disparities: Measurement and data needs. Panel on DHHS collection of race and ethnicity data. In M. Ver Ploeg & E. Perrin (Eds.), *Committee on National Statistics, Division of Behavioral and Social Sciences and Education*. Washington, D.C: The National Academies Press.

NationMaster.com. (2011). Encyclopedia > *on the shoulder of giants* webpage. Retrieved August 21, 2011, from http://www.nationmaster.com/encyclopedia/On-the-shoulders-of-giants.

Nguyen, G. T., & Bellamy, S. R. (2006). Cancer information seeking preferences and experiences: Disparities between Asian Americans and whites in the Health Information National Trends Survey (HINTS). *Journal of Health Communication, 11*, 173–180.

Notani, P. N. (2001). Global variation in cancer incidence and mortality. *Current Science, 81*(5), 465–474.

Office of Management and Budget (OMB), Executive Office of the President (EOP). (1994). *Appendix, Directive no. 15: Race and Ethnic Standards for Federal Statistics and Administrative Reporting (as adopted May 12, 1977)*. Federal Register, June 9, 1994. Retrieved June 29, 2011, from http://www.whitehouse.gov/omb/fedreg_notice_15.

OMB, EOP. (1997). *Revisions to the Standards for the Classification of Federal Data on Race and Ethnicity, October 30, 1997*. Federal Registry (62 FR 58782-58790). Washington, D.C.: Government Printing Office. Retrieved June 29, 2011, from http://www.whitehouse.gov/omb/fedreg_1997standards.

OMB, EOP. (2000). *Provisional Guidance on the Implementation of the 1997 Standards for Federal Data on Race and Ethnicity, Tabulation Working Group, Interagency Committee for the Review of Standards for Data on Race and Ethnicity, December 15, 2000*. (See the December 15, 2000 "Note to Readers" from Katherine K. Wallman, Chief Statistician, Executive Office of the President, OMB). Retrieved June 29, 2011, from http://www.whitehouse.gov/sites/default/files/omb/assets/information_and_regulatory_affairs/re_guidance2000update.pdf.

Papa Ola Lokahi. (2007). *Threads in the human tapestry. The disaggregation of the API identifier and the importance of having the NHOPI (Native Hawaiian and Other Pacific Islander) category in data collection, analysis, and reporting*. Honolulu: Papa Ola Lokahi. Retrieved June 29, 2011, from http://www.papaolalokahi.org/coconut/news/pdf/Disaggregation_API_AAPI.pdf.

Parker, S. L., Davis, K. J., Wingo, P. A., Ries, L. A. G., & Heath, C. W., Jr. (1998). Cancer statistics by race and ethnicity. *CA: A Cancer Journal for Clinicians, 48*(1), 31–48.

Pourat, N., Kagawa-Singer, M., Breen, N., & Sripipatana, A. (2010). Access versus acculturation: Identifying modifiable factors to promote cancer screening among Asian American women. *Medical Care, 48*(12), 1088–1096.

President's Cancer Panel. (2011). *2009–2010 Annual Report. America's demographic and cultural transformation: Implications for cancer*. Bethesda, MD: National Cancer Institute.

Radley, A., & Bell, S. E. (2007). Artworks, collective experience and claims for social justice: The case of women living with breast cancer. *Sociology of Health & Illness, 29*(7), 366–390.

Richmond Unified School District (RUSD). (1972). *Asian American Studies Project: The Chinese American experience and the Japanese American experience. Elementary guide intermediate grades*. Teaching Curriculum (ED106438). Richmond, CA: RUSD. Retrieved June 29, 2011, from http://www.eric.ed.gov/PDFS/ED106438.pdf.

Schleicher, E. (2007). *Immigrant women and cervical cancer prevention in the United States*. Baltimore, MD: Women's and Children's Health Policy Center, Johns Hopkins Bloomberg School of Public Health.

Shinagawa, S. M. (1999). API women get breast cancer too: Myth of the model health minority (Testimony). *In: Agenda for research on women's health for the 21st century. A report of the Task Force on the NIH Women's Health Research Agenda for the 21st Century, Vol. 6. Differences among populations of women*. Scientific meeting and public hearing, Santa Fe, New Mexico, July 1997. Bethesda, MD: National Institutes of Health. NIH Publication No. 99-4390, pp. 257–280. Retrieved June 29, 2011, from http://orwh.od.nih.gov/pubs/agenda_book_6.pdf.

Shinagawa, S. M., Kagawa-Singer, M., Chen, M. S., Jr., Tsark, J. U., Palafox, N. A., & Mackura, G. (1999). Cancer registries and data for Asian Americans and Native Hawaiians and Pacific Islanders: What registrars need to know. *Journal of Registry Management, 26*(4), 128–141.

Shinagawa, S. M. (2000). The excess burden of breast cancer in minority and medically underserved communities: Application, research and redressing institutional racism. *In: Proceedings of the National Action Plan on Breast Cancer Workshop on the Multicultural Aspects of Breast Cancer Etiology, Washington, D.C., March 17–19, 1999. Cancer (Suppl), 88*(5),1217–1223.

Shinagawa, S. M. (2010). Time traveler (unabridged article). *Asian & Pacific Islander National Cancer Survivors Network newsletter*. Retrieved June 29, 2011, from http://www.apiahf.org.

Shinagawa, S. M. (2011, August 22). Personal communication.

Sobero, R. A., Giraldo, G. P., Strode, M. L., Rosa, L. A., & DeLuca, G. V. (2003). Using a culturally competent framework to increase annual breast cancer screening rates among low-income Latinas: A case study of the Orange County Cancer Detection Partnership. *California Journal of Health Promotion, 1*(2), 101–117.

Susan G. Komen for the Cure. (2007) (originally published 1996, updated Apr 2005). *Asians or Pacific Islanders: Developing effective cancer education print materials*. Dallas: Susan G. Komen for the Cure.

Tabár, L., Vitak, B., Chen, T. H.-H., Yen, A. M.-F., Cohen, A., Tot, T., et al. (2011). Swedish two-county trial: Impact of mammographic screening on breast cancer mortality during 3 decades. *Radiology, 260*(3), 658–663.

Tucker, C. & Taylor, D. (2011). Good science: Principles of community-based participatory research. Race, Poverty & the Environment website. *A Journal of Environmental Justice*. Project of Urban Habitat. Retrieved August 21, 2011, from http://urbanhabitat.org/node/159.

U.S. Bureau of the Census, Racial Statistics Branch, Population Division. (1993a). *We the Americans: Pacific Islanders (WE-4)*. Washington, D.C.: U.S. Government Printing Office.

U.S. Bureau of the Census, Racial Statistics Branch, Population Division. (1993b). *We the Americans: Asians (WE-3)*. Washington, D.C.: U.S. Government Printing Office.

U.S. Cancer Statistics Working Group. (2010). *2007 Cancer types grouped by race and ethnicity* webpage. *United States Cancer Statistics: 1999–2007. Incidence and Mortality Web-based Report*. Atlanta: U.S. Department of Health and Human Services, Centers for Disease Control and Prevention and National Cancer Institute. Retrieved September 24, 2011, from http://apps.nccd.cdc.gov/uscs/cancersbyraceandethnicity.aspx.

U.S. Preventive Services Task Force. (2009a). Screening for breast cancer: U.S. Preventive Services Task Force recommendation statement. *Annals of Internal Medicine, 151*(10), 716–726. W-236.

U.S. Preventive Services Task Force. (2009b). *Screening for breast cancer* website (updated December 2009). Retrieved September 15, 2011, from http://www.uspreventiveservicestaskforce.org/uspstf09/breastcancer/brcanrs.htm.

Vainshtein, J. (2008). Disparities in breast cancer incidence across racial/ethnic strata and socioeconomic status: A systematic review. *Journal of the National Medical Association, 100*(7), 833–839.

Ziegler, R. G., Hoover, R. N., Pike, M. C., Hildesheim, A., Nomura, A. M. Y., West, D. W., et al. (1993). Migration patterns and breast cancer risk in Asian-American women. *Journal of the National Cancer Institute, 85*, 1819–1827.

Ziegler, R. G., Hoover, R. N., Nomura, A. M. Y., West, D. W., Wu-Williams, A. H., Pike, M. C., et al. (1995). Relative weight, weight change, height, and breast cancer risk in Asian-American women. *Journal of the National Cancer Institute, 88*, 650–660.

The Versailles Social Movement and Implications for Asian American Environmental Health In Post-Katrina New Orleans

30

Maureen Lichtveld and Vy Thuc Dao

Introduction

Less than a month after Hurricane Katrina collapsed much of the city of New Orleans, an otherwise unknown Vietnamese American community began to systematically recover from the wreckage of its flooded neighborhoods. Located 12 miles in relative isolation from the colorful distractions of the historic French Quarter and even further from the oak lined avenues of the Garden District and Uptown, the area in the east known as Versailles had been largely described by locals as a culturally remote and physically secluded community that was home to one of the most concentrated populations of Vietnamese American in the South (Airriess & Clawson, 1999; Zhou & Bankston, 1999).

Media coverage heralded the story as inspirational and praised Versailles residents as exemplars of independent resiliency. Indeed, this impression of the Vietnamese American community as a well-recovered neighborhood became indelible when, five months after the storm, a national waste disposal company re-opened a

M. Lichtveld (✉)
Freeport McMoRan Chair of Environmental Policy,
Environmental Health Sciences Department, Tulane
University School of Public Health and Tropical
Medicine, New Orleans, LA, USA
e-mail: mlichtve@tulane.edu

V.T. Dao
Department of Sociology, Tulane University,
New Orleans, LA, USA
e-mail: vdao@tulane.edu

municipal landfill to dispose hurricane debris within two miles of residents' homes. Issued through Mayor Ray Nagin by an emergency executive order, the 100 acre landfill bordering the Chef Menteur highway would be the depository of over 2.6 million tons of debris (Eaton, 2006). East New Orleans residents warned that the moldering site posed a significant toxic risk to their community despite assurances from the Louisiana Fish and Wildlife Service and pressure from the Army Corp of Engineers that the landfill was both safe and necessary (Choi, Bhatt, & Chen, 2006). Immediately, the Vietnamese American community went on the offensive and partnered with a coalition of scientists, national environmental agencies, and city council members to effectively shut down the landfill on August 15th, 2006.

To some essayists, this demonstrates an empowered ethnic enclave (Kromm, 2006; Schwinn, 2006), to Asian American scholars, the successful grassroots campaign from a community previously unknown for its political activism offers intriguing questions regarding the future of environmental justice and Asian Americans. Why Louisiana? Why now? And what are the implications for the broader Asian American Environmental Justice movement?

In this chapter, we will explore how the early Environmental Justice movement developed as a response to the more conservative goals of the general Environmental movement, and then we will examine the trajectory of the Asian American Environmental Justice Movement (AAEJM) through

G.J. Yoo et al. (eds.), *Handbook of Asian American Health*,
DOI 10.1007/978-1-4614-2227-3_30, © Springer Science+Business Media, LLC 2013

the initial establishment of organizations and objectives. The future of the AAEJM is examined through the lens of Hurricane Katrina and the subsequent development of an activist community in Southern Louisiana. Specifically, we will hear from members of the community in their own words as they describe how community activism and media command played a major role in the social justice movement and hurricane recovery for the New Orleans Vietnamese American community. Lastly, this chapter will examine the transformational opportunities for the AAEJM in the aftermath of the April 2010 Mexican oil spill in the Gulf.

Environmental Risk, Vulnerability and the Growth of the Modern EJ Movement

The contemporary Environmental Justice movement can only be understood in the context of the modern environmental movement. Before there was a deep articulation of social justice for the marginalized, the initial objectives of the movement sought to conserve, protect and appreciate natural capital. Prior to the 1960s, the approach of conservationists had been one that emphasized human stewardship of natural resources rather than an activist rising of consciousness. In this paradigm, human beings are framed as moral heroes ordained to protect and conserve natural resources, a tradition exemplified by dynamic early twentieth century figures such as Theodore Roosevelt and John Muir (Shabecoff, 2003). This romantic framing of individuals as exuberant participants in the veneration of nature quickly dissipated in the second half of the twentieth century as swelling urban centers and growing corporate interests created power differentials that increasingly resulted in environmental inequality.

Far from the concern of protecting natural reserves of beauty, the public began to realize the imminent dangers of toxic dumping, the contamination of air and water, and the abject plundering of natural resources. The threat of roiling pollution emerged during a time of increasing public outrage against institutionalized racism and sexism in the

1960s. Civil and social rights movements provided a model for environmental organization which some scholars suggest merged with the conservationist, protectionist attitudes of early environmental activists to form the foundation of the modern Environmental Justice movement (Agyenman, 2005; Bullard, 2000; Cole & Foster, 2001).

Yet it became apparent early on that this burgeoning activism failed to address ethnic and minority interests (Sandler & Pezzullo, 2007). A significant reason for this exclusion can be explained by the institutionalization, and what critics describe as a bureaucratization of the movement. From the turbulent events and rhetoric of the 1960s, the beginning of 1970 saw the establishment of the Environmental Protection Agency (EPA) which dependent on Congressional support, cultivated an agenda focused on regulatory projects, ecological protections and scientific research rather than recognizing environmental injustice (Powell, 1999). Throughout the 1970s and into the 1980s, groups began to document the significantly disproportionate hazards distributed across low-income and ethnic minority peoples.

Two powerful milestones for the Environmental Justice Movement include a major protest event and a seminal investigative study of racism and toxicity. In Warren County, North Carolina, in the summer of 1982, hundreds of protestors organized by the National Black Caucus gathered en masse to restrict the opening of a landfill which would have held tons of Poly Chlorinated Biphenyls (PCB)-contaminated soil close to several communities of color. This marks the first time that citizens created a significant, organized and sustained disturbance against inequitable toxic dumping (Agyenman, 2005; Bullard, 2000). Then, in 1987, Charles Lee's report entitled *Toxic Wastes and Race in the United States* presented cogent evidence of health disparities based on race and provided the catalyst for scientists and community residents to collectively organize. Leaders based within vulnerable communities spoke openly about the everyday dangers that ranged from higher exposures to pests, pesticides, low quality air, polluted water, and greater contact with toxins as a result of living in substandard conditions and too little advocacy from protective institutions. African American communities, particularly those in the rural South, drew on their momentum originating from Civil Rights campaigns to create the groundbreaking work for the contemporary Environmental Justice movement (Bullard, 2000; Cole & Foster, 2001).

The Asian American Environmental Justice Movement Finds a Voice

The phrase *environmental racism*, coined by African American environmental activist, Benjamin Cavis in 1981, describes the inequitable distribution of risk along racial and economic lines. Thus, clearly differentiating the divide between simple human assaults on the environment versus the systemic environmental destruction of vulnerable communities. It would be within this foundation of grassroots organization and advocacy that the Asian American Environmental Justice Movement would find its momentum (Adalberto & Lio, 2008; Sze, 2004). The movement to propel environmental health awareness has met with challenges that stem from benign impressions that the Asian American community does well for itself. For example, Silicon Valley's high percentage of Asian professionals has helped to reinforce model minority stereotypes. While well-educated researchers, developers and entrepreneurs occupy upper middle strata for income and status, rank and file factory workers who make microchips, hardware and circuit boards are routinely exposed to over 700 potentially toxic chemicals (Pellow, 2002).

In 1991, the organization of a national summit to address the environmental inequities experienced by racial and economic minorities was convened in Washington DC. The People of Color Environmental Summit articulated the principles of social justice and established objectives to guide the movement's collective actions for redressing environmental exploitation of minorities. From this initial gathering, the Asian Pacific Environmental Network (APEN) formed in 1993 to specifically champion the needs of Asian

American and Asian immigrant communities. The headquarters in Oakland, California provide a sustainable institution that supports the large West Coast population of Asians. For nearly two decades, APEN, along with other Asian American groups endeavor to protest all manner of environmental problems affecting their communities such as sweat shop hazards, illegal dumping, poor air and water quality within their neighborhoods, and differential toxic effects in occupational settings.

In one of their earliest substantive projects, APEN focused on the large numbers of Korean immigrants who worked in ubiquitous sweat-shops. At high risk for wage and health exploitation, workers toiled for long hours in shut-in warehouses with little ventilation amid dyes, fumes and other toxic chemicals. APEN focused on calling attention to these conditions as violations of basic human and civil rights. Their work with the Vietnamese American community in Northern California advocated for fishermen who made their livelihoods and fed their families by fishing in the San Francisco Bay, where they may have been exposed to high levels of toxins after ingesting polluted fish.

One of their most significant projects centers on Laotians in one of the most environmentally compromised areas of Contra Costa, CA. In 1995, buoyed by research that estimated that nearly half of Asian Americans were living near uncontrolled toxic waste sites (Dowie, 1995), APEN helped to establish the Laotian Organizing Project (LOP). Laotian immigrants living near and working in the nearly 350 toxic industrial sites had grown increasingly alarmed at the encroaching presence of chemical operations into already impoverished and environmentally compromised regions of Richmond, California. In particular, issues such as limited English and relative cultural isolation proved hazardous to the community members when they would receive little warning from fires or breakdowns at nearby chemical sites. APEN began programmatic initiatives that promoted leadership, cultural competence and grassroots organization of Laotian and Asian residents of Richmond and Oakland. The APEN and LOP's campaign to empower the vulnerable community sought to develop leadership among residents by instructing them in strategic organization and to promote an all-inclusive approach. In 2007, after 12 years of laying the groundwork for community cohesiveness and winning victories against oil refineries, the Environmental Protection Agency awarded $50,000 for a two year Environmental Justice development entitled the Richmond Environmental Justice Community Leadership Project.

Yet to the surprise of many Asian American political activists, the first Vietnamese American United States Congressman sworn in on January 6th 2009 did not come from this region. The foreign born Anh "Joseph" Quang Cao is the first native Vietnamese to work in the federal legislative branch, serving under a historically significant administration during a time of enormously volatile economic conditions. There were many paradoxical turns. The fact that he represented the Democratic stronghold of Louisiana's 2nd District as a Republican, and that he did not hail from California, with its large Asian population, or from New York, with its long history of Asian American activism, or even the economically rich state of Texas with a large proportion of Asian entrepreneurs and professionals (Kim, 2007), raises fascinating questions on the state of contemporary Asian American mobilization. What are the circumstances that would lead to this major advancement for social justice?

Black, White, and Some In-Between: Culture, Settlement and the Racial Binary

Arguably, New Orleans has retained one of the most unique racial and cultural reputations of any American City. The meshing of French, Spanish, African, Latin American and Native American influences combine for a distinctive social layering that influence how race and race relations are seen today. Due to its position as a port city, New Orleans developed its local economy, particularly at the turn of the twentieth century, around river-based commerce, cotton trading with the eventual

move in the mid-1950s toward ship building, petroleum, chemical industries and the cultivation of tourism, leisure and gaming (Dawdy, 2008; Gotham, 2007). However, the fact that New Orleans operated one of the most sophisticated and expansive slave trades in the new country (Sublette, 2009) created an unusual situation where many different African and West Indian slave influxes mingled with European and Latin Americans peoples, thus funneling an otherwise highly nuanced population to a simple but powerful racial binary of Whites and non-Whites.

In the wake of Katrina, this racial binary became emphasized to the extent that many Americans seeing the devastation of New Orleans through a hyperbolic media gaze assumed only that those suffering the most were black. Dyson (2006) illustrates the issue clearly:

> Many colors were present in this multicultural stew of suffering, but the dominant color was black. From the sight of it, this was the third world…the suffering on the screen created cognitive dissonance; it suggested that this must be somewhere in India…This surely couldn't be the United States of America (p. 2).

The disparate images of poor African Americans conflating with the uncomfortable notion of third-world suffering was enhanced by the use of the term "refugee" to describe storm evacuees in dire straits (Masquelier, 2007). Members of the media noted that the term was both technically accurate and evocatively appropriate in describing the wholesale devastation of one's home and livelihood, while others found the term undignified at best, or at worst, a sinister obfuscation of racist labeling. In short, the word *refugee* carried a "heavy semantic load" (Masquelier, 2007, p. 736). Few saw the irony that among those swimming in this "multicultural stew of suffering," was one relatively overlooked group, the Vietnamese, who could offer a most unique perspective on the use of "refugee" given their migratory background. In other words, if anyone can give a unique perspective of the notion on the nature of disaster, disruption and displacement, it is the Vietnamese.

The Making of Versailles: The Settlement of Vietnamese in New Orleans East

The settlement of Asians to Southern Louisiana is a fairly recent event. While there are reports of Filipino sailors arriving as early as 1763 to the Gulf Coast, and groups of Chinese workers in the late 1800s, the bulk of Asians in New Orleans consists of Vietnamese and other Southeast Asians arriving en masse during the 1970s and 1980s as war refugees. United States resettlement programs placed war refugees in an area of New Orleans East known as Versailles (Zhou & Bankston, 1999).

Located 13 miles from the Central Business District, this area of New Orleans had been a prosperous suburban retreat for New Orleanians during the 1960s as the petroleum and aerospace industries grew. NASA's establishment of an assembly plant in the region during this time brought further prosperity but due to the nature of highly specialized production, could offer little in the way for non-specialized labor. A deep economic downturn in the mid-1970s initiated a slow disintegration of the east. Over time, poor African Americans, who had been especially affected by the collapse of manufacturing, building and other industries, began to settle in these decaying communities. The isolation of the area, which had been a luxury for well-to-do Whites, served only to increase the segregation and poverty of African Americans.

In this region, several factors coincided to suddenly create a space for a highly concentrated Vietnamese settlement during the late 1970s. First, American dispersal strategy had been to settle the several "waves" of Vietnamese into every state in the country so that they would not overwhelm major metropolitan or urban centers (Pham, 2005). In fact, this was a short-sighted strategy as those fleeing Vietnam were a heterogeneous group depending on approximately which year they left. Earlier groups consisted of the well-educated, professional Vietnamese who had greater familiarity with American culture and naturally gravitated toward central cities despite initial placement (Rutledge, 1992). This type of secondary migration also applied to subsequent waves of Vietnamese, with many migrating where established Vietnamese had gathered. Despite these preferences, the efforts of voluntary agencies (VOLAGS) such as the U.S. Catholic Conference settled refugees in non-traditionally Asian receiving area such as the Gulf Coast cities of Biloxi and New Orleans (Zhou & Bankston, 1999).

In the case of New Orleans, the influential refugee director for Associated Catholic Charities, Elise Cerniglia, intuitively felt that recovery for incoming Vietnamese would be enhanced by locating them close to one another. At this time, several tracts of apartments known as the Versailles Arms, a Housing and Urban development subsidized by the government, became available after the neighboring NASA industry cut back on employee retention, thus opening a prime area for widespread settlement. Over time, this community grew rapidly to a concentrated population of nearly 5,000 in 1990 to just over 7,000 in the mid-2000s. Airriess (2006) contends that the ethnic-Vietnamese commercial enclave consists of roughly 7,118 Vietnamese packed tightly into an approximate three mile radius around the Mary Queen of Vietnam Catholic Church (MQVNC), ringed on the periphery by African American neighbors. This creates a highly centralized core for this enclave which supports a local ethnic marketplace of 93 different businesses (grocery stores, dry goods supplies, restaurants, jewelry, medical and dental services, etc.).

Despite the rapid growth, there had been some decline of the breakneck population expansion in Versailles due to an increasing suburban exodus to New Orleans Westbank region where Gretna and Algiers, LA are located, thus creating something of a bimodal distribution of Vietnamese American residents within the city. Thus, it is important to remember that the distribution of the Vietnamese American community in New Orleans is not monolithic, and that not every Vietnamese community member resides only in Versailles. However, during the aftermath of the storm, the community of Versailles received considerable attention for its timely evacuation, orderly management of evacuees in Houston and subsequent return to New Orleans as one of the first groups to do so.

Grassroots Grown from Disaster: Asian American Mobilization After Hurricane Katrina

> You should have seen the church, people were everywhere, cooking, giving out food, talking to one another. There were so many families, but it wasn't sad or anything, it was no concentration camp; it was people who wanted some good food, some news. Even if they had a place to go, they wanted to stay around to help
>
> (T. Nguyen, Personal Communication, December 28, 2009).

In New Orleans, Mary Queen of Vietnam Catholic Church (MQVNC) looms as the most socially, religiously and in recent years, politically important entity for the Vietnamese. Established in the late 1970s, Mary Queen of Vietnam Catholic Church is situated within a network of overlapping neighborhoods and residential areas and acts as a spatial and social hub. Over 4,000 parishioners live within a mile of the Church (Dunbar, 2006) and media stories of evacuation, mobilization and recovery centered around Father Vien Nguyen's pastoral command.

In New Orleans, preliminary reports indicate that the Catholic Church and its non-profit arm established exclusively to respond to Katrina in 2006, the Mary Queen of Vietnam Community Development Corporation (MQVN CDC), provided a systematic evacuation of their congregation (Leong et al., 2007; Li, 2008). And later, as citizens were allowed re-entry into the city, MQVN CDC principally spearheaded the recovery process of the New Orleans Vietnamese American community. In the early coverage of the storm, the Vietnamese American in New Orleans commanded a great deal of attention. Popular national news outlets such as USA Today and special ABC News reports describe the successful rebuilding in New Orleans with quotes from pastors of Mary Queen of Vietnam Catholic Church that describe their community as 80% returned by 2006 and nearly 90% in 2007 (Do, 2007; Jervis, 2007).

Many other trumpeted this positive assessment of recovery describing Versailles as "the Katrina-ravaged district has transformed itself back into a livable neighborhood. Its rapid development stands in contrast to the glacial pace of rebuilding in the surrounding areas" (Howley, 2007). And many others, relied upon interviews with representatives from the church, gave glowing accounts of supportive relationship cemented between MQVN and the community, and by extension, positively contributing to the high return rate (Allen, 2007; Hill, 2006; Zucchinoi, 2005). What is striking about this front-line literature is that it indirectly weaves a narrative of Vietnamese American recovery that promotes themes of self-reliance, defiance, survival and ethnic community cohesiveness:

> Q: "What did you hear about the Vietnamese community in New Orleans?"
> A: "Oh it was great! I never saw so much about us before, they were interviewing at Mary left and right. Also, there was a documentary film maker that came down…"
> Q: "Why do you think that is? What story were they telling?"
> A: "About how strong we are."
> Q: "Tell me more about that…"
> A: "We as a group have been through everything, look at me, I still do my job and that is to survive. Some people around here, they been back and forth across Vietnam; the older people especially know what it is like to lose everything. So, it's something they done before, they were, not prepared or anything like that, but they knew what it could be like. So rebuilding is normal."
>
> (T. Leong, Personal Communication, February 6, 2010)

The Oil Spill-Driven Transformation

On April 2010, the Gulf of Mexico became engulfed with unprecedented quantities of volatile organic compounds representing varying mixtures of oil and dispersants. Communities, scientists, and policy makers were confronted with a number of "firsts": unique mixtures of environmental contamination affecting multiple environmental media including air, surface water, soil- resulting in multiple potential exposure routes – inhalation, dermal contact, ingestion – affecting an equally unique population: Bayou and Vietnamese fisher folk, men and women- turned environmental clean-up workers. To address the myriad of data gaps and mounting community health concerns, the Institute of Medicine (IOM) convened two Gulf Coast workshops related to the Gulf of Mexico Oil spill.

Lessons learned in the aftermath of Hurricane Katrina indeed were influential. Beyond the traditional issues of science, IOM members specifically emphasized the community perspective, the need to take a holistic, rather than a silo-driven approach to addressing health issues and a strong focus on the immediate and longer term psychosocial consequences of the disaster (Institute of Medicine [IOM], 2010a, b). At the 2010 meeting of the Gulf long-term follow-up worker study, Tap Bui, an MQVNC leader, was invited to speak about major concerns (ION, 2010b). Similarly, MQVN CDC invited the leadership of the National Institute of Environmental Health Sciences to participate in community workshops so they could learn firsthand the Vietnamese fisher folks' concerns. This first transformation from a retrospective social movement to a prospective stand has already influenced the science agenda: seafood consumption and pregnant women have been identified as priority research gaps to be addressed. Perhaps even more profound is the second transformation – from an advocacy role to one of effector. MQVN CDC is increasingly the lead partner in several community-based participatory research studies currently underway not only to fingerprint the potential impact of the oil spill on the Vietnamese fisher folk and their families but to actively intervene and protect. From operating community health clinics to assisting with oil spill claim submissions, the organization has become an inseparable component of not only the Vietnamese community, but that of the City of New Orleans, State of Louisiana, the Gulf Coast Region, and indeed our nation.

In this chapter we explored Hurricane Katrina as the singular catastrophic event that raises the political consciousness of the Vietnamese living in New Orleans East. In the wake of the historic storm, we examined the development of an activist community in Southern Louisiana, understood their place within the multicultural context of New Orleans, and we examined the pivotal events that marked Versailles, which debuted onto the national scene as a major political and environmental player. In summary we discussed how a social justice movement evolved not only in strategic positioning from a reactive enterprise to a prospective one, but also as a transdisciplinary force influencing science, policy and practice.

The inextricable link between ecosystem health and human health which characterizes the early AAEJM is confronting us again (Goldstein, Osofsky, & Lichtveld, 2011). This time however, it is not about terminology-driven action – activism, justice, or equity- but about serving as a change agent, often leading disparate coalitions to protect communities in a holistic fashion. Unlike post-Hurricane Katrina, the affected Vietnamese American community is no longer an obscure vulnerable population; rather one who is frequently sought after for answers, approaches, and as a trusted source of information. This strategic positioning may well signal a new era for the AAEJM and a new responsibility: assuring science and policy work for communities in a deliberately pro-active manner and MQVN CDC are leading the way.

Future endeavors to strengthen the environmental justice movement must take both an aggressive tack toward promoting parity yet simultaneously, aggressively pursue increasingly sophisticated political and activist agendas with innovative strategies. In this chapter we have discussed how early social movements primarily addressed existing disparities. Whether the issues concerned an isolated immigrant group in Southeast Louisiana affected by a natural disaster, or garment workers laboring in dangerous conditions, or residents battling to ensure their health in mixed zoning neighborhoods, vulnerable individuals had to transform into politicized and mobilized activists. With the passage of time however, a movement matures and what were once merely protests must become platforms with leaders not only rallying campaigns but helping communities articulate their visions for the future and with the use of the most innovative technology.

In the future, the AAEJM will continue to organize grass roots protests and mount local campaigns for social fairness, but will do so with the use of social media and networking. It will also tap into the growing reserves of young, well educated Asian Americans, emerging future politicians, scholars and public intellectuals who will craft missions that take into account the increasingly global views on the nature of fairness and sustainability – these will be our future policy makers. We will see these new faces on the steps of any given city hall rallying a crowd as well as inside the building creating new policies to advance social justice. Let us not lose this momentum.

References

Adalberto, A., Jr., & Lio, S. (2008). Spaces of mobilization: The Asian American Pacific Islander struggle for social justice. *Social Justice, 35*(2), 1–17.

Agyenman, J. (2005). *Sustainable communities and the challenges of environmental justice.* New York: New York University Press.

Airriess, C. (2006). Scaling central place of an ethnic-Vietnamese enclave. In D. H. Kaplan & W. L. Lanham (Eds.), *Landscapes of the ethnic economy* (pp. 17–33). Lanham, MD: Rowman and Littlefield Publishers.

Airriess, C. A., & Clawson, D. L. (1994). Vietnamese market gardens in New Orleans. *Geographical Review, 84*(1), 16–31.

Allen, G. (2007, March 27). Retrieved November 15, 2009, from http://www.npr.org/templates/story/story.php?storyId=9163113.

Bullard, R. D. (2000). *Dumping in Dixie: Race, class and environmental quality* (3rd ed.). Boulder, CO: Westview Press.

Choi, J., Bhatt, A., & Chen, F. (2006). In the aftermath of Hurricane Katrina: The Chef Menteur landfill and the effects of the Vietnamese American community. Asian American Justice Center. August Report.

Cole, L. W., & Foster, S. R. (2001). *From the ground up: Environemental racism and the rise of the environmental justice movement.* New York: New York University Press.

Conaway, C., Ross, J., Looker, R., Mason, R., & Flegal, R. (2007). Decadal mercury trends in San Francisco estuary sediments. *Environmental Research, 105*(1), 53–66.

Dawdy, S. L. (2008). *Building the devil's empire: French colonial New Orleans.* Chicago: The University of Chicago Press.

Do, S.(2007). By pulling together, community rebuilds and residents return. USA Today. June 19. A12.

Dowie, M. (1995). *Losing ground: American environmentalism at the close of the twentieth century.* Cambridge, MA: MIT Press.

Dunbar, T. (2006). Update from New Orleans: The people's approach. *Social Policy, 40*, 1.

Dyson, M. E. (2006). *Come hell or high water: Hurricane Katrina and the color of disaster.* New York: Basic Civitas.

Eaton, L. (2006, August 16). New Orleans mayor closes a disputed landfill used for debris from Hurricane. *The New York Times*, Section A.

Goldstein, B. D., Osofsky, H. J., & Lichtveld, M. Y. (2011). The gulf oil spill. *The New England Journal of Medicine, 364*, 14.

Gotham, K. (2007). Authentic New Orleans: Race, Culture and Tourism in the Big Easy. New York: NYU Press.

Hill, L. (2006, January 23). The miracle of Versailles: New Orleans Vietnamese community rebuilds. *New Orleans Louisiana Weekly.*

Howley, K. (2007). Vietnamese Resistance: God and government in New Orleans. *Reason, 38*(8), 1–6.

Institute of Medicine. (2010a). *Assessing the effects of the Gulf of Mexico oil spill on human health.* Washington, DC: National Academies press.

Institute of Medicine. (2010b). *Review of the proposal for the gulf long-term follow up study: Highlights from the September workshop.* Washington, DC: National Academies press.

Jervis, R. (2007). Many in Mississippi still lack homes after '05 storms; some uprooted by hurricanes live in woods. The Sun Herald September 25, 2009. News Pg 3A.

Kim, T. P. (2007). *The racial logic of politics: Asian Americans and party competitions.* Philadelphia, PA: Temple University Press.

Kromm, C. (2006, September 18). Grassroots gumbo. *The Nation*, pp. 22–26.

Leong, K. J., Airriess, C. A., Li, W., Chia-Chen Chen, A., & Keith, V. M. (2007). Resilient history and the rebuilding of a community: The Vietnamese American community in New Orleans East. *Journal of American History, 94*(3),770–779.

Li, W., Airriess, C. A.. Chia-Chen Chen, A., Leong, K. J., Keith, V. M., & Adams, K. L. (2008). Surviving katrina and its aftermath: Evacuation and community mobilization by Vietnamese Americans and African Americans. *Journal of Cultural Geography, 25*(3), 263–286.

Masquelier, A. (2007). Why Katrina's victims aren't refugees: Musings on a "dirty" word. *American Anthropologist, 108*(4), 735–743.

Pellow, D. N. (2002). *Garbage wars: The struggle for environmental justice in Chicago.* Cambridge, MA: MIT Press.

Pham, A. (2005, September 18). Vietnamese lose all, this time to Katrina. *USA Today*, p. 11A.

Powell, M. R. (1999). *Science at EPA: Information in the regulatory process.* Washington, DC: Resources for the Future.

Rutledge, P. J. (1992). *The Vietnamese experience in America.* Bloomington, IN: Indiana University Press.

Sandler, R., & Pezzullo, P. (2007). Working together and working apart. In R. Sandler & P. Pezullo (Eds.), *Environmental Justice and Environmentalism: The Social Justice Challenge to the Environmental Movement* (pp. 309–320). Cambridge: MIT Press.

Schwinn, E. (2006). Charity coalition helps shut down landfill. *The Chronicle of Philanthropy, 18*(21), 11–11.

Shabecoff, P. (2003). *A fierce green fire: The American environmental movement*. Washington, DC: Island Press.

Sublette, N. (2009). *The world that made New Orleans: From Spanish silver to Congo Square*. Chicago: Lawrence Hill Books.

Sze, J. (2004). Asian American activism for environmental justice. *Peace Review, 16*(2), 149–156.

Zhou, M., & Bankston, C. L., III. (1999). *Growing up American: How Vietnamese children adapt to life in the United States*. New York: Russell Sage Foundation.

Zucchinoi, D. (2005, May 16). Searchers wade through the thick of it. *Los Angeles Times*.

Ted Fang and Jason Liu

Kate was the fifth of six children. Immigrating originally from China, her family shared everything. Family dinners were frequent, and as her sisters married, the number of seats at the table kept growing. Each person was full of life and energy. All were blessed with good health. Her grandmother lived a century and no family member had any major sickness or even injury. But on a routine trip to the doctor, the whole family's life was shattered when her father was diagnosed with liver cancer.

Kate knew her father had a virus called hepatitis B (HBV). But everyone assumed it was harmless. Now the family was catapulted into a state of shock and paralysis. They learned that HBV was a major cause of fatal liver cancer. After the diagnosis, her father, 65, went from hope to despair to depression. The doctor insisted all family members get tested. Five of the six children, including Kate, were HBV positive. Family dinners were no longer comfortable. Kate felt cheated. Anger was her first reaction – she had done nothing wrong to deserve a lifetime of disease. Then sadness overtook her, as she thought

of the health of her own future children. Kate and her family felt they were destined to die from the infection.

After two years, Kate's father did succumb to cancer. The family is still learning to live without him. But the disease, rather than being a fearful or foreign concept, became very much a part of their lives. In the most ironic twist, HBV taught them to take care of one another, to make sure they followed treatment plans and adhered to healthy lifestyle changes. What started out as routine day-to-day discussions, turned into regular medical check-ups. Everyone in the family was able to get their HBV infection under control with no signs of liver cancer. Kate herself took things a step further. She wanted to have a degree of control over the disease and wondered what she could do to prevent the epidemic in the next generation. Kate became an active patient advocate. She visited schools, offices of U.S. Senators, hospitals and community groups. At every visit, she shared her story and asked people to remind each other to take HBV seriously.

But the truth is there have been woefully few efforts to address HBV disease and liver cancer. The reality is that liver cancer is still the deadliest cancer in the United States with the most deaths per capita. It is also the greatest health disparity for Asian Americans. These are the facts:

- Hepatitis B (HBV) infection is the leading cause of liver cancer in the world.
- HBV infection is the most common untreated disease in the world.

T. Fang (✉)
Asian Week Foundation, San Francisco Hep B Free,
San Francisco, CA, USA
e-mail: tedyfang@gmail.com

J. Liu
San Francisco Hep B Free, San Francisco, CA, USA

G.J. Yoo et al. (eds.), *Handbook of Asian American Health*,
DOI 10.1007/978-1-4614-2227-3_31, © Springer Science+Business Media, LLC 2013

- Asians are 100 times more likely to be infected with HBV and are most likely to die from liver cancer.
- HBV infection and liver cancer are the greatest health disparities for Asian and Pacific Islander Americans.
- A vaccine can prevent Hep B infection and is considered the first anti-cancer vaccine.
- Effective treatments can prevent liver cancer from developing from HBV infection.

HBV is a top health issue for Asian Americans, as well as a top global issue. Research indicates the virus appeared 1,500 years ago in Africa (Zhou & Holmes, 2007). Today, Asia has the most cases of HBV infection and the most cases of liver cancer (Pfizer, 2008). However, it has been in America, where virtually all the medical tools for preventing and treating HBV infection have been discovered. This chapter studies how these multi-national roots and other factors affected mobilization around HBV disease to become a formative moment for Asian Americans. It focuses on the national and global Hep B Free (HBF) movement begun in San Francisco to address the first major Asian American issue not emanating from nor led by the legal or civil rights arenas. The community itself brought forth the issue of HBV and has been both the leader and the driver to stop the disease.[1]

Through key informant interviews[2] conducted of key partners and leaders in the Hep B Free movement, this chapter also documents how the Asian American community coalesced, developed and implemented the San Francisco Hep B Free Campaign. Based on findings of these key informant interviews and an analysis of process and activities of this movement, this chapter examines four themes most prominent in this campaign. First, that Hep B Free (HBF) is an Asian American movement – starting from the community, growing with the community, focusing on a top community issue, and having bi-cultural attributes of the community. Second, that the overriding characteristic of this Asian American effort is collaboration – the ability to sustain a wide-ranging and full spectrum cooperation of partners and supporters. Third and fourth, that dual tactics of "extravagance and necessity" are used to keep the collaboration together and to spur action forward. "Extravagance" here alludes to the grand vision and desire by community members to "do things they had thought beyond their capabilities", such as making an entire city free of hepatitis B disease (Takaki, 1993, p. 11). "Necessity" is referring to the need of dealing with practical difficulties such as the necessity of securing funds, communicating in multiple languages, and dealing with bureaucratic institutions. The combination of activating those two forces magnify the community's impact and capacity to make change. The analysis concludes by placing the HBF effort in the context of Asian

---

[1] Community Based Participatory Research (CPBR) require that community involvement abide by prescribed institutional project frameworks limited to the resources of the sponsoring agency (Nguyen et al., 2006). Hep B Free's (HBF), provides a wider conception of community based participatory research that employs resources and participation that exceed what can be measured. Rather, we propose an alternative analysis of community-based research that has been used in HBF based on Ethnic Studies theory (Deleuze & Guattari, 1980; Espiritu, 1992; Takaki, 1993; Turner, 1974; Van Gennep, 1960) which points out broader ways of utilizing Asian American assets and the larger public to engage community members.

[2] To document and assess how the Asian American community in the San Francisco coalesced, developed and implemented the San Francisco Hep B Free Campaign, twenty three semi-structured key informant interviews were conducted with key partners and leaders in 2010. Those interviewed included community members and also health care providers, media and political leaders, and leaders of community organizations serving the Asian American community. During these in-depth interviews, questions were asked their involvement in the campaign, what resources they brought to the campaign, gaps and challenges in the campaign, messages that have resonated with Asian Americans and their thoughts on the effectiveness of specific aspects and best practices of the campaign. Findings of these key informant interviews are used throughout this chapter (Yoo, 2010; Yoo, Fang, Zola, & Dariotis, 2011).

American history to reflect on how health interventions and other causes can be made more effective when they are built on and tap into the changing strengths and characteristics of Asian Pacific America.

Background

The number of people suffering from chronic HBV in Asia is almost equal to the entire population of the United States. Nearly two-thirds of the 350–400 million chronic hepatitis B patients worldwide are found in Asia (Custer, Hazlet, Iloejo, Veenstra, & Kowdley, 2004; World Health Organization [WHO], 2008). China alone accounts for one-third of all global cases with 120–130 million chronically infected (Liu & Fan, 2007). Correspondingly, Asia carries the highest rates of liver cancer worldwide. Three fourths of new liver cancer cases in males and two thirds in females occur in Asia. Liver cancer has the highest incidence of any cancer in Laos, Mongolia, Taiwan, and Thailand (Pfizer, 2008).

The United States accounts for only 0.4% of liver cases worldwide (Centers for Disease Control [CDC], 2011; WHO, 2008). While chronic HBV appears in 1 out of 12 Asian and Pacific Islander Americans, for the general population it occurs in less than 1 out of 1,000 (Cohen et al., 2008). Despite being over 100 times less prevalent in America (CDC, 2011), all of the major medical breakthroughs for HBV prevention and treatment have been discovered in the United States. In 1964, it was Dr. Baruch Blumberg, a New Yorker, who discovered the hepatitis B virus. He and his team then developed a test to screen for the virus and invented the first hepatitis B vaccine. The link between hepatitis B and liver cancer meant this was the first anti-cancer vaccine, and in 1976 Blumberg won the Nobel Prize in Medicine for his achievements.

But discovery of the virus and vaccine were only the first steps. Because most chronic hepatitis B shows no symptoms, initial efforts focused on cases of acute hepatitis B, which often do manifest intense short-term symptoms. Although chronic HBV causes up to 80% of all liver cancers, this was not understood until decades later when mass screenings came into use and epidemiological data was collected. This later data also showed that acute HBV among adults was not a major cause of liver failure. Thus, the introduction of the HBV anti-cancer vaccine was a public health failure, and rates of liver cancer continued to increase. Initial vaccination campaigns overlooked the at-risk population of Asian/Pacific Islanders as well as the primary mode of chronic HBV, which is from mother to baby during birth (WHO, 2008).

Asian American Roots of Hep B Free Campaign

Misinformation, stigma, lack of sanitary health procedures and lack of resources have made HBV epidemic on the Asian continent. Many Asians have wrongly believed infection occurs through casual contact, causing patients to be ostracized (Clements et al., 2006; Gust, 1996). Governments in Asia have been reluctant to institute widespread screening programs because identifying a wave of new patients could cause public panic. Progress has been made, however. China, for example, took steps towards ending HBV employment discrimination in 2009, as well as expanding vaccination programs for children under 15 (Liu, 2009).

Early U.S. public health efforts to end chronic HBV were mostly started by Asian Americans working in medicine. In 1991, Timothy and Joan Block started the Hepatitis B Foundation in Pennsylvania as the first non-profit to focus on hepatitis B (HBV) research. Dr. Samuel So founded the Asian Liver Center at Stanford University in 1996 devoted to the ailment in Asians and Asian Americans, and introduced the Jade Ribbon as a symbol for HBV activism. In 1997, Dr. Moon Chen started the National Task Force on Hepatitis B: Focus on Asian Americans and Pacific Islanders, with the U.S. Centers for Disease Control. Then in 2000, Chinese Hospital in San Francisco became the first medical institution in America to do community screenings for HBV.

The first attempt to take a coordinated systemic approach emerged from the Asian American community itself with the Hep B Free campaign launched in San Francisco in 2007. Initial discussions of (SFHBF) sprung from activities at the Asian Heritage Street Celebration the year prior when four Asian Americans of widely different backgrounds collaborated to conduct the largest ever 1-day screening for HBV in the United States: public relations expert Grace Niwa, a who conceived the event, Paul Chen, a young executive at pharmaceutical giant Glaxo Smith Kline who funded the event, Ted Fang, a veteran media and community leader who led the event, and Dr. So, and an international expert on HBV disease who ran the screening program. With lines going around the block, 536 people were screened in 5 hours, including high profile public officials such as San Francisco Mayor Gavin Newsom and Congressman Mike Honda, the highest-ranking Asian American in the U.S. House of Representatives. Asian media in many languages provided extensive coverage.

The unexpectedly huge community interest prompted Fang and So to begin talking about a universal approach toward ending HBV on a jurisdictional level. They broadened the discussion and reached out to the San Francisco Department of Public Health (SFDPH) and Fiona Ma, then a San Francisco Supervisor. These four formed the initial steering committee, and SFDPH came to be represented by veteran health educator Janet Zola. Chinese Hospital became an honorary steering committee member. The co-founders brought in different and necessary elements of health systems, medical expertise, business experience, community organizing, public policy, and public spokespersons. SF Hep B Free's (SFHBF) collaborative model soon attracted a broad network of Asian Pacific American community groups, and the most intensive coalition of non-Asian partnerships ever to assemble together around an Asian American concern. SFHBF Free pioneered ways for motivating greater Asian American involvement and for propelling increased participation from general society.

Model collaborations and partnerships include:

The Asian American community as a venue for releasing nationwide U.S. health guidelines. In

2008, the head of Viral Hepatology for the U.S. Centers for Disease Control flew to San Francisco to feature the work of SFHBF and announced new national guidelines calling on all doctors to screen Asian and at-risk patients for HBV. The new guidelines later served as the basis for the SF Hep B Free Clinician Honor Roll which has the goal of recruiting 90% of San Francisco doctors to sign a pledge that they will fulfill the CDC guidelines of screening Asian patients for HBV (Pang, 2008, 2009).

The Asian American community as a platform for launching national healthcare reform efforts. After introducing Health Care Reform legislation in the U.S. Congress, the first public appearance by then Speaker of the U.S. House of Representatives Nancy Pelosi was at a press conference in San Francisco's Chinatown promoting Hep B Free. Pelosi articulated how HBV is a concern for all Americans as an issue of national health equity and as an example of the need for implementing health prevention principles. The event received nationwide news coverage and was attended by over a dozen officials including the head of the U.S. Office of Minority Health (Zheng, 2009).

Federal recognition by U.S. Department of Health and Human Services. In 2011 the U.S. Department of Health and Human Services issued the nation's first National Action Plan for Viral Hepatitis, with specific reference to the success of the community-based model of HBF (United States Department of Health and Human Services [USDHHS], 2011). CDC officials declared HBF "one of the finest examples of community mobilization" (Picture, 2008, para. 25).

Major league sports partnerships to support an Asian American cause. In 2008, the San Francisco Giants hosted their first San Francisco Hep B Free Night and Asian Heritage Week. Activities included designating a Giants player as a Hep B Free champion to participate in (1) a home plate ceremony, (2) a scoreboard video, and (3) a baseball card with Hep B prevention facts on the back. The Giants also donated a portion of ticket revenues and spurred the Oakland Raiders football team and the

Golden State Warrior basketball team to institute similar major league sponsored San Francisco Hep B Free sports events (Swing, 2008).

Private sector partnerships to promote Asian American issues. In May 2011, Nordstrom held a month long event promoting HBV education for Asian Americans. Signage was posted in all stores, full-page announcements appeared in Nordstrom's mail-order catalogue, and an educational web-based survey was promoted through Asian community media. A donation was made to Hep B Free for each survey completed up to a maximum of $75,000. Other private sector support included the donation of a car by Subaru of America, painted with the Hep B Free colors and used as a moving promotional billboard. Walgreens printed 100,000 HBV awareness fliers and distributed them through their locations in San Francisco.

Major market advertising campaigns utilizing all Asian models. SFHBF's second ad campaign, entitled "Which One Deserves to Die,?" highlighted that one in ten Asian Americans might die from liver cancer due to HBV. Ten people were featured in six different ad themes on television, billboards, buses, metro stations, newspapers, and online. Images included a multi-generational Filipino family, a pan-Asian group of ten physicians, and other Asian settings. All 60 models were volunteers from the community, and numerous businesses donated nearly $1 million in cash, services and media. The campaign was presented in English and four Asian languages. Though somewhat controversial, the ads generated huge interest in the Asian American community as the first major market advertising campaign to feature all Asian models. It drew national attention from The New York Times, National Public Radio, PBS News Hour, and many media outlets (McKinley, 2010; Spencer, 2010; Varney, 2010).

Full Spectrum Collaboration

The strength of San Francisco Hep B Free (SFHBF) has stemmed from its depth and breadth of community support, totaling more than 150 organizations in the city. The Asian American leadership involvement has been self-evident with steering committee members, more than half of the actively participating partners, more than 70 percent of community supporters, and a large majority of attendees at monthly planning meetings having roots in the Asian American community. Simultaneously, active participation in the campaign has cut across all aspects of society from the city's local health department to the Speaker of the United States House of Representatives. Medical involvement has ranged from top international liver specialists to community health clinics serving the uninsured. Private sector support has included Chinatown merchants all the way up to Fortune 500 corporations. The list of more than three dozen actively participating partners has been led by all the major hospitals in San Francisco. Spokespersons have included the second highest ranking member of the California Assembly and local television network news anchor Alan Wang. "It is an important venture," stated Dr. Edward Chow, the longest serving member of San Francisco's Health Commission. "It has galvanized an entire city. Not just the health community – to help place on the map an important public health issue that seldom gets that same type of attention".

This community-based collaboration of SF Hep B Free reflects the broad vision of a larger Asian American community consisting of both Asians themselves, as well as interactions with mainstream society. This vision defines what organizers at the AsianWeek Foundation have labeled a full-spectrum strategy towards organizing Asian Pacific America. This full spectrum strategy is the core principle of Hep B Free. It looks for ways to make all aspects of society become stakeholders in a combined endeavor. For analysis, these aspects of society can be categorized into four groups: the Asian American community, the healthcare systems, the public sector, and the private sector. The tactics and processes of Hep B Free have revolved around keeping these four groups active and engaged toward the singular goal of eliminating HBV (see Fig 31.2 San Francisco Hep B Free Asian Community Model).

San Francisco Hep B Free Logic Model

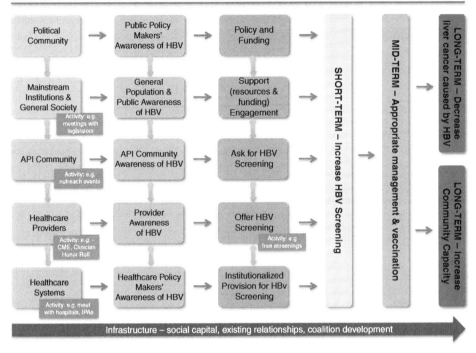

Fig. 31.1 San Francisco Hep B Free Logic Model

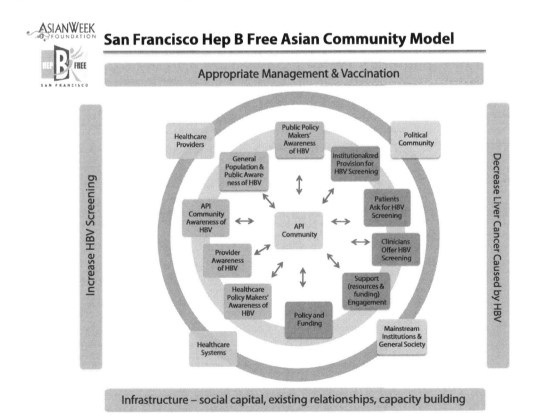

Fig. 31.2 San Francisco Hep B Free Asian Community Model

Extravagant Hopes and Dreams

The first of two fundamental tactics was to paint a grand vision for Hep B Free that would encompass all the different players. In this sense, San Francisco Hep B Free (SFHBF) strategically did not position itself as a screening program or patient support program or even an advocacy program. Rather, HBF represented a holistic perspective for a comprehensive program to educate the public, to educate and change the practice patterns of health providers, and to link patients to adequate care. This full spectrum philosophy not only welcomed the participation of all, but in fact, fed on itself. By inviting more stakeholders to participate, the increasing number fed into the energy of the campaign, creating more enthusiasm which attracted more participants and supporters. "I get inspired because people are so excited about it," enthused Ma, who was the first high profile person to openly speak about her HBV and has become a national poster child for the cause. "It just kind of inspires me that people (who aren't even infected) feel this passion about it – then we must be doing something right." After attending a few planning meetings, Lisa Tang, a physician at Kaiser Permanente in San Francisco, was motivated to lead a working group to outreach to other doctors. She later became Chairperson of the National Hep B Taskforce. Tang felt that she became part of a bigger mission: "I think as a physician, I make a difference in patients' lives kind of one life at a time. Doing this, I can really impact the community."

The concept of SFHBF is a dream – to become the first city to "eradicate" hepatitis B and to lead the eradication of the deadly virus globally. The San Francisco Chronicle's front page story in 2010 got the headline right – "Lofty goal: Stamp out silent killer hepatitis B (Allday, 2010)". SF Hep B Free's ambitions have indeed been lofty. Ron Smith, Senior Vice President of the Northern California Hospital Council, conveyed the exuberance of Tom Hennessy, CEO of St. Francis Hospital saying: "We eliminated smallpox [and] we can do the same with hepatitis B." That would make HBV only the second disease in the history of human medicine to be eliminated. The sheer scope and size of the cause has made it a rallying point for the Asian American community. The campaign captures what Dr. Stewart Cooper, lead hepatologist at the California Pacific Medical Center, called "the good side of human nature," the part of people that is "prepared to share a bit of what you have, so that even if nothing happens to you, your neighbor can be helped."

One might ask, however, if this passion of hopes and dreams can be sustained. HBF's solution has been to build on an infrastructure of existing resources and medical tools and then channeling them into continuous practical steps. Many of the techniques used, such as free screening clinics, existed prior to the campaign. But without the lofty ideals, it was difficult to bring their efforts together. HBF has allowed these collective passions to resonate off of one another.

Tamiko Wong, who helped organize many SFHBF events and meetings reported how the monthly planning meetings exemplify a rare expansive collaboration: "There's not just one voice; there's not just one interest; there's not just one plan; there's not just one type of organization". Janet Zola, co-founder of SFHBF affirmed this: "People come together (and) they leave their competing missions at the door." Though informal in structure, there is a strong sense of belonging to an important cause. And as Zola's comments imply, the process strives to be non-confrontational where every idea is considered within the realm of possibility – including the choice to pursue this passion or not. Without any formal requirement or obligation for participation, each person and organization takes ownership of their course of action to achieve the common goal.

The organization's title, San Francisco, Hep B Free (SFHBF) did not just name a goal, but an extravagant idea. Zola expounded: "The bigger picture of the process, [other] than the task piece of the process, which is eliminating the disease, [is] more about bringing people together – bringing the community together." As Dr. So emphasizes, "We only work with people who are passionate." This is not so much because partners are tested for their resolve, but because these are the types of people that SFHBF attracts. Abby Yant, Vice President at St. Francis Hospital, elaborates: "the coalition itself, I think, is phenomenal. I go there to get energy."

Dealing with Necessities

The campaign's second fundamental tactic was to be practical and pragmatic toward the challenges and reality of working with each of the four full-spectrum groups mentioned. These groups correspond to the four categories depicted as working together to form the outer ring of the Asian Community Model diagram which included the following actions: (1) To make change in the healthcare system to include prevention practices for HBV and liver cancer, (2) To fund project activities, the private sector was looked to for partnerships and support, (3) To actively appeal to policy makers to get the government to recognize and act on the need to end liver cancer and health disparities and (4) To mobilize community and to activate all the other areas for mobilizing the target population to take action in protecting their own health.

Messaging Asian Americans

SFHBF organizers looked to the unique characteristics of the Asian American community for developing tactics, rather than trying to import methodologies that worked in other communities and applying them to Asian Americans. Four practical mechanisms were consistently effective:
1. Emphasizing the appreciation of differences within the Asian American community and refraining from conventional calls for more unity.
2. For the one-third of Asian Americans who immigrated to America as adults, some of whom may feel more comfortable communicating in their native language, materials were available in Chinese, Vietnamese, Tagalog and Korean.

3. For the two-thirds of Asians in America who were born or raised in the United States, outreach was conducted in English, but with Asian cultural sensitivities. And these English-dominant Asian Americans were used as a key bridge to communicate with Asian-language-dominant immigrants (Shinagawa & Kim, 2008).
4. Understanding the family unit as a means of communication.

Mary Jung, a corporate manager and community activist, noted the thoughtful tone of the SFHBF messaging: "They've been really respectful. They've done their best to get their message out. But they haven't been intrusive. It's sort of like, they're out there, but you can come to them." Jeanette Tam, an administrator at Chinese Community Health Plan, also noted the informational nature of SFHBF when she brought up the subject with a friend: "So the movement … provides you with information that people can access right away." David Chiu, President of the San Francisco Board of Supervisors portrayed Hep B Free messaging as balanced: "Not necessarily putting it in their face but being aggressive at talking about taboo issues."

SFHBF's aggressive inclusiveness for community participation across political divides and ethnic differences spread nationally to include organizations like Organization of Chinese Americans (OCA), the largest Asian American membership organization with over 80 chapters. By the end of 2010, the Hep B Free model was replicated in 14 sites in the United States including Hawaii. That breadth of community support also helped make HBV one of the priorities for the White House Initiative on Asian Americans and Pacific Islanders and helped get HBV included in remarks by President Barack Obama recognizing Asian Pacific Heritage month in May of 2009, the first time that a United States president included hepatitis B in his comments.

HBF was successful in de-stigmatizing HBV as a fatal sickness and transforming the issue into a topic of community discourse. Targeted population surveys directed by the San Francisco Department of Public Health two years after the start of the campaign found that 85% of Asian respondents in San Francisco recognized the term hepatitis B; 68% of those screened did so since the campaign began; and 40% specifically recognized the SFHBF advertising campaign (Henne Group, 2009).

Mayoral aide Francis Tsang helped with efforts to educate new immigrant populations, remarking "it's harder to reach them because they are not as plugged into the community." One tactic the campaign developed was to match speakers from each linguistic community to specific media outlets. Another was enlisting community leaders to help turn the media outlets into partners providing not only editorial coverage, but also advertising space. In another area, community awareness presentations spawned an innovative translation program for training community members to make presentations in various Asian languages. This speakers bureau program was begun by the Hep B Collaborative and evolved into the Volunteer Health Interpreters Organization, run collaboratively by students from the University of California, Berkeley alongside medical school students from the University of California, San Francisco. These students learned medical interpretation skills in Cantonese, Mandarin, Korean, Vietnamese, and with plans to add Lao, Cambodian and Thai. The use of younger Asian Americans to reach non-English speakers was a key practice. "They become youth ambassadors," said Fiona Ma, who was elected to the California Assembly in 2006, adding: "These young people are able to go back and ask their aunts or ask their mother, uncles, whether they've been tested for it." The campaign also successfully utilized English-dominant Asian Americans as influencers for non-English dominant Asian Americans. "It's important for people to understand that even though you're English-speaking and may have been born here, your association with others – with the sibling … with informing the older generation – that is important," detailed Dr. Ed Chow who is Chief Medical Officer of Chinese Community Health Plan.

SFHBF employed a multi-pronged approach towards community awareness that can be called the "dinner table strategy." This focused on the family unit as the place where major decisions were made and tapped into the pan-Asian custom of shared family meals. "Even though there may be a lot of stresses on the family, it's a unit that is still a very key, key part of peoples' lives," outlined Sandy Mori, a long-time community leader and former secretary to the San Francisco Health Commission. With the dinner table strategy, just one person would bring up the topic of HBV at the dinner table. However, enough participation from others would also be necessary to sustain a discussion and engage the whole family unit. This group strategy required organizers to use multiple techniques and languages to reach the different generations, with the goal of these messages being shared and reinforced at the dinner table setting. "Yeah, because we're Asian we can sit around the dining table and talk about it over food," commented Tsang. Businesswoman Celia Wang pictured the scene: "Back home at the family dinner or something, they talk about, hey, what did you learn today?"

Political Community

Hep B Free's (HBF) approach towards public policy was also pragmatic. Its success was far-reaching, all the way up to the White House and entries into the Congressional Record (Eshoo, 2011). Its impact was wide too at the local level. In May 2009, 14 elected and appointed officials attended a press conference on the eve of Mother's Day to highlight mother-to-infant transmission as the most frequent mode of infection for Asians. Participants included Chief Administrative Officer Ed Lee, who in 2010 was appointed the first Asian American Mayor of San Francisco. But campaign leaders gave tacit acknowledgment to the fact that the Asian American community did not have many of the more effective tools used by others to pressure public policy changes such as a disinclination by the community to use its constitutional right to gather and protest. "We're not going to be like HIV where we are going to act out and be really wild about it and go out and express our feelings," related Dr. Stuart Fong representing

Chinese Hospital as Honorary Steering Committee member. But public policy makers nonetheless played a vital role by utilizing the highly symbolic value they customarily have with Asians. "Public officials, I think those are important … to be able to show a solidarity that this is an important issue for that community," proclaimed Dr. Chow. Particularly effective was the ubiquitous Ma who served as Hep B Free's Honorary Chairperson. Celia Wang talked about the effect on her: "Wow, they're a community leader and they have a vulnerable side as well, and this could happen to anyone. It could happen to me."

Initially, HBF did not engage public officials to aggressively pursue legislative routes, but utilized these leaders to make connections and to open doors. Ron Smith of the Hospital Council recalled one situation where it was the symbolic value that made the difference: "Fiona Ma called and said, could she come and present on hepatitis B? Obviously, we're not going to say no to an Assemblywoman." As it turned out, Ma was delayed in Sacramento on legislative business. HBF representatives Fang and So spoke to the group. That presentation without Assemblywoman Ma nonetheless convinced every hospital CEO in San Francisco to support and commit available resources to the campaign. The campaign also strategically balanced the dynamic relationship between elected officials and their community constituents. "A big lesson is the importance of community involvement. We have a lot of elected officials who support us, who come to press conferences. … I think truly the reason that they want to be involved is, it's votes. It's votes from this large community that they represent. And it's the right thing to do," explained Zola.

Private Sector and General Society

SFHBF went to the San Francisco hospital CEO's to seek their financial backing. However, the community did not present a traditional social services or charity care rationale. Rather, they developed a business case for the hospitals, citing the overall higher rates of Asian Americans having health insurance (California Health Interview Survey, 2003). This appreciation of

business realities helped hospitals to take it upon themselves to build HBV programs that fit their own operational plans. This ensured sustainability rather than having to constantly raise funds for medical services. Smith praised the campaign for "doing it right, in that they appreciate that everyone's contribution is different." He added: "Each hospital has its own way of dealing with it. But they're all actively involved. And they've all given money to the project as well as what they themselves were doing." SFHBF also leveraged the economic strength of the Asian American community to help community members in need. Hospitals not only created programs for insured patients, but also were asked to take responsibility for those segments of the Asian American community, such as Korean Americans, which have lower rates of health insurance coverage (Kaiser Family Foundation [KFF], 2008). All hospitals agreed informally with the San Francisco health department to jointly distribute ownership of the HBV care for uninsured patients.

This practical attitude of raising funds as needed and in different modes, was highly successful for SFHBF, but not replicable for any institution needing funds to sustain operations. In its first 4 years, SFHBF and its partners raised $5 million in about even amounts of cash and in-kind contributions. Almost all resources were raised from the private sector, with no significant revenue from philanthropic foundations or government sources. About 25% came from pharmaceutical companies (SFDPH, 2009). Much of the revenue came from major corporations wishing to develop or deepen relationships with the Asian American market. SFHBF successfully recruited the first national retailer, Nordstrom, and the first automotive manufacturer, Subaru, to take on sponsorships of an Asian American health issue. Organizers were always able to raise funds, but did not raise more than needed, for reserve funds, or for future operations.

Healthcare Systems

In the final analysis, Hep B Free activities were geared toward the ultimate goal of improving healthcare delivery. The campaign's tag-line, "Be a hero. See a doctor who tests for Hep B," was designed to drive people into the healthcare system. But this strategy required that healthcare providers offer proper HBV screening and care. Thus, the campaign used multi-faceted connections to engage all of the large healthcare institutions in the county from top-down approaches, such as talking with executives and decision makers, to bottom-up grassroots organizing of patients and hospital workers, as well as other pathways from peer-to-peer relationships to business-to-business associations. Josh Adler, Chief Medical Officer of the University of California San Francisco Medical Center articulated his institution's multiple motivations for participating: "It's a worthy endeavor, and so that was probably number one. ... Second, our CEO is on the Bay Area Hospital council, and at the time may have even been the chair of the council and thus was interested in a city-wide collaboration, ... third, and very important, was the fact that UCSF has a student organization" that was engaged with SFHBF participating in educational outreach. Janet Zola gave another example of how using multiple entry points helped compel hospitals to action: "It's much easier for a project manager to decide to go ahead and do something like this when the CEO has said we want to do this, (rather) than when that project manager has to go back and somehow convince their superiors this is a good idea."

Ching Wong, health educator at the UCSF Vietnamese Community Health Promotion Project, characterized the SFHBF organization as being "very tight", meaning all of the messaging and all of the activities revolved around only one axis: making San Francisco free of HBV. The campaign avoided distractions by competitive, political or other concerns. Adler stressed this approach: "They have sent a sense of community. In other words, all the hospitals are involved, but we're not there alone. ... This is not the Department of Public Health's project. This is not the hospitals' project. This is everybody's project. I think that's the key to replicate. ... Bringing us together to pull in one direction at the same time I think is a tremendous success. In my roughly 20 years in San Francisco providing healthcare, I've never

seen or been part of anything that's been quite this good. Or even nearly as good, on that score."

A Community Movement in the Development of Asian America

The story of Asians in America is different from the story of Asian Americans. Journalist and author Helen Zia points out the convergence of immigration, politics and changing times that spawned the emergence of Asian Americans as a group in the 1960s and 1970s. Legal scholar and university chancellor Frank Wu goes further, claiming that "Asian Americans are uniquely Americans," adding that "Our concerns about self-realization, racial dynamics, minority status and the related matters arising from our status arise here; they do not bother Asians overseas (Wu, 2003, p. 310)."

But how has Asian America evolved? The exploration of an Asian American identity and community – inclusive of Asian Pacific American identity and community – has been a topic of intellectual pursuit since the civil rights era. Zia and Yen Le Espiritu cite the civil rights trials in the killing of Vincent Chin as formative for the development of the Asian American community (Espiritu, 1992; Zia, 2001). In his observations on American civil rights and discrimination law in regards to Asian Americans, Kenji Yoshino wishes that he "could live in an America that would not force (him) to surrender (his) ethnicity." (Yoshino, 2006, p. 141). We are still searching to define our identity and the boundaries of Asian Pacific America. Where does our Americanness end, and our Asianness begin? Part of this evolution is discovering matters that concern Asian Americans but do not arise from our status as Americans, issues that also bother Asians overseas, and methodologies for action that are as much Asian as American. Hepatitis B is one such concern, the greatest cause of liver cancer. This widespread health epidemic was transferred to us from our Asian roots, while the medical tools to end this deadly disease were discovered here in America.

In describing themselves as "community-based", Asian American organizers of SFHBF

inserted their own multiplistic meaning to community: "When you talk about the community
title, you also talk about other forces that link
your community together to become a more visible sense of political crowd, connecting business,
cultural – and all these things have to link together
to make a community strong," explained Ching
Wong. And though all the work of SFHBF was
local, Asian Americans also exhibited a global
sense of community and an awareness of their
roles to link Asians in America to Asians in Asia.
"There is open communication, dialogue between
our country and Asia through the people who
have ties and families over there," pointed out
mayoral aide Tsang. "Some day, hopefully we
can pass this word on hepatitis B all the way back
to the Asian Pacific rim so that all of the Asian
people in Asia should be aware … among the
people in China, among the people in Vietnam
and all the different Pacific rim countries," added
Ron Lee, Commander of the Cathay Post,
Veterans of Foreign Wars #384. Peter Swing
specified the role of Asian Americans: "I think
that Asian Americans can be the conduit, the link
of providing that knowledge to other Asians."
As a diverse hybrid, hyphenated people with multiple identities, HBF has been empowering for
Asian Americans to realize this role of bridging,
of being a possible key to bringing the two worlds
of Asia and America together in understanding
one another.

This sense of Asian Americans as providing
the link between America and Asia, between older
and younger generations and between the community and general society, was necessary to facilitate collaborations in SFHBF. Like hepatitis B
disease itself, many of the tactics and qualities of
the HBF campaign were rooted in the community's Asian heritage. But the key characteristic of
connectivity, of being able to link different groups,
was felt to arise from a Yin and Yang like duality
of being Asian in America. "In Asia itself …
there's a lot less of a Pan-Asian kind of spirit so
the power of what's happening in America is that
it reaches across to these different ethnic groups,"
observed Darrell Chiang, Executive Director of
the Asian American Theatre Company. Tsang

commented that Asian Americans like himself are
"kind of between the cultures."

The concept of Asian Americans as being
"betwixt and between" was used by America's
pre-eminent multicultural historian Ronald
Takaki of UC Berkeley to illuminate how Asian
Americans, and Americans of color generally,
live their lives between the two cultures of modern American life and the heritage from the land
of their ancestors (Takaki, 1998, 1993). It is also
reflected in the way Asian Americans seem to
operate between the poles of "extravagance and
necessity" in developing themselves and contributing back to society (Takaki, 1998, p. 18). Asian
American author Maxine Hong Kingston first
introduced the concept of extravagance and
necessity in her memoir, Woman Warrior
(Kingston, 1989). Sau-ling Wong deconstructed
the concepts with her insightful analysis of
Kingston's work, and Takaki popularized them in
his comparative history of Asian Americans,
Strangers from a Different Shore (Wong, 1993;
Takaki, 1998). Takaki's book recounts the community's "dynamic and dialectical" nature, and
"the yielding of old-world memories to new-
world experiences". He used the term "liminal-
ity" to express the ability of Asian Americans to
operate as "in-between Americans", whether
linking the different cultures in their lives or connecting the various stakeholders in Hep B Free
(Gennep, 1960; Takaki, 1998; Turner, 1974).
"Asian Americans have been transforming America
and also finding themselves being transformed by
America," Takaki writes. "The men and women of
our story made decisions about their lives and
communities, though usually in circumstances not
of their choosing (Takaki, 1998, p. 504)."

What does it mean to be Asian American?
Actually, "there are no Asians in Asia" – in Asia
there are only Chinese, Japanese, Korean, and so
forth. We become classified as Asians when we
come to America (Takaki, 1998, p. 502). But our
concerns as Asian Americans are expansive. Says
Takaki: "Statistics do not stir insightful or imagi-
native thinking about what will happen to Asian
Americans in the coming century. … Numbers
cannot capture and convey dynamic movements

and changes, or extravagant as well as dashed dreams, or thoughts and feelings in ferment (Takaki, 1998, p. 493)." This chapter takes a look at the dreams, thoughts and feelings, as well as the actions of the Asian American community as they began the HBF movement in San Francisco. If this groundbreaking health intervention is part of a move by the Asian American community into new issue areas such as community-specific health issues and private sector partnerships, then the community will need additional methodologies for making progress in these arenas. And if indeed the broader-based concerns and full-spectrum approaches of HBF indicate a new phase of increasing contributions of Asian Americans to the progress and development of the United States, then the strategies and tactics introduced through SFHBF are only some of the new and innovative approaches with more yet to come.

Notes

The origins of the endemicity of HBV in Asia is not clearly understood, although the lack of modern health prevention practices is certainly the reason it remains epidemic in Asia today. High rates of HBV are also endemic in Sub Saharan Africa, the Amazon basin and eastern Europe (Clements et al., 2006; Gust, 1996; Zhou & Holmes, 2007).

The authors use the terms "Asian American", "Asian Pacific American", and "Asian Pacific Islander American" interchangeably. The terms are meant to include Americans with heritage from East Asia, Southeast Asia, South Asia and the Pacific Islands.

References

Allday, E. (2010). Lofty goal: Stamp out silent killer hepatitis B. *SF Chronicle*. Retrieved June 22, 2011, from http://www.sfgate.com.

California Health Interview Survey. (2003). *2003 California health interview survey*. Los Angeles: Author. Retrieved June 22, 2011, from http://www.chis.ucla.edu/.

Centers for Disease Control. (2000). *Hepatitis B vaccination coverage among Asian and Pacific Islander children – United States, 1998*. Atlanta, GA: Author.

Retrieved June 22, 2011, from http://www.cdc.gov/mmwr/preview/mmwrhtml/mm4927a3.htm.

Centers for Disease Control. (2011). *Hepatitis B FAQs for health professionals*. Atlanta, GA: Author. Retrieved June 22, 2011, from http://www.cdc.gov/hepatitis/HBV/HBVfaq.htm#overview.

Clements, C. J., Baoping, Y., Crouch, A., Hipgrave, D., Mansoor, O., Nelson, C. B., et al. (2006). Progress in the control of hepatitis B infection in the Western Pacific region. *Vaccine, 24*, 1975–1982.

Cohen, C., Evans, A., London, W., Block, J., Conti, M., & Block, T. (2008). Underestimation of chronic hepatitis B virus infection in the United States of America. *Journal of Viral Hepatitis, 15*(1), 12–13.

Custer, S. S., Hazlet, T., Iloejo, U., Veenstra, D., & Kowdley, K. (2004). Global epidemiology of hepatitis B virus. *Journal of Clinical Gastroenterology, 38*(10 Supp. 3), S158–S168.

Deleuze, G., & Guattari, F. (1980). *A thousand plateaus: Capitalism and schizophrenia*. New York: Continuum.

Eshoo, A. G. (2011). A tribute in honor of Asian Pacific American heritage month and the Hep B free campaign. *Congressional Records*. Retrieved June 22, 2011, from http://www.gpo.gov/fdsys/pkg/CREC-2011-05-13/pdf/CREC-2011-05-13-pt1-PgE900-2.pdf.

Gennep, A. V. (1960). *The rites of passage*. Chicago: University of Chicago.

Gust, I. D. (1996). Epidemiology of hepatitis B infection in the Western Pacific and South East Asia. *Gut, 38*, S18–S23.

Henne group. (2009). San Francisco Hep B Free Public Awareness Evaluation Projects, Unpublished report.

Kaiser Family Foundation. (2008). Health care coverage and access to care among Asian Americans, native Hawaiians and Pacific Islanders. Kaiser Family Foundation. Retrieved August 03, 2011, from http://www.kff.org/minorityhealth/upload/7745.pdf.

Kingston, M. H. (1989). *The woman warrior: Memoirs of a girlhood among ghosts*. New York: Vintage Books.

Le Espiritu, Y. (1992). *Asian American panethnicity: Bridging institutions and identities*. Pennsylvania: Temple University Press.

Liu, A. (2009). Health ministry to cancel hepatitis B tests for employment and school enrollment. *China Today*. Retrieved June 22, 2011, from http://english.cctv.com/program/chinatoday/20091230/101108.shtml.

Liu, J., & Fan, D. (2007). Hepatitis B in China. *The Lancet, 369*(9573), 1582–1583.

McKinley, J. (2010). In ads, plea for Asians to get test for hepatitis. *The New York Times*. Retrieved June 22, 2011, from http://www.nytimes.com/2010/05/03/us/03hepatitis.html.

Michels, S. (2010). PBS newshour: Vaccination, education key to stemming Asian hepatitis outbreaks. *PBS Newshour*. Retrieved June 22, 2011, from http://www.pbs.org/newshour/bb/health/jan-june10/hepatitis_06-03.html.

Nguyen, T. T., McPhee, S. J., Bui-Tong, N., Luong, T.-N., Ha-laconis, T., Nguyen, T., et al. (2006). Community-based participatory research increases cervical cancer screening among Vietnamese-Americans. *Journal of Health Care for the Poor and Underserved, 17*(2), 41–54.

Office of Minority Health. (2011). *National hepatitis B initiative for Asian Americans and Pacific Islanders.* Rockville, MD: Author. Retrieved June 22, 2011, from http://minorityhealth.hhs.gov/templates/browse. aspx?lvl=2&lvlID=190.

Pang, A. (2008). CDC Announces new testing recommendations. *AsianWeek.* Retrieved June 22, 2011, from http://www.asianweek.com/2008/09/23/cdc-announces-new-testing-recommendations/.

Pang, A. (2009). Hep B honor roll names clinicians preventing liver cancer. *AsianWeek.* Retrieved June 22, 2011, from http://www.asianweek.com/2009/10/15/hep-b-honor-roll-names-clinicians-preventing-liver-cancer/.

Pfizer. (2008). The burden of cancer in Asia. *Pfizer Incorporated.* Retrieved June 22, 2011, from http://www.pfizer.com/files/products/cancer_in_asia.pdf.

Picture, B. (2008). Many heroes and heroines at SF's Hep B free campaign. *AsianWeek.* Retrieved June 22, 2011, from http://www.asianweek.com/2008/10/31/many-heroes-and-heroines-at-sf%E2%80%99s-hep-b-free-campaign/.

SFDPH. (2009). San Francisco Hep B Free: Campaign Activities and Evaluation Summary April 2007 – June 2009, Unpublished report.

Shinagawa, L. H., & Kim, D. Y. (2008). *A portrait of Chinese Americans: A national demographic and social profile of Chinese Americans.* College Park, MD: OCA and University of Maryland Asian American Studies Program.

Swing, P. (2008). SF giants go to bat for SF Hep B Free. *AsianWeek.* Retrieved June 22, 2011, from http://www.asianweek.com/2008/05/09/sf-giants-go-to-bat-for-sf-hep-b-tree/.

Takaki, R. T. (1993). *A different mirror: A history of multicultural America.* New York: Little, Brown.

Takaki, R. T. (1998). *Strangers from a different shore: A history of Asian American.* New York: Little, Brown.

Turner, V. (1974). *Dramas, fields, and metaphors: Symbolic action in human society.* Ithaca, NY: Cornell University Press.

Varney, S. (2010). Hepatitis B campaign targets Asians in San Francisco. *NPR.* Retrieved June 22, 2011, from http://www.npr.org/templates/story/story. php?storyId=127409718.

Wong, S-L. (1993). Necessity and extravagance in Maxine Hong Kingston's the woman warrior: Art and the ethnic experience. *MELUS*, 15(1), 3–26, Ethnic Women Writers V (Spring, 1988). Published by: The Society for the Study of the Multi-Ethnic Literature of the United States (MELUS).

World Health Organization. (2008). *Hepatitis B fact sheet N*204.* Geneva: Author. Retrieved June 22, 2011, from http://www.who.int/mediacentre/factsheets/fs204/en/.

Wu, F. H. (2003). *Yellow: Race in America beyond black and white.* New York: Basic Books.

Yoo, G. (2010). *Mobilizing Asian Americans: Understanding the San Francisco Hep B Free Movement.* Retrieved from http://www.sfhepbfree.org/files/publications/YOO_Grace_Bestpractices120410.pdf.

Yoo, G. J., Fang, T., Zola, J., & Dariotis, W. M. (2011). Destigmatizing hepatitis B in the Asian American community: Lessons learned from the San Francisco Hep B free campaign. *Journal of Cancer Education.* Retrieved July 20, 2011, from http://www.springer-link.com/content/h802400242mh25u2/.

Yoshino, K. (2006). *Covering: The hidden assault on our civil rights.* New York: Random House.

Zheng, C. (2009). Speaker Pelosi says hepatitis B prevention at core of healthcare reform. *AsianWeek.* Retrieved June 22, 2011, from http://www.asianweek. com/2009/11/04/speaker-pelosi-says-hepatitis-b-prevention-at-core-of-healthcare-reform/.

Zhou, Y., & Holmes, E. C. (2007). Bayesian estimates of the evolutionary rate and age of hepatitis B virus. *Journal of Molecular Evolution, 65,* 197–205.

Zia, H. (2001). *Asian American dreams: The emergence of and American people.* New York: Farrar, Straus and Giroux.

About the Editors and Contributors

Alvin N. Alvarez, PhD is the associate dean of the College of Health and Human Services and professor of counseling at San Francisco State University. He was the former president of the Asian American Psychological Association. His research and publications focus on Asian Americans, their racial identity development and their experiences with racism.

Emily Avera, MPhil, MA has research interest in the social and cultural aspects of transplant medicine, expert knowledge networks, and diversity awareness in various international contexts. Starting as an intern at the Asian American Donor Program in 2003, she has continued to be an advocate of the organization ever since.

Roshan Bastani, PhD is professor of health services and associate dean for research in the University of California, Los Angeles (UCLA) School of Public Health. She is co-director of the UCLA Kaiser Permanente Center for Health Equity and also director of Cancer Disparities Research at the UCLA Jonsson Comprehensive Cancer Center.

Nancy J. Burke, PhD is an associate professor in the Department of Anthropology, History, and Social Medicine and Helen Diller Comprehensive Cancer Center at the University of California, San Francisco. Her research and publications focus on the critical study of inequalities in cancer prevention, treatment and survivorship. Specifically, her work utilizes theoretical and methodological insights from medical anthropology to improve research on social inequalities in health, and to address cancer disparities.

Moon S. Chen, Jr., PhD, MPH is a professor of internal medicine and associate director for cancer control, University of California, Davis Cancer Center. He is principal investigator of "Liver Cancer Control Interventions for Asian Americans," a program research grant funded by the National Cancer Institute, and lead principal investigator of AANCART.

Serena Chen, MPH received her degree from the Columbia University Mailman School of Public Health, in the Department of Sociomedical Sciences. She hopes to pursue research to address health disparities in Asian American and immigrant communities.

G.J. Yoo et al. (eds.), *Handbook of Asian American Health*,
DOI 10.1007/978-1-4614-2227-3, © Springer Science+Business Media, LLC 2013

Ricky Y. Choi, MD, MPH, FAAP is the department head of pediatrics at Asian Health Services Community Health Center in Oakland, CA. There he provides primary care for children and adolescents from families who speak any of the ten Asian languages. Dr. Choi has degrees from the University of Chicago, Medical University of South Carolina, and Harvard University and completed his internship and residency at the University of California, San Francisco.

Vy Thuc Dao, MA is completing her PhD in sociology at Tulane University. Her areas of research center upon the study of formal organizations, social networks, and ethic organizations. Currently, she proposes to conduct a comparative study of the economic, social and organizational patterns of recovery and rebuilding by the Vietnamese communities in post-Katrina New Orleans and the Gulf Coast of Mississippi.

Roderick Raña Daus-Magbual, MA, Ed.D is the associate director of curriculum development of the Pin@y Educational Partnerships (PEP) in San Francisco, CA and an instructor at Skyline Community College.

Kira Donnell, MA is doctoral student in University of California, Berkeley's Ethnic Studies program where her research focuses on advocacy of adult international Korean adoptees. Kira's writing – both creative and academic – has appeared in a number of publications including *Journal of Korean Adoption Studies*, *Korean Quarterly*, and *More Voices: A Collection of Works from Asian Adoptees*.

Ted Fang is founder of the AsianWeek Foundation and a co-founder of the Hep B Free campaign begun in San Francisco. Fang is a student of diversity, with research and practice interests in assembling community and identity. He is a pioneer in the media industry, a successful businessman and a respected community activist. He built the largest non-daily newspaper in the entire country and was the first Asian American to run a major metropolitan daily newspaper. He is also founder of the Asian Heritage Street Celebration, the largest gathering of Asians in America.

Linda A. Gerdner, PhD, RN, FAAN is an ethnogeriatric specialist at Stanford Geriatric Education Center, through Stanford University School of Medicine. Her overall focus of research is family caregiving issues of persons with dementia. In 2001, she began focusing her research efforts on the perception and care of Hmong American elders with dementia. She has over 70 scholarly publications and is the primary author of *Grandfather's Story Cloth*, a bilingual picture book to help Hmong American children and their family who know or live with an elder who has Alzheimer's disease.

Deborah A. Goebert, DrPH is an associate professor and associate director of research at the Department of Psychiatry, John A. Burns School of Medicine, University of Hawaii. She is also co-principal investigator for school-based interventions at the Asian/Pacific Islander Youth Violence Prevention Center. Her research interests include social epidemiology, youth development, culture, and family.

Fang Gong, PhD is an assistant professor in the Department of Sociology at Ball State University. Her main research and teaching interests are medical sociology, mental health, race and ethnicity, life course research and social statistics. She has published in several journals including Journal of Health and Social Behavior, American Journal of Public Health, Public Health Report, Journal of Community Psychology, and Journal of Behavioral Medicine.

Ariel T. Holland is a research assistant in the Health Policy Research Department at the Palo Alto Medical Foundation Research Institute. Ms. Holland graduated with a bachelor's degree in psychology from the University of Virginia, with a minor in Biology. She has previous experience working with vital statistics data and researching the health of Asian Americans. Ms. Holland recently co-authored a paper with Dr. Palaniappan examining cause-specific mortality of Asian Indians in California.

Laureen D. Hom, MPH is the senior research & evaluation associate at the Charles B. Wang Community Health Center. She has experience in health disparities and health services research that include HIV/AIDS, breast cancer, and hepatitis B, and her professional interests include Asian American health disparities and urban community health. She received her MPH from Mailman School of Public Health at Columbia University in sociomedial sciences, with a specialization in urbanism & the built environment.

Nadia Islam, PhD is an assistant professor at NYU School of Medicine. She is the principal investigator of several community health worker interventions designed to prevent and manage cardiovascular disease disparities in Asian American communities. Dr. Islam is also the deputy director of the NYU Center for the Study of Asian American Health and the research director of the NYU Prevention Research Center. She specializes in community based participatory research and immigrant health.

Su Yeong Kim, PhD is an assistant professor in the Department of Human Development and Family Sciences at the University of Texas at Austin. She studies the role of family and cultural contexts in the development of Asian American and Latino adolescents in the U.S. She is a 2010 early career award winner from the Asian American Psychological Association and the International Society for the Study of Behavioral Development.

Caroline Kuo, DPhil completed interdisciplinary training in social policy and development studies at Oxford University and is currently a postdoctoral research fellow in the Department of Psychiatry and Alpert Medical School at Brown University. Her work examines the impacts of HIV/AIDS among families and children, with a specific focus on children who have been orphaned in the context of the global HIV/AIDS epidemic. She has led the largest known study of families affected by HIV/AIDS in South Africa.

Simona C. Kwon, DrPH, MPH is the director of the NYU B Free CEED, 1 of 18 CDC-funded Centers of Excellence in the Elimination of Health Disparities and an associate investigator of the NIH-funded Center for the Study of Asian American Health, and the NYU Health Promotion and

Prevention Research Center. Her research focus is on the application of a community-based participatory approach to address the socio-cultural factors influencing health behaviors and outcomes among Asian American, and other minority and underserved communities. Her current research includes identifying evidence-, and practice-based strategies across the social determinants of health to eliminate hepatitis B and other health disparities.

Mai-Nhung Le, DrPH, MPH is an associate professor in the Asian American Studies Department at San Francisco State University. She has extensive knowledge of women's health issues among the Asian American population, and has conducted a significant amount of research on the spread of sexually transmitted diseases in both Vietnam and the United States. In recent years, she has shifted her area of research to Asian Americans and cancer, focusing on the area of cancer survivorship. She also has developed a strong interest in understanding social, cultural, and health issues in racial and ethnic minority populations.

Thao N. Le, PhD, MPH was an associate professor at Colorado State University prior to joining the faculty in Department of Family and Consumer Sciences at the University of Hawaii at Manoa. Her research interests include developing, evaluating, and collaborating with community-based partners on programs related to preventing maladpative behaviors, as well as fostering positive youth development. She is also interested in multiculturalism, mindfulness, and working with underserved, ethnically diverse populations.

Jonathan Leong is the founder and an executive board member of the Asian American Donor Program (AADP). He is also the founder of several Bay Area businesses, including commercial insurance firms that serve the Port of Oakland and Bay Area Rapid Transit (BART).

Maureen Lichtveld, MD, MPH has a 30 year career in public health and currently is professor and chair of the Department of Global Environmental Health Science at the Tulane University School of Public Health and Tropical Medicine. Her research interests are environmentally-induced disease, including asthma and cancer, health disparities, environmental health policy, community-based participatory research, cultural competence, and disaster preparedness. She holds an endowed chair in environmental policy and is associate director of population sciences at the Louisiana Cancer Research Consortium. Her current research includes addressing the public health implications of the Gulf of Mexico Oil spill on vulnerable populations in Louisiana including the Vietnamese fisher folk and their families.

Russell F. Lim, MD, MEd is a health sciences clinical professor and director of diversity education and training at the UC Davis School of Medicine, Department of Psychiatry and Behavioral Sciences. He is the editor of the *Clinical Manual of Cultural Psychiatry*, APPI, 2006. He has been the course director of a Continuing Medical Education (CME) course at the American Psychiatric Association's Annual Meeting on cultural psychiatry for the last 16 years.

Jason Liu, MS is a member of SF Hep B Free and the Asian American Network for Cancer Awareness Research and Training, he is currently contributing to efforts to address the hepatitis B healthcare disparities affecting the Asian American community. He is a graduate student, and has contributed to research on brain tumors and on the role of small RNA in maintaining stem cell fate.

Francis G. Lu, MD is the Luke & Grace Kim Endowed Professor in cultural psychiatry, director of cultural psychiatry, and associate chair for medical student education in the Department of Psychiatry & Behavioral Sciences at the UC Davis Health System. He is also the assistant dean for faculty diversity at the UC Davis School of Medicine.

Richard Sean Magbual, MD is a board certified physician in general internal medicine and hospital medicine. He completed his formal residency training at Loma Linda University Medical Center with a focus in diabetic research. He is presently a full time hospitalist at a large medical center in Southern California.

Annette E. Maxwell, DrPH is a professor in the School of Public Health at the University of California, Los Angeles. She is engaged in a research program broadly focused on cancer health disparities in diverse populations, especially among several Asian American groups. Her research in cancer prevention and control has ranged from cancer screening to follow-up of breast abnormalities, dissemination of evidence-based interventions and smoking.

Ranjita Misra, PhD, CHES, FMALRC is a well known health disparities researcher with investigation of clinical and non-clinical risk factors (individual, psychosocial, environmental/contextual) that impact disparities in prevalence and management of diabetes, metabolic syndrome, and cardiovascular disease in multi-ethnic populations (Asians, Hispanics, and African Americans). She has also implemented several community- and clinic-based diabetes and nutrition education programs that are literacy- and culturally-appropriate among African Americans, South Asians, and Mexican Americans in the US, India and Mexico.

Heather Ngai, MPH is a public health analyst in the Office of Quality and Data, Bureau of Primary Health Care of the Health Resources and Services Administration. She coordinates and manages the Uniform Data System (UDS), a standardized reporting system that provides demographic, clinical and other data on Community Health Center, Migrant Health Center, Homeless, and Public Housing patients. Prior to joining HRSA, Heather studied public health at the University of Washington in Seattle, WA and was a community health specialist at Asian Health Services in Oakland, CA.

Quyen Ngo-Metzger, MD, MPH is data branch chief in the Bureau of Primary Health Care at HRSA, Dr. Ngo-Metzger's current work involves evaluating clinical quality of care, access, and cost of care for approximately 19 million patients seen at over 8,000 federally-qualified community health center sites. She has oversight of the Uniform Data System (UDS), a standardized reporting system that provides data on Community Health Centers, Migrant Health Centers, and Homeless and Public Housing patients.

Giang T. Nguyen, MD, MPH, MSCE is an assistant professor of family medicine and community health at the University of Pennsylvania, where he leads the Penn Asian Health Initiatives. His research focuses on immigrant health, cancer control, health communication, and community-based participatory research. He also sees primary care patients; teaches medical students, residents, and graduate public health students; and does public health outreach to Asian immigrant communities. He serves on several community boards, including the National Advisory Council of the Asian and Pacific Islander National Cancer Survivors Network.

Tung T. Nguyen, MD is director of the Vietnamese Community Health Promotion Project and a professor of Medicine at the University of California, San Francisco. He is a principal investigator of the Asian American Network for Cancer Awareness, Research, and Training (AANCART), a national center to reduce cancer health disparities.

Tu-Uyen Nguyen, PhD, MPH is an assistant professor in Asian American Studies at California State University, Fullerton. Her current research focuses on effective cancer education strategies for diverse Asian American and Pacific Islander communities; program evaluation using qualitative and mixed research methods; community-based health navigation; community and organizational capacity building strategies; linguistic-cultural competency in health promotion programs.

Alan Y. Oda, PhD is a professor of undergraduate psychology at Azusa Pacific University, Azusa, California. His research includes parenting and family relations, adolescence, Asian American and other minority American populations, and faith development. He served as the executive director of the Asian American Christian Counseling Service (AACCS) and continues as a member of the agency's board of directors.

Don Operario, PhD is a behavioral/social scientist in the Program in Public Health at Brown University. His research addresses the social context of HIV transmission and the social sequelae of HIV/AIDS in affected communities, with an emphasis on developing and evaluating theory-based social and behavioral interventions in high-risk groups. He conducts research addressing both U.S. domestic and international public health issues.

Latha P. Palaniappan, MD, MS is an associate investigator at the Palo Alto Medical Foundation Research Institute (PAMFRI), adjunct assistant professor at the Stanford University School of Medicine, and clinical assistant professor at the University of California San Francisco. She is also a graduate of Stanford's clinical epidemiology master's program, funded by the Clinical Research Curriculum Award (K30). She is board certified in general internal medicine, augmented by further clinical training in Preventive Cardiology.

Shilpa Patel, MPH is a doctoral student in Public Health at New York University and a research fellow at the NYU School of Medicine Health Promotion and Prevention Research Center. She earned her BS from Rutgers University with a double major in public health and psychology, and her MPH from Columbia University, with a concentration in effectiveness and outcomes research. Shilpa is interested in research that evaluates how health services and policies affect health outcomes, particularly among vulnerable populations.

Tazuko Shibusawa, MSW, PhD is an associate professor of social work at the New York University Silver School of Social Work. Dr. Shibusawa's research focuses on aging among vulnerable populations, including intimate violence among older couples, life experiences of people with co-occurring substance use and mental illness, and psychological well being of Asian-American elders. Dr. Shibusawa's clinical experiences have been in the areas of geriatric, psychiatric and school social work. She is a Hartford Geriatric Social Work Faculty Scholar.

Jaeyoun Shin, MS, NCC received her master's degree in counseling with the specialization of marriage and family therapy from San Francisco State University. Her clinical and research interests include Asian American immigrants, multicultural issues, racial discrimination, domestic violence, and ethnic minority children and adolescents. She is currently working at a nonprofit counseling organization as a full-time clinician and is in the process of pursuing a doctorate in counseling psychology.

Susan Matsuko Shinagawa is co-founder & former chair of the Asian & Pacific Islander National Cancer Survivors Network and the past chair of the Intercultural Cancer Council Spring Valley (San Diego County), California

Dara H. Sorkin, PhD is an associate adjunct professor in the Division of General Internal Medicine and a research fellow in the Health Policy Research Institute at the University of California, Irvine. Trained as a developmental psychologist, the focus of her research has been on examining racial/ethnic disparities in indicators of both mental and physical health among older adults, and designing interventions that leverage patients' social networks and personal resources to promote health in later life and to address these disparities.

Susan Stewart, PhD is an associate adjunct professor of medicine at the University of California, San Francisco and a member of the UCSF Helen Diller Family Comprehensive Cancer Center Biostatistics Core.

Angela Sun, PhD has devoted her career to increase health literacy on various health topics for the Asian community particular the Chinese immigrant community utilizing current evidence based venues and continues to explore effective health communication methods. Through the Chinese Community Health Resource Center (CCHRC), Dr. Sun has developed culturally and linguistically competent preventive health, disease management, and research programs.

Jeanelle J. Sugimoto-Matsuda, MS is a research investigator and program manager at the University of Hawai'i Manoa, John A. Burns School of Medicine, Department of Psychiatry. Her research interests focus mainly on behavioral and mental health, and this has included work with the Asian/Pacific Islander Youth Violence Prevention Center (APIYVPC). She is currently pursuing her doctorate in public health, with an emphasis in health policy and violence/injury prevention.

David T. Takeuchi, PhD is a sociologist and currently professor in the School of Social Work and the Department of Sociology at the University of Washington. He is also the associate dean for research in the School of Social Work. He is a sociologist with postdoctoral training in epidemiology and health services research. His research focuses on investigating the social, structural, and cultural contexts that are associated with different health outcomes, especially among racial and ethnic minorities.

Judy Tan, PhD is a social and health psychologist and postdoctoral research fellow at the Center for AIDS Prevention Studies, UCSF. Her main research areas are in social and health inequality, the psychological experience and social outcomes of stigmatized group members, and HIV/AIDS interventions with minority populations. She has specific interests in HIV/AIDS in racial/ethnic minority groups, particularly among Asian Americans.

Cathy J. Tashiro, PhD, MPH, RN is an associate professor in the nursing program at the University of Washington Tacoma. She has several published articles and book chapters on mixed race identity, mixed race and health disparities, and the meaning of race in healthcare and research. She is the author of the book "Standing on Both Feet: Voices of Older Mixed Race Americans," based on interviews with older people of mixed race.

Vicky Taylor, MD, MPH is a Member in the Cancer Prevention Program at Fred Hutchinson Cancer Research Center and a Research Professor in the Department of Health Services at the University of Washington.

Khatharya Um, PhD is an associate professor of Asian American and Asian Diaspora Studies at the University of California Berkeley. Her research and teaching interests focus simultaneously on Southeast Asia and Southeast Asian American communities and include refugee, diaspora and transnational studies, postcolonial and genocide studies, and the politics of memory.

Stephen Vong, MS is a research associate at San Francisco State University for the Cancer Disparities Research Group. He is currently in a post-baccalaureate program at San Francisco State University and is in the process of applying to medical school.

May C. Wang, DrPH is an associate professor in the Department of Community Health Sciences at the School of Public Health, University of California, Los Angeles. She is interested in addressing social disparities in the health and well-being of ethnic minority and immigrant families, with a focus on childhood obesity and bone health. She currently leads several interdisciplinary studies of the contributions of physical and social environments to food behavior and obesity development.

Yijie Wang, MA is a graduate student in the Department of Human Development and Family Sciences at the University of Texas at Austin. She is interested in the family dynamics that influence adolescent development within a cross-cultural context. Her current research is on parenting practices and adolescent adjustment in Chinese immigrant families in the U.S.

Isha Weerasinghe, MSc is the program coordinator for the NYU B Free CEED, the National Center of Excellence in the Elimination of Hepatitis B Disparities. She currently works in health policy and community-based participatory research, working to eliminate disparities in hepatitis B and promote health equity for AANHPIs.

Evaon Wong-Kim, PhD, MPH, LCSW is chair and professor at the Department of Social Work, California State University, East Bay. Dr. Wong-Kim has been a well recognized advocate and researcher for minority and low-income cancer patients, especially the Asian immigrant and Pacific Islander population. Her publications include studies on issues relating to survivorship, community attitude towards cancer and quality of life confronting immigrant Chinese cancer patients.

Sachiko Wood, MA is a research associate with the cancer disparities research group at San Francisco State University. Her research interests include Asian Americans, mixed heritage identity and health.

Gwen Yeo, PhD was the founding director of Stanford Geriatric Education Center, Stanford University School of Medicine, which helped develop the field of ethnogeriatrics, or health care for elders from diverse backgrounds. Her current work focuses on development of educational resources in ethnogeriatrics.

Grace J. Yoo, PhD, MPH is a sociologist and professor of Asian American Studies in the College of Ethnic Studies at San Francisco State University. Her research interests are understanding social support needs on a wide range of health care issues impacting Asian Americans including cancer control and cancer survivorship, management of chronic illnesses and health care access.

Lixin Zhang, PhD, MS practiced integrative medicine for 3 years before pursuing her graduate studies in the United States. She received her master's and doctoral degree in health services research, policy and administration. Her research interest includes the use of complementary and alternative medicine and health disparities among minority and immigrant populations.

Wei Zhang, PhD is an assistant professor of sociology at the University of Hawaii at Manoa. Her major areas of expertise include medical sociology, social epidemiology, social gerontology and research methods. Many of her studies have examined how socioeconomic factors were related to health and well-being of Asian Americans, multi-ethnic population in Hawaii, and the elder in China.

Index